The Influenza Viruses and Influenza

Contributors

William J. Bean, Jr.
D. Bucher
Purnell W. Choppin
Richard W. Compans
R. Gordon Douglas, Jr.
W. R. Dowdle
B. C. Easterday
E. D. Kilbourne
Hans-Dieter Klenk
W. Graeme Laver
P. Palese
Marcel W. Pons
G. C. Schild
Christoph Scholtissek
J. L. Schulman
Irene T. Schulze
Robert W. Simpson
Akira Sugiura
Robert G. Webster

The Influenza Viruses and Influenza

Edwin D. Kilbourne

Department of Microbiology
Mount Sinai School of Medicine
of the City University of New York
New York, New York

ACADEMIC PRESS   New York   San Francisco   London   1975

A Subsidiary of Harcourt Brace Jovanovich, Publishers

ACADEMIC PRESS, INC.
111 Fifth Avenue, New York, New York 10003

United Kingdom Edition published by
ACADEMIC PRESS, INC. (LONDON) LTD.
24/28 Oval Road, London NW1

Library of Congress Cataloging in Publication Data
Main entry under title:

The Influenza viruses and influenza.

    Bibliography: p.
    Includes index.
    1.   Influenza.   2.   Influenza viruses.   I.   Kilbourne,
Edwin D.   [DNLM: 1.   Influenza.   2.   Influenza Viruses.
QW160.I4 I43]
RC150.I48   616.2'03'0194   75-13091
ISBN 0−12−407050−7

PRINTED IN THE UNITED STATES OF AMERICA

Contents

1 The Influenza Viruses and Influenza—An Introduction
E. D. Kilbourne

2 The Structure of Influenza Virus
Purnell W. Choppin and Richard W. Compans

3 The Biologically Active Proteins of Influenza Virus: The Hemagglutinin
Irene T. Schulze

4   The Biologically Active Proteins of Influenza Virus: Neuraminidase
D. Bucher and P. Palese

5   The Biologically Active Proteins of Influenza Virus: Influenza Transcriptase Activity of Cells and Virions
Robert W. Simpson and William J. Bean, Jr.

6   Influenza Virus RNA(s)
Marcel W. Pons

7   Influenza Virus Genetics
Akira Sugiura

8   Influenza Virus Replication
Christoph Scholtissek and Hans-Dieter Klenk

9   Laboratory Propagation of Human Influenza Viruses, Experimental Host Range, and Isolation from Clinical Materials
W. R. Dowdle and G. C. Schild

10   Antigenic Variation of Influenza Viruses
Robert G. Webster and W. Graeme Laver

11   Influenza Virus Characterization and Diagnostic Serology
G. C. Schild and W. R. Dowdle

List of Contributors

Numbers in parentheses indicate the pages on which the authors' contributions begin.

William J. Bean, Jr. (125), Waksman Institute of Microbiology, Rutgers University, New Brunswick, New Jersey

D. Bucher (83), Department of Microbiology, Mount Sinai School of Medicine of the City University of New York, New York, New York

Purnell W. Choppin (15), The Rockefeller University, New York, New York

Richard W. Compans (15),* The Rockefeller University, New York, New York

R. Gordon Douglas, Jr. (395), Departments of Medicine and Microbiology, University of Rochester School of Medicine and Dentistry, Rochester, New York

W. R. Dowdle (243, 315), World Health Organization, Collaborating Center for Influenza, Virology Division, Center for Disease Control, Atlanta, Georgia

B. C. Easterday (449), Department of Veterinary Science, University of Wisconsin, Madison, Wisconsin

E. D. Kilbourne (1, 483), Department of Microbiology, Mount Sinai School of Medicine of the City University of New York, New York, New York

Hans-Dieter Klenk (215), Institut für Virologie, Justus Liebig-Universität, Giessen, Germany

W. Graeme Laver (269), John Curtin School for Medical Research, Australian National University, Canberra City, Australia

P. Palese (83), Department of Microbiology, Mount Sinai School of Medicine of the City University of New York, New York, New York

* Present address: Department of Microbiology, University of Alabama, Birmingham, Alabama.

Marcel W. Pons (145), Department of Virology, The Public Health Research Institute of the City of New York, New York, New York

G. C. Schild (243, 315),* World Health Organization, World Influenza Center, National Institute for Medical Research, Mill Hill, London, England

Christoph Scholtissek (215), Institut für Virologie, Justus Liebig-Universität, Giessen, Germany

J. L. Schulman (373), Department of Microbiology, Mount Sinai School of Medicine of the City University of New York, New York, New York

Irene T. Schulze (53), Department of Microbiology, St. Louis University School of Medicine, St. Louis, Missouri

Robert W. Simpson (125), Waksman Institute of Microbiology, Rutgers University, New Brunswick, New Jersey

Akira Sugiura (171), The Institute of Public Health, Minato-ku, Tokyo, Japan

Robert G. Webster (269), Laboratories of Virology and Immunology, St. Jude Children's Research Hospital, Memphis, Tennessee

* Present address: National Institute of Biological Standards and Control, Holly Hill Hamstead, London, England.

Preface

To the biased beholder and student of influenza, it is always an appropriate time to consider its chameleon complexities and review the vagaries of its protean virus. With the present decennial periodicity of pandemics of the disease, it is always just after, between, or just before major changes in the virus.

But now does seem to be a particularly propitious time for a collation of the increasingly abundant data from many laboratories on the biochemistry, structure, and function of the influenza viruses. Not because all the questions have been answered but because the problems have been isolated and better defined—and that is prelude to progress. And although the control of no infectious disease has yet depended upon a definitive understanding of the molecular biology of its causative agent, influenza may well be the first exception. Influenza vaccines, imperfect as they are, are the first to deliberately exploit genetic manipulation in their production. The epidemiology and immunity of the disease are already better understood through the recent clear definition of two discrete viral glycoproteins through which the virion interacts with the host and its environment. Studies of influenza viral structure are well advanced, and understanding of replication is progressing rapidly. On this understanding depends the development of rational approaches to chemoprophylaxis and therapy.

In a real sense, this book began in Madison, Wisconsin in September, 1971, with the first of a series of workshops on influenza sponsored by the National Institute of Allergy and Infectious Diseases. At this first informal conference (with international representation) most of the authors of this book were present, and many also attended the subsequent six conferences during the next three years. At these workshops we got to know each other well and to understand and respect each other's work. The fortunate result has been a continuing active international communication and even collaboration, as is the case with this effort to present a comprehensive view of the influenza viruses and the results of their existence.

Influenza transcends national boundaries so that this present international collaboration seems particularly appropriate.

Edwin D. Kilbourne

1

The Influenza Viruses and Influenza—An Introduction

E. D. Kilbourne

I. Introduction—Influenza, an Unvarying Disease Caused by a Varying Virus

The extraordinary attention that influenza and its causative viruses have received during the period of modern virology deserves comment in view of the very ordinary symptomatology of this generally uncomplicated infection of the human respiratory tract. The influenza virus replicates in straightforward fashion as a productive infection, without apparent recourse to latency, neoplastic induction, or other subtleties of virus–host relationship, to produce an acute inflammatory disease focused in the trachea that is attended by severe but briefly sustained fever and prostration. The disease in the typical patient has been essentially unvarying during at least the past 400 years, while, paradoxically, it has smoldered as a nuisance, or recurrently has aroused terror as the last great plague of man (Kilbourne, 1963). Paradoxically, also, the disease continues to defy control by artificial immunization despite the proved immunogenicity of specific vaccine

1

almost 40 years age (Chenoweth *et al.,* 1936). In 1947, with the appearance of the H1N1 strains (Table 1.2), it was first appreciated that the magnitude of antigenic variation of influenza A virus might be so great as to circumvent previously acquired immunity to antecedent strains. Thus, the unvarying disease appears to be caused by a varying virus—indeed, by a virus unique among infectious agents in its antigenic variability. Coincident with the growing evidence of the epidemiologic complexity of influenza, its virus has proved increasingly interesting as an object of laboratory study—the first virus for which hemagglutination was demonstrated (Hirst, 1941; McClelland and Hare, 1941), the animal virus first shown to undergo "recombination" (Burnet and Lind, 1949), the virus first demonstrated to contain an enzyme as a structural protein (Hirst, 1942; Rafelson *et al.,* 1963; Kilbourne and Laver, 1966; Drzeniek *et al.,* 1966), and the virus first shown to reproduce by budding from the plasma membrane of the host cell (Murphy and Bang, 1952). Yet remarkably, research on the virus rarely has been isolated or segregated from research on the disease. The seminal early investigations of the "first generation" of scientists interested in influenza, Shope, Andrewes, Smith, Laidlaw, Stuart-Harris, Hoyle, Mulder, Burnet, Hirst, Francis, Horsfall, and Smorodintsev, have been conducted alternately at the bench and in the field, gaining lessons first from one source and then the other. This tradition has continued to the present so that many of the authors of this book could have written effectively about other aspects of influenza viruses or influenza than those assigned for their special consideration.

The last 10 years have witnessed an accelerated advance in understanding of the structure, replication, and immunology of the virus that has been in part dependent on the application of techniques widely used in molecular biology and in part upon the development of special systems and techniques for study of influenza virus. The latter include the development of plaquing and cloning systems that have facilitated genetic and antigenic studies of the virus (Simpson and Hirst, 1961; Sugiura and Kilbourne, 1965), techniques for isolation and purification of the viral polypeptides (Laver, 1963; Eckert, 1966; Compans *et al.,* 1970; Haslam *et al.,* 1970; Schulze, 1970; Skehel and Schild, 1971), the development of animal models for investigation of pathogenesis and immunity (Shope, 1931; Loosli, 1949; Schulman and Kilbourne, 1963; Nayak *et al.,* 1965; Webster *et al.,* 1971; Potter *et al.,* 1973), and the application of new serologic techniques to viral antigenic analysis and field investigations (see Schild and Dowdle, Chapter 11). The result of this activity has been a considerable increase in knowledge of the nature of the virus, a marked improvement in epidemiologic surveillance, the design of novel approaches to the fabrication of new vaccines (Chapter 15), and, as yet, no substantial impact on the incursions of the disease.

II. Taxonomy of the Influenza Viruses

The influenza viruses are relatively large enveloped viruses that contain RNA in divided or segmented form as genome. The single-stranded RNA molecules are of nonmessage polarity ["negative" in Baltimore's terminology (Baltimore, 1971)] and accordingly contain an RNA-dependent RNA transcriptase within the virion. Transcripts of the five to seven RNA segments code (probably as monocistronic messengers) for the production of five to seven virion structural proteins and possibly cell associated nonstructural protein(s) as well (see Chapters 2, 6, and 8).

As orthomyxoviruses, the influenza viruses bear certain striking similarities to the larger parainfluenza viruses of the paramyxovirus genus (Table 1.1), including the possession of negative stranded RNA and a virion transcriptase, an external envelope that contains glycoprotein spikes bearing

Table 1.1 Taxonomic Relationship of Influenza Viruses (Orthomyxoviruses) to Other RNA Animal Viruses[a]

Family	Genus	"Species"[c]
Picornaviridae	*Enterovirus*	
	Rhinovirus	
	Calicivirus	
Togaviridae	*Alphavirus*	
	Flavivirus	
—[b]	*Orthomyxovirus*	Influenza (type) A
		Influenza (type) B
		Influenza (type) C
—[b]	*Paramyxovirus*	
—[b]	*Coronavirus*	
—[b]	*Arenavirus*	
—[b]	*Bunyamwera* "supergroup" (genus provisional)	
—[b]	*Leukovirus* ("oncornavirus"; "RNA tumor viruses")	
—[b]	*Rhabdovirus*	
Reoviridae	*Reovirus* *Orbivirus*	"Diplornavirus" suggested

[a] Based on 1971 report of International Committee on Nomenclature of Viruses (ICNV), Wildy (1971) and Fenner *et al.* (1975).
[b] No family designation recognized.
[c] Species designation seems appropriate on basis of absent complementation and recombination among influenza A, B, and C viruses.

Table 1.2 Taxonomy of Influenza Viruses

Family	Genus	"Species" (type)	Subtype[a] (human)	Prevalence	Antigenic variant[b] (within subtype)
None defined	*Orthomyxovirus*	Influenza A	H0N1	(?1929–1947)	Several (not listed)
			H1N1	(1946–1957)	Several (not listed)
			H2N2	(1957–1968)	Several (not listed)
			H3N2	(1968–)	Hong Kong/1/68[d]
					England/42/72
					Port Chalmers/1/73
					Scotland/840/74
			(animal)		
			Hsw1N1[c]		[e]
			Heq1Neq1, etc.		
		Influenza B	No true subtypes but antigenic variation may be equivalent to that observed within an influenza A subtype (e.g., H3N2)		
		Influenza C	None		Significant variation has not been defined

[a] Major antigenic variant with respect to hemagglutinin and/or neuraminidase external virion antigens. Chronologic transition from one subtype to another constitutes antigenic "shift" and is usually associated with pandemic disease.

[b] Minor antigenic variant within a subtype, probably resulting from series of point mutations and selection. May effectively challenge subtype-specific immunity within an interpandemic period. Antigenic "drift."

[c] Probable human prototype strain of 1918–1929.

[d] Strain designation is A/Hong Kong/1/68 (H3N2) [*Bull. W.H.O.* **45**, 119 (1971)].

[e] See Tables 14.1 and 14.2.

hemagglutinating and neuraminidase activity, and respiratory tract patho-genicity. Unlike the parainfluenza viruses, however, the influenza viruses possess a segmented genome, undergo high frequency genetic recombination or reassortment (Chapter 7), have a nuclear actinomycin D-susceptible rep-lication phase, demonstrate no cell fusing or hemolytic properties, appear to contain hemagglutinin and neuraminidase activities in separate proteins, and have not been convincingly shown to cause persistent infections experi-mentally or in nature.

Influenza viruses exist as three biologically similar, but antigenically heterologous types, A, B, and C (Table 1.2). These viruses share no virus-coded antigens in common, differ in epidemiology and probably to some degree in the severity of illness that they cause. Genetic recombination, or complementation, among these types has not been verified. Therefore, the types appear to deserve identification as separate viral species (see footnote *c* to Table 1.1), *Subtypes* of influenza A virus comprise the major antigenic variants that when they first appear are associated with pandemics. Only one such subtype is present in the human population at any one time—each being superseded by the next in turn. In the case of animal influenza viruses, antigenically different subtypes can coexist (Chapters 9 and 15).

In man, significant variation in both neuraminidase and hemagglutinin antigens of a subtype is recognized every two to three years during inter-pandemic periods. Such variants probably exist as a continuum based on sequential point mutations of the original prototype strain (Chapter 10). However, rapid strain selection in nature plus inadequacies of sampling creates a picture of rather limited variation which, however, is sufficiently different among strains for their categorical definition. In each period of subtype prevalence such recognizable minor variants have appeared. Table 1.2 lists only the four minor variants of the contemporary H3N2 (Hong Kong) subtype that have thus far been associated with significant wide-spread epidemic disease. Such variants possess some antigenic determinants in common, but differ completely with respect to others (Laver *et al.*, 1974). The revised taxonomy of influenza virus strain designations appears in Table 1.3.

III. A Comparison of Influenza A, B, and C Viruses— Similarities and Differences

Soon after the isolation of influenza A virus from human disease, it be-came evident that not all cases of influenza were associated with that virus. In 1940, Francis (1940) and Magill (1940) independently isolated a virus

Table 1.3 Antigenic Characteristics of Reference Influenza A Viruses[a,b]

Neuraminidase subtypes	H0	H1	H2	H3	Hsw1	Heq1	Heq2	Hav1	Hav2	Hav3	Hav4	Hav5	Hav6	Hav7	Hav8
N1	1	2			5										
N2			3	4									14		
Neq1						6		8	10						
Neq2							7							15	
Nav1										11	12				
Nav2												13			
Nav3								9							
Nav4															16
Nav5													17		

The column group "H0 H1 H2 H3 Hsw1 Heq1 Heq2 Hav1 Hav2 Hav3 Hav4 Hav5 Hav6 Hav7 Hav8" is headed **Hemagglutinin subtypes**.

[a] Revised from tabulated data from *Bull. W.H.O.* **45**, 119 (1971).

[b] Previous designations:

1 = AO/PR/8/34	7 = A/equine-2/Miami/63
2 = A1/FM/1/47	8 = A/FPV/Dutch/27
3 = A2/Singapore/1/57	9 = A/turkey/England/63
4 = A2/Hong Kong/1/68	10 = A/chicken/Germany N/49
5 = A/swine/Wisconsin/15/30	11 = A/duck/England/56
6 = A/equine-1/Prague/56	12 = A/duck/Czech./56

13 = A/tern/South Africa/61
14 = A/turkey/Mass./65
15 = A/duck/Ukraine/1/63
16 = A/turkey/Ontario/6118/68
17 = A/Shearwater/E. Australia/1/72

from human influenza that differed completely antigenically from influenza A virus. This virus, which resembled influenza A viruses in host range and biological behavior, was termed influenza B virus. Still later, in 1947, Taylor (1949) recovered a hemagglutinating virus from a subject suffering from mild upper respiratory tract infection. "Strain 1233" was originally thought to be a sporadic isolation of a virus of little public health importance, but Francis and his associates (1950) later isolated an antigenically identical virus from an epidemic of respiratory disease in children. Subsequently, the association of this virus with other episodes of mild influenza-like illness appeared to justify designation of the virus as influenza C. Difficulties in developing adequate tissue culture systems for replication of the virus and the infrequency of its demonstrable association with human disease have curtailed its study, so that much less information is available concerning its properties than is the case with influenza A and B viruses. At this writing, the presence of a viral neuraminidase has not been verified (Kendal and Kiley, 1974), nor has any other glycosidase been related to destruction of its cellular receptors (Table 1.4) that follows hemagglutination reactions. It seems probable that neuraminidase or other glycosidase activity will be found when appropriate experimental conditions have been defined.

The order of discovery of influenza A, B, and C viruses is also the rank order of these viruses with respect to their human and animal virulence, their host range in cell culture, the magnitude and frequency of antigenic variation, their optimal replication temperature, and their epidemiologic importance (see Table 1.4). Influenza A viruses differ importantly from B and C in their existence and serial transfer in lower animal species and in their association with pandemic disease—two factors that may be associated (Chapters 10 and 15). An interesting unexplained susceptibility to amantadine also differentiates influenza A from influenza B and C viruses, although some amantadine derivatives are reported to affect influenza B virus (Indulen et al., 1974). An actinomycin D-sensitive step early in influenza A viral replication (indicative of a need for cellular DNA transcription) has not yet been unequivocally established for influenza B or C viruses.

Perhaps reflecting its lesser virulence and apparent predilection for the upper respiratory tract, influenza C virus differs from influenza A and B viruses in replicating (at least in the chick embryo or in vitro infection) most efficiently at less than mean human body temperature (37°C). Possibly this virus, and to some extent influenza B virus, are "shut off" from replication at the higher temperature of the human lung in a manner similar to selected temperature-sensitive mutants of influenza A virus (Mills and Chanock, 1971) and consequently are reduced in primary human pathogenicity.

Table 1.4 Comparison of Influenza A, B, and C and Their Causative Viruses[a]

	A	B	C
Virus first isolated	1900[b]	1940	1947
Viral structure	5–7 negative strand RNA segments; 5–7 structural proteins including RNA polymerase-enveloped virus	Probably same as A, but less studied	Possession of viral neuraminidase is uncertain
Antigenic variation	Major and minor	Minor	Very minor
Replication and inhibition	Actinomycin D-sensitive step, inhibited by amantadine	? (but mitomycin C inhibition)[c] Not inhibited by amantadine	? ?
Optimal replication temperature	37°C	35°C	32°C
Genome and genetics	Segmented; high frequency recombination	Probably segmented; high frequency recombination	Nature of genome and frequency of recombination not known
Host range (experimental)	Chick embryo, ferret, hamster, subhuman primates, mice, abortive (neurovirulent) replication in mouse brain; chick embryo, avian, primate, and bovine cell cultures	Same as A except for lack of demonstrated experimental neurovirulence	Chick embryo, ferret, hamster, monkey; chick embryo, and primate cell cultures
Host range in nature	Man, various other vertebrates[d]	Man (rarely and sporadically others)	Man
Disease in man	Principally middle respiratory tract, possibly more virulent than B and C in adult	Principally middle respiratory tract, possibly more severe than A or C in child, as in Reyes syndrome	Principally upper respiratory tract, less severe than A or B
Epidemiology	Pandemic, epidemic, and endemic forms in all age groups	Epidemic and endemic phases; disease most common in older children	Subclinical or endemic infection must be common
	Present in man at least since 1889[e]	Present in man at least since 1935[e]	Present in man at least since 1936[e]
	May exist and persist in sub-human mammals and birds		

[a] Note that some of the apparent differences among influenza A, B, and C viruses may simply reflect less adequate study of B and C.
[b] First recovery of fowl plague virus from chickens (Stubbs, 1965). First isolation of a probable human virus was from swine in 1931 (Shope) and from man in 1933 (Smith, Andrewes, and Laidlaw).
[c] Nayak and Rasmussen (1966).
[d] See Chapter 14.
[e] Based on serologic studies.

IV. Structural and Functional Relationship of Influenza Viruses to Other RNA Viruses

Answers to the riddles of antigenic variation and single subtype prevalence of influenza virus must reside ultimately in the structure and function of the virion. In other words, the unique biologic behavior of the virus may be correlated with uniqueness in molecular composition or structure. If influenza viruses are compared with other RNA animal viruses (Table 1.5), it is evident that they share in common with the closely related paramyxoviruses and the quite unrelated togaviruses and rhabdoviruses external envelopes derived from host cell plasma membranes. In common with the other enveloped RNA viruses listed, influenza viruses bud from the cell surface

Table 1.5   Structural and Functional Similarities of Influenza Viruses to Certain Other RNA Viruses of Animals

	In-fluenza viruses	Para-myxo-viruses[a]	Toga-viruses	Rhabdo-viruses	Reo-viruses	Leuko-viruses
"Negative-stranded" RNA of nonmessage polarity	+	+	0	+	+[b]	0
Virion contains RNA-dependent RNA polymerase	+	+	0	+	+	0
Replication dependent on functional host DNA	+	0	0	0	0	0
Segmented genome	+	0	0	0	+	+
High frequency recombination	+	0	0	0	+	+
Enveloped virus budded from cell surface with incorporation of host lipid	+	+	+	+	0	+
Spike-like external virion polypeptides	+	+	+	+	0	+
Phenotypic mixing with influenza viruses reported	−	+	0	+	0	0
Viral neuraminidase present	+	+	0	0	0	0
Neuraminic acid present in viral envelope	0	0	+	+	−	+
Antigenic variation in nature	+	0	0	0	0	0
Respiratory tract pathogen	+	+	0	±	±	0

[a] Parainfluenza and mumps viruses.
[b] Virion RNA is double stranded.

in the final assembly-release step, incorporating host lipid in the process. Glycosylation of the virus coated "spike" external polypeptides with carbohydrate produced by host enzymes occurs before this final replication step (see Chapters 2 and 8).

The relative nonspecificity of the budding process is evidenced by the fact that phenotypic mixing or substitution of viral envelope components to produce viral pseudotypes can follow dual infection of cells with influenza and parainfluenza (Granoff and Hirst, 1954) or even influenza and rhabdoviruses (Zavada and Rosenbergova, 1972).

As the only other viruses that contain virus-coded neuraminidases, the parainfluenza and mumps viruses bear a striking superficial similarity to the influenza viruses, possessing also hemagglutinating activity, affinity for same cell receptors and capacity for replication to high titer in the allantoic sac of the chick embryo, and pathogenic predilection for cells of the respiratory tract. But critical differences beween ortho- and paramyxoviruses include differences in the replication, genomes, and genetics of the viruses. Most striking of these are the nuclear phase and host DNA-dependent replication step of influenza virus and its segmented genome and capacity for high frequency recombination or genetic reassortment. With respect to this latter capacity, resemblances may be seen to reoviruses (Fields and Joklik, 1969) and possibly to the RNA tumor viruses (leukoviruses) (Vogt, 1971), although these viruses differ considerably in complexity of structure and in replication from influenza virus. Reoviruses contain double-stranded segmented RNA, and leukoviruses uniquely possess an RNA-dependent DNA polymerase.

If antigenic variability is somehow related to the capacity of influenza viruses for genetic reassortment, it must be explained why similar variability has not been demonstrated with reoviruses. As discussed elsewhere (Kilbourne, 1973), inactive or defective reovirus particles do not participate in genetic reassortment (Fields, 1971) unlike similar influenza virus particles, so that this avenue of mutational amplification is not available to them. The apparent incapacity of influenza viruses to become stably or persistently associated with the host cell or its genome, or an external reservoir, may have dictated its need for continual antigenic change as a survival mechanism.

V. Antigenic Variation of Influenza Viruses Contrasted with Antigenic Variation in Other Infectious Agents

For most organisms the antigenicity of their protein or carbohydrate components is such a stable property that it serves as a taxonomic standard.

Minor antigenic variants of viruses can be selected for in the laboratory and identified by such refined methods of antigenic analysis as kinetic neutralization or plaque size reduction in the continued presence of anti-serum (Wecker, 1960). Such minor intratypic variation (as with polio-viruses) are insufficient to affect cross-immunity among strains appreciably and serve more to emphasize than to refute the concept of antigenic stability as an almost universal characteristic of infective agents.

Notable exceptions to this rule (in addition to the influenza viruses) may be organisms of the genus *Borrelia* that purportedly undergo significant anti-genic change even during infection of a single host. Indeed, the relapsing fever of the disease that *Borrelia* sp. cause in mammalian hosts has been explained as due to the repeated emergence of antigenically distinct organisms during illness (reviewed by Felsenfeld, 1965). Such recurrences, some suffered weeks after the initial attack, if related to antigenic variation of the spirochete, suggest mutations of almost incredible rate and degree. Although at least one study has described the development of multiple *Borrelia* variants in rats following inoculation of a single organism (Schuhardt and Wilkerson, 1951), as many as nine *Borrelia* variants have been found in a single tick vector (Cunningham and Frazier, 1935), suggesting the possibility that *preexisting* antigenic variants multiplying at different rates may be responsible for relapses. In view of the inadequacy of present methods for the antigenic analysis of *Borrelia* and the fact that "it has not yet been possible to characterize and differentiate strains on the basis of their antigenic reactivity" (Turner, 1965), comparison with the well-documented studies of influenza viruses is not instructive at present.

Antigenic variation during the course of infection has been described in natural and experimental trypanosomiasis and malaria. This variation has been correlated with occurrence of the febrile relapses that characterize these diseases. Present evidence suggests that in the case of the trypanosomes anti-genic variation is induced as a phenotypic modification of a surface glyco-protein of the parasite, and that in essence, the organism has a replaceable coat (Vickerman, 1969; Vickerman and Luckins, 1969). These surface anti-gens are lost when the protozoan is subjected to artificial cultivation, and reversion to a basic antigenic type occurs after the metacylic trypanosome develops in the vector (Vickerman, 1969). Thus, stable antigenic genotypes do not seem to be derived by mutation and selection in the manner of the influenza viruses. Similarly, the variation of merozoite surface antigens in experimental simian malaria may also be an induced phenomenon not re-lated to immunoselection. Rather, it may reflect "phenotypic regulation by specific immune globulins" (Brown, 1973). Furthermore artificial immuniza-tion with a merozoite vaccine produces immunity that is broader and less specific than that resulting from infection (Mitchell *et al.,* 1974), suggesting the possession of common antigenic determinants by the immunologic variants.

Limited evidence suggests that the unclassified RNA virus of equine infectious anemia may undergo stable antigenic variation in assocation with febrile relapses of the disease (Kono *et al.,* 1973). However, the authors of this report cautiously admit that their cloning procedures were not ideal; thus, this interesting system must receive further study before its comparability with influenza virus variation is established.

Other nonpersistent organisms (notably those that infect the respiratory tract) seem to have met the problem of survival by representation through divergent microevolution of multiple, apparently stable antigenic types that exist and circulate contemporaneously (rhinoviruses, adenoviruses, pneumococci, and streptococci). In the case of rhinoviruses, for example, intertypic competition for the same host substrate may preserve through interference an adequate number of susceptible hosts for maintenance of each viral type. It is in the *disappearance* of variants and subtypes and the *restricted prevalence of a single subtype* that influenza virus appears to be unique. It may be surmised that influenza viruses exist in a delicately balanced, even tenuous relationship with man, in which fierce competition occurs among variants for ascendancy.

VI. Unanswered Questions

It is the primary function of this book to summarize and to present critically and in perspective the present state of knowledge of influenza and its causative viruses. Much has been learned about the virus and its replication in recent years. Much less has been learned recently about the disease or its epidemiology, although newer information about the nature of the virion has led to some reasonable and intriguing hypotheses about the origin of new strains (Chapters 10 and 15). Much still remains unanswered, however, about the nature of the virus and its replication, as well as the pathogenesis of the disease. The details of the replicative process require definition, especially the mechanisms of transcription and translation and the kind of evidence provided for reoviruses that each RNA segment is responsible for a monocistronic message. The mystery of the host DNA-dependent step must be unraveled, and the location and function of the P polypeptides (Chapter 2) defined. The precise structure of the genome within the virus is unknown, as is the occurrence and importance of true intramolecular recombination.

The apparent selective inhibition of influenza A viruses by amantadine deserves further exploration, as does the apparent absence of a neuraminidase from influenza C virus.

The clinical puzzle of a prostrating disease with systemic symptoms and the absence of demonstrable viremia in most cases should be resolved by a search for *antigenemia* and examination of the toxicity of purified virion polypeptides.

Why of the orthomyxoviruses do only the influenza A viruses persist and cause epidemics in lower animals and birds, and what ecologic factors permit simultaneous prevalence of multiple subtypes in these species? Will prospective studies reveal clear evidence for the first time of the source of the next great pandemic? Is influenza, unique as it is, also uniquely susceptible to eradication by the proper strategy and tactics of artificial immunization?

References

Baltimore, D. (1971). *Bacteriol. Rev.* **35**, 235.

Brown, K. N. (1973). Nature (*London*) **242**, 49.

Burnet, F. M., and Lind, P. E. (1949). *Aust. J. Sci.* **12**, 109.

Chenoweth, A., Waltz, A. D., Stokes, J., Jr., and Gladen, R. G. (1936). *Amer. J. Dis. Child.* **52**, 757.

Compans, R. W., Klenk, H. D., Caliguiri, L. A., and Choppin, P. W. (1970). *Virology* **42**, 880.

Cunningham, J., and Frazier, A. G. L. (1935). *Indian J. Med. Res.* **22**, 595.

Drzeniek, R., Seto, J. T., and Rott, R. (1966). *Biochim. Biophys. Acta* **128**, 547.

Eckert, E. A. (1966). *J. Bacteriol.* **92**, 1430.

Felsenfeld, O. (1965). *Bacteriol. Rev.* **29**, 46.

Fenner, F., Pereira, H. G., Porterfield, J. D., Joklik, W. K., and Downie, A. W. (1974). *Intervirology* **3**, 193.

Fields, B. (1971). *Virology* **46**, 142.

Fields, B., and Joklik, W. K. (1969). *Virology* **37**, 335.

Francis, T., Jr. (1940). *Science* **92**, 405.

Francis, T., Jr., Quilligan, J. J., and Minuse, E. (1950). *Science* **112**, 495.

Granoff, A., and Hirst, G. K. (1954). *Proc. Soc. Exp. Biol. Med.* **86**, 84.

Haslam, E. A., Hampson, A. W., Egan, J. A., and White, D. O. (1970). *Virology* **42**, 555.

Hirst, G. K. (1941). *Science* **94**, 22.

Hirst, G. K. (1942). *J. Exp. Med.* **76**, 195.

Indulen, M. K., Kanele, I. A., Dzeguze, D. P., Ryasantseva, G. M., and Kalninya, V. A. (1974). *Proc. Symp. Antiviral Substances, Bratislava,* 1974.

Kendal, A. P. (1975). *Virology* **65**, 87.

Kilbourne, E. D. (1963). *In* "Preventive Medicine and Public Health" (W. G. Smillie, ed.), p. 192. Macmillan, New York.

Kilbourne, E. D. (1973). *J. Infect. Dis.* **128**, 668.

Kilbourne, E. D., and Laver, W. G. (1966). *Virology* **30**, 493.

Kono, Y., Kobayashi, K., and Fukunaga, Y. (1973). *Arch. Virusforsch.* **41**, 1.

Laver, W. G. (1963). *Virology* **20**, 251.

Laver, W. G., Downie, J. C., and Webster, R. G. (1974). *Virology* **59**, 230.

Loosli, C. G. (1949). *J. Infec. Dis.* **84**, 153.

McClelland, L., and Hare, R. (1941). *Can. Pub. Health J.* **32**, 530.

Magill, T. P. (1940). *Proc. Soc. Exp. Biol. Med.* **45**, 162.

Mills, J., and Chanock, R. M. (1971). *J. Infec. Dis.* **123**, 145.

Mitchell, G. H., Butcher, G. A., and Cohen, S. (1974). *Nature (London)* **252**, 311.

Murphy, J. S., and Bang, F. B. (1952). *J. Exp. Med.* **95**, 259.

Nayak, D. P., Twiehaus, M. J., Kelley, G. W., and Underdahl, N. R. (1965). *Amer. J. Vet. Res.* **26**, 1271.

Nayak, D. P., and Rasmussen, A. F., Jr. (1966). *Virology* **30**, 673.

Potter, C. W., Jennings, R., and McLaren, C. (1973). *Arch. Gesamte Virus Forsch.* **42**, 285.

Rafelson, M. E., Schneir, M., and Wilson, V. W. (1963). *Arch. Biochem. Biophys.* **103**, 424.

Schuhardt, V. T., and Wilkerson, M. (1951). *J. Bacteriol.* **62**, 215.

Schulman, J. L., and Kilbourne, E. D. (1963). *J. Exp. Med.* **118**, 257.

Schulze, I. T. (1970). *Virology* **42**, 890.

Shope, R. E. (1931). *J. Exp. Med.* **54**, 373.

Simpson, R. W., and Hirst, G. K. (1961). *Virology* **15**, 436.

Skehel, J. J., and Schild, G. C. (1971). *Virology* **44**, 396.

Smith, W., Andrewes, C. H., and Laidlaw, P. P. (1933). *Lancet* **2**, 66.

Stubbs, E. L. (1965). *In* "Diseases of Poultry" (H. E. Biester and L. H. Schwarte, eds.), 5th ed., p. 813. Iowa State Univ. Press, Ames.

Sugiura, A., and Kilbourne, E. D. (1965). *Virology* **26**, 478.

Taylor, R. M. (1949). *Amer. J. Pub. Health* **39**, 171.

Turner, T. (1965). *In* "Bacterial and Mycotic Infections of Man" (R. Dubos and J. Hirsch, eds.), 4th ed. Lippincott, Philadelphia, Pennsylvania.

Vickerman, K. (1969). *J. Cell Sci.* **5**, 163.

Vickerman, K., and Luckins, A. G. (1969). *Nature (London)* **224**, 1126.

Vogt, P. K. (1971). *Virology* **46**, 947.

Webster, R. G., Campbell, C. H., and Granoff, A. (1971). *Virology* **44**, 317.

Wecker, E. (1960). *Virology* **10**, 376.

Wildy, P. (1971). *Monogr. Virol.* **5**, 49.

Zavada, J., and Rosenbergova, M. (1972). *Acta Virol. (Prague)* **16**, 103.

2

The Structure of Influenza Virus

Purnell W. Choppin and Richard W. Compans

I. Introduction

Studies on influenza virus have long been in the forefront of work on virus structure. The influenza virus was one of the first to be studied in the electron microscope (Taylor *et al.*, 1943), and it was with influenza virus that it was first demonstrated that certain viruses were assembled by budding from the cell membrane (Murphy and Bang, 1952). The application of negative staining to viruses provided an enormous impetus to the study of virus structure, and influenza virus was the object of some of the earliest and most striking work (Horne *et al.*, 1960; Hoyle *et al.*, 1961) which revealed both the presence of an envelope covered with surface projections and a helical internal component of nucleocapsid. In recent years

15

the virus has been investigated by a variety of physical and chemical techniques, and as a result, the influenza virus is one of the best understood of the enveloped viruses from the standpoint of structure.

The value of such knowledge concerning the structure and assembly of influenza virus is great because of the biological importance of the disease that the various influenza viruses produce in man and animals. There is also the added benefit that influenza and other enveloped viruses serve as excellent models for study of the structure of cell membranes. This is because the virus possesses a membrane which is morphologically similar to, and assembled in continuity with, cell membranes. The advantages of the use of membrane-enclosed viruses are that they are simple and manipulable models which can be obtained in highly purified and homogeneous form for chemical, physical, and biological studies. They possess only a few proteins which are virus-coded, and thus can be varied by selection of different virus strains and mutants, and these proteins can in many instances be isolated in biologically active form. The lipid and carbohydrate content of the viral membrane can be varied by changing the host cell, since these components of the viral membrane are determined largely by the host. The value of viruses as model membranes has been emphasized previously (Choppin et al., 1971, 1972; Choppin and Compans, 1975; Compans and Choppin, 1975; Lenard and Compans, 1974).

This chapter will describe the overall composition and morphology of the virus, and the interrelationship of the various components. Other chapters (i.e., Chapters 3, 6, 10, and 12) will deal in detail with the biological and immunological properties of the various components, as well as elaborate on the structure of the nucleic acid and some of the individual proteins. Other recent reviews have dealt with the structure and assembly of influenza virus (Compans and Choppin 1971, 1973, 1975; Choppin et al., 1972; Schulze, 1973; Laver, 1973; Choppin, 1975; White, 1974).

II. Composition of the Virus Particle

A. Overall Composition and Mass

The chemical composition of influenza virions cannot be given with absolute precision because of the heterogeneity of the virus population and the fact that, as discussed below, the composition of the virion is in part dependent on the host cell with regard to lipids and carbohydrates. Approximate compositions, however, have been determined: 0.8–1.1% RNA, 70–75% protein, 20–24% lipid, and 5–8% carbohydrate (Ada and Perry, 1954; Frommhagen et al., 1959; Blough et al., 1967). Influenza virus particles grown under most conditions consist largely of noninfectious "incomplete" virus particles; thus the above value for RNA content represents a low estimate for an infectious particle containing a full complement of RNA. Careful analyses of virus particles grown in the MDBK line of bovine kidney cells, which produce a high yield of infectious particles and fewer incomplete particles relative to other cells (Choppin, 1969), and purified by means designed to select for complete particles on the basis of density should yield a more accurate figure for RNA content.

The exact molecular weight of the influenza virion is also uncertain due to the heterogeneity of the population, and estimations have varied widely. On the basis of electron microscopy and sedimentation properties, estimates of 270×10^6 to 290×10^6 daltons have been obtained (Lauffer and Stanley, 1944; Sharp *et al.*, 1945; Schramm, 1954). A lower value of 151×10^6 daltons was obtained for fowl plague virus on the basis of sedimentation and diffusion coefficients (Schäfer *et al.*, 1952; Schramm, 1954), and a higher estimate of 360×10^6 daltons was obtained based on protein determination and electron microscopic particle counts (Reimer *et al.*, 1966). Because of the variation in size of the virus particle, it is not possible to obtain a value which will apply to all particles, and in addition the techniques such as particle counting and sedimentation coefficients are difficult to apply with accuracy to enveloped virus particles which vary in shape and are susceptible to disruption. Although the exact value for the mass of influenza virus particles will of necessity vary, and no precise value can be given, there is now relatively good agreement among various laboratories concerning the various species of RNA's and proteins contained in the virus particle.

B. RNA

The RNA content of the influenza virion has been reported to be 0.8–1.1% (Ada and Perry, 1954; Frisch-Niggemeyer and Hoyle, 1956; Frommhagen *et al.*, 1959). Since the purity of the virus preparations used was not conclusively established, these values are subject to some uncertainty. The fact that Frisch-Niggemeyer and Hoyle (1956) also reported an RNA content of 5.3% for the isolated influenza viral ribonucleoprotein, whereas more recent studies yielded values of 10–12% (Pons *et al.*, 1969; Krug, 1971), suggests that the early estimates of RNA content of the virion may also be on the low side. The early chemical estimates of RNA content suggested that the size of the viral genome was about 2×10^6 daltons (Frisch-Niggemeyer, 1956), which is also considerably lower than recent estimates of 4×10^6 to 5×10^6 daltons based on gel electrophoresis of viral RNA.

The available biological and biochemical evidence indicates that influenza viral RNA occurs in the form of multiple segments in the virion. This evidence will not be reviewed in detail here, since extensive discussion of the viral RNA is presented in Chapter 6. In polyacrylamide gels of viral RNA, six or seven species appear to be present, ranging in molecular weight from

3.5×10^5 to 10×10^5 daltons (Skehel, 1971; Lewandowski *et al.*, 1971; Bishop *et al.*, 1971). The discrete size classes observed and the studies of RNA termini (Young and Content, 1971; Lewandowski *et al.*, 1971, indicate that the RNA segments are not the result of fragmentation or cleavage by nuclease. Estimates of the total genome size, obtained by adding the molecular weights of the segments, are in the range of 4×10^6 to 5×10^6 daltons. The sizes of the individual RNA segments correlate well with the estimated molecular weights of virus-coded polypeptides, suggesting that each genome segment codes for one viral polypeptide. The viral RNA is contained in a helical ribonucleoprotein internal component, and, as discussed below, distinct size classes of ribonucleoproteins are found which contain different viral RNA segments.

No convincing evidence has been obtained for linkage or specific aggregation of viral RNA segments, either in the virion or the infected cell. An aggregate structure of $\sim 3 \times 10^6$ daltons has been obtained when RNA was extracted from virions in the presence of divalent cations, and was converted to slower-sedimenting structures by heat treatment (Agrawal and Bruening, 1966; Pons, 1967). One electron microscopic study reported the observation of RNA molecules with estimated molecular weights up to 3×10^6 daltons, which were dissociated into smaller molecules at pH 3 (Li and Seto, 1971). However, the heterogeneity in the observed length distribution did not support the view that a specific aggregate of all viral genome segments had been obtained.

Variation in the RNA profiles of influenza virus has been detected. Serial undiluted passage of influenza virus leads to the production of noninfectious particles and is reflected in a low infectivity to hemagglutinin ratio (von Magnus, 1954). Such virus is termed "incomplete" virus and is characterized by a lack of the largest RNA species, and an increase in the amount of small heterogeneous RNA (Pons and Hirst, 1968; Duesberg, 1968; Choppin and Pons, 1970). Some variation in RNA sedimentation patterns has been reported among different virus strains, and also in virus of the same strain when prepared at different times of harvest or multiplicities of infection (Barry *et al.*, 1970). Such variation may reflect unequal rates of synthesis of different virion RNA segments, with smaller RNA species replicating more rapidly than larger RNA's.

C.   Protein

1. THE NUMBER AND DESIGNATIONS OF POLYPEPTIDES

The various polypeptides found in the virion will be described briefly here, and their arrangement within the virion will be discussed in Section III.

In addition, the properties of some of these proteins, particularly the hemagglutinin and neuraminidase, will be discussed in detail in subsequent chapters [synthesis (Chapter 8), chemical and biological properties (Chapter 3), and immunological properties (Chapters 10 and 12)]. Although the influenza virion is assembled by budding from the plasma membrane of the host cell, host cell polypeptides are not present as structural proteins of the virion. This lack of host proteins in the virion has been shown by a variety of lines of evidence. These include the failure to detect prelabeled cellular polypeptides in the virion (Holland and Kiehn, 1970), the presence of the same polypeptides in virions grown in different cell types (Compans et al., 1970a; Schulze, 1970), and the failure to find common peptides in influenza virus and other enveloped virus grown in the same cell type. In addition, all of the influenza virion polypeptides can be found as newly synthesized species in infected cells (Lazarowitz et al., 1971; Skehel, 1972; Klenk et al., 1972b; Compans, 1973a).

Because three virion proteins could be identified immunologically, i.e., the nucleocapsid protein, hemagglutinin, and neuraminidase (see Chapters 10 and 12), attention was focused on these proteins throughout the 1960's, and early electrophoretic studies also revealed three major polypeptides which were equated with these three antigens. However, with the development of improved resolution of polyacrylamide gels and labeling with both amino acids and sugars to identify the proteins and glycoproteins, it was found that there were as many as 7 structural polypeptides present in the virion. These ranged in size from $\sim$25,000 to $\sim$94,000 daltons (Compans et al., 1970a; Schulze, 1970). There is now general agreement regarding the protein composition of the virion (Haslam et al., 1970a; Compans et al., 1970a; Schulze 1970; Skehel and Schild, 1971; Lazarowitz et al., 1971, 1973a; Klenk et al., 1972a). Figure 2.1 shows the polypeptides of the WSN strain of influenza A virus grown in primary rhesus monkey kidney cells. Table 2.1 lists the polypeptides whose existence has been well established, and gives their functions and location within the virion, where this is known. The designations are those adopted in 1971 at a Workshop on Influenza (Kilbourne et al., 1972).

2. The P Polypeptides

The function and exact location of the largest virion proteins, molecular weights 81,000–94,000 daltons, designated P_1 and P_2 have not been established. However, these proteins are internal components of the virion; they are probably associated with the nucleocapsid and may be involved in the RNA transcriptase activity of the virion (Compans et al., 1970a; Schulze

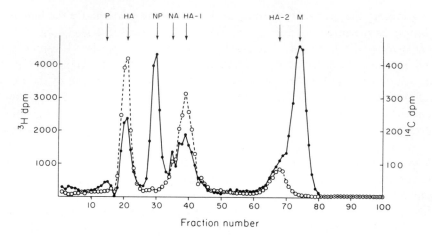

Fig. 2.1. Polyacrylamide gel electropherogram of the polypeptides of the WSN strain of influenza A virus doubly labeled with a [^{14}C]amino acid mixture (solid line) and [^{3}H]fucose (dashed line). The virus was grown in primary rhesus monkey kidney cells. The properties of the polypeptides are described in the text. Some of the hemagglutinin (HA) polypeptides have been cleaved to yield HA$_1$ and HA$_2$. (Modified from Compans et al., 1970a).

1970; Klenk et al., 1972a; Skehel, 1971; Bishop et al., 1972; Caliguiri and Compans, 1974).

3. The Hemagglutinin

The largest glycoprotein, HA, molecular weight 75,000–80,000 daltons, is the receptor binding protein or hemagglutinin of the virus. It is synthesized as a single primary gene product, but under certain conditions may be cleaved proteolytically to yield two polypeptides, HA$_1$ and HA$_2$, molecular weights ~50,000 and 28,000 daltons, respectively (Lazarowitz et al., 1971). The extent of this cleavage, which may vary from none to complete cleavage of all molecules, depends on the host cell, the virus strain, and the presence or absence of plasminogen or other proteolytic enzymes in the cell culture medium or other host system, such as the allantoic sac of the chick embryo (Lazarowitz et al., 1971, 1973a,b; Rifkin et al., 1972; Klenk et al., 1972b; Skehel, 1972; Stanley et al., 1973). Complete cleavage usually occurs in the chick embryo (Lazarowitz et al., 1973a), and this accounts for the earlier finding of two hemagglutinin polypeptides (Laver, 1971; Stanley and Haslam, 1971), originally termed the heavy and light polypeptides and now designated HA$_1$ and HA$_2$. These HA$_1$ and HA$_2$ portions of the HA protein are held together by disulfide bonds (Laver, 1971). The cleavage of the HA molecule is not required for assembly of the virus particle or for expres-

Table 2.1   The Proteins of the Influenza Virion

Designation[a]	Molecular weight (daltons)	Location in virion	Function	Comments
P₁, P₂	81,000–94,000	Internal	Involved in RNA transcription?	Two polypeptides have been resolved in some, but not all strains
HA	75,000–80,000	Spikes on surface	Binding to cellular receptors	Glycoprotein. May be cleaved to yield HA₁ and HA₂
NP	55,000–65,000	Internal	Subunit of nucleocapsid	Strains of the same type share a common nucleoprotein antigen
NA	55,000–70,000	Spikes on surface	Neuraminidase	Glycoprotein
HA₁	49,000–58,000	Spikes on surface	Binding to cellular receptors	Glycoproteins, derived from HA by proteolytic cleavage and linked by disulfide bonds
HA₂	25,000–30,000	Spikes on surface		
M	21,000–27,000	Beneath lipid bilayer in envelope	Major structural component of envelope	Nonglycosylated membrane protein

[a] The designations of the various proteins are those adopted at Influenza Virus Workshop I, Madison, Wisconsin, October, 1971 (see Kilbourne *et al.*, 1972).

sion of its hemagglutinating activity (Lazarowitz *et al.*, 1973a; Stanley *et al.*, 1973), and, under certain conditions, virions are assembled in which there has been no cleavage of any of the HA molecules (Lazarowitz *et al.*, 1973a,b; Choppin *et al.*, 1975), emphasizing the nonessential nature of this event. Figure 2.2 shows the lack of cleavage of the HA polypeptide of WSN virions grown in the absence of serum plasminogen, and complete cleavage in the presence of this enzyme. Recently it has been found with strains of both influenza A and B viruses that the infectivity of virions, which have no detectable cleaved HA molecules, can be enhanced by cleavage with trypsin (P. W. Choppin and S. G. Lazarowitz, unpublished experiments; H.-D. Klenk and R. Rott, personal communication). The exact mechanism of this enhancement of infectivity is at present unknown, but presumably involves some early step in virus–cell interaction other than adsorption.

As will be discussed in detail in Chapters 3, 10, and 12, the hemagglutinin and neuraminidase polypeptides of different strains vary greatly in amino

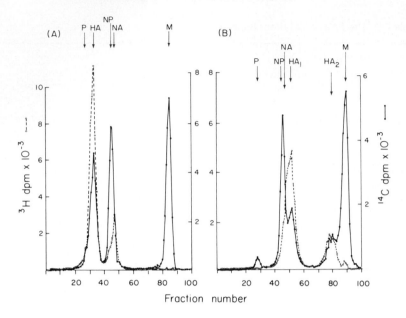

Fig. 2.2. Effect of the presence of plasminogen in the growth medium on the cleavage of the HA polypeptide of the WSN strain of influenza A virus. Poly-acrylamide gel electropherogram of the polypeptides of virions grown in MDBK cells in reinforced Eagle's medium without serum in the presence or absence of plasminogen, and labeled with [^{14}C]amino acid mixture and [^{3}H]glucosamine. (A) Virions grown in the absence of plasminogen showing no cleavage of the HA polypeptide. (B) Virions grown in the presence of plasminogen, 3.5 μg/ml, show-ing complete cleavage of the HA polypeptide. (From Lazarowitz et al., 1973b).

acid sequence and antigenicity. These surface glycoproteins are responsible for the strain-specific immunological properties of the virions.

4. The Neuraminidase

The neuraminidase polypeptide (NA) is a glycoprotein, the subunit of which has a molecular weight reported to be in range of 50,000 to 65,000 daltons, depending on the virus strain and conditions of isolation in various laboratories (Haslam et al., 1970b; Webster, 1970; Skehel and Schild, 1971; Gregoriades, 1972; Lazdins et al., 1972). Two different sizes of neuramini-dase polypeptides from the same virus have been reported (Webster, 1970; Skehel and Schild, 1971; Bucher and Kilbourne 1972; Lazdins et al., 1972). Lazdins et al. (1972) found a major component of 63,000 daltons and a minor component with 56,000 daltons, but only the smaller component was found in neuraminidase preparations obtained by trypsin treatment of the virus. This suggested that the smaller component was derived from the larger native subunit by proteolytic cleavage. The smaller molecule did not aggregate, suggesting that the portion removed contained a hydrophobic region. The electron microscopic studies of Wrigley *et al.* (1973) showed that trypsin removed the stalk of the mushroom-shaped neuraminidase spike, and activity remained indicating that the oblong head of the spike contains the active site of the enzyme. As will be discussed in Chapter 3, there is much evidence which suggests that the enzyme is present in the virion in the form of a tetramer with a molecular weight of 200,000–250,000 daltons (Kendal and Eckert, 1972; Bucher and Kilbourne, 1972; Lazdins *et al.*, 1972; Wrigley *et al.*, 1973).

5. THE NUCLEOCAPSID PROTEIN

The NP polypeptide is the protein subunit of the helical nucleocapsid (Duesberg, 1969; Joss *et al.*, 1969; Pons *et al.*, 1969). The estimates of the size of this protein from many different laboratories and in different strains of virus have ranged from 55,000 to 65,000 daltons, with 60,000 daltons usually being quoted as the approximate size. It contains no carbohydrate, and is the type-specific antigen upon which the classification into types A, B, and C is based (see Chapter 12). Amino acid analyses of NP protein from type A and B strains have revealed significant differences (Laver and Baker, 1972). The NP protein shows an affinity for influenza virus RNA *in vitro,* both virion and complementary RNA strands (Scholtissek and Becht, 1971).

6. THE MEMBRANE PROTEIN

The most plentiful protein in the influenza virion is the membrane or matrix protein (M). This is the smallest protein in the virion with an estimated molecular weight of 21,000–28,000 daltons (Compans *et al.*, 1970a; Schulze, 1970, 1972; Haslam *et al.*, 1970b; Skehel and Schild, 1971; Klenk *et al.*, 1972a). Peptide maps of M protein purified by filtration on an agarose column in the presence of 8 *M* guanidine indicated that the protein was distinct from a slightly smaller nonstructural protein (NS), molecular weight 25,000 daltons (Lazarowitz *et al.*, 1971). Gregoriades (1973) compared peptide maps of the M protein extracted from virions by acidic chloroform–methanol and of a protein with similar electrophoretic mobility from infected cells, and found that they were similar. In this study the M and NS proteins were not resolved on electrophoresis. The explanation for the apparent discrepancy between these two reports is not clear, but one possibility is that the acid chloroform–methanol extracted only the M protein from cells and not NS. Alternatively, there could be a relationship between M and NS, but this seems less likely tin view of the differences between the two obtained in the previous analyses of proteins separated and purified by agarose filtration (Lazarowitz *et al.,* 1971), and the lack of a precursor–product relationship in long pulse-chase experiments (Meier-Ewert and Compans,1974). Amino acid analyses of the M protein of several strains of influenza virus have been reported (Laver and Baker, 1972).

Schild (1972) examined the M proteins of influenza A and B virus strains in immunodiffusion studies and found that they possessed type-specific antigenicity, but were not related to the NP protein which also possesses type specificity. Since the M protein is not on the virion surface, and therefore not exposed to antibody, the lack of the strain-specific antigenic variation which characterizes the surface glycoproteins is not surprising.

7. Amounts of Polypeptides in the Virion

Because of heterogeneity in the size of influenza virions and also strain variation, any calculation of the number of molecules of the various polypeptides present in the virion is necessarily difficult. Furthermore, the HA and its cleavage product, HA_1 and HA_2, may vary markedly depending on the extent of cleavage of the HA molecule, and this cleavage, as described above, depends on a variety of conditions. Finally, the total amount of the HA and the NA glycoproteins on the virion of a given strain may vary with the host cell (Lazarowitz *et al.,* 1973a; Choppin *et al.,* 1975). Thus, any estimate of the number of polypeptides is only an approximation of those present in the average virion under a given set of conditions. Table 2.2 lists the range of values obtained in several laboratories which are in fairly good agreement. For a more complete listing of values obtained by a number of workers using different strains, the reader is referred to the extensive review of influenza virus proteins by White (1974).

8. Influenza B and C Viruses

Most of the studies on the chemistry and structure of the virion and its proteins have been done on influenza A strains; however sufficient work has been done with the Lee strain of influenza B virus to indicate that it is in general similar in structure and composition to the type A viruses (Haslam *et al.,* 1970b; Lazdins *et al.,* 1972; Laver and Baker, 1972; Oxford, 1973; Tobita and Kilbourne, 1975). However, some small but significant differences have been found with the GL/1760/54 strain of influenza B (Choppin *et al.,* 1975). Examination of the proteins of this virus grown in hamster kidney cells revealed no detectable P protein, and coelectrophore-

Table 2.2 Approximate Amounts of the Various Polypeptides
in the Influenza Virion

Polypeptide	Percent of total protein[a]	Number of molecules per virion[b]
P_1, P_2	1.5–2.7	30–60
HA	0–24	640–930
NP	17–26	500–940
NA	3–7	110–240
HA_1	0–21	—
HA_2	0–12	—
M	33–46	2500–3120

[a] The values in this table represent the ranges obtained in studies by Compans *et al.* (1970a), Schulze (1970), Skehel and Schild, (1971), and Lazarowitz *et al.* (1973a,b). The great variation in the percent of HA, HA_1, and HA_2 reflects differences in the extent of cleavage of HA to yield and HA_1 and HA_2.

[b] The estimate given for HA represents the sum of uncleaved HA molecules plus the HA_1 + HA_2 complexes. The relative number of each varies with the extent of cleavage. The estimates are based on a total protein content of 2.0×10^8 daltons per virion.

sis of the proteins of this strain and the WSN strain of influenza A revealed that the HA, NP, and NA proteins of GL/1760 were slightly larger, with molecular weights of 82,000, 66,000, and 64,000 daltons, respectively, whereas the M protein of GL/1760, with a molecular weight of 24,000 daltons, was slightly smaller than the WSN M protein. Figure 2.3 shows a polyacrylamide gel pattern of the proteins of the B/GL/1760 strain.

A striking finding with the GL/1760 strain was the complete lack of cleavage of the HA protein when grown in hamster kidney cells. However the HA polypeptide could be cleaved *in vitro* with trypsin to yield HA_1 and HA_2, and it was found that whereas NA and HA_1 contained fucose residues, HA_2 did not, although it did contain glucosamine. Thus there is an absence of a sugar, which is usually located distally on the carbohydrate chains, on the HA_2 portion of the hemagglutinin spike. This is the portion by which the spike attaches to the membrane, and the absence of fucose on HA, and its presence on HA_1 and NA of this strain and on HA_2 of other strains, suggests that there may be a more intimate relationship between the HA_2 molecule of this strain and the membrane, and that this may interfere with completion of glycosylation on the membrane.

Another interesting finding with the GL/1760 strain was that early and late labeling with radioactive amino acids showed that the membrane pro-

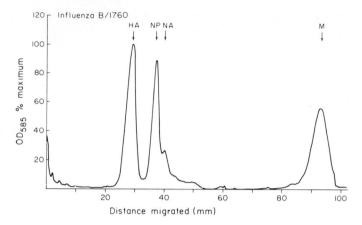

Fig. 2.3. Polyacrylamide gel electropherogram of the polypeptides of the GL/1760/54 strain of influenza B virus grown in the HKCC line of hamster kidney cells. There has been no cleavage of the HA polypeptide, and no P protein is seen. The gel was stained with Coomassie blue, and the profile of absorbance of the stained gel determined at 585 nm in a Gilford recording spectrophotometer. (From Choppin *et al.,* 1975.)

tein was synthesized relatively late in the growth cycle, and that NP protein made early in infection is incorporated into virions which contain M protein synthesized later (Choppin *et al.,* 1975). Similar results have recently been obtained with the WSN strain (Meier-Ewert and Compans, 1974). These results are compatible with the previous suggestion that the synthesis of M protein is tightly controlled and may be a rate-limiting step in virus production (Lazarowitz *et al.,* 1971).

Relatively little work has been done on the composition of influenza C viruses; however a recent preliminary report indicates that the virion has a protein composition which showed general similarities to that of the influenza A and B viruses. However the virus lacked neuraminidase activity, and it was suggested that it may possess another type of glycosidase capable of destroying receptors for the virus (Kendal and Kiley, 1974).

D. Lipid

The lipids present in the influenza virion are located in the viral membrane and, as described below, appear to be present in the form of a bilayer. Of the 20–24% of the mass of the virion which lipids comprise, most is represented by phospholipids (10–13%) and cholesterol (6–8%), and a small but perhaps important part is glycolipid (1–2%). (Frommhagen *et al.,* 1959; Kates *et al.,* 1961; Blough and Merlie, 1970; Klenk *et al.,* 1972a; H.-D. Klenk and P. W. Choppin, unpublished experiments). Early studies indicated that prelabeled cellular lipids were incorporated into influenza virions (Wecker, 1957), and that the lipids of virions grown in different cells resembled those of the host (Kates et al., 1961). This early work suggested that the host cell played a significant role in determining the lipid composition of the virus. Later Blough and co-workers analyzed the lipids of different strains of influenza virions grown in the chick embryo (Tiffany and Blough, 1969; Blough, 1971; Blough and Tiffany, 1973). On the basis of differences observed, they proposed that the viral envelope proteins determine the lipid composition of the virion by selective association of these proteins with lipids. However, these differences were observed largely in the fatty acids of neutral lipids. Because these represent a small proportion of the total lipids, and because in general the fatty acids of the polar lipids were similar among the various strains, the significance of these differences is not clear. These analyses were done on virions grown in the chicken embryo under multiple cycle conditions; strains may vary in their kinetics of growth and effects on cellular metabolism, and therefore the lipid composition of the host membrane may vary. In addition, analyses done on virions grown at different times in different lots of eggs are difficult to evaluate.

Examination of virions grown under the more controlled conditions of cell culture has obvious advantages. Extensive comparison of the lipids of enveloped virions and of the plasma membrane of different host cells have been carried out, including detailed analyses of phospholipids, cholesterol, glycolipids, and fatty acids (Klenk and Choppin, 1969, 1970a,b; Choppin et al., 1971; Renkonen et al., 1971; Quigley et al., 1971; Laine et al., 1972; McSharry and Wagner, 1971). Although minor differences were observed in some instances, in most cases the lipid composition reflects very closely that of the plasma membrane of the host cell. Concentrations of phospholipids in a given virus strain may vary as much as threefold depending on the host cell, and host-specific qualitative differences in glycolipids were also observed (Klenk and Choppin, 1969, 1970b). Further, the fatty acid composition could be varied as much as fourfold by changing the composition of the medium (Klenk and Choppin, 1970b). These results indicate that, although under certain conditions there may be minor variations in lipid composition which might be affected by the viral proteins, the major determining influence on viral lipid composition is the host cell, and that the lipids of the viral membrane closely resemble those of the plasma membrane of the host cell.

It should be emphasized that the finding of a similarity between the lipids of the viral membrane and the plasma membrane of the host cell and the conclusion that the host is the major determinant of the lipids of the virus do not imply that all the lipids incorporated into the virus are present in the cell at the time of infection. Indeed, the fact that with many enveloped viruses, virus production continues over a long period, requires that some newly synthesized lipids are incorporated into virions. The recent report (Blough, 1974) that newly synthesized lipids are incorporated into virus thus does not indicate these lipids are specified by the virus, but only that the biosynthesis of lipids which become part of the viral membrane does not cease after infection, and that newly synthesized lipids as well as preexisting lipids are utilized in virus assembly.

The major qualitative exception to the similarity between virus and host membrane lipids is that there are no neuraminic acid-containing glycolipids, i.e., gangliosides, found in influenza virions, nor is there neuraminic acid bound to the glycoproteins of the virion (Klenk and Choppin, 1970b; Klenk *et al.*, 1970b). The absence of neuraminic acid residues on the virion is due to the incorporation of the viral enzyme neuraminidase into those areas of membrane which become the viral envelope. Enveloped virions which lack neuraminidase, such as vesicular stomatitis virus, contain the same gangliosides as the plasma membrane of the host cell (Klenk and Choppin, 1971).

The subject of lipids in the membrane of influenza virus and other enveloped viruses has been recently reviewed by several authors (Choppin *et al.*, 1971; Choppin and Compans, 1975; Compans and Choppin, 1975; Blough and Tiffany, 1973; Klenk, 1973, 1974; Lenard and Compans, 1974.)

E. Carbohydrates

In addition to ribose present in the viral RNA, about 5–8% of the mass of the influenza virion is carbohydrate (Frommhagen *et al.*, 1959). Most, if not all of the carbohydrate is bound covalently to glycoprotein or glycolipid. Galactose, mannose, glucosamine, and fucose are present in the virion, and the composition of the component sugars is similar to that of host cell mucoproteins (Ada and Gottschalk, 1956). The isolated HA_1 polypeptide of the hemagglutinin of the BEL strain grown in the chick embryo contained 9.4% N-acetylglucosamine, and about 20% of its total mass was estimated to be carbohydrate (Laver, 1971, 1973). The carbohydrate represents a host cell-specific antigen which has been found in purified virions (Knight, 1946; Smith *et al.*, 1953) and is covalently linked to viral glycoprotein (Harboe, 1963; Laver and Webster, 1966; Lee *et al.*, 1969). Carbohydrate components have been isolated from membranes of uninfected cells (Laver and Webster, 1966) and from chick allantoic fluid (Haukenes *et al.*, 1965; Lee *et al.*, 1969) which are antigenically related to the host antigen of purified virions. The allantoic antigen is a mucopolysaccharide sulfate free of uronic or neuraminic acid, which resembles the keratan sulfate class of polysaccharides in composition (Haukenes *et al.,* 1965). Recently it was found that the virion glycoproteins are selectively labeled with radioactive sulfate, which appears to be linked to the carbohydrate as a sulfate ester (Compans and Pinter, 1975). In addition, sulfate is incorporated into a high molecular weight component which appears to be a mucopolysaccharide derived from the host cell, and which may correspond to the host cell antigen that has been found in association with purified virions.

Incorporation of the radioactive precursors glucosamine and fucose into the virion glycoproteins, hemagglutinin and neuraminidase, indicates that the carbohydrate portions of these molecules are newly synthesized after infection (Compans *et al.,* 1970a; Schulze, 1970). Whether newly synthesized or preexisting cellular carbohydrates are present in virion glycolipids has not been established.

The available evidence indicates that the sequence and composition of the carbohydrates of viral glycoproteins and glycolipids are specified by the host cell. In addition to the host cell-specific antigenic properties of the carbohydrates described above, differences in electrophoretic mobilities of glycoproteins of virions grown in different cell types suggest that the amount of carbohydrate incorporated into the glycoproteins may be host cell determined (Haslam *et al.,* 1970a; Compans *et al.,* 1970a; Schulze, 1970). At least four specific transferases would be required for synthesis of the carbohydrate side chains of glycoproteins, and the virus does not appear to contain sufficient genetic information to code for these transferases. Glycosylation of the hemagglutinin polypeptide appears to occur in association with endoplasmic reticulum membranes, a process analogous to the synthesis of the carbohydrates of cellular glycoproteins (Compans, 1973b; Hay, 1974).

Neuraminic acid residues are absent from influenza virions, presumably as a result of the viral neuraminidase (Klenk and Choppin, 1970b; Klenk *et al.,* 1970a,b; Palese *et al.,* 1974). Parainfluenza virions, which also contain a neuraminidase, similarly lack neuraminic acid residues in their glycoproteins and glycolipids (Klenk and Choppin, 1970b; Klenk *et al.,* 1970a,b), whereas enveloped viruses of other major groups possess no neuraminidase and contain neuraminic acid residues. A neuraminidase appears to be required by those enveloped viruses which bind to neuraminic acid-containing receptors, as discussed further in Chapter 3. Cells infected with temperature-sensitive influenza virus mutants which lack neuraminidase yield virus particles which contain neuraminic acid residues, and form large aggregates at the cell surface (Palese *et al.,* 1974). This aggregation is prevented by addition of neuraminidase, indicating that neuraminic acid incorporated into virions can serve as receptor for the influenza virus hemagglutinin, resulting in aggregation and low yields of infectious virus. Thus the lack of neuraminic acid in influenza and parainfluenza virions is· a virus-specific modification of its carbohydrate that is essential for the normal release of virus from the infected cell.

In the presence of the abnormal metabolite 2-deoxy-D-glucose or high concentrations of glucosamine, the normal glycosylation process of viral glycoproteins is inhibited, and in infected cells a nonglycosylated or partially glycosylated precursor of the HA polypeptide is detected (Klenk *et al.*, 1972b; Gandhi *et al.*, 1972). The aberrant glycoproteins produced in the presence of these inhibitors are found in smooth and rough endoplasmic reticulum membranes and are incorporated into progeny virus particles (Klenk *et. al.*, 1974; Compans *et al.*, 1974). These virus particles, however, possess reduced infectivity and hemagglutinating activity. Thus the normal carbohydrate components do not appear to be required for association of glycoproteins with cytoplasmic membranes; however the yield of mature virions is reduced, and glycosylation appears to be necessary for full biological activity of the virion.

III. Morphology and Arrangement of Components in the Virion

A. Size and Shape

Early ultrafiltration and electron microscopic studies indicated that the influenza virions examined had an average diameter of 80–120 nm and were roughly spherical (Elford *et al.*, 1936; Taylor *et al.*, 1943). With the application of negative contrast techniques to influenza virus, it was found that the surface of the virion was covered with closely spaced projections or spikes 10–12 nm long, and that the nucleocapsid enclosed within the viral envelope was helical (Horne *et al.*, 1960; Hoyle *et al.*, 1961). The negative staining technique also revealed heterogeneity and pleomorphism within the population of virions. However, much of the pleomorphism is due to the preparative procedures and can be minimized by fixing the virus before staining (Choppin *et al.*, 1961). Figures 2.4 and 2.5 show negatively stained influenza virions.

Although most laboratory-adapted strains are roughly spherical in shape, shadowed whole-mount preparations of the Japan/305 strain of influenza A revealed a slightly elongated or bacillary shape (Choppin *et al.*, 1960), and when seen in thin section newly formed influenza virions often appear to be slightly elongated (Fig. 2.6) (Compans and Dimmock, 1969; Compans *et al.*, 1970b; Bächi *et al.*, 1969). The nucleocapsid of sectioned particles is seen as electron-dense strands arranged parallel to the long axis of the particle, and the envelope consists of a membrane with a layer of projections on the outer surface. (Figs. 2.5–2.8).

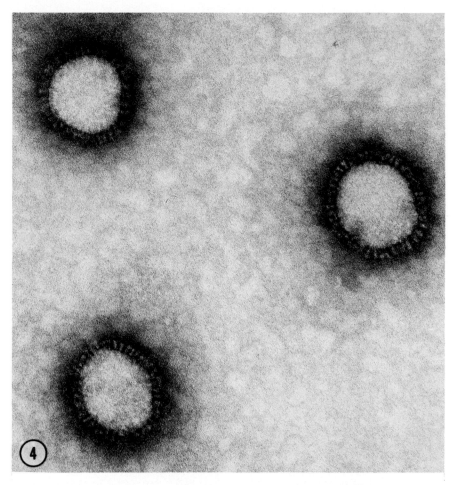

Fig. 2.4. Influenza virions of the AO/WSN strain, negatively strained with sodium phosphotungstate. The particles appear roughly spherical, about 100–120 nm in diameter, with a distinct layer of spikes on their surfaces. × 200,000.

In addition to the roughly spherical or slightly elongated virions that are usually seen, long filamentous forms are sometimes found. These filaments are covered with surface projections and have a diameter similar to that of the spherical forms, i.e., 80–100 nm, but may be very long, with lengths up to 4 μm having been observed (Mosely and Wyckoff, 1946; Chu *et al.*, 1949; Choppin *et al.*, 1960, 1961). Figure 2.5 shows a negatively stained influenza virus filament. The filamentous particles predominate in newly isolated strains (Chu *et al.*, 1949; Choppin *et al.*, 1960). It is possible that filamentous forms also predominate in human infections of the respiratory

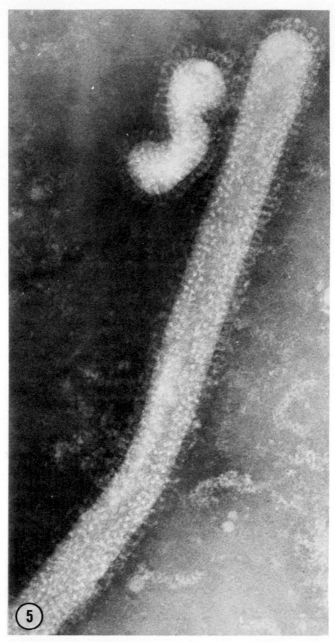

Fig. 2.5. Negatively stained virions of the A2 RI/4⁻ strain of influenza virus. Part of a long, filamentous particle is shown with spikes covering its entire surface. × 280,000. (From Choppin et al., 1961).

tract, since on the first passage in the egg, the virus population is highly filamentous, but on serial passages, a spherical population is selected (Choppin *et al.*, 1960). It seems unlikely that one passage in the egg would select for filaments from a predominantly spherical population in the human infection, and then on a further passage in the egg a spherical form would again be selected. However, the nature of the morphology of the virions produced in human infections remains to be established by examination of sufficiently large amount of virus obtained directly from man. The specific infectivity of filaments has been examined and found to be higher than that of spherical virions, and they contain more RNA per particle than do the spheres (Ada *et al.*, 1958).

The production of filaments is a genetic trait which can be exchanged by recombination (Kilbourne and Murphy, 1960; Kilbourne, 1963; Choppin, 1963). Recombination of spherical A0 strains with filamentous A2 strains resulted in the production of spherical A2 and highly filamentous A0 strains. Filamentous morphology can thus be used as a marker in genetic studies. This genetically determined variation in virion morphology suggests a difference in the structure or rate of synthesis of an envelope protein, possibly the M protein. Preliminary studies on spherical and filamentous virions of the same strain have not revealed differences in their overall protein composition (P. W. Choppin, unpublished experiments); however more detailed studies are needed.

Surface-active agents, such as vitamin A alcohol, have been shown to induce the formation of filaments and large pleomorphic particles in strains which usually are spherical (Blough, 1963). Although these studies show that the shape of the virus can be affected by the presence of such agents, they are not in conflict with the studies cited above showing genetic control of filament formation in the absence of surface-active agents.

A high degree of structural regularity was observed when influenza virions were examined by freeze drying or freeze etching (Nermut and Frank, 1971). Some of the particles cast angular shadows, and it was suggested that the virions may have icosahedral symmetry. Regular hexagonal arrangements on the surface of the virion have also been observed (Archetti *et al.*, 1967; Almeida and Waterson, 1967; Nermut and Frank, 1971), and influenza C virions have been observed to have what appeared to be a hexagonal lattice underlying the surface (Waterson *et al.*, 1963; Flewett and Apostolov, 1967). It has been suggested that the M protein of the virus forms an icosahedral shell beneath the lipid layer, and thus functions as a kind of capsid for the virus (Schulze, 1973). However, the observations made to date do not establish icosahedral symmetry for the virion, and indeed there are reasons for thinking such an arrangement unlikely. Although there are other examples of virions with icosahedral symmetry which may

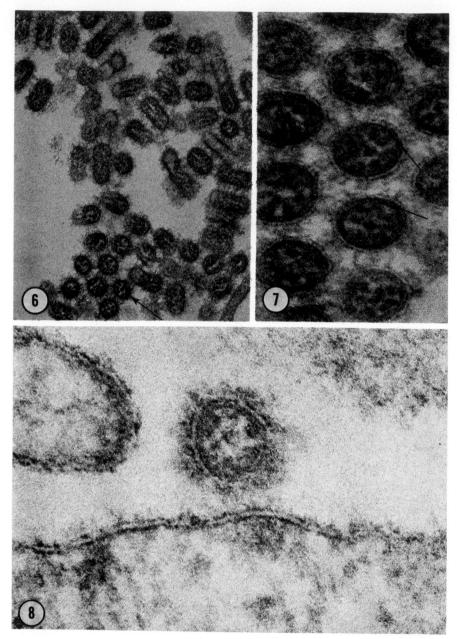

Figs. 2.6–2.8

exist in long tubular arrangements as well as in icosahedra, the spherical influenza virions occur in a wide range of sizes, and there is no precedent for packing identical subunits into icosahedral capsids in a continuum of sizes. Most virions observed do not show outlines suggesting icosahedral symmetry, and the angular outlines sometimes seen could be due to distortion. Further evidence is needed to determine conclusively whether there is icosahedral symmetry in the viral envelope.

B. Spikes

The hemagglutinin and neuraminidase will be discussed in detail in Chapters 3 and 10, and therefore only the structural features will be reviewed briefly here.

1. THE HEMAGGLUTININ

As indicated above, the hemagglutinin spike is formed by glycoprotein subunits with a molecular weight of $\sim$75,000–80,000 daltons. These may be present as a continuous polypeptide chain, HA, or as a complex formed by the products of proteolytic cleavage, HA_1 and HA_2, which are still held together by disulfide bonds.

Early studies using ether to disrupt the virions indicated that a subviral component with hemagglutinating activity could be released from the virus (Hoyle, 1952; Schäfer and Zillig, 1954), and negative staining of ether-released hemagglutinin particles revealed rosette-like structures 300–500 Å in diameter, in which spikes identical to those present on the virus surface were arranged radially (Hoyle *et al.*, 1961; Choppin and Stoeckenius, 1964). Laver and Valentine (1969) isolated spikes using a strain in which

---

Fig. 2.6.   Influenza virions in thin section. Many of the particles are elongated and are sectioned longitudinally, whereas others (arrow) are circular cross sections in which the internal ribonucleoprotein strands are also cut in cross section, appearing as electron-dense dots. × 90,000.

Fig. 2.7.   High magnification of influenza virions in thin section, illustrating the unit membrane of the viral envelope and the dense inner layer (arrows) which is thought to be composed of the M polypeptide. The particles in Figs. 2.6 and 2.7 are temperature-sensitive mutants of the A0/WSN strain which are defective in neuraminidase production, and which therefore produce virions in large aggregates, as described further in the text and in Chapter 3. × 200,000.

Fig. 2.8.   Thin section of an influenza virion (A0/WSN strain) adjacent to a region of the surface of an MDBK cell. The unit membrane is clearly visible on the cell surface, and the sectioned virion contains a similar unit membrane with an additional dense inner layer. × 300,000. (From Compans and Choppin, 1973).

the hemagglutinin was resistant to sodium dodecyl sulfate (SDS). These hemagglutinating spikes were ~40 Å in diameter and 140 Å long. After removal of SDS, the spikes aggregated by one end, suggesting that the base of the spike was hydrophobic in nature. On the basis of the dimensions of the hemagglutinin spikes as seen in the electron microscope, Laver and Valentine (1969) suggested that the molecular weight of a spike was at least 150,000 daltons. When it became clear that the structure was composed of proteins with a molecular weight of 75,000–80,000 daltons, it was suggested that two such proteins, consisting of $HA_1 + HA_2$ complexes, formed the spike (Laver, 1971; Stanley and Haslam, 1971; Skehel and Schild, 1971). Later an estimate of 215,000 daltons was made on the basis of sedimentation (Brand and Skehel, 1972), and electron microscopic studies showed a triangular shape for the spike when viewed end-on (Laver, 1973; Griffith, 1975). It was therefore suggested that each spike is a trimer composed of three HA polypeptides, or $HA_1 + HA_2$ complexes.

The hydrophobic nature of the base of the spike suggested that this region was involved in binding of the spike to the viral membrane (Laver and Valentine, 1969). Subsequently it was found that on treatment with protease particles could be obtained which retained HA_2, but had no hemagglutinin activity and no identifiable spikes (Compans et al., 1970a). This suggested that the HA_2 portion of the HA molecule was involved in binding, and this was supported by the finding of Brand and Skehel (1972) that hemagglutinin spikes could be solubilized by protease treatment, and these spikes had lost only a small portion of the HA_2 polypeptide. Such spikes did not aggregate and could be crystallized. Thus the evidence suggests clearly that the HA_2 portion of the HA protein contains a hydrophobic region and is involved in the binding of the spike to the membrane. The exact mechanism of binding of the spike is not yet known. However as will be discussed below, the lipid in the viral membrane is in the form of a bilayer, and the available suggests that no major part of the spike penetrates deeply into the bilayer, although small peptides enriched in hydrophobic amino acids appear to remain associated with the particle after protease treatment (R. Compans, unpublished observations). Protease treatment does not significantly disturb the structure of the lipid bilayer, and the structure of the lipid phase appears to be determined more by lipid–lipid interactions than by interactions between the glyproteins and lipid (Compans et al., 1970a; Landsberger et al., 1971, 1973).

2. THE NEURAMINIDASE

In the same study cited above in which hemagglutinin spikes were isolated (Laver and Valentine, 1969), spikes with different morphology and neuraminidase activity were also isolated from a different strain of virus. This provided evidence that there were two different kinds of spikes on the influenza virion. The neuraminidase spikes had oblong heads of $\sim 50 \times 85$ Å attached to a fiber ~ 100 Å long, with a small knob 40 Å in diameter at the end. In the absence of detergents, these spikes also aggregated by their ends to form rosettes, suggesting that they also had hydrophobic bases. Although two types of spikes have been isolated from virions with detergents, it has not been possible to resolve them clearly on untreated virions, possibly because of the close packing of spikes. This may also be due to difficulty in identifying the neuraminidase spikes among the more numerous hemagglutinin spikes.

As discussed above, the molecular weight of the neuraminidase monomer is in the range of 55,000–65,000 daltons, and there is biochemical and morphological evidence that the neuraminidase spike consists of a tetramer with a molecular weight of 200,000–250,000 daltons (Kendal and Eckert, 1972; Bucher and Kilbourne, 1972; Lazdins *et al.*, 1972; Wrigley *et al.*, 1973). Electron microscopic examination of neuraminidase after treatment with trypsin revealed a structure composed of four spheres 4 nm in diameter in coplaner square array (Wrigley *et al.*, 1973). This tetramer when viewed on edge appears to correspond to the oblong knob seen in the neuraminidase spikes isolated by detergent. The trypsin treatment removed the stalk of the spike.

As in the case of the hemagglutinin spike the mechanism of attachment of the neuraminidase spike to the membrane is not clear. However, like the HA spike, the NA spike apparently has a hydrophobic base which is involved in the attachment, and which is susceptible to protease attack under certain conditions.

C. Lipid Bilayer

Since the influenza virus particle forms by a process of budding at the plasma membrane, and the lipid of the virion is derived from the plasma membrane in this process, it is likely that the arrangement of lipids in the viral envelope closely reflects that of the cellular plasma membrane. The available evidence indicates that the viral lipids are arranged in a bilayer structure. Electron spin resonance (ESR) studies using stearic acid derivative spin label molecules have provided evidence for a bilayer structure in influenza virus (Landsberger *et al.*, 1971, 1973). A flexibility gradient, which is characteristic of a bilayer structure (McConnell and McFarland, 1972), was observed in spin-labeled influenza virions. Thus a nitroxide-containing spin label group attached close to the polar head group of a stearic acid molecule is held in a highly rigid environment, whereas a similar group attached further down the hydrocarbon side chain is in a relatively fluid environment. Figure 2.9 illustrates a comparison of ESR spectra of influenza virions spin-labeled with stearic acid and steroid derivatives and human erythrocytes labeled with the same derivatives; there is a high degree of similarity in the spectra of the two membranes.

Based on their reactivity with a surface-labeling reagent, it has been suggested that the arrangement of phospholipids is asymmetric in cell surface membranes, with choline-containing molecules located predominantly in the outer half of the bilayer, and aminophospholipids in the inner monolayer (Bretscher, 1972, 1973). Whether such an arrangement is present in viral envelopes remains to be established; however existing data on the lipid composition of parainfluenza viruses (Klenk and Choppin, 1969, 1970a,b) do not support the conclusion that phosphatidylethanolamine and phosphatidyl-

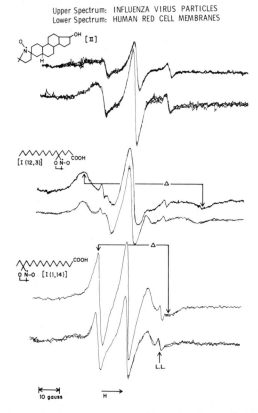

Fig. 2.9. ESR spectra of influenza virions and human erythrocyte membranes labeled with the same spin label molecules. The splitting between the high and low magnetic field peaks, denoted Δ, is markedly greater for the spin label I (12,3) than for I (1,14), as is characteristic of a bilayer structure. (From Landsberger et al., 1971).

serine are always located in the inner half of the bilayer and phosphatidyl-choline in the outer half. The ratios of aminophospholipids to choline-containing phospholipids vary widely in viruses grown in different cell types, reflecting the ratios in the corresponding host cells. Since these parainfluenza viruses all contain the same envelope proteins, the suggestion that protein may replace lipid in part of the bilayer (Bretscher, 1973) cannot account for differences in phospholipid composition. It is therefore likely that differences in lipid composition are reflected in a different distribution of individual phosopholipid species between the internal and external halves of the bilayer.

The influenza virion possesses a characteristic membrane structure when seen in thin section, which is morphologically similar to the membrane structure on the host cell surface (Figs. 2.6–2.8). The appearance of the viral envelope depends on the cell type in which the virus is grown, as well as on the electron microscopic staining procedure (Compans and Dimmock, 1969). Whenever a unit membrane is seen on the cell surface, a membrane of similar appearance is found in the viral envelope. The outer surface of the viral membrane is covered with surface projections, and an additional electron-dense layer is found on the inner surface of the viral membrane, which is not found in the normal cellular membrane. As described below, it is likely that this layer corresponds to the location of the M protein on the internal surface of the bilayer.

The distribution of stain after osmium fixation of membranes may reflect the location of aminophospholipids (Bretscher, 1973). Using osmium fixation and the same staining procedure, both the inner and outer leaflets of the unit membrane are clearly stained in the MDBK cell, but only the cytoplasmic side is stained in BHK21-F cells or chick embryo fibroblasts. These differences are reflected in the envelopes of influenza virions grown in these cells. The staining of the outer leaflet in MDBK-grown influenza virions correlates with a higher content of aminophospholipids in these cells (Klenk and Choppin, 1970a), and in such circumstances it is possible that aminophospholipids are distributed in both halves of the bilayer, whereas they may be restricted to the inner half of the bilayer in BHK21-F cells.

Glycolipids are present in influenza virions, and their exposure at the outer surface of the bilayer has been demonstrated by agglutination of virions with specific lectins (Klenk et al., 1972a). In the intact virion the glycolipids are not exposed, but they become accessible to lectins upon removal of spikes by protease treatment.

D. Membrane Protein

As mentioned above, when stained thin sections of influenza virions are examined in the electron microscope an additional electron-dense layer can be resolved on the inner surface of the viral envelope (Figs. 2.7 and 2.8), which is not present in normal cellular plasma membranes (Apostolov and Flewett, 1969; Apostolov *et al.,* 1970; Kendal *et al.,* 1969; Compans and Dimmock, 1969; Bächi *et al.,* 1969). There are now several lines of evidence which suggest that this layer is composed of the smallest and most plentiful protein in the virion, which is designated the membrane or matrix, protein (M). The evidence includes the following. (1) The glycoprotein spikes can be removed proteolytically leaving the M protein and the electron-dense layer unchanged (Compans *et al.,* 1970a; Schulze, 1970, 1972; Kendal *et al.,* 1969). The only other proteins remaining after such treatment are the nucleocapsid protein and the P proteins, neither of which could be responsible for the electron-dense layer. The few molecules of P proteins present could not possibly account for such a layer, and the nucleocapsid protein is present in the interior of the virion in the helical nucleocapsid. (2) Calculations reveal that the M protein is the only one that is present in sufficient quantity to form such a structure, and that it could form a shell 4–6 nm thick beneath the bilayer (Compans *et al.,* 1972; Schulze, 1972). (3) After lipid extraction of fixed, spikeless virions a shell remained which could only be formed by the M protein (Schulze, 1972). (4) Iodination experiments with chloramine T indicated that the M protein, though not on the surface of the virion, was external to the nucleoprotein (Stanley and Haslam, 1971). (5) Fluorescence transfer experiments have indicated that there is transfer from this protein to a fluorescent probe incorporated into the lipid bilayer (Lenard *et al.,* 1974).

The above evidence indicates a close association of the M protein with the under side of the membrane, but this protein does not appear to penetrate through the bilayer to the outside. This is indicated by the lack of effect of proteolytic enzymes on this protein (Compans *et al.,* 1970a; Schulze, 1970; Klenk *et al.,* 1972a), by the failure of the M protein to react with reagents specific for external proteins (Stanley and Haslam, 1971; Rifkin *et al.,* 1972), and by the failure to find intramembraneous particles in freeze-fracture studies of the influenza virus membrane (Bächi *et al.,* 1969).

From the location of the M protein in a shell beneath the lipid layer and the fact that the spike glycoproteins do not play a major role in maintaining the shape or integrity of the viral membrane, it appears likely that the M protein plays the major structural role in the viral envelope. In addition there are other functions that are suggested by its location and properties. During the assembly process of enveloped viruses, the nucleocapsid aligns specifically beneath those areas of plasma membrane which contain viral envelope proteins, implying that recognition occurs between the nucleocapsid and those areas of membranes. Further, during the assembly and budding process, the viral membrane is continuous with the remainder of the plasma membrane, and yet no host proteins are found in the virion, in spite of the increasing body of evidence that proteins can migrate in the plane of the cell membrane. This implies that the virus has a mechanism for maintaining a localized domain within the plasma membrane which contains viral proteins, and from which cellular proteins are excluded. As suggested previously, the most likely candidate for both providing a recognition site for the viral nucleocapsid and maintaining a localized domain within the membrane is the M protein (Choppin et al., 1972; Choppin and Compans, 1975; Compans and Choppin, 1975; Choppin, 1975).

E. Nucleocapsid

The internal structure of influenza virions is revealed only rarely in negatively stained preparations, and most information on the structure of the internal ribonucleoprotein has been obtained in studies of isolated ribonucleoproteins or thin sections of virus particles. There is general agreement that the ribonucleoprotein is in the form of discrete segments, each of which contains one molecule of viral RNA, multiple copies of the NP polypeptide, and probably one or more P polypeptides.

The ribonucleoproteins (RNP's) can be isolated in a density gradient from virions which have been disrupted with detergents, such as deoxycholate or NP40, or by ether treatment. When examined by negative staining with uranyl acetate or phosphotungstate, the structures obtained by these procedures (Figs. 2.10 and 2.11) appear as strands 10–15 nm in diameter which vary in length from ~30 to 110 nm (Pons et al., 1969; Schulze et al., 1970; Compans et al., 1972). The strands sometimes exhibit loops on one end, and a periodicity consisting of alternating major and minor grooves, which suggests that the structure is formed by a strand that is folded back on itself and then coiled into a double helix. The model depicted in Fig. 2.12 indicates the suggested structure of the ribonucleoproteins.

The ribonucleoproteins can be separated into distinct size classes by sedimentation in velocity gradients, reflecting the sizes of the RNA's which they contain (Duesberg, 1969; Pons, 1971). The separated fractions contain structures of similar diameter, which differ considerably in length (Compans et al., 1972). The length distributions of isolated RNP's have been determined using positive staining with uranyl acetate, which binds preferentially to the nucleic acid (Fig. 2.11). The most rapidly sedimenting RNP's have a peak in length distribution at 90–110 nm; the medium-sized RNP's at 60–90 nm, and the smallest RNP's at 30–50 nm. These lengths can be correlated with the molecular weights of the nucleic acids contained in the various size classes. Thus the large RNP's contain the largest viral RNA molecules of about 10^6 daltons (see Section II,B and Chapter 6). The RNP's contain

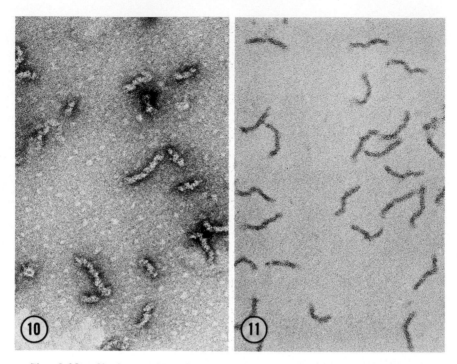

Fig. 2.10. Nucleocapsids of influenza virus, negatively stained with uranyl acetate. The strands vary in length from ~30 nm to over 100 nm, and are about 15 nm in diameter. × 110,000. (From Compans and Choppin, 1973).

Fig. 2.11. Nucleocapsids positively stained with uranyl acetate. The stain binds preferentially to the viral RNA, and the strands have a uniform width of ~10 nm. × 100,000. (From Compans and Choppin, 1973).

10–12% RNA with the balance almost entirely consisting of NP protein subunits (Pons *et al.*, 1969; Krug, 1971). One can calculate from these data that there are about 150 protein subunits with a molecular weight of 60,000 daltons in the 100 nm RNP strand, or about 12 subunits per single helical turn, and 20 nucleotides per protein subunit (Compans *et al.*, 1972).

Thin sections of influenza virions are compatible with the conclusion that the viral ribonucleoprotein is arranged in the virion as multiple short segments (Compans and Dimmock, 1969; Bächi *et al.*, 1969; Compans *et al.*, 1970b; Schulze, 1973). Virus particles in the process of budding are generally slightly elongated, and internal strands are arranged parallel to the long axis of the particle (Compans and Dimmock, 1969). Negative staining of protease-treated spikeless particles with uranyl acetate revealed multiple internal strands similar in morphology to the ribonucleoproteins isolated after detergent treatment (Schulze, 1973). Thus different preparative procedures, in which the internal structure is revealed in most virus particles in a population, yield images which are compatible with the view that the ribonucleoprotein is segmented in the virion.

In an occasional virion in negatively stained preparations, large, rigid coiled structures are observed (Apostolov and Flewett, 1965; Almeida and Waterson, 1970; Schulze *et al.*, 1970). It has been considered that such structures may represent "intact" nucleocapsids of influenza virions, and that the ribonucleoproteins isolated from virions are fragmentation products (Almeida and Waterson, 1970). However, the finding of terminal loops on one end of the isolated ribonucleoprotein strands, as well as the fact that lengths of the strands have a discrete range of sizes (Compans *et al.*, 1972), indicates that they are not direct products of fragmentation of a larger structure. In addition, as described above, thin sections of virus preparations in which the internal structure can be resolved in most particles indicate that such large coils are present very rarely if at all. Occasionally structures similar to the large rigid coils are found in infected cells, and it remains to be established whether they have any relationship to the viral ribonucleoproteins. This will probably not be possible unless the coiled structures are isolated and their composition determined.

It has been proposed that RNP's are incorporated randomly into virions from an intracellular pool (Hirst, 1962), which leads to the high frequency of recombination observed with influenza viruses (see Chapter 7). Whereas it might be argued that such a random process would only rarely result in virions containing all of the genome segments required for infectivity, the proportion of infective virions in a population is increased significantly if virions contain extra pieces of RNA (Compans *et al.*, 1970b). Evidence in favor of random incorporation of RNA segments is provided by the observation of Hirst and Pons (1973) that aggregates of influenza virions which are found normally, or are produced artifically with nucleohistone, have enhanced infectivity. These results suggest complementation by two or more virus particles, each of which alone lacks one or more of the RNA segments required for infectivity.

Several properties of the ribonucleoproteins of influenza virus distinguish them from the helical nucleocapsids of paramyxoviruses. The RNA in the ribonucleoprotein is susceptible to ribonuclease (Duesberg, 1969; Kingsbury and Webster, 1969; Pons *et al.*, 1969), whereas RNA in paramyxovirus nucleocapsids is resistant (Compans and Choppin, 1968). Treatment of the ribonucleoprotein with polyvinyl sulfate results in displacement of the RNA, with the protein subunits binding to the polyvinyl sulfate in a structure that is morphologically very similar to the ribonucleoprotein (Pons *et al.*, 1969; Goldstein and Pons, 1970). Paramyxovirus nucleocapsids are unaffected by such treatment (Goldstein and Pons, 1970). Thus the nature of the

RNA–protein interaction differs considerably in the two structures, with the RNA apparently more exposed in the influenza viral ribonucleoprotein structure.

The ribonucleoprotein structure is also susceptible to degradation with protease (Pons *et al.*, 1969). At low concentrations of pronase, the ribonucleoprotein retained its sedimentation characteristics, whereas prior treatment with ribonuclease followed by pronase caused degradation (Duesberg, 1969). These observations suggest that pronase can degrade the bonds between protein subunits, with the structural integrity being maintained by means of bonding between protein subunits and RNA.

The minor P polypeptides appear to be associated with ribonucleoproteins isolated from virions (Bishop *et al.*, 1972) or infected cells (Caliguiri and Compans, 1974). Because only a few P polypeptides may be present in each RNP strand, they are unlikely to play a role in determining the structural properties of the ribonuclcoprotein, and their exact location remains to be determined. The P proteins appear to be attached to the ribonucleoprotein less firmly than NP polypeptides, because the former can be removed during purification (Schulze, 1973). These minor polypeptides may function as components of the virion transcriptase (Bishop *et al.*, 1972) or as initiators in the encapsidation of virion RNA by the nucleocapsid protein.

IV. Assembly (see also Chapter 8)

The assembly of influenza virions occurs by a process of budding at the plasma membrane. This process will be discussed in Chapter 8 and has been reviewed in detail not only for influenza viruses, but also other viruses which form by budding at cellular membranes (Compans and Choppin, 1971, 1973, 1975; Choppin *et al.*, 1971, 1972; Lenard and Compans, 1974; Compans *et al.*, 1974; Klenk, 1973, 1974; Choppin and Compans, 1975), and will only be summarized briefly here. The ribonucleoprotein is assembled in the cytoplasm, and aligns under regions of the cell surface which contain viral envelope proteins. The virion then is formed by a process of budding and detachment from the plasma membrane. During the process of budding, the unit membrane structure in the emerging virion is continuous with that found on the surface of the host cell (Compans and Dimmock, 1969; Bächi *et al.*, 1969). The glycoproteins appear to arrive first at the plasma membrane, following their association with intracellular membranes (Compans, 1973a,b; Stanley *et al.*, 1973; Klenk *et al.*, 1974; Hay, 1974), and can be detected by specific adsorption of erythrocytes to plasma membranes of infected cells (Compans and Dimmock, 1969). The M polypeptide then appears to associate with the inner surface of the plasma membrane, forming a distinct electron-dense layer (Apostolov and Flewett, 1969; Compans and Dimmock, 1969; Bächi *et al.*, 1969). The glycoproteins as well as the M protein are found associated with plasma membranes after a short pulse label (Lazarowitz *et al.*, 1971). The presence of the M polypeptide presumably forms a binding site for the ribonucleoprotein, which is then incorporated into virions by budding. The shape change at the plasma membrane which leads to budding may result from asymmetric expansion of the outer half of the bilayer by the spike proteins, in a manner analogous to that suggested by Sheetz and Singer (1974) for amphipathic drugs which induce shape changes in cell membranes. The assembly process is completed by the sealing by fusion of both the viral membrane and the cell membrane at the site where the budding particle pinches off. Either spherical or filamentous virions are formed by this process and the mechanism by which the viral genome controls the morphology of the virions remains to be elucidated.

V. Summary—A Model of the Influenza Virion

Figure 2.12 shows a schematic diagram of the structure of the influenza virion based on existing knowledge. This model of necessity reflects well-established structural features, and also some interpretations of data that are still uncertain. As discussed above, there have been alternative suggestions by others for some features of the virion. Not all of the fine structural features are illustrated on this model, such as the oligomeric nature of the spikes, but these are discussed in the text and illustrated in Chapters 3 and 10. The available evidence suggests that the virion proteins are all specified by the viral genome, but that the lipid composition and the sequence of the carbohydrate chains linked to glycoproteins or glycolipids of the viral membrane are determined largely, if not entirely, by the host cell. The virions may exist as roughly spherical particles 80–120 nm in diameter, or as filamentous particles of the same diameter and varying lengths.

The surface of the virion is covered with projections or spikes. These spikes are oligomeric structures composed of glycoproteins which possess hemagglutinating (HA) or neuraminidase (NA) activities. The hemagglutinin spikes consist of three HA polypeptides, molecular weight ~80,000 daltons, which form a rod ~14 nm long. Under certain conditions, the HA polypeptide may be cleaved proteolytically to yield two polypeptides, HA_1 and HA_2, which are linked by disulfide bonds. This cleavage is not required for assembly nor for hemagglutinating activity. The HA_2 portion of the HA

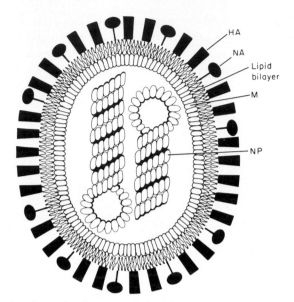

Fig. 2.12.   A schematic diagram of the structure of the influenza virion. Two types of glycoprotein surface projections or spikes, which differ morphologically and possess hemagglutinating and neuraminidase activities, are attached to a lipid bilayer. The hemagglutinin spikes are thought to consist of trimers of the HA polypeptide (see Fig. 10.2, Chapter 10), and the neuraminidase spike is a tetramer of the NA polypeptide. The numbers of the two kinds of spikes shown here are not meant to indicate the exact ratio or distribution of these spikes on the virion. The relative numbers of the two kinds of glycoproteins may vary in different strains. The mechanism of attachment of the spikes to the lipid bilayer is unknown, but each has a hydrophobic base. On the inner surface of the bilayer is a layer of nonglycosylated membrane protein (M) which is thought to be the major structural protein of the viral envelope. Within the envelope are segments of double helical nucleocapsids of different lengths containing different-sized pieces of the segmented single-stranded RNA genome. The protein subunit of the nucleocapsid is the NP polypeptide. Also located within the virion, and presumably associated with the nucleocapsid are the P polypeptides. These are not shown here because their arrangement in the virion is unknown. (See also Fig. 10.1, Chapter 10). (From Compans and Choppin, 1975.)

polypeptide is hydrophobic and contains the region of the molecule which is in contact with the viral membrane.

The neuraminidase spike is composed of four NA polypeptides, molecular weight ~55,000 daltons. These have terminal knobs ~4 nm in diameter which form a planar array that gives an oblong appearance when viewed from the side. These knobs are connected to a fiberlike stalk ~8 nm long which is attached to the viral membrane.

The exact mechanism of attachment of the spikes to the viral membrane is unknown. Both the hemagglutinin and neuraminidase spikes have hydrophobic bases that could be involved in hydrophobic interactions with the viral lipids, which are present in the form of a bilayer. However, the spikes do not appear to penetrate through the lipid bilayer, or deeply into it, although some penetration may exist. The spikes can be removed without destroying the integrity of the viral membrane.

On the inner surface of the lipid bilayer, there is a layer of protein formed by a nonglycosylated protein, M, molecular weight $\sim$25,000 daltons. This protein is thought to play the major structural role in the viral envelope, providing stability and perhaps determining the shape of the envelope. It is also suggested that this protein may serve as the recognition site for the nucleocapsid during virus assembly at the cell membrane, and may play an important role in the maintenance, during the assembly process, of a domain within the plasma membrane which contains only virus-specific proteins.

Within the viral envelope are contained multiple pieces of the nucleocapsid. These are double helical structures of various lengths which are formed by a single species of protein, NP, molecular weight $\sim$60,000 daltons, and which contain the different pieces of the segmented single-stranded RNA genome. Also located within the envelope, and probably associated with the nucleocapsids in as yet an unknown manner, are the P proteins, molecular weight $\sim$90,000 daltons; the function of these proteins is not certain, but they may be involved in the RNA transcriptase activity of the virus.

Acknowledgments

Research by the authors was supported by Research Grants AI-05600 and AI-10884 from the National Institute of Allergy and Infectious Diseases, and GB-43580 from the National Science Foundation.

References

Ada, G. L., and Gottschalk, A. (1956). *Biochem. J.* **62**, 686.
Ada, G. L., and Perry, B. T. (1954). *Aust. J. Exp. Biol. Med. Soc.* **32**, 453.
Ada, G. L., Perry, B. T., and Abbot, A. (1958). *J. Gen. Microbiol.* **19**, 23.
Agrawal, H. O., and Bruening, G. (1966). *Proc. Nat. Acad. Sci. U.S.* **55**, 818.
Almeida, J. D., and Waterson, A. P. (1967). *J. Gen. Microbiol.* **46**, 107.
Almeida, J. D., and Waterson, A. P. (1970). *In* "The Biology of Large RNA Viruses" (R. D. Barry and B. W. J. Mahy, eds.), pp. 27–51. Academic Press, New York.
Apostolov, K., and Flewett, T. H. (1965). *Virology* **26**, 506.
Apostolov, K., and Flewett, T. H. (1969). *J. Gen. Virol.* **4**, 365.
Apostolov, K., Flewett, T. H., and Kendall, A. P. (1970). *In* "The Biology of

Large RNA Viruses" (R. D. Barry and B. W. J. Mahy, eds.), pp. 3–26. Academic Press, New York.

Archetti, I., Jamelo, A., and Steve-Bocciarelli, D. (1967). *Arch. Gesamte Virusforsch.* **20**, 133.

Bächi, T., Gerhard, W., Lindenmann, J., and Mühlethaler, K. (1969). *J. Virol.* **4**, 769.

Barry, R. D., Bromley, P. A., and Davies, P. (1970). *In* "The Biology of Large RNA Viruses" (R. D. Barry and B. W. J. Mahy, eds.), pp. 279–300. Academic Press, New York.

Bishop, D. H. L., Obijeski, J. F., and Simpson, R. W. (1971). *J. Virol.* **8**, 74.

Bishop, D. H. L., Roy, P., Bean, W. J., Jr., and Simpson, R. W. (1972). *J. Virol.* **10**, 689.

Blough, H. A. (1963). *Virology* **19**, 349.

Blough, H. A. (1971). *J. Gen. Virol.* **12**, 317.

Blough, H. A. (1974). *Nature (London)* **251**, 333.

Blough, H. A., and Merlie, J. (1970). *Virology* **40**, 685.

Blough, H. A., and Tiffany, J. M. (1973). *Advan. Lipid Res.* **11**, 267.

Blough, H. A., Weinstein, D. B., Lawson, D. E. M., and Kodicek, E. (1967). *Virology* **33**, 459.

Brand, C. M., and Skehel, J. J. (1972). *Nature (London), New Biol.* **238**, 145.

Bretscher, M. (1972). *Nature (London), New Biol.* **236**, 11.

Bretscher, M. (1973). *Science* **181**, 622.

Bucher, D. J., and Kilbourne, E. D. (1972). *J. Virol.* **10**, 60.

Caliguiri, L. A., and Compans, R. W. (1974). *J. Virol.* **14**, 191.

Choppin, P. W. (1963). *Virology* **21**, 278.

Choppin, P. W. (1969). *Virology* **38**, 130.

Choppin, P. W. (1975). *Proc. Miles Int. Symp., 8th, 1974* (in press).

Choppin, P. W., and Compans, R. W. (1975). *In* "Comprehensive Virology" (H. Fraenkel-Conrat and R. R. Wagner, eds.), Vol. 4, pp. 95–178. Plenum, New York.

Choppin, P. W., and Pons, M. W. (1970). *Virology* **42**, 603.

Choppin, P. W., and Stoeckenius, W. (1964). *Virology* **22**, 482.

Choppin, P. W., Murphy, J. S., and Tamm, I. (1960). *J. Exp. Med.* **112**, 945.

Choppin, P. W., Murphy, J. S., and Stoeckenius, W. (1961). *Virology* **13**, 548.

Choppin, P. W., Klenk, H.-D., Compans, R. W., and Caliguiri, L. A. (1971). *Perspect. Virol.* **7**, 127.

Choppin, P. W., Compans, R. W., Scheid, A., McSharry, J. J., and Lazarowitz, S. G. (1972). *In* "Membrane Research" (C. F. Fox, ed.), pp. 163–185. Academic Press, New York.

Choppin, P. W., Lazarowitz, S. G., and Goldberg, A. R. (1975). *In* "Negative Strand Viruses" (R. D. Barry and B. W. J. Mahy, eds.). Academic Press, New York (in press).

Chu, C. M., Dawson, I. M., and Elford, W. J. (1949). *Lancet* **1**, 602.

Compans, R. W. (1973a). *Virology* **51**, 56.

Compans, R. W. (1973b). *Virology* **55**, 541.

Compans, R. W., and Choppin, P. W. (1968). *Virology* **35**, 289.

Compans, R. W., and Choppin, P. W. (1971). *In* "Comparative Virology" (K. Maramorosch and E. Kurstak, eds.), pp. 407–432. Academic Press, New York.

Compans, R. W., and Choppin, P. W. (1973). *In* "Ultrastructure of Animal Viruses and Bacteriophages: An Atlas" (J. A. Dalton and F. Hagnenau, eds.), pp. 213–237. Academic Press, New York.

Compans, R. W., and Choppin, P. W. (1975). *In* "Comprehensive Virology" (H. Fraenkel-Conrat and R. R. Wagner, eds.), Vol. 14, pp. 179–252. Plenum, New York.

Compans, R. W., and Dimmock, N. J. (1969). *Virology* 39, 499.

Compans, R. W., and Pinter, A. (1975). *Virology* (in press).

Compans, R. W., Klenk, H.-D., Caliguiri, L. A., and Choppin, P. W. (1970a). *Virology* 42, 880.

Compans, R. W., Dimmock, N. J., and Mier-Ewert, H. (1970b). *In* "The Biology of Large RNA Viruses" (R. D. Barry and B. W. J. Mahy, eds.), pp. 87–108. Academic Press, New York.

Compans, R. W., Content, J., and Duesberg, P. H. (1972). *J. Virol.* 10, 795.

Compans, R. W., Landsberger, F. R., Lenard, J., and Choppin, P. W. (1972). *Int. Virol.* 2, 130.

Compans, R. W., Meier-Ewert, H., and Palese, P. (1974). *J. Supramol. Struct.* 2, 496.

Duesberg, P. H. (1968). *Proc. Nat. Acad. Sci. U.S.* 59, 930.

Duesberg, P. H. (1969). *J. Mol. Biol.* 42, 485.

Elford, W. J., Andrewes, C. H., and Tang, F. F. (1936). *Brit. J. Exp. Pathol.* 17, 51.

Flewett, T. H., and Apostolov, K. (1967). *J. Gen. Virol.* 1, 297.

Frisch-Niggemeyer, W. (1956). *Nature (London)* 178, 307.

Frisch-Niggemeyer, W., and Hoyle, L. (1956). *J. Hyg.* 54, 201.

Frommhagen, L. H., Knight, C. A., and Freeman, N. K. (1959). *Virology* 8, 176.

Gandhi, S. S., Stanley, P., Taylor, S. M., and White, D. O. (1972). *Microbios* 5, 41.

Goldstein, E. A., and Pons, M. W. (1970). *Virology* 41, 382.

Gregoriades, A. (1972). *Virology* 49, 333.

Gregoriades, A. (1973). *Virology* 54, 369.

Griffith, I. P. (1975). *In* "Negative Strand Viruses" (R. D. Barry and B. W. J. Mahy, eds.). Academic Press, New York (in press).

Harboe, A. (1963). *Acta Pathol. Microbiol. Scand.* 57, 488.

Haslam, E. A., Hampson, A. W., Egan, J. A., and White, D. O. (1970a). *Virology* 42, 555.

Haslam, E. A., Hampson, A. W., Radiskevics, I., and White, D. O. (1970b). *Virology* 42, 566.

Haukenes, G., Harboe, A., and Mortensson-Egnund, K. (1965). *Acta Pathol. Microbiol. Scand.* 64, 534.

Hay, A. J. (1974). *Virology* 60, 398.

Hirst, G. K. (1962). *Cold Spring Harbor Symp. Quant. Biol.* 27, 303.

Hirst, G. K., and Pons, M. W. (1973). *Virology* 56, 620.

Holland, J. J., and Kiehn, E. D. (1970). *Science* 167, 202.

Horne, R. W., Waterson, A. P., Wildy, P., and Farnham, A. E. (1960). *Virology* 11, 79.

Hoyle, L. (1952). *J. Hyg.* 50, 229.

Hoyle, L., Horne, R. W., and Waterson, A. P. (1961). *Virology* 13, 448.

Joss, A., Gandhi, S. S., Hay, A. J., and Burke, D. C. (1969). *J. Virol.* 4, 816.

Kates, M., Allison, A. C., Tyrrell, D. A., and James, A. T. (1961). *Biochim. Biophys. Acta* 52, 455.

Kendal, A. P., and Eckert, E. A. (1972). *Biochim. Biophys. Acta* **258**, 484.

Kendal, A. P., and Kiley, M. P. (1974). *Abstr. Amer. Soc. Microbiol.* p. 222.

Kendal, A. P., Apostolov, K., and Belyavin, G. (1969). *J. Gen. Virol.* **5**, 141.

Kilbourne, E. D. (1963). *Progr. Med. Virol.* **5**, 79.

Kilbourne, E. D., and Murphy, J. S. (1960). *J. Exp. Med.* **111**, 387.

Kilbourne, E. D., Choppin, P. W., Schulze, I. T., Scholtissek, C., and Bucher, D. L. (1972). *J. Infec. Dis.* **125**, 447.

Kingsbury, D. W., and Webster, R. G. (1969). *J. Virol.* **4**, 219.

Klenk, H.-D. (1973). *In* "Biological Membranes" (D. Chapman and D. F. H. Wallach, eds.), Vol. 2, pp. 145–183. Academic Press, New York.

Klenk, H.-D. (1974). *Curr. Top. Microbiol. Immunol.* **68**, 29.

Klenk, H.-D., and Choppin, P. W. (1969). *Virology* **38**, 255.

Klenk, H.-D., and Choppin, P. W. (1970a). *Virology* **40**, 939.

Klenk, H.-D., and Choppin, P. W. (1970b). *Proc. Nat. Acad. Sci. U.S.* **66**, 57.

Klenk, H.-D., and Choppin, P. W. (1971). *J. Virol.* **7**, 416.

Klenk, H.-D., Caliguiri, L. A., and Choppin, P. W. (1970a). *Virology* **42**, 473.

Klenk, H.-D., Compans, R. W., and Choppin, P. W. (1970b). *Virology* **42**, 1158.

Klenk, H.-D., Rott, R., and Becht, H. (1972a). *Virology* **47**, 579.

Klenk, H.-D., Scholtissek, C., and Rott, R. (1972b). *Virology* **49**, 723.

Klenk, H.-D., Wöllert, W., Rott, R., and Scholtissek, C. (1974). *Virology* **57**, 28.

Knight, C. A. (1946). *J. Exp. Med.* **83**, 281.

Krug, R. M. (1971). *Virology* **44**, 125.

Laine, R., Kettungen, M.-L., Gahmberg, C. G., Kääräinen, L., and Renkonen, O. (1972). *J. Virol.* **10**, 433.

Landsberger, F. R., Lenard, J., Paxton, J., and Compans, R. W. (1971). *Proc. Nat. Acad. Sci. U.S.* **68**, 2579.

Landsberger, F. R., Compans, R. W., Choppin, P. W., and Lenard, J. L. (1973). *Biochemistry* **12**, 4498.

Lauffer, M. A., and Stanley, W. M. (1944). *J. Exp. Med.* **80**, 531.

Laver, W. G. (1971). *Virology* **45**, 275.

Laver, W. G. (1973). *Advan. Virus Res.* **18**, 57.

Laver, W. G., and Baker, N. (1972). *J. Gen. Virol* **17**, 61.

Laver, W. G., and Valentine, R. C. (1969). *Virology* **38**, 105.

Laver, W. G., and Webster, R. G. (1966). *Virology* **30**, 104.

Lazarowitz, S. G., Compans, R. W., and Choppin, P. W. (1971). *Virology* **46**, 830.

Lazarowitz, S. G., Compans, R. W., and Choppin, P. W. (1973a). *Virology* **52**, 199.

Lazarowitz, S. G., Goldberg, A. R., and Choppin, P. W. (1973b). *Virology* **56**, 172.

Lazdins, I., Haslam, E. A., and White, D. O. (1972). *Virology* **49**, 758.

Lee, L. T., Howe, C., Meyer, K., and Choi, H. U. (1969). *J. Immunol.* **102**, 1144.

Lenard, J., and Compans, R. W. (1974). *Biochim. Biophys. Acta* **344**, 51.

Lenard, J., Wong, C. Y., and Compans, R. W. (1974). *Biochim. Biophys. Acta* **332**, 341.

Lewandowski, L. J., Content, J., and Leppla, S. H. (1971). *J. Virol.* **8**, 701.

Li, K. K., and Seto, J. T. (1971). *J. Virol.* **7**, 524.

McConnell, H. M., and McFarland, B. G. (1972). *Ann. N.Y. Acad. Sci.* **195**, 207.

McSharry, J. J., and Wagner, R. R. (1971). *J. Virol.* **7**, 59.
Meier-Ewert, H., and Compans, R. W. (1974). *J. Virol.* **14**, 1083.
Mosley, V. M., and Wyckoff, R. W. G. (1946). *Nature (London)* **157**, 263.
Murphy, J. S., and Bang, F. B. (1952). *J. Exp. Med.* **95**, 259.
Nermut, M. V., and Frank, H. (1971). *J. Gen. Virol.* **10**, 37.
Oxford, J. S. (1973). *J. Virol.* **12**, 827.
Palese, P., Tobita, K., Ueda, M., and Compans, R. W. (1974). *Virology* **61**, 397.
Pons, M. W. (1967). *Virology* **31**, 523.
Pons, M. W. (1971). *Virology* **46**, 149.
Pons, M. W., and Hirst, G. K. (1968). *Virology* **34**, 386.
Pons, M. W., Schulze, I. T., and Hirst, G. K. (1969). *Virology* **39**, 250.
Quigley, J. P., Rifkin, D. B., and Reich, E. (1971). *Virology* **46**, 106.
Reimer, C., Baker, R., Newlin, T., and Havens, M. L. (1966). *Science* **152**, 1379.
Renkonen, O., Kääräinen, L., Simons, K., and Gahmberg, C. (1971). *Virology* **46**, 318.
Rifkin, D. B., Compans, R. W., and Reich, E. (1972). *J. Biol. Chem.* **247**, 6432.
Schäfer, W., and Zillig, W. (1954). *Z. Naturforsch. B* **9**, 779.
Schäfer, W., Munk, K., and Armbruster, O. (1952). *Z. Naturforsch. B* **7**, 29.
Schild, G. C. (1972). *J. Gen. Virol.* **15**, 99.
Scholtissek, C., and Becht, H. (1971). *J. Gen. Virol.* **10**, 11.
Schramm, G. (1954). "Die biochemie der Viren." Springer-Verlag, Berlin and New York.
Schulze, I. T. (1970). *Virology* **42**, 890.
Schulze, I. T. (1972). *Virology* **47**, 181.
Schulze, I. T. (1973). *Advan. Virus Res.* **18**, 1.
Schulze, I. T., Pons, M. W., and Hirst, G. K. (1970). *In* "The Biology of Large RNA Viruses" (R. D. Barry and B. W. J. Mahy, eds.), pp. 324–246. Academic Press, New York.
Sharp, D. G., Taylor, A. R., McLean, I. W., Beard, D., and Beard, J. W. (1945). *J. Biol. Chem.* **159**, 29.
Sheetz, M. P., and Singer, S. J. (1974). *Proc. Nat. Acad. Sci. U.S.* **71**, 4457.
Skehel, J. J. (1971). *J. Gen. Virol.* **11**, 103.
Skehel, J. J. (1972). *Virology* **49**, 23.
Skehel, J. J., and Schild, G. C. (1971). *Virology* **44**, 396.
Smith, W., Belyavin, G., and Sheffield, F. W. (1953). *Nature (London)* **172**, 669.
Stanley, P., and Haslam, E. A. (1971). *Virology* **46**, 764.
Stanley, P., Gandhi, S. S., and White, D. O. (1973). *Virology* **53**, 92.
Taylor, A. R., Sharp, D. G., Beard, D., Beard, J. W., Dingle, J. H., and Feller, A. E. (1943). *J. Immunol.* **47**, 261.
Tiffany, J. M., and Blough, H. A. (1969). *Science* **163**, 573.
Tobita, K., and Kilbourne, E. D. (1975). *Arch Virol.* **47**, 367.
von Magnus, P. (1954). *Advan. Virus Res.* **2**, 59.
Waterson, A. P., Hurrell, J. M. W., and Jensen, K. E. (1963). *Arch. Gesamte Virusforsch.* **12**, 487.
Webster, R. G. (1970). *Virology* **40**, 643.
Wecker, E. (1957). *Z. Naturforsch. B* **12**, 208.
White, D. O. (1974). *Curr. Top. Microbiol. Immunol.* **63**, 1.
Wrigley, N. G., Skehel, J. J., Charlwood, P. A., and Brand, C. M. (1973). *Virology* **51**, 525.
Young, R. J., and Content, J. (1971). *Nature (London), New Biol.* **230**, 140.

3

The Biologically Active Proteins of Influenza Virus: The Hemagglutinin

Irene T. Schulze

I. Introduction

The observation that the influenza viruses can agglutinate erythrocytes has had a profound effect on the development of our image of these viruses. Hemagglutination has proven to be an extremely valuable technique for virus identification, quantitation and purification. In addition, from the time that hemagglutination was first observed about 35 years ago (Hirst, 1941; McClelland and Hare, 1941), it has been assumed that adsorption of influenza viruses to host cells and to erythrocytes are analogous reactions. Consequently, our concepts of how these virions initiate infection have been strongly influenced by information about their interaction with erythrocytes.

Within a few years of the original observation, the essential features of the hemagglutination reaction had been elucidated by Hirst (1941, 1942a,b). It was demonstrated that hemagglutination could be used not only to detect the presence of virus but also to quantitate it, that proportionality existed between the hemagglutinating activity and lethal dosage for mice, and that adsorption of allantoic fluid with erythrocytes brought about concomitant reduction of egg infectious units and hemagglutinin titer. It was also shown that convalescent sera which neutralized infectivity also prevented hemagglutination. Thus, highly specific, simple and rapid methods for the quantitation of influenza viruses and of specific antibodies became available.

Hirst also observed that virus which was adsorbed to erythrocytes would elute at 37°C and that the eluted virus could readsorb to new erythrocytes. The cells from which the virus had been released could, however, no longer be agglutinated by the same strain of virus. Mild heat treatment destroyed the ability of the virus to elute without altering its hemagglutinating activity. These experiments suggested that a specific receptor on the cell was destroyed by a virion-associated enzyme. An investigation into the nature of this receptor (Hirst, 1948a,b, 1949a,b) revealed that it was a mucoprotein similar to the soluble hemagglutination inhibitors which had by then been found in normal sera (Hirst, 1942b; McCrea, 1946; Burnet and McCrea, 1946; Francis, 1947).

Hirst's experiments provided the first evidence for the existence of the virion-associated neuraminidase which is described in Chapter 4. Since they showed that virions are unaltered by the elution process, they also provided a method for purifying and concentrating influenza viruses. Techniques employing cycles of adsorption and elution were rapidly developed (Hare *et al.*, 1941, 1942; Francis and Salk, 1942) and are still in use today.

Shortly after its discovery hemagglutination was used to start another important chapter in the history of viruses. Disparity between infectivity titers and hemagglutination end points led von Magnus (1951) to recognize the existence of genetically incomplete virions now known as von Magnus virus or defective interfering particles.

We now know that the structures responsible for the hemagglutinating activity of the influenza viruses are evenly spaced, radial surface projections which are composed of glycoprotein subunits (see Chapter 2). When these structures are removed, both infectivity and hemagglutinating activity are lost. Interaction of the hemagglutinin with the cell membrane must therefore be the first step in the infectious cycle. However, as will be discussed in Section IV, conditions can be established in which virions will initiate infection although they will not agglutinate erythrocytes. It is the purpose of this chapter to describe all of the biological activities of the virion-associated hemagglutinin and to relate these activities to its structure. In the process, the analogy between adsorption of virions to host cells and to erythrocytes will be reevaluated. In order to do this, the hemagglutination reaction itself will be described, current information on the structure of the hemagglutinin will be reviewed, and its biological activities *in situ* and after removal from the virion will be discussed.

II. The Hemagglutination Reaction

A. Composition of the Receptor Substance from Human Erythrocytes

Influenza viruses cause hemagglutination because they attach to a specific sialic acid-containing glycoprotein which is a component of the erythrocyte membrane. This virus receptor has been isolated from human red cell stroma, and its composition and physical properties have been well characterized by Winzler and co-workers (see Winzler, 1969a,b). It is a glycoprotein which contains M and N blood group antigens (Kathan and Winzler, 1963; Morawiecki, 1964; Kathan and Adamany, 1967). When isolated from the cell, it is a potent inhibitor of influenza virus hemagglutination. Table 3.1 presents the properties of the isolated receptor and of a sialoglycopeptide which can be released from the amino terminal end of the molecule by trypsin. The released glycopeptide has no inhibitory activity, although it contains most of the sialic acid, hexose, and hexosamine originally associated with the virus receptor (Winzler *et al.*, 1967). The polypeptide moiety constitutes only 18% of the sialoglycopeptide. Serine and threonine account for almost half of the amino acid residues. The carbohydrate is attached to these two amino acids by O-glycosidic and to asparagine by N-glycosidic linkage. Sialic acid residues occupy terminal positions on the carbohydrate chains and can be released from the receptor by viral neuraminidase (Kathan and Winzler, 1963). Removal of sialic acid from this molecule destroys its hemagglutination inhibition activity as well as its M and N blood group activities (Springer and Ansell, 1958). Polymerization of the intact molecules occurs readily in the absence of detergents and produces aggregates with molecular weights as high as 590,000. Inhibitory activity and M and N blood group activities increase with polymerization (Springer, 1967). This tendency to polymerize is thought to be due to the hydrophobic nature of the carboxyl terminal portion of the receptor. Polypeptides, which are composed predominantly of hydrophobic residues and are insoluble in aqueous medium,

Table 3.1 Physical Properties and Composition of Influenza Virus Receptor from Human Erythrocytes[a]

Physical properties	Virus receptor from erythrocyte stroma		Trypsin released sialoglycopeptide	
$s_{20,w}$	2.1		1.5	
M.W.	31,400		10,100[b]	
Chemical composition	% of dry wt.	moles/ 31,000 gm	% of dry wt.	moles/ 10,000 gm
Hexose	15.8	27	23.8	13
Fucose	1.2	2	1.8	1.1
Acetylhexosamine	19.7	27	17.3	8.3
N-Acetylneuraminic acid	27.8	28	37.4	12.1
Amino acids	35.7	105	18.4	15.2

[a] From Winzler (1969b). In "Red Cell Membrane Structure and Function" (G. A. Jamieson and T. J. Greenwald, eds). Lippincott, Philadelphia, Pennsylvania. Reproduced by permission.

[b] Average of values obtained from sedimentation and diffusion data (9500) and by the approach to equilibrium (Archibald) method (10,700).

can be cleaved from the C-terminal region of the molecule by trypsin (Winzler, 1969a) or by cyanogen bromide (Marchesi et al., 1972).

Winzler (1969a,b) proposed that the virus receptors are attached to the erythrocyte membrane via hydrophobic regions near their carboxyl ends and that the sialopeptides at the amino terminal ends extend out into the aqueous environment where they can react with influenza virus, with antibodies against the M and N antigens and with trypsin. Based on the amount of sialic acid released from cells by trypsin treatment, he calculated that each human erythrocyte has about 10^6 sialopeptides on its surface. However, the number of receptor sites on the erythrocyte is probably smaller than the number of receptor molecules. Howe et al. (1970) have found that ferritin-conjugated antibody to purified receptor binds to discrete sites on the membrane of intact cells; it is not evenly distributed over the cell surface. Thus, clusters of these receptor molecules appear to constitute the virus-binding sites on erythrocytes.

B. Interaction of Influenza Viruses with Erythrocytes

Sialic acid on erythrocytes appear to be essential for the adsorption of influenza viruses, since complete removal of these residues makes cells resistant to agglutination (Hirst, 1950). Virus particles also fail to bind to artificial membranes composed of phosphatidylcholine and glycoproteins unless the glycoproteins are sialylated (Tiffany and Blough, 1971). The amount of sialic acid required for binding does, however, differ from strain to strain. Virus strains can, in fact, be arranged in a series according to their capacity to agglutinate erythrocytes from which other strains have eluted (Burnet *et al.*, 1946).

The importance of sialic acid residues in the attachment process has also been emphasized by the experiments of Suttajit and Winzler (1971). The polyhydroxyl side chains of the sialic acid residues in glycoproteins can be shortened by one or two carbons by mild periodate oxidation followed by reduction with sodium borohydride. These altered glycoproteins exhibit greatly reduced capacity to prevent hemagglutination.* Methylation of the carboxyl group of sialic acid also reduces the inhibitory activity (see Kilbourne *et al.*, 1972b). Thus, the charge properties of the glycoprotein as well as other factors which determine its overall configuration appear to influence binding.

Sialic acid-containing components other than the specific virus receptors described above may also be involved in binding virus to some species of erythrocytes. Winzler (1969a) has observed that influenza viruses can still agglutinate human erythrocytes from which the sialopeptides have been removed by trypsin. Since liposomes which contain gangliosides can bind Sendai virus, a paramyxovirus (Haywood, 1974), it is likely that sialylated glycolipids on the surface of the erythrocyte will also bind influenza viruses. Haywood suggests that receptor sites need not contain any glycoproteins if gangliosides are present. She proposes that these glycolipids, when properly oriented on the membranes, can provide the orderly array of sialic acid molecules needed for virus receptor activity. Free sialic acid, free gangliosides, and small sialylated carbohydrates do not inhibit hemagglutination (Haywood, 1974; see also Hughes, 1973).

There is also some evidence that molecules which lack sialic acid residues may play a role in binding virus particles to cells. Some strains of virus do not elute although they release sialic acid from the cells to which they are bound (Tsvetkova and Lipkind, 1966), and, conversely, viruses can elute from some cells in the absence of detectable sialic acid release (Tamm, 1954). Were binding determined only by the sialic acid content of the receptor, the amount of neuraminidase activity associated with the virus particle should determine its rate of elution. This is not always the case (Choppin and Tamm, 1959, 1960; Tsvetkova and Lipkind, 1966).

Taken together these observations suggest that agglutination requires interaction with cell membrane components in addition to the sialic acid resi-

* This modification also inactivates the M blood group substance, providing additional evidence that the erythrocyte glycoprotein has both blood group and virus-receptor activity (Liao *et al.*, 1973).

dues of the virus receptors. The avidity with which viruses and erythrocytes interact appears to depend on the overall structure of the binding sites on the cell as well as on the structure of the viral hemagglutinin. Thus, a sufficient number of sialic acid residues at a given site and structural complementarity between the cell membrane and the viral hemagglutinin seem to be required for hemagglutination (Fazekas de St. Groth and Gottschalk, 1963; Springer *et al.,* 1969).

C. Assay Procedures Based on Hemagglutination

1. QUANTITATIVE HEMAGGLUTINATION

In view of the large number of receptor molecules on the surface of erythrocytes, it is not surprising that large amounts of influenza virus can be bound to each cell. It has been estimated that one guinea pig erythrocyte can accommodate as many as 7000 virus particles (Bateman *et al.,* 1955). However, when a limited amount of virus is present, virus particles and erythrocytes form aggregates in which the two components are present at ratios ranging from 1 to 20 virus particles per erythrocyte (Tyrrell and Valentine, 1957; Seto *et al.,* 1961; see also Hoyle, 1968).

The amount of hemagglutination observed with a given amount of virus depends on the species of erythrocytes; on the strain of virus; and on the temperature, pH, and ionic components of the reaction. The type of cell used is of major importance in determining whether agglutination will be observed. Vertebrate erythrocytes of avian, amphibian, and mammalian origin can be used (see Hoyle, 1968). The agglutinability of cells as well as the amount of virus which they will adsorb varies from species to species and from one member to another within the species.

Virus particles also differ in their ability to cause agglutination. Quantitative interpretation of the hemagglutination reaction therefore requires detailed information about all components of the system used. For example, virus particles of newly isolated strains of influenza (i.e., strains which have been grown for only a few passages in the laboratory), are frequently filamentous in shape, whereas those of established laboratory strains are usually sperical. Filamentous virus particles can, theoretically, bind large numbers of erythrocytes; thus, the amount of agglutination observed does not necessarily reflect the number of virus particles present.

With all virus strains, the observed amount of agglutination depends on two opposing reactions, adsorption and elution. Since adsorption requires that collisions between erythrocytes and virus particles occur, the rate of this reaction is determined by the concentration of the reactants and is almost completely independent of temperature. In contrast, elution usually results from the enzymatic destruction of the receptor and is, therefore, highly dependent on temperature. Virus strains with low neuraminidase activity can be assayed for hemagglutinating activity at 20°C. With virus strains possessing high neuraminidase activity, elution may be sufficiently rapid at 20°C so that agglutination does not occur. Agglutination by these viruses can be observed at 4°C or at 20°C after destruction of the virus-associated neuraminidase by mild heat treatment (Hirst, 1948b; Stone, 1949).

Various techniques for the detection of influenza virus-induced hemagglutination have been developed. Dilutions of virus are incubated with standard erythrocyte suspensions and the mixtures are examined for agglutination by direct observation (Salk, 1944) or by densitometry. In the latter case, photometric measurements of undisturbed virus–cell mixtures are made after a standard incubation period and settling time (Hirst and Pickels, 1942; Levine et al., 1953; Horsfall, 1954; Drescher, 1957). More recently a procedure has been developed whereby agglutination is quantitated by measuring hemoglobin released from the fraction of cells not agglutinated by a given dilution of virus (Cohen and Belyavin, 1966). The amount of hemoglobin is estimated and recorded by an automatic analyzer. Techniques for the quantitation of hemagglutinin subunits have also been developed (Drescher, 1966, 1967).

Of all of the above-mentioned procedures, the direct observation of dilution end points by the agglutination pattern method is the most frequently used. Chicken erythrocytes are commonly used in this technique. Twofold dilutions in test tubes or in plastic trays in which the reaction can be carried out in small volumes are usually employed. When more precise estimations are needed, the fractional dilution procedure of Horsfall and Tamm (1953) can be used or end points can be determined by densitometry. Standard deviations of mean virus titers determined by the fractional dilution method are about 17% (Horsfall and Tamm, 1953). Drescher (1957) has reported standard deviations as low as 3% when photometric techniques were employed.

2. HEMADSORPTION

Since influenza virions emerge from the cell by a budding process, viral hemagglutinin can be detected on the surface of infected cells prior to virion release. Virus can be quantitated by using erythrocyte binding to cells to determine titration end points (Shelokov et al., 1958), by counting foci of erythrocyte-coated cells within a monolayer (Hotchin et al., 1960), by determining the fraction of suspended cells which will bind erythrocytes (White *et al.,* 1965), or by measuring the hemoglobin from erythrocytes bound to the infected cells (Finter, 1964). The latter two techniques do not require that progeny virus be produced by the infected cells. They have been used to detect hemagglutinin on the surface of HeLa cells abortively infected with influenza virus (Wong and Kilbourne, 1961; White *et al.,* 1965), and to detect hemagglutinin synthesis by temperature-sensitive mutants at nonpermissive temperatures (Mackenzie and Dimmock, 1973).

3. Hemagglutination Inhibition

The hemagglutination reaction is inhibited by antibodies specific for the viral hemagglutinin and also by a number of soluble glycoproteins found in serum and other body fluids. Hemagglutination inhibition (HI), due either to specific antibody or to nonspecific inhibitors, is quantitated by mixing a standard amount of virus with dilutions of the serum to be tested. Erythrocytes are then added and titers are determined from the highest dilution of serum which prevents agglutination.

Nonspecific inhibitors of hemagglutination are present in varying amounts in most sera and must be removed or destroyed before specific antibody can be measured. Combinations of heat, neuraminidase, trypsin, and periodate treatment are used for this purpose. These inhibitors can also be removed by ion exchangers (see Kilbourne *et al.,* 1972b). Since these treatments may also reduce the level of specific antibody, the procedure used must be designed for the specific virus strain and type of serum under investigation.

D. Interaction of Influenza Viruses with Nonspecific Inhibitors of Hemagglutination

Although nonspecific inhibitors add complexity to the task of determining the amount of specific antibody present in serum, they are useful because they block hemagglutination and can be used to investigate virus–erythrocyte interactions. They have been classified as α, β, and γ inhibitors, depending on their chemical composition and properties (see review by Krizanova and Rathova, 1969). Of these the α, or "Francis inhibitor" (Francis, 1947) is the most thoroughly characterized. It is a sialylated glycoprotein which inhibits hemagglutination but does not prevent infection. Its activity is destroyed by neuraminidase, but not by heating for 30 minutes at 56°C. The β or "Chu inhibitor" (Chu, 1951) is apparently not sialyated; it is inactivated by heat (56°C for 30 minutes) but not by neuraminidase, and does neutralize infectivity. The γ inhibitor, first recognized as a nonspecific inhibitor of an Asian strain of influenza A (Shimojo *et al.*, 1958; Cohen and Belyavin, 1959), resembles α inhibitors in most but not all properties.

Whether α and γ inhibitors are sufficiently different to justify their separation into two classes is a matter of controversy (see Kilbourne *et al.*, 1972b). According to the classification reviewed by Krizanova and Rathova (1969), α inhibitors are destroyed by neuraminidase whereas γ inhibitors are not. However, neuraminidase may destroy the activity of a given inhibitor against one virus strain without altering its activity against another strain. In addition, a given glycoprotein may inhibit hemagglutination of two virus strains while destroying the infectivity of only one of the two. Thus, the type of inhibition observed depends partially on the strain of virus used to test inhibitory activity. Since a variety of strains have been used as test virus, the distinction between α and γ inhibition is at present somewhat arbitrary. Choppin (see Kilbourne *et al.*, 1972b) has suggested that these inhibitors be identified by source and, when known, by distinguishing chemical and physical properties rather than by the type of inhibition observed with a given virus strain.

A great deal of confusion presently surrounds the role of these inhibitors in virus neutralization. Since it is assumed that receptors on host cells and on erythrocytes are similar in composition, inhibitors of hemagglutination should also neutralize infectivity. Charge repulsion as well as steric effects should prevent virions with α inhibitor molecules attached to them from adsorbing to sialylated sites on host cell membranes. However, since virions are infectious in the presence of α inhibitor, it has been postulated that adsorption occurs after the particle-associated neuraminidase has liberated the virion from the inhibitor (see Krizanova and Rathova, 1969). One would expect α inhibitors to reduce the infectivity of virus strains with low neuraminidase activity if this were the case. As will be described in Section IV, the infectivity of virions that have no detectable neuraminidase activity is increased by at least one sialylated hemagglutination inhibitor. Something other than the neuraminidase activity of the virion is, therefore, responsible for the differences observed when virions are exposed to erythrocytes and to host cells. Our present attempts at visualizing host cell receptors through the use of hemagglutination inhibitors may be analogous to trying to put together a picture puzzle without knowing if all of the available pieces should be used. We may, indeed, have already used some pieces in wrong places. For example, perhaps we should not consider sialic acid residues to be an essential part of the structure of host cell receptors until we have used host cells instead of erythrocytes to investigate the requirements for virus binding.

III. Structure of the Hemagglutinin

General aspects of influenza virus structure, including the polypeptide composition of the virion have been presented in Chapter 2. Specific aspects of the hemagglutinin structure will be described here. In order to do this, the methods used to purify this glycoprotein will be presented, the composition of the subunits which make up the hemagglutinin will be reviewed, and the three-dimensional structure of the active hemagglutinin molecule will be described.

A. Isolation and Purification of the Hemagglutinin

A variety of detergents including Nonidet-P-40, Triton X-100, sodium deoxycholate, Sarkosyl NL 30 and sodium dodecyl sulfate (SDS) have been used to disrupt influenza viruses. The critical micellar concentration of the first four of these detergents is low and thus their effective concentration in aqueous solutions is insufficient to denature most proteins. SDS, on the other hand, reaches a sufficiently high concentration in aqueous solutions so that denaturation of most proteins does occur. However, the hemagglutinin from some strains of virus remains active when exposed to SDS (Laver, 1963). The first procedure for the separation of the hemagglutinin from the neuraminidase without the use of proteases took advantage of this unusual stability (Laver, 1964). Virus proteins other than the hemagglutinin were denatured by SDS and migrated as anions at pH 9.0, whereas the hemagglutinin migrated as a cation. The hemagglutinin could therefore be purified by electrophoresis on cellulose acetate. Purified hemagglutinin from the Bel strain of influenza virus was prepared in this manner and has been used to obtain much of the information to be presented in Sections III,B, and III,C.

Unfortunately, this technique cannot be used with all strains of influenza virus. The hemagglutinin of many strains is denatured by SDS. With others, neither the neuraminidase nor the hemagglutinin are denatured, and they are not separated by electrophoresis. The hemagglutinin from these strains can be isolated only after a recombinant is made which has a SDS-sensitive neuraminidase. Isolation of the hemagglutinin from most strains of virus by this technique is therefore cumbersome.

The hemagglutinin from the X-31 strain, an H0N1-H2N2 recombinant with both the neuraminidase and hemagglutinin from the H2N2 parent (Kilbourne, 1969), has been removed from the virus by bromelain and has been purified by velocity sedimentation (Brand and Skehel, 1972). The glycoprotein so purified forms crystals when concentrated by vacuum dialysis against distilled water. The procedure works with some strains of both influenza A and B. However, pure proteins obtained in this manner are apparently altered in both structure and function (see Section III,B).

Recently, two techniques have been developed which use nondenaturing detergents to disrupt the virus and DEAE-cellulose chromatography in the presence of low levels of detergent to separate the components (Gregoriades, 1972; Stanley *et al.*, 1973b). These techniques have not as yet been put to extensive use but should be superior to SDS disruption and electrophoresis on theoretical grounds. They can be expected to work with a large number of strains, neuraminidase can also be recovered from the same sample of virus, and they can be used for large scale purification.

B. The Chemical Composition of the Hemagglutinin Subunit

The hemagglutinin represents from 25 to 35% of the virion protein. These values are based on polyacrylamide gel electrophoresis profiles of the polypeptides from four strains of influenza virus A grown in a variety of host cells (see Schulze, 1973). About 6% of the dry weight of the virus is carbohydrate (Ada and Perry, 1954; Frommhagen *et al.*, 1959), most of which is associated with the hemagglutinin. Thus, the hemagglutinin is a glycoprotein in which carbohydrate comprises 15 to 20% of the dry weight.

The hemagglutinin is composed of glycoprotein subunits of approximately 80,000 daltons which have been designated HA (Kilbourne *et al.*, 1972a; see Chapter 2). Since the composition of the oligosaccharides attached to the virions is determined by the host cell, virions from different hosts have different-sized hemagglutinin molecules (Compans *et al.*, 1970b; Haslam *et al.*, 1970; Schulze, 1970).

Under certain conditions of virus growth two glycopeptides, HA_1 and HA_2, are produced from the HA subunit by proteolytic cleavage. The factors which determine whether this cleavage occurs are discussed in Chapters 2 and 8. Cleavage is not essential for the formation of a functional spike, nor does it destroy hemagglutinating activity or infectivity (Lazarowitz *et al.*, 1971, 1973a; Stanley *et al.*, 1973a). In cleaved subunits the two glycopeptides are held together by disulfide bonds and can be dissociated from each other by SDS and reducing agents (Laver, 1971).

Molecular weight measurements of HA_1 and HA_2 from a number of preparations of virus grown in one host indicate that these glycopeptides vary in size from preparation to preparation no more than do the intact HA subunits (see Schulze, 1970). However, the HA_1 and HA_2 bands in SDS-polyacrylamide gels are usually wider than the HA band, indicating that in every preparation there is some heterogeneity in the size of the cleavage products. The sizes of HA_1 and HA_2 obtained from two strains of virus grown in one host can also differ (Klenk *et al.*, 1972; Stanley *et al.*, 1973a). Thus, differences in the amino acid sequence of the HA polypeptide can change either the position of the cleavage site or the distribution of the oligosaccharides along the polypeptides. Cleavage apparently occurs in the same limited number of places in the polypeptide chain each time virus is prepared under a given set of conditions. HA_1 and HA_2 can be readily obtained by treating virions with trypsin (Schulze, 1970; Lazarowitz *et al.*, 1971, 1973a) or plasmin (Lazarowitz *et al.*, 1973b; see also Chapter 2). Under these conditions cleavage must produce either HA_1 or HA_2 molecules with arginine or lysine residues at their C-terminal ends.

1. Chemical Composition of the Isolated Glycopeptides

Proteolytic cleavage of the HA subunit is useful to virologists even if it proves to be of little importance to the virus, since it permits us to analyze the two parts of the molecule separately and to ascribe functions to each. HA_1 and HA_2 from the A_0/Bel H0N1 and B/Lee strains grown in chick embryos have been separated from each other by velocity sedimentation using sucrose gradients containing guanidine hydrochloride and dithiothreitol (Laver, 1971; Laver and Baker, 1972). As shown in Table 3.2, the amino acid composition of HA_1 is similar to that of HA_2 except that HA_1 is higher in proline and lower in methionine than is HA_2. However, tryptic peptide maps of HA_1 and HA_2 from A_0/Bel virus show distinct differences, indicating that their amino acid sequences are not the same (Laver, 1971; see also Chapter 11 for tryptic peptide maps of HA_1 and HA_2 of other strains of virus).

Laver and Webster (1972, 1973) have used peptide mapping to look for the molecular basis of the antigenic variation of the hemagglutinin. Working with only those tryptic peptides which are soluble at pH 6.5, they have compared maps of the two glycopeptides from a number of different strains of influenza A. In antigenically distinct strains, they find large differences in amino acid sequence in both HA_1 and HA_2, whereas in closely related strains, only small differences are observed. The genetic implications of these experiments will be discussed in Chapter 10. With respect to the structure of the hemagglutinin, it is clear from the variety of maps which have been obtained that glycopeptides with distinctly different amino acid sequences are capable of assuming the proper configuration to form an active hemagglutinin. This is presumably why this virus is so capable of undergoing changes in antigenicity. Were the structural requirements for the biological activities of the hemagglutinin exceedingly stringent, large variations in its

Table 3.2 Amino Acid Composition[a] of the
Hemagglutinin Glycopeptides from
the A_0/Bel Strain of Influenza Virus

Amino acid	HA_1	HA_2
Lysine	5.6	7.3
Histidine	2.6	1.8
Arginine	4.4	2.3
Aspartic acid	11.7	13.8
Threonine	7.0	4.6
Serine	8.6	8.2
Glutamic acid	10.8	12.2
Proline	5.6	2.0
Glycine	7.7	9.2
Alanine	5.1	5.2
Cysteine[b]	2.2	2.0
Valine	5.7	5.9
Methionine[c]	0.7	2.2
Isoleucine	6.5	6.0
Leucine	8.2	8.3
Tyrosine	4.3	4.9
Phenylalanine	3.3	4.0
Tryptophan	ND[d]	ND

[a] Calculated from data of Skehel and Waterfield (1975). Values are moles of amino acid per 100 moles after correction for degradation during hydrolysis.
[b] As cysteic acid.
[c] As methionine sulfone.
[d] ND, not determined.

amino acid sequence could not be tolerated. As a consequence, mutations in the hemagglutinin would be lethal instead of beneficial to the virus.

Most of the carbohydrate of the HA subunit appears to be associated with the HA_1 glycopeptide. In the case of A_0/Bel virus, about five times as much glucosamine is associated with HA_1, as with HA_2, although the two segments differ only twofold in protein content (Laver, 1971). Thus, the carbohydrate moiety comprises a larger fraction of HA_1 than of HA_2. In addition to glucosamine, fucose, galactose, and mannose are present in HA_1 (Laver, 1971). Sialic acid appears to be absent from the virion (Klenk and Choppin, 1970; Klenk et al., 1970), but can be enzymatically added to both segments of the HA subunits of the A_0/WSN strain after the virions are assembled (Schulze, 1973a,b; see also Section IV). About five times as many residues have been added to HA_1 as to HA_2. The enzyme used transfers sialic acid from cytidine 5′-monophosphate sialic acid to terminal galactose residues on glycoproteins (Bartholomew and Jourdian, 1966). Whether the terminal galactoses on the hemagglutinin are produced by removal of sialic acid by viral neuraminidase or by incomplete carbohydrate chain termination is not known. Fucose, another sugar which is frequently found at the terminus of glycoprotein oligosaccharides, is not incorporated into the HA_2 segment of some virus strains whereas glucosamine is (see Chapter 2). Whether fucose can be added onto assembled virus particles *in vitro* has not been tested.

As indicated in Table 3.2, HA_1 and HA_2 contain about the same mole fraction of tyrosine. Stanley and Haslam (1971) have, however, observed that HA_2, the smaller of the two glycopeptides, can be more extensively iodinated than can HA_2. Thus, the three-dimensional configuration of the hemagglutinin must restrict the availability of tyrosyl residues in HA_1.

Finally, the amino acid composition of the hemagglutinin from the B/Lee strain of influenza virus has been shown by Laver and Baker (1972) to be similar to that of A_0/Bel. Their results indicate that 90% of the proline of the hemagglutinin is in the HA_1 glycopeptide. Since this amino acid prevents α-helix formation, its uneven distribution between the two portions of the HA subunit could have important structural consequences.

2. Antigenic Properties of the HA_1 Glycopeptide

Since the HA_1 region of the hemagglutinin extends out into the aqueous environment surrounding the virion, one might expect that it would contain the site (or sites) which interact with erythrocytes, host cells, soluble inhibitors, and antibodies. Information concerning this point is still sparse. However, a hemagglutinin binding antigen (HABA) which appears to be a dimer of HA_1 has been isolated from the PR8 (H0N1) strain of influenza virus (Eckert, 1966, 1969, 1973). This molecule does not cause hemagglutination but does react with antibodies specific for the viral hemagglutinin. When treated with detergent and dithiothreitol, it dissociates into molecules with molecular weights of about 40,000. This material quantitatively removes HI antibodies from antisera prepared against whole virus. It also induces HI and neutralizing antibodies. The amino acid composition of HABA resembles that of the HA_1 glycopeptide from the A_0/Bel strain of virus. However, as indicated above, HA_1 and HA_2 from the Bel strain are similar in amino acid composition except for their proline content and can be clearly distinguished only by techniques which show differences in amino acid sequence.

The experiments of Brand and Skehel (1972) also suggest that HA_1 may contain antigenic determinants which induce specific antibodies against the hemagglutinin. Bromelain-released crystalline hemagglutinin forms a single precipitin line with antisera against whole virus or against HA_1. A preciptin line was observed with anti-HA_2 sera only after reducing agents were added to the crystalline antigen. The results suggest that the functioning antigenic site of the intact hemagglutinin is on the HA_1 glycopeptide and that an additional site on HA_2 is unmasked by dissociating HA_1 from HA_2. However, it has recently been observed that HA subunits contain multiple antigenic determinants and that one of these determinants is missing from bromelain-released hemagglutinin (Laver *et al.,* 1974; see also Chapter 10). Some antigenic sites are apparently contained entirely within the HA_1 region, whereas others may include regions from the HA_2 glycopeptide, or be located entirely within it. The effect of cleavage of the HA subunit on the antigenic activity of these sites remains to be determined.

3. Hydrophobic Properties of the HA_2 Glycopeptide

The HA subunits isolated from detergent disrupted virus have some hydrophobic properties. For example, removal of the detergent from disrupted virus results in the formation of large aggregates with hemagglutinating activity (see Section III,C). The HA_2 glycopeptide appears to be responsible for this tendency of the HA subunit to polymerize. When separated from HA_1 by detergents and reducing agents, HA_2 molecules form aggregates even in the presence of guanidine hydrochloride and dithiothreitol (Laver, 1971). However, HA subunits removed from the virus by bromelain do not aggregate (see Laver, 1973). Such subunits will not hemagglutinate but will react with antisera prepared against hemagglutinin released from the same strain of virus by SDS. They contain HA_2 glycopeptides which are smaller by about 5000 daltons than are those obtained from detergent-released hemagglutinin. Thus, bromelain apparently removes from HA_2 a hydrophobic region which is responsible for the tendency of the HA subunit to aggregate.

It was pointed out earlier by Laver (1973) that the amino acids which comprise the hydrophobic region of HA_2 must be located at one (or both) end of the molecule since their removal does not reduce HA_2 to small fragments. Very recently Skehel and Waterfield (1975) have shown that HA_2 and bromelain-modified HA_2 have identical amino-terminal amino acid sequences. The amino acids released by bromelain must therefore come from the carboxyl terminus of HA_2. This segment, approximately 50 amino acids long, contains half of the serine residues of HA_2. Twenty-one of these fifty residues can be considered to be hydrophobic.

4. Structure of the HA Subunit

A diagram of the HA subunit based on the information just reviewed is presented in Fig. 3.1. It depicts the molecule as consisting of one glyco-

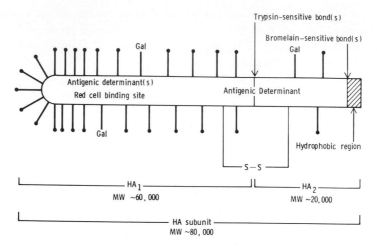

Fig. 3.1. A diagram of the HA subunit. The HA subunit is depicted as a molecule of approximately 80,000 daltons which can be cleaved by trypsin to form two glycopeptides, HA₁ and HA₂. These two are held together by one or more disulfide bonds (see text). Bromelain removes a hydrophobic region from one end of the HA₂ polypeptide. Both HA₁ and HA₂ are glycosylated, with most of the oligosaccharides (indicated by short lines extending out from the structure) attached to the HA₁ region. These oligosaccharides are presumably attached to serine, threonine, and asparagine residues in the polypeptide chain. No information is presently available about their size or structure except that glucosamine, galactose, mannose, and fucose are present. Some oligosaccharides on both HA₁ and HA₂ terminate in galactose and can be sialylated. The red cell binding site and one antigenic determinant is in the HA₁ region, whereas a second antigenic determinant is located at least partially in HA₂ (see text).

peptide of about 80,000 daltons with a trypsin-sensitive bond approximately one-third the length of the molecule from one end. A hydrophobic region is shown to be at one end of the HA subunit. Cleavage of the trypsin-sensitive bond(s) produces the two glycopeptides, HA₁ and HA₂, which are connected by a disulfide bridge. Based on the cysteic acid content of the HA₂ glycopeptides reported in Table 3.2, there can be up to four disulfide bonds connecting it to HA₁.* Reducing agents separate the cleaved subunits into two glycopeptides, HA₁ and HA₂. HA₁ contains most of the carbohydrate and HA₂ has hydrophobic properties. Some of the oligosaccharides attached to both HA₁ and HA₂ terminate in galactose and can be sialylated. One or more antigenic site is depicted as being located entirely within the HA₁ glycopeptide, and an additional site is shown to extend into the HA₂ region. The red cell binding site is also shown to be in HA₁, although the HA₂

* The molecular weight of the polypeptides moieties of HA₁ and HA₂ were assumed to be approximately 50,000 and 19,000, respectively.

region of the molecule may be required for the HA subunits to form active oligomers (see Section III,C).

When cleavage of HA occurs, HA_2 is apparently released from the carboxyl end of the molecule (Skehel and Waterfield, 1975); thus, the amino-terminal end of HA_2 and the carboxyl-terminal end of HA_1 are generated by cleavage. Skehel and Waterfield have compared the sequence of the first 10 amino acid residues at the amino terminus of HA_1 derived from three antigenically distinct human A strains. Highly similar sequences, with substitutions at positions one or two, were observed. A single amino acid sequence was also found at the amino-terminal end of HA_2 derived from antigenically distinct hemagglutinins. Five strains representative of human influenza A subgroups as well as one strain of influenza B have been examined. This sequence is composed largely of hydrophobic amino acids. It contains a palindrome of 7 amino acids which Skehel and Waterfield (1975) suggest could be a recognition sequence for these proteases which cleave the HA subunit to form HA_1 and HA_2.

These results, together with the variations in tryptic peptide maps reported by Laver and Webster (1972, 1973), suggest that amino acid sequences in certain parts of the hemagglutinin are tightly conserved in nature whereas others are not. Presumably, those regions which can vary in sequence are responsible for antigenic variation whereas those which cannot, maintain the three-dimensional structure of the active hemagglutinin. The size of the variable region(s) and the fraction of the total amino acid sequence which can be varied without destroying the structure and function of the HA subunit can presumably be determined by more extensive sequence analysis.

5. Antigenic Homogeneity of HA Subunits

As will be described in Section III,C, the active hemagglutinin is composed of more than one HA subunit. This fact, along with the evidence that some virus strains contain several distinct antigenic sites within the hemagglutinin, makes it important to determine whether one virus strain can have HA subunits with distinctly different amino acid sequences. This question has special significance with the influenza viruses because their genomes are segmented (see Chapter 6), and it has been proposed that random packaging of the virion RNA may produce particles with extra copies of some genome segments (Compans et al., 1970a). Since these particles would be partial diploids, one virus strain could contain the genetic information for the synthesis of two different HA subunits, if both alleles were perpetuated through multiple cycles of virus replication.

One way to detect that a virus population contains more than one kind of HA subunit would be to compare the number of distinct tryptic peptides obtained from the HA subunit with that expected from the number of arginine and lysine residues in each molecule. This analysis cannot be made at this time since the entire hemagglutinin molecule has not been analyzed by peptide mapping (see Section III,B).

Another approach is to see whether antigenic determinants can be physically separated by specific antisera. Using these techniques, Laver *et al.* (1974) have found that antisera prepared against either of two determinants associated with the HA subunits will precipitate both determinants. The experiments provide preliminary evidence that these antigenic determinants are physically linked (i.e., located on the same HA subunit). They also suggest that the strains examined by Laver *et al.* did not synthesize two antigenically distinct HA subunits.

C. The Structure of the Hemagglutinin Spike

1. THE MONOVALENT HEMAGGLUTININ

The isolated 80,000 dalton HA subunits have no hemagglutinating activity. The smallest active molecule is an oligomer composed either of HA subunits or of its cleavage products, HA_1 and HA_2. This "monovalent" hemagglutinin was first released from the virion by SDS (Laver, 1964; Laver and Valentine, 1969). It adsorbs to erythrocytes but does not cause hemagglutination. It has a sedimentation coefficient of approximately 7.5 S in the presence of SDS (Laver and Valentine, 1969) and is a rod-shaped molecule about 40×140 Å. Its morphology is shown in Fig. 10.2 (Chapter 10).

According to the first estimates, each monovalent hemagglutinin was thought to have a molecular weight of about 150,000 and to be composed of two HA subunits (Laver and Valentine, 1969). This value was based on the dimensions of the monovalent hemagglutinin obtained from electron microscopy, the molecular weight of the HA subunit as determined by SDS-polyacrylamide gel electrophoresis, the sedimentation coefficient of the monovalent hemagglutinin, and an assumed partial specific volume of 0.73 cm^3/gm. More recent work has shown, however, that the monovalent hemagglutinin is probably a trimer. Its molecular weight has been estimated from equilibrium sedimentation data to be approximately 215,000 (J. J. Skehel and P. A. Charlwood, personal communication). Thus, it is approximately three times the size of the HA subunit. In addition, electron micrographs of partially disrupted virions occasionally show triangular structures of the proper size to be hemagglutinin spikes viewed from the end (see

Laver, 1973; Schulze, 1972, 1973). This view of the molecule has now been clearly shown by mixing crystalline catalase with highly purified hemagglutinin released from A_0/Bel virus by SDS (Fig. 10.2, Chapter 10). Under these conditions, the hemagglutinin molecules pack together in an orderly fashion so that virtually all of them are viewed end-on. When negatively stained, each molecule is triangular in shape, again suggesting that each spike is composed of three HA subunits.

The morphology and dimensions of the spike layer on intact virus along with the properties of the isolated hemagglutinin strongly suggest that monovalent hemagglutinin molecules represent single spikes which have been released from the lipid bilayer. Release can be accomplished either by providing detergent molecules with which the hydrophobic region of the spike can interact, or by removing the hydrophobic region from the HA_2 portion of the subunit by proteolysis. Approximately 300 to 450 spikes are present on a single virus particle (see Schulze, 1973) and are attached to the virion lipid by the HA_2 regions of each trimer. Some strains of virus appear to contain less than one HA_1 molecule for each molecule of HA_2 (see Schulze, 1973). Thus, some of the spikes on virions with cleaved hemagglutinin subunits may be incomplete in structure.*

2. Aggregation and Dissociation of the Monovalent Hemagglutinin

As indicated above, hemagglutination requires multivalent molecules which can be formed *in vitro* only if the HA_2 portion of the subunit is intact. Such aggregates are shown in Fig. 10.3 (Chapter 10). Since they are composed of different numbers of hemagglutinin spikes, they vary in size.

The dissociation of the hemagglutinin spike and its aggregation to form hemagglutinating particles is diagrammed in Fig. 3.2. The spike is represented as a trimer with the hydrophobic region of each of the three HA subunits inserted into the lipid bilayer of the virus. These hydrophobic regions are removed from protease-released hemagglutinin (Fig. 3.2A). The molecules are therefore no longer capable of forming multivalent aggregates. The trypsin-sensitive bonds (see Fig. 3.1) are also cleaved so that no intact HA subunits are observed when these molecules are treated with SDS and reducing agents. In detergent-released hemagglutinin (Fig. 3.2B), the hydrophobic regions of the molecules are intact. When detergent is removed, these regions interact and produce aggregates of various sizes which can agglutin-

---

* Errors in molecular weight determinations could also cause an apparent discrepancy between the number of HA_1 and HA_2 glycopeptides associated with the virion. If such is the case, a systematic error is present, since the same glycopeptide is always in molar excess.

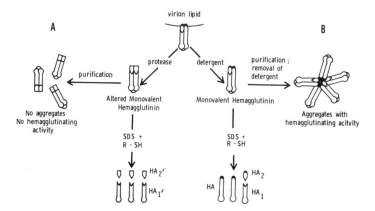

Fig. 3.2. Aggregation and dissociation of the monovalent hemagglutinin. The virion spike is depicted as consisting of a trimer which can be removed from the virion by protease (A) or by detergents (B). In (A) the protease-altered monovalent hemagglutinin is shown to lack that part of the HA_2 region (dark area) which is necessary for the formation of aggregates. All subunits are shown to be composed of two glycopeptides, designated HA_1' and HA_2' which can be dissociated by SDS and reducing agents. These glycopeptides differ from intact HA_1 and HA_2 as indicated in the text. In (B) detergent-released monovalent hemagglutinin molecules are shown to aggregate and to acquire hemagglutinating activity when the detergent is removed. Dissociation of the detergent-released monovalent hemagglutinin by SDS and reducing agents yields either HA subunits, or the two glycopeptides HA_1 and HA_2, depending on whether the trypsin-sensitive bonds in the subunit have been cleaved. One of the subunits within the spike is shown to be cleaved. [Based on models previously proposed by Laver and Valentine (1969) and Schulze, 1972, 1973).]

ate erythrocytes. Further treatment of the monovalent hemagglutinin with SDS and reducing agents dissociates the molecules into either HA subunits or its cleavage products HA_1 and HA_2 depending on whether the trypsin-sensitive bonds depicted in Fig. 3.1 were cleaved prior to releasing the spikes from the virus particles.

This model is based on information obtained from a number of strains of virus; however, not all of its features are demonstrable with every strain. For example, large differences in the susceptibility of virus strains to proteases have been observed (see Schulze, 1973). Proteases inactivate and presumably degrade the hemagglutinin of many strains of virus (see Kilbourne, 1963); yet, with some strains, inactivation by proteases does not appear to involve only the hemagglutinin. Kilbourne and associates have observed that sensitivity to protease can be segregated from HA antigen during genetic recombination (see Kilbourne et al., 1972a). These observations also point out the dangers involved in predicting structural changes from changes in biological activity. Finally, the model implies that bromelain-released hemagglutinin is unaltered except for the removal of its hydrophobic region. However, bromelain-released hemagglutinin from some strains of virus will not bind to erythrocytes (Laver *et al.*, 1974), suggesting that the structure of the hydrophilic region of the HA subunit (i.e., HA_1), has also been changed. Since these alterations may be quite small, they could easily go undetected by the physical methods employed thus far.

IV. Functions of the Hemagglutinin

Two important aspects of the viral hemagglutinin were obvious long before a detailed analysis of the virion structure was possible. With the influenza epidemic of 1947, it became clear that the virion surface antigens could undergo major changes in composition so that strains of virus with a common internal antigen would show little cross-reactivity in virus neutralization and HI tests (Francis *et al.*, 1947). Subsequently, it was shown that the hemagglutinin constitutes the major surface antigen and that it alone stimulates synthesis of antibodies which neutralize infectivity and inhibit hemagglutination (Drzeniek *et al.*, 1966; Laver and Kilbourne, 1966). Thus, it could be concluded that the hemagglutinin is responsible for the attachment of virus to host cells as well as to erythrocytes, and that it undergoes major changes in antigenic composition.

As shown in Section III, some of these properties remained with the hemagglutinin when it was physically separated from the rest of the virus. Isolated hemagglutinin can adsorb to erythrocytes and, if conditions are such that multivalent aggregates can form, it can also cause hemagglutination. The hemagglutinin stimulates the formation of HI and neutralizing antibody, even when detergent-treated molecules with no detectable hemagglutinating activity are used as antigens. These isolated molecules exhibit a high degree of antigenic specificity so that strain differences which are detectable in intact virions can be even more precisely analyzed by using subunit antigens.

As the structure of the virion was elucidated, the so-called "host antigen" activity of purified virions was also explained. This antigen, detected in purified preparations of virus (Knight, 1944; Harboe *et al.*, 1961; Harboe, 1963), is now known to be the carbohydrate moiety of the surface glycoproteins. When obtained from the host, it is a glycoprotein which lacks sialic acid residues (Haukenes *et al.*, 1966; Laver and Webster, 1966). It reacts with antibodies against the hemagglutinin and will block their HI activity.

These cross-reactions occur because the hemagglutinin contains oligosaccharides which have been synthesized by host enzymes from the available sugar nucleotide pool and are therefore similar to those found in host glycoproteins.

Information about the isolated hemagglutinin has been extremely valuable in evaluating structural relationships within the HA spike, and in determining which parts of the spike are capable of binding to lipid bilayers and which can associate with cell receptors. However, understanding the role of the hemagglutinin spike in the attachment of virions to erythrocytes and to host cells requires that the hemagglutinin be studied *in situ*. Attempts have therefore been made to alter the hemagglutinin while it is still on the virion so that changes in structure can be correlated with changes in function.

Structural evidence that the HA_1 glycopeptide is required for infectivity has been obtained in this manner. Virions were subjected to controlled proteolysis and changes in their biological activities were correlated with the disappearance of the virion glycopeptides (Table 3.3). Removal of the HA_1 glycopeptide results in loss of both hemagglutinating activity and infectivity.

Attempts have also been made to study the effects of less drastic modification of the HA subunit. One approach which has proved fruitful is to covalently attach sialic acid residues to intact virions (Schulze, 1973, 1975a,b). The hemagglutinin glycopeptides as well as the uncleaved HA on A_0/WSN virions can be sialylated *in vitro* by sialyltransferase (Fig. 3.3). Sialic acid is attached to the two glycopeptides concomitantly, but approximately 5 times as many residues are put onto HA_1 as onto HA_2 (Schulze, 1975b). Virions freed of neuraminidase activity by trypsin will accept at least 2500

Table 3.3   Effects of Proteases on the Biological Activities and Glycoprotein Composition of Influenza Virus

Treatment of virus	% of initial activity			Glycoproteins remaining on virions after treatment
	PFU	HA	Neuraminidase	
—	100	100	100	HA, HA_1, HA_2, NA
Trypsin[a]	120	100	<0.2	HA_1, HA_2
Bromelain[b]	0.012	0.10	0.5	HA_2
Chymotrypsin[a]	0.001	0.01	<0.2	none

[a] The A_0/WSN strain of virus was incubated at 37°C with trypsin, 0.01 mg/ml, for 20 minutes or chymotrypsin, 1.0 mg/ml, for 18 hours. (From Schulze, 1970.)

[b] Virus was incubated at 37°C for 2 to 4 hours with 1.3 mg of bromelain. (From Compans *et al.*, 1970b.)

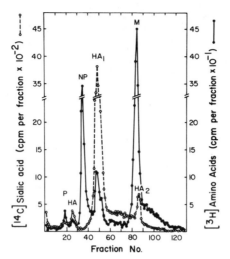

Fig. 3.3. Polypeptide profile of sialylated influenza virus. 102,400 hemagglutinating units of [³H]amino acid labeled influenza virus of the A₀/WSN strain were incubated with 0.4 μCi CMP-[¹⁴C]sialic acid and sialyltransferase for 3 hours in 1.0 ml of 0.1 M KPO₄, pH 6.9, containing 0.05 M NaCl, and 5×10^{-4} M EDTA. The sialylated virions were separated from the reaction mixture by centrifuging them to equilibrium in a sucrose density gradient. They were then solubilized and subjected to SDS-polyacrylamide gel electrophoresis as described by Schulze (1970). Mobility is from left to right. (From Schulze, 1975a.)

sialic acid residues per particle or five residues per spike. Whether the residues are in fact evenly distributed over all spikes is not known.

The rather surprising biological consequences of *in vitro* sialylation of the hemagglutinin are summarized in Fig. 3.4. The hemagglutinating activity is lost; the neuraminidase activity remains the same as that of incubated control virus; and the infectivity is significantly stimulated. The amount of stimulation observed depends on the amount of sialic acid added, on the cells used to measure infectivity, and on whether the virus has been treated with trypsin to remove its neuraminidase prior to sialylation.

Sialic acid residues attached to intact virus *in vitro* can be removed by the neuraminidase of the sialylated virions if conditions are made optimum for this enzyme (Schulze, 1975a,b). It seems likely, therefore, that the viral neuraminidase does remove sialic acid residues put onto the virion hemagglutinin by host sialyltransferases. Evidence that this may be the case has been presented by Palese *et al.* (1974) and will be described in Chapter 4. Covalent linkage of sialic acid to virion glycoproteins or to a precursor molecule *in vivo* has, however, not been demonstrated.

The mechanism by which sialylation increases the infectivity is presently under investigation. Since the amount of stimulation observed depends

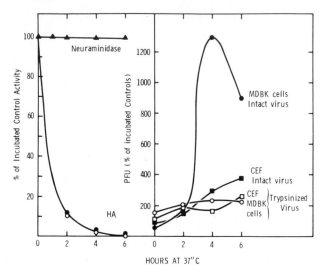

Fig. 3.4 Effects of sialylation on the biological activities of influenza virus. Purified virus of the A$_0$/WSN strain was incubated with CMP-sialic acid and sialyltransferase. At the times indicated, aliquots were assayed for hemagglutinating and neuraminidase activity and for infectivity. Neuraminidase activity was determined from the rate of release of sialic acid from fetuin using the colorometric assay described by Aminoff (1961). Infectivity was measured by plaque production on MDBK (Madin and Darby, 1958) and chick embryo fibroblast (CEF) monolayers. Virus particles with neuraminidase removed by trypsin treatment (see Table 3.3) were also incubated and assayed in the same manner. Controls consisted of intact or trypsinized virus incubated in the complete reaction mixture minus CMP-sialic acid. After 6 hours at 37°C, these controls retained full hemagglutinating activity, and approximately 60 and 10% of the initial infectivity and neuraminidase activity. Open symbols indicate trypsinized virus. (From Schulze, 1975b.)

partly on the cell used to assay infectivity, it seems likely that sialylation increases the binding of virions to some cell receptors. It is interesting in this respect that in preliminary experiments sialylated virions which do not hemagglutinate appear to bind to fowl erythrocytes as well as to control virions (I. T. Schulze, unpublished observations). The results point out that under some conditions hemagglutination is a poor indication of whether virions can interact with receptors on erythrocytes, let alone with those on host cells.

Similar changes in activity can be induced by treating influenza virus with fetuin, a sialylated glycoprotein (Der and Schulze, 1975). Exposure of virions to fetuin destroys hemagglutinating activity and increases the infectivity of the preparation (Table 3.4). In order to prevent destruction of the inhibitor by the virion-associated neuraminidase, virus samples were

Table 3.4　Effects of Fetuin and Desialofetuin on Influenza Virus[a]

			% of control activity	
Virus	Conc. HAU/ml	Treatment (5 μg/HA)	HA	Infectivity
Intact	70	Fetuin	5	600
		Desialofetuin	100	109
Trypsin-treated	70	Fetuin	4	1100
		Desialofetuin	100	282

[a] The A_0/WSN strain of virus was used. Intact or trypsin-treated virus (see Table 3.3) were incubated with fetuin or desialofetuin for 1 hour at 37°C. Infectivity was assayed as described in Fig. 3.4.

treated with trypsin before they were incubated with fetuin. These trypsin-treated preparations which lack neuraminidase activity also lose hemagglutinating activity and show substantial increases in infectivity when incubated with fetuin. Removal of the sialic acid residues from fetuin greatly reduces its stimulatory effect and eliminates inhibition of hemagglutination, indicating that these residues must be involved in both changes in activity. The results suggest that binding of virions to host cells can be aided by some soluble sialoglycoproteins. This increase in infectivity, as well as that obtained by sialylating virions, could also be due to the formation of aggregates which initiate infection as clumps of incomplete but complementary particles (see Hirst and Pons, 1973). Independent of which of these alternatives proves to be the case, we will need to reevaluate the role of sialoglycoproteins in the infectious process, since some of these molecules can apparently foster infection instead of interfering with it.

Whatever the mechanism involved in loss of hemagglutinating activity and stimulation of infectivity, the experiments clearly show that sialylation of the hemagglutinin or interaction of the virus with a sialylated glycoprotein produces infectious but nonhemagglutinating particles. Infectious influenza virus which does not hemagglutinate has been observed in persistently infected cultures (Gavrilov et al., 1972), following chemotherapy in mice (Magrassi et al., 1966), and during adaptation of an A_2 strain of virus to growth in a new host cell (Thibon et al., 1967). Since none of these nonhemagglutinating viruses has been investigated after purification, the mechanism by which hemagglutination is inhibited is not known. It was suggested by Thibon et al. (1967) that in their experiments the hemagglutinin was present on the virion but masked, since it stimulated the synthesis of HI antibodies. Inhibitors of A_2 virus could not be detected in the culture medium.

V. Concluding Remarks

Most of the information about the influenza viruses presented here has been obtained from studies using strains of influenza A. Although little data is available from other than A strains, the structure of the hemagglutinin of influenza B appears to closely resemble that of influenza A (see Chapter 2; and Section III,B). Influenza C has not been mentioned here because no information about the molecular structure of its hemagglutinin is available.

Only a few aspects of the interactions between the viral hemagglutinin and erythrocytes merit further discussion. From what we now know about the molecular structures of the receptor on erythrocytes and the viral hemagglutinin, we can conclude that hemagglutination results from interactions between molecules which are similar in composition and structure but which are vastly different in charge properties. Both the viral hemagglutinin and virus receptors on red cells are low molecular weight glycoproteins which have a tendency to aggregate when isolated; in their native configuration both have specific sites at which they can be cleaved by trypsin; both have a hydrophobic region at the carboxyl end of the molecule and a hydrophilic region at the amino terminus. These properties may well be shared by most membrane-associated glycoproteins. The difference in the two molecules is their sialic acid content. Whereas sialic acid constitutes 27% of the weight of the erythrocyte glycoprotein, it is absent from the virion glycoprotein. Since the carboxyl group of sialic acid is ionized at physiological pH, the ionic shell surrounding the erythrocyte must be vastly different from that of the virion.

Many of the properties of the virus–erythrocyte interaction may stem from these charge differences. In this respect, it is important to point out that adsorption of viruses to erythrocytes should not be equated with hemagglutination. Although attachment of virus to the erythrocyte receptor is a prerequisite for hemagglutination, it need not be the limiting step in the production of a lattice or aggregate. A different overall view of how influenza viruses interact with red cells would undoubtedly have developed had we been able to investigate independently virus binding and hemagglutination. In much of the literature, binding has been equated with hemagglutination because no other techniques for measuring binding were available.

It is also important for us to recognize that we know little about the composition of virus receptors on host cells which are susceptible to infection. It is legitimate to assume, however, that they differ significantly from those on erythrocytes. The human erythrocyte glycoprotein has a higher sialic acid content than do most plasma membrane glycoproteins (see Spiro, 1973), and it constitutes a larger fraction of the total membrane protein than does any single glycoprotein in other plasma membranes (see Hughes, 1973). Whereas all of the sialic acid residues can be readily removed from the surface of the erythrocyte membrane by neuraminidase (Eylar *et al.*, 1962), on other cells some of these residues are inaccessible to neuraminidase (Glick *et al.*, 1970). These inaccessible residues are thought to be attached to glycolipids (Glick *et al.*, 1970) and could be involved in virus binding and in penetration (Haywood, 1974). Attachment of virus to host cells has in most cases been monitored by measuring the infectivity of a virus suspension. As with hemagglutination, the assay employed requires that processes in addition to binding be operative. Binding of virus to host cells and to erythrocytes could therefore involve two independent processes, neither of which has been investigated by techniques appropriate for the answers which we seek.

In view of these observations, I would like to suggest that we have named the major surface glycoprotein of influenza virus rather unwisely. It is to us a hemagglutinin because that is the function which we have measured; to the virus it serves other functions. Although our naming this glycoprotein inaccurately cannot change its function, it has already influenced our perception of how it interacts with cells. The characterization of the hemagglutinin presented here is derived largely from experiments designed to test its hemagglutinating activity. Techniques are now available for more direct examination of the interaction between the virion and both host cells and erythrocytes. Since we cannot depend on serendipity to provide us again with unearned insights, we are more likely to understand the function of that surface glycoprotein which we call "the hemagglutinin" if we do not pursue too strict an analogy between the way it interacts with erythrocytes and with host cells.

Acknowledgments

Work from the author's laboratory reported here was supported in part by Grant AI-10097 from the National Institute of Allergy and Infectious Disease, U.S. Public Health Service. The author wishes to thank Barbara Morgan Detjen and Drs. Subir K. Bose, Arnold Kaplan, and Norman E. Melechen for helpful suggestions during the preparation of this manuscript.

References

Ada, G. L., and Perry, B. T. (1954). *Aust. J. Exp. Biol. Med.* **32,** 453.
Aminoff, D. (1961). *Biochem. J.* **81,** 348.
Bartholomew, B. A., and Jourdian, G. W. (1966). *In* "Methods in Enzymology"

(E. F. Newfeld and V. Ginsburg, eds.), Vol. 8, pp. 368–372. Academic Press, New York.

Bateman, J. B., Davis, M. S., and McCaffrey, P. A. (1955). *Amer. J. Hyg.* **62**, 349.

Brand, C. M., and Skehel, J. J. (1972). *Nature (London), New Biol.* **238**, 145.

Burnet, F. M., and McCrea, J. F. (1946). *Aust. J. Exp. Biol. Med. Sci.* **24**, 277.

Burnet, F. M., McCrea, J. F., and Stone, J. D. (1946). *Brit. J. Exp. Pathol.* **27**, 228.

Choppin, P. W., and Tamm, I. (1959). *Virology* **8**, 539.

Choppin, P. W., and Tamm, I. (1960). *J. Exp. Med.* **112**, 921.

Chu, C. M. (1951). *J. Gen. Microbiol.* **5**, 739.

Cohen, A., and Belyavin, G. (1959). *Virology* **7**, 59.

Cohen, A., and Belyavin, G. (1966). *Abstr. Int. Congr. Microbiol., 9th, 1966* p. 379.

Compans, R. W., Dimmock, N. J., and Meier-Ewert, H. (1970a). *In* "The Biology of Large RNA Viruses" (R. D. Barry and B. W. J. Mahy, eds.), pp. 87–108. Academic Press, New York.

Compans, R. W., Klenk, H. -D., Caliguiri, L. A., and Choppin, P. W. (1970b). *Virology* **42**, 880.

Der, C. -L., and Schulze, I. T. (1975). In preparation.

Drescher, J. (1957). *Zentralbl. Bakteriol., Parasitenk., Infektionskr. Hyg., Abt. 1: Orig.* **169**, 314.

Drescher, J. (1966). *Amer. J. Epidemiol.* **84**, 167.

Drescher, J. (1967). *Amer. J. Epidemiol.* **86**, 451.

Drzeniek, R., Seto, J. T., and Rott, R. (1966). *Biochim. Biophys. Acta* **128**, 547.

Eckert, E. A. (1966). *J. Bacteriol.* **92**, 430.

Eckert, E. A. (1969). *J. Immunol.* **102**, 1105.

Eckert, E. A. (1973). *J. Virol.* **11**, 183.

Eylar, E. H., Madoff, M. A., Brody, O. V., and Oncley, J. L. (1962). *J. Biol. Chem.* **237**, 1992.

Fazekas de St. Groth, S., and Gottschalk, A. (1963). *Biochim. Biophys. Acta* **78**, 248.

Finter, N. B. (1964). *Virology* **24**, 589.

Francis, T. (1947). *J. Exp. Med.* **85**, 1.

Francis, T., and Salk, J. E. (1942). *Science* **96**, 499.

Francis, T., Salk, J. E., and Quilligan, J. J., Jr. (1947). *Amer. J. Pub. Health* **37**, 1013.

Frommhagen, L. H., Knight, C. A., and Freeman, N. K. (1959). *Virology* **8**, 176.

Gavrilov, V. I., Asher, D. M., Vyalushkina, S. D., Ratushkina, L. S., Zmieva, R. G., and Tumyan, B. G. (1972). *Proc. Soc. Exp. Biol. Med.* **140**, 109.

Glick, M. C., Comstock, C., and Warren, L. (1970). *Biochim. Biophys. Acta* **219**, 290.

Gregoriades, A. (1972). *Virology* **49**, 333.

Harboe, A. (1963). *Acta Pathol. Microbiol. Scand.* **57**, 317.

Harboe, A., Borthne, B., and Berg, K. (1961). *Acta Pathol. Microbiol. Scand.* **53**, 95.

Hare, R., Curl, M., and McClelland, L. (1941). *Can. J. Pub. Health* **37**, 284.

Hare, R., McClelland, L., and Morgan, J. (1942). *Can. J. Pub. Health* **38**, 325.

Haslam, E., Hampson, A. W., Egan, J. A., and White, D. O. (1970). *Virology* **42**, 555.

Haukenes, G., Harboe, A., and Mortensson-Egnund, K. (1966). *Acta Pathol. Microbiol. Scand.* **66**, 510.

Haywood, A. M. (1974). *J. Mol. Biol.* **83**, 427.

Hirst, G. K. (1941). *Science* **94**, 22.

Hirst, G. K. (1942a). *J. Exp. Med.* **75**, 47.
Hirst, G. K. (1942b). *J. Exp. Med.* **76**, 195.
Hirst, G. K. (1948a). *J. Exp. Med.* **87**, 301.
Hirst, G. K. (1948b). *J. Exp. Med.* **87**, 315.
Hirst, G. K. (1949a). *J. Exp. Med.* **89**, 223.
Hirst, G. K. (1949b). *J. Exp. Med.* **89**, 233.
Hirst, G. K. (1950). *J. Exp. Med.* **91**, 161.
Hirst, G. K., and Pickels, E. G. (1942). *J. Immunol.* **45**, 273.
Hirst, G. K., and Pons, M. W. (1973). *Virology* **56**, 620.
Horsfall, F. L. (1954). *J. Exp. Med.* **100**, 135.
Horsfall, F. L., and Tamm, I. (1953). *J. Immunol.* **70**, 253.
Hotchin, J. E., Deibel, R., and Benson, L. M. (1960). *Virology* **10**, 275.
Howe, C., Spiele, H., Minio, F., and Hsu, K. C. (1970). *J. Immunol.* **104**, 1406.
Hoyle, L. (1968). *In* "The Influenza Viruses" (S. Gard, C. Hallauer, and K. F.
    Meyer, eds.), Virol. Monogr., p. 81. Springer-Verlag, Berlin and New York.
Hughes, R. C. (1973). *Progr. Biophys. Mol. Biol.* **29**, 191.
Kathan, R. H., and Adamany, A. (1967). *J. Biol. Chem.* **242**, 1716.
Kathan, R. H., and Winzler, R. J. (1963). *J. Biol. Chem.* **238**, 21.
Kilbourne, E. D. (1963). *Progr. Med. Virol.* **5**, 79.
Kilbourne, E. D. (1969). *Bull. W.H.O.* **41**, 643.
Kilbourne, E. D., Choppin, P. W., Schulze, I. T., Scholtissek, C., and Bucher, D. L.
    (1972a). *J. Infec. Dis.* **125**, 447.
Kilbourne, E. D., Coleman, M., Choppin, P. W., Dowdle, W. R., Schild, G. C., and
    Schulman, J. L. (1972b). *J. Infec. Dis.* **126**, 219.
Klenk, H. -D., and Choppin, P. W. (1970). *Proc. Nat. Acad. Sci. U.S.* **66**, 57.
Klenk, H. -D., Compans, R. W., and Choppin, P. W. (1970). *Virology* **42**, 1158.
Klenk, H. -D., Rott, R., and Becht, H. (1972). *Virology* **47**, 579.
Knight, C. A. (1944). *J. Exp. Med.* **80**, 83.
Krizanova, O., and Rathova, V. (1969). *Curr. Top. Microbiol. Immunol.* **47**, 125.
Laver, W. G. (1963). *Virology* **20**, 251.
Laver, W. G. (1964). *J. Mol. Biol.* **9**, 109.
Laver, W. G. (1971). *Virology* **45**, 275.
Laver, W. G. (1973). *Advan. Virus Res.* **18**, 56.
Laver, W. G., and Baker, N. (1972). *J. Gen. Virol.* **17**, 61.
Laver, W. G., and Kilbourne, E. D. (1966). *Virology* **30**, 493.
Laver, W. G., and Valentine, R. C. (1969). *Virology* **38**, 105.
Laver, W. G., and Webster, R. G. (1966). *Virology* **30**, 104.
Laver, W. G., and Webster, R. G. (1972). *Virology* **48**, 445.
Laver, W. G., and Webster, R. G. (1973). *Virology* **51**, 383.
Laver, W. G., Downie, J. C., and Webster, R. G. (1974). *Virology* **59**, 230.
Lazarowitz, S. G., Compans, R. W., and Choppin, P. W. (1971). *Virology* **46**, 830.
Lazarowitz, S. G., Compans, R. W., and Choppin, P. W. (1973a). *Virology* **52**, 199.
Lazarowitz, S. G., Goldberg, A. R., and Choppin, P. W. (1973b). *Virology* **56**, 172.
Levine, A. S., Puck, T. T., and Sagik, B. P. (1953). *J. Exp. Med.* **98**, 521.
Liao, T. -H., Gallop, P. M., and Blumenfeld, O. O. (1973). *J. Biol. Chem.* **248**,
    8247.
McClelland, L., and Hare, R. (1941). *Can. Pub. Health J.* **32**, 530.
McCrea, J. F. (1946). *Aust. J. Exp. Biol. Med. Sci.* **24**, 283.
Mackenzie, J. S., and Dimmock, N. J. (1973). *J. Gen. Virol.* **19**, 51.
Madin, S. H., and Darby, N. B., Jr. (1958). *Proc. Soc. Exp. Biol. Med.* **98**, 574.

Magrassi, F., Altucci, P., Jori, G. P., Lorenzutti, G., Sapio, U., and Tarro, G. (1966). *Arch. Gesamte Virusforsch.* **18**, 422.

Marchesi, V. T., Tillack, T. W., Jackson, R. L., Segrest, J. P., and Scott, R. E. (1972). *Proc. Nat. Acad. Sci. U.S.* **69**, 1445.

Morawiecki, A. (1964). *Biochim. Biophys. Acta* **83**, 339.

Palese, P., Tobita, K., Veda, M., Compans, R. W. (1974). *Virology* **61**, 397.

Salk, J. E. (1944). *J. Immunol.* **49**, 87.

Schulze, I. T. (1970). *Virology* **42**, 890.

Schulze, I. T. (1972). *Virology* **47**, 181.

Schulze, I. T. (1973). *Advan. Virus Res.* **18**, 1.

Schulze, I. T. (1975a). *In* "Negative Strand Viruses" (R. D. Barry and B. W. J. Mahy, eds.) Academic Press, New York (in press).

Schulze, I. T. (1975b). In preparation.

Seto, J. T., Nishi, T., Hickey, B. J., Rasmussen, A. F. (1961). *Virology* **13**, 13.

Shelokov, A., Vogel, J. E., and Chi, L. (1958). *Proc. Exp. Biol. Med.* **97**, 802.

Shimojo, H. A., Sugiura, A., Akao, J., and Enomoto, C. (1958). *Bull. Inst. Pub. Health, Tokyo* **7**, 219.

Skehel, J. J., and Waterfield, M. D. (1975). *Proc. Nat. Acad. Sci. U.S.* **72**, 93.

Spiro, R. G. (1973). *Advan. Protein Chem.* **27**, 350.

Springer, G. F. (1967). *Biochem. Biophys. Res. Commun.* **28**, 510.

Springer, G. F., and Ansell, N. J. (1958). *Proc. Nat. Acad. Sci. U.S.* **44**, 182.

Springer, G. F., Schwick, H. G., and Fletcher, M. A. (1969). *Proc. Nat. Acad. Sci. U.S.* **64**, 634.

Stanley, P., and Haslam, E. A. (1971). *Virology* **46**, 764.

Stanley, P., Gandhi, S. S., and White, D. O. (1973a). *Virology* **53**, 92.

Stanley, P., Crook, N. E., Streader, L. G., and Davidson, B. E. (1973b). *Virology* **56**, 640.

Stone, I. D. (1949). *Aust. J. Exp. Biol. Med. Sci.* **27**, 337.

Suttajit, M., and Winzler, R. J. (1971). *J. Biol. Chem.* **246**, 3398.

Tamm, I. (1954). *J. Immunol.* **73**, 180.

Thibon, M., Reculard, P., and Cateigne, G. (1967). *Ann. Inst. Pasteur, Paris* **113**, 731.

Tiffany, J. M., and Blough, H. A. (1971). *Virology* **44**, 18.

Tsvetkova, I. V., and Lipkind, M. A. (1966). *Abstr. Int. Congr. Microbiol., 9th, 1966* p. 387.

Tyrrell, D. A. J., and Valentine, R. C. (1957). *J. Gen. Microbiol.* **16**, 668.

von Magnus, P. (1951). *Acta Pathol. Microbiol. Scand.* **28**, 278.

White, D. O., Day, H. M., Batchelder, E. J., Cheyne, I. M., and Wansbrough, A. J. (1965). *Virology* **25**, 289.

Winzler, R. J. (1969a). *In* "Cellular Recognition" (R. T. Smith and R. A. Good, eds.), p. 11. Appleton, New York.

Winzler, R. J. (1969b). *In* "Red Cell Membrane, Structure and Function" (G. A. Jamieson and T. J. Greenwald, eds.), p. 157. Lippincott, Philadelphia, Pennsylvania.

Winzler, R. J., Harris, E. D., Pekas, D. J., Johnson, C. A., and Weber, P. (1967). *Biochemistry* **6**, 2195.

Wong, S. C., and Kilbourne, E. D. (1961). *J. Exp. Med.* **113**, 95.

4

The Biologically Active Proteins of Influenza Virus: Neuraminidase

D. Bucher and P. Palese

I. Introduction

The existence of neuraminidase was first suggested by the now classical observation of Hirst (1942), who observed that red blood cells agglutinated by influenza virus would disagglutinate, and on the addition of fresh virus could not be reagglutinated. The eluted virus, however, would reagglutinate fresh cells. Something had changed the surface of the red cells. His astute observation that an enzyme must be functioning on the virion was in opposition to the generally held view of that day which stated that viruses differed from bacteria primarily by their absolute lack of enzymes.

Until the early 1960's, it was uncertain whether or not the neuraminidase was a separate and distinct entity from the hemagglutinin. It was postulated by Hirst (1942) that hemagglutination was a reflection of the enzyme binding to substrate, and both functions, agglutination and release, could be explained on the basis of the existence of a single enzyme. Hirst (1942) suggested the analogy of the reaction with the interaction of enzymes and substrate. The combination of enzyme and substrate, the ES complex, would be equivalent to hemagglutination. When the substrate is chemically altered, enzyme and substrate dissociate and the enzyme is free to adsorb to and alter more substrate. Hirst proposed that the substrate corresponded to the substance at the receptor site on the red blood cell and was destroyed during agglutination. Burnet (1951) further supported the viewpoint that the hemagglutination and enzymic sites of the virion were identical.

With the separation of neuraminidase from hemagglutinin, first by proteolytic action with trypsin (Mayron et al., 1961; Noll et al., 1962) and later by detergents such as SDS (Laver, 1963), it became clear that these were indeed separate proteins. Probably absolute proof came with the ability to segregate antigenically distinct viral neuraminidases and hemagglutinins by genetic recombination and show their biochemical and antigenic distinctiveness (Laver and Kilbourne, 1966). Ada and Lind (1961) had suggested that neuraminidase might be a host enzyme incorporated into the virion, since uninfected chick cells contained neuraminidase activity and antisera to viral neuraminidase grown in ovo inhibited chick cell neuraminidase. However, later work showed the viral enzyme to be antigenically the same whether the virus was grown in ovo or in calf kidney cells; the cross-reaction between avian and viral neuraminidase was probably mediated by a common host determinant of a carbohydrate nature (Ada et al., 1963).

II. Specificity of Neuraminidase

Gottschalk (1957) and Blix et al. (1957) established that the enzyme of influenza virus hydrolytically cleaves the glycosidic bond joining the keto group of N-acetylneuraminic acid to D-galactose or D-galactosamine and possibly other sugars. Neuraminidase has come to be the accepted name for the enzyme (Gottschalk, 1957). Sialidase is also frequently used as a designation for this enzyme and refers to its cleavage of *substituted* neuraminic acids or sialic acids (Heimer and Meyer, 1956). The systematic name for neuraminidase is mucopolysaccharide N-acetylneuraminylhydrolase, EC 3.2.1.18, according to Enzyme Nomenclature (1965). The enzyme hydrolyzes cleavage of the linkage between terminal sialic acid and an adjacent α-linkage to a sugar molecule. Comprehensive review articles on the properties of bacterial and viral neuraminidases have been written by Drzeniek (1972, 1973) and Gottschalk and Drzeniek (1972).

Naturally occurring *neuraminic* acid is always substituted at the amino group of carbon atom 5 by an N-acetyl or N-glycolyl group, and is sometimes O-acetylated at hydroxyl group(s) (Blix *et al.,* 1957; Gottschalk, 1960). O-Acetyl groups are formed at the hydroxyls in either the 4, 7, or 8 position and are easily split off by dilute acid or alkali treatment. In most mammals, N-acetyl- and N-glycolylneuraminic acids occur together with the ratio differing in various species and in various tissues and secretions of the same species (Gottschalk, 1960). The specificity of neuraminidases is dependent on the N-substitution of the sialic acid of the substrate; the N-acetyl form is cleaved much more rapidly than N-glycolylneuraminic acid by influenza viral neuraminidases (Flockton and Hobson, 1970). Influenza viral neuraminidase have been found to be highly specific with a specificity different from that of bacterial neuraminidases (Drzeniek, 1972). Using synthetic neuraminic acid derivatives it was shown that the presence of a free carboxyl group is an absolute requirement for hydrolysis by neuraminidases (Meindl and Tuppy, 1966a). Substitution of the N-acetyl group by bulkier groups such as benzoyl, butyryl, or benzyloxycarbonyl groups makes neuraminic acid-containing substrates resistant to hydrolysis by bacterial neuraminidases (Meindl and Tuppy, 1966b; Faillard *et al.,* 1969). Susceptibility of substrates to viral neuraminidases is markedly reduced after oxidative removal of carbon atom 9 or carbon atom 8 and 9 of the neuraminic acid backbone, demonstrating the strict structural requirements of neuraminidase (Suttajit and Winzler, 1971).

The nature of the linkage of neuraminic acid to the carbohydrate moiety (aglycon) is important to the specificity of viral neuraminidase. From its behavior with natural substrates, most of which have an α-linkage between the neuraminic acid and the aglycon, it was suggested that neuraminidase cleaves only the α-linkage (Gottschalk, 1957, 1958; Kuhn and Brossmer, 1958). Using synthetic substrates Meindl and Tuppy (1966a,b) showed definitively that the enzyme will not hydrolyze neuraminic acid with a β-linkage. The aglycon itself appears to be relatively unimportant as noted by Schauer and Faillard (1968).

Carbon atom 2 of neuraminic acid is either linked to carbon atom 3, 6, and possibly 4 of galactose; carbon atom 6 of N-acetylgalactosamine, carbon atom 6 of N-acetyl-D-glucosamine or carbon atom 8 of a second neuraminic acid molecule (Drzeniek, 1973). Neuraminic acid is always terminal unless linked to a second neuraminic acid (α, $2 \rightarrow 8$) (Gottschalk and Drzeniek, 1972). Bacterial neuraminidases act upon most α-ketosidic linkages, (α, $2 \rightarrow 3$), (α, $2 \rightarrow 4$), (α, $2 \rightarrow 6$), and (α, $2 \rightarrow 8$), whereas viral neuraminidases, such as Newcastle disease virus and fowl plague viral neuraminidases, preferentially hydrolyze $2 \rightarrow 3$ linkages (Drzeniek, 1967, 1972, 1973). Both viral neuraminidase are relatively inactive against $2 \rightarrow 4$ and $2 \rightarrow 6$ linkages (Huang and Orlich, 1972; Drzeniek, 1967), and $2 \rightarrow 8$ linkages are split by NDV neuraminidase but not by the fowl plague enzyme (Drzeniek and Gauhe, 1970).

III. Neuraminidase Substrates

A. Assay for N-Acetylneuraminic Acid

The assay generally used for measuring neuraminic acid release involves production of a chromophore with the addition of thiobarbituric acid as developed by Warren (1959, 1963) and modified by Aminoff (1959, 1961). This assay permits measure of liberated neuraminic acid without interference by bound N-acetylneuraminic acid. If the reaction of N-acetylneuraminic acid in the assay is set at 100%, then production of chromophore by related neuraminic acids such as N-glycolylneuraminic acid is 63%, N-acetyl-4-O-acetylneuraminic acid is 100%, N-acetyl-8-O-acetylneuraminic acid is 47%, and N-acetyl-7-O-acetylneuraminic acid is 0% (Drzeniek, 1972).

B. Natural Substrates

Neuraminidase is unique in its ability to attack substrates of a very wide range of size (Cinader, 1967). Its range extends from the relatively small sialyllactose (MW 633), to orosomucoid (MW 44,000) and fetuin (MW 48,400) to urinary glycoprotein (MW 7×10^6). A summary of commonly used substrates, their characteristics, and sources of isolation is presented in Table 4.1.

Substrates can be grouped into two categories, small and large. The small natural substrates are best typified and perhaps limited by the example of N-acetylneuraminyllactose or sialyllactose (see Fig. 4.1). N-Acetylneuraminyllactose was isolated from bovine colostrum by Kuhn and Brossmer

Table 4.1 Natural Substrates for Neuraminidase[a]

	MW	% NANA[b]	N-Substitution	Source	Preparation
Sialyllactose (N-acetylneuraminyllactose)	633	49%	N-Acetyl	Bovine colostrum	11, 17
Orosomucoid (α_1 acid glycoprotein)	44,100[1]	12%[1]	—	Human plasma	3, 13
Fetuin	48,400[6]	9%[6]	N-Acetyl (93%)[6], N-Glycoyl (7%)[6]	Fetal calf serum	2, 6, 14
Ovomucin	110,000[7]	6%[1]	N-Glycoyl[7]	Hen egg	2
Submaxillary mucin (porcine)	830,000[18]	15%[1]	N-Acetyl	Porcine submaxillary gland	10
Submaxillary mucin (ovine)	1.0×10^6[19]	25%[1]	O,N-Diacetyl[5,7]	Sheep submaxillary gland	4
Submaxillary mucin (bovine)	—	21%[1]	N-Acetyl, N-Glycoyl, O,N-Diacetyl[5,7]	Bovine submaxillary gland	9
Urinary glycoprotein[15,16] (human)	7.0×10^6[16]	9%[1]	O,N-Diacetyl[8]	Human urine	15
Collocallia mucoid	—	8%[1]	—	Edible bird's nest	12
Meconium glycoprotein	—	10%[1]	—	Human meconium	—
Ovarian cyst glycoprotein	—	18%[7]	—	Human ovarian cyst fluid	—
Stroma glycoprotein	—	23%[7]	—	Human erythrocyte stroma	—

[a] Key to references:
1. Sober, H. A., ed. (1968). "Handbook of Biochemistry," p. C-40–46. Chem. Rubber Publ. Co., Cleveland, Ohio.
2. Mahadevan S., *et al.* (1967). *J. Biol. Chem.* **242**, 4409.
3. Bezkorovainy, A., and Winzler, R. J. (1961). *Biochim. Biophys. Acta* **49**, 559.
4. Tettamanti, G., and Pigman, W. (1968). *Arch. Biochem. Biophys.* **124**, 41.
5. White, A., Handler, P., and Smith, E. L. (1968). "Principles of Biochemistry," p. 34. McGraw-Hill, New York.
6. Spiro, R. G. (1960). *J. Biol. Chem.* **235**, 2860.
7. Gottschalk, A., Belyavin, G., and Biddle, F. (1972). *In* "The Glycoproteins" (A. Gottschalk, ed.) Chapter 9. Elsevier, Amsterdam.
8. Kathan, R. H., and Weeks, D. I. (1969). *Arch. Biochem. Biophys.* **134**, 572.
9. Heimer, R., and Meyer, K. (1956). *Proc. Nat. Acad. Sci. U.S.* **42**, 728.
10. Gibbons, R. A. (1963). *Biochem. J.* **89**, 380.
11. Kuhn, R., and Brossmer, R. (1956). *Angew. Chem.* **70**, 25.
12. Howe, C., Lee, L. T., and Rose, H. M. (1961). *Arch. Biochem. Biophys.* **95**, 512.
13. Eylar, E. H., and Jeanloz, R. W. (1962). *J. Biol. Chem.* **237**, 622.
14. Graham, E. R. B. (1961). *Aust. J. Sci.* **24**, 140.
15. Tamm, I., and Horsfall, F. L. (1950). *Proc. Soc. Exp. Biol. Med.* **74**, 108.
16. Tamm, I., and Horsfall, F. L. (1952). *J. Exp. Med.* **95**, 71.
17. Schneir, M. L., and Rafelson, M. E. (1966). *Biochim. Biophys. Acta* **130**, 1.
18. Tamm, I., Burgher, J. C., and Horsfall, F. L. (1955). *J. Biol. Chem.* **212**, 125.
19. Hashimoto, Y., Hashimoto, S., and Pigman, W. (1964). *Arch. Biochem. Biophys.* **104**, 282.
20. Gottschalk, A., and McKenzie, H. A. (1961). *Biochim. Biophys. Acta* **54**, 226.

[b] NANA N-acetylneuraminic acid.

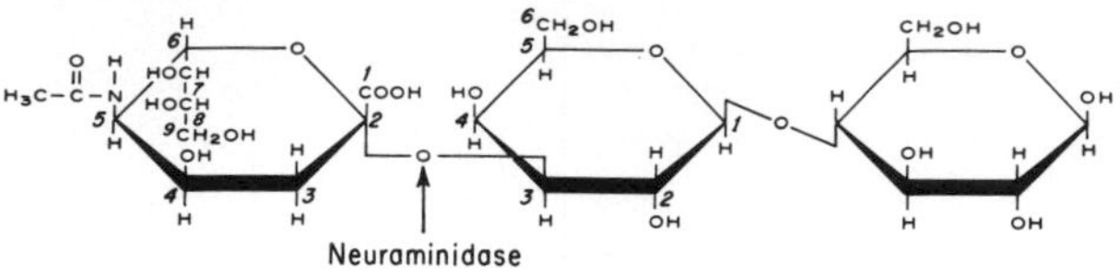

N-acetyl neuraminyl (α,2→3) lactose
(3'-sialyl lactose)

Fig. 4.1. N-Acetylneuraminyl(α, 2 → 3)lactose is a commonly used low molecular weight substrate for influenza viral neuraminidase. The preparation as isolated from bovine colostrum also contains 8–14% of N-acetylneuraminyl(α, 2 → 6)lactose (Schneir and Rafelson, 1966; Ohman and Hygstedt, 1968).

(1958) and contains about 8–14% of the (α, 2 → 6) linkage with 72% being the (α, 2 → 3) form (Schneir and Rafelson, 1966; Ohman and Hygstedt, 1968). The (α, 2 → 6) form is separable from the (α, 2 → 3) form by ion exchange chromatography as reported by Schneir and Rafelson (1966). Ideally, (α, 2 → 3) N-acetylneuraminyllactose should be used as substrate for influenza viral neuraminidase; however, generally the substrate as used is a mixture of both isomers. Small synthetic substrates have also been employed and will be discussed later.

Many "large" molecular weight sialic acid containing substrates exist in nature. In determining the suitability of a substrate for assay of influenza viral neuraminidase the homogeneity and purity of the substrate must be considered. The type of sialic acid, such as N-acetyl-N-glycolyl- or O, N-diacetylneuraminic acid, present in the substrate is important. The linkage existing between neuraminic acid and the aglycon whether (α, 2 → 3), (α, 2 → 6), or (α, 2 → 8) also will determine the value of a substrate for viral neuraminidases. Many sialic acid containing glycoproteins and mucoproteins have been employed as substrates, but few have been biochemically characterized.

Fetuin, an α_2 glycoprotein of fetal calf serum, has come to be the large substrate primarily used for assay of influenza viral neuraminidase. Spiro (1960) was able to isolate fetuin with a yield of 17% of the total protein concentration from fetal calf serum. Sialic acid represented 8.7% of the total weight of the polypeptide, which has a molecular weight of 48,400. Sialic acid is present primarily as the N-acetyl form, with N-glycolylneuraminic acid approximately 7% of the total sialic acid. The conditions for assay of viral neuraminidase with fetuin as substrate have been standardized for determination of anti-neuraminidase antibodies (Aymard-Henry et al., 1973).

Submaxillary mucins have frequently been employed as substrates for neuraminidase. Depending on the source, the content of N-glycolyl or N-acetylneuraminic acid may vary (Gottschalk *et al.*, 1972). Whereas ovine submaxillary mucin contains mainly *N*-acetylneuraminic acid, porcine submaxillary mucin possesses primarily *N*-glycolylneuraminic acid and bovine submaxillary mucin contains both *N*-glycolyl- and *N*-acetylneuraminic acids. Since influenza viral neuraminidase cleaves the *N*-acetyl form of neuraminic acid much more efficiently than the *N*-glycolyl form (see Section II), ovine submaxillary mucin would be the substrate of choice.

Collocalia mucoid, isolated from edible bird's nest, was proposed as a viral neuraminidase substrate by Howe and associates (1961). Neuraminic acid represents approximately 9–13% of the total weight. However, a large percentage of the acetyl groups are present as the *O*-acetyl rather than the *N*-acetyl form of neuraminic acid (Kathan and Weeks, 1969). Orosomucoid, the α_1 acid glycoprotein of human serum, has also been used as a substrate for influenza viral neuraminidase (Rafelson *et al.*, 1963a).

In a comparison of rates of cleavage of *N*-acetylneuraminic acid from several large substrates, Rafelson *et al.* (1963a) found the relative amounts of neuraminic acid released for collocalia mucoid, 26%; haptoglobin 1-1, 23%; haptoglobin 2-2, 22%; orosomucoid, 17%; stromal inhibitor, 10%; and urinary glycoprotein, 5%, as compared to 100% for sialyllactose. However, even though there was wide variation in *rates* of release, the absolute quantities of neuraminic acid released given sufficient time ranged from 58–85% for the above substrates as compared with 100% for sialyl lactose.

Little is known about the actual substrates that are attacked during influenza virus replication *in vivo*. It is known that viral neuraminidases remove neuraminic acid from the influenza virus receptor protein at the surface of red blood cells during elution from these cells. This receptor protein, a glycoprotein of a molecular weight of about 31,000 daltons, has been isolated and possesses M and N blood group substance activity (Kathan and Winzler, 1963; for review, see Winzler, 1972). Comparable glycoproteins from other cell membranes have not been studied to the same extent.

C. Synthetic Substrates

Many synthetic substrates for neuraminidase have been synthesized by coupling aliphatic and aromatic alcohols to carbon atom 2 of different neuraminic acid derivatives (for review, see Tuppy and Gottschalk, 1972). These synthetic compounds can be prepared with high purity and have provided insight into the specificity of different neuraminidases. Meindl and Tuppy (1967) described the use of the phenylketoside of *N*-acetylneuraminic acid, 2-phenyl-*N*-acetylneuraminic acid, as a convenient crystalline neuraminidase substrate. The liberated phenol is assayed by the Folin phenol test. Priwalowa and Khorlin (1969) described the synthesis of 2-*p*-nitro-phenyl-*N*-acetylneuraminic acid which is a convenient chromogenic neuraminidase substrate. A similar substrate, 2-(3′-methoxyphenyl)-*N*-acetylneuraminic acid (MPN) (Tuppy and Palese, 1969), can also be used to determine viral neuraminidases using the Folin phenol test (Palese *et al.*, 1973). An alternate procedure using MPN as substrate was described by Sedmak and Grossberg (1973). After enzymatic hydrolysis of MPN the liberated 3-methoxyphenol (MP) is measured as a solubilized MP-diazonium salt complex. Protein at high concentrations interferes with the Folin method for assay of liberated phenol (Palese *et al.*, 1973) but not with the MPN-diazonium salt method (Sedmak and Grossberg, 1973), thus permitting assay of neuraminidase activity of crude viral preparations. MPN has also been used to visualize neuraminidase activity on polyacrylamide gels and cellulose acetate strips (Tuppy and Palese, 1969; Bucher and Kilbourne, 1972), and has aided in the development of a plaque assay for neuraminidase-containing viruses (Palese *et al.*, 1970, 1973). For the plaque assay, monolayers are infected with influenza or parainfluenza viruses and an agar overlay is made. After a suitable incubation period the substrate MPN and the diazonium salt of 4-amino-2,5-dimethoxy-4-nitroazobenzene is added and allowed to diffuse through the agar. At sites of virus replication the substrate is hydrolyzed and forms an insoluble red dye with the diazonium salt (see Fig. 4.2). Infectious virus can be isolated from these foci.

Recently a fluorometric substrate 4-methylumbelliferyl-*N*-acetyl-neura-

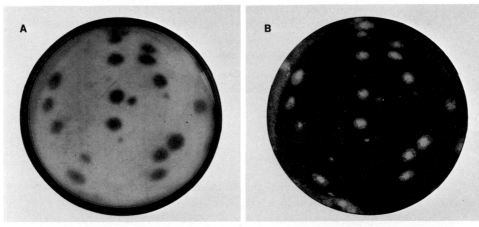

Fig. 4.2. Specific staining of influenza X-7 (HON2) virus plaques with 2-(3′-methoxyphenyl)-*N*-acetylneuraminic acid (MPN). MPN and diazonium salt is incorporated into the agar overlay (Palese *et al.*, 1973). At the site of virus replication dark red foci appear as a result of the viral neuraminidase activity (A). After removal of the agar overlay, the same dish was stained with crystal violet (B). Picture by P. Palese and E. D. Kilbourne, unpublished.

minic acid (P. Palese, unpublished results) has been synthesized which provides a rapid and sensitive way to determine neuraminidase activity. Development of similar substrates should facilitate research into the properties of neuraminidase and aid in its isolation and quantitation. Custom design of substrates should aid in further probing of the nature of the active site.

IV. Chemical Properties of the Enzyme

A. The Michaelis Constant

The Michaelis constant (K_m) provides a measure of the affinity of an enzyme for substrate and gives a parameter for comparison of viral neuraminidase from different strains. The K_m for different influenza virus strains using N-acetylneuraminyllactose $(\alpha, 2 \rightarrow 3)$ as substrate are as follows: PR-8 (N1) $K_m = 1.0 \times 10^{-3}$ M, pH optimum = 7.0: A2/Japan/ 305/57 (N2) $K_m = 2.0 \times 10^{-4}$ M, pH optimum = 6.5; fowl plague virus $K_m = 4.0 \times 10^{-4}$ M, pH optimum = 6.0; and B/Lee $K_m = 2.0 \times 10^{-4}$ M, pH optimum = 6.8 (as summarized in Gottschalk and Drzeniek, 1972). Both the pH optimum and K_m are substrate dependent.

Utilizing the synthetic substrate, MPN, at pH 5.8, Sedmak and Grossberg (1973) found the K_m of A_o/NWS/39 neuraminidase (N1) to be 3.5×10^{-3} M, whereas the K_m for the neuraminidase derived from A_2/R15+/57, X-7 or X-7 (F1) (N2) had a value of 6.5×10^{-4} to 6.9×10^{-4} M, representing a fivefold difference in substrate affinity between the two types of neuraminidases. With both sialyllactose and MPN, the N2 neuraminidase showed a fivefold greater affinity for substrate than N1. However, the absolute affinity of both N1 and N2 neuraminidases for substrate (K_m) was three times greater for sialyllactose than for MPN.

B. pH Optima

The pH optima has been found to vary with strains and be substrate dependent. Generally the pH optima for influenza viral neuraminidases are more basic and closer to neutrality than the rather acidic optima found for the bacterial and mammalian neuraminidases. Kendal and Madeley (1969) found a range from pH 6.4 to 7.0 for a number of viral strains including those of A_0 and A_1 (N1), A_2 (N2), B, and avian A strains with sialyllactose as substrate. The pH optima is also dependent on the type of linkage being cleaved. Schneir and Rafelson (1966) found a maximal rate of cleavage for neuraminidase (N2) for the $(\alpha, 2 \rightarrow 3)$ linkage at pH 6.5, whereas the

(α, $2 \to 6$) linkage was cleaved at maximal rate at pH 4.5. However, the maximal velocity for the (α, $2 \to 6$) N-acetylneuraminyllactose was only 6% of the V_{max} for the (α, $2 \to 3$) form.

C. Product Inhibition

Influenza viral neuraminidase shows competitive inhibition with its product, N-acetylneuraminic acid, although relatively high levels of neuraminic acid are required. Walop et al. (1960) found a K_i of 5.0×10^{-3} M for neuraminidase of A_2/57/Sing (N2) strain when N-acetylneuraminyllactose is the substrate. Rafelson et al. (1963b) determined a K_i of 2×10^{-2} M for the PR8 strain (N1) and 4×10^{-3} M for the Asian strain (N2) at pH optima of 7.0 and 6.5, respectively. This represents a fivefold greater affinity of the N2 strain for product than for the N1 strain, the same ratio that exists between N2 and N1 for substrate affinity (K_m) see above.

D. Heat Stability and the Ca^{2+} Requirement

Although these two topics might seem considerably different, in fact we find a recurrent observation of interplay between the two. Burnet and Stone (1947) observed that *Vibrio cholerae* neuraminidase had an inactivation point 8°C higher in the presence of Ca^{2+} as compared with the absence of Ca^{2+}, and that a similar effect could be demonstrated for the enzyme of B/Lee influenza virus. Boschman and Jacobs (1965) observed that the neuraminidase of FMI (N1), A_2/Japan (N2) and B/Joh became very heat sensitive following treatment with EDTA. The sensitivity to heat and the requirement for Ca^{2+} has been found to vary with the strain (Boschman and Jacobs, 1965; Dimmock, 1971). A_0 (WSN) (N1) possessed no detectable neuraminidase activity after heating in the absence of Ca^{2+} (Dimmock, 1971). If Ca^{2+} was present, 35% of the activity survived. Mg^{2+} could not substitute for Ca^{2+} to produce this stabilizing effect. The Ca^{2+} effect could be reversed by EDTA.

The requirement for Ca^{2+}, apart from the factor of heat stabilization, was a matter of dispute for several years. Although enhancement of activity could be seen, it had been difficult to find an absolute requirement. After removal of Ca^{2+} by Sephadex gel filtration or addition of EDTA to thoroughly chelate minimal concentrations present, Wilson and Rafelson (1967) found a reduction in activity to about 20% of the original for N2 neuraminidase; maximal activity could be obtained by addition of 0.1 mM Ca^{2+}. A near absolute requirement for Ca^{2+} was found by Dimmock (1971) for WSN

(N1) neuraminidase. In the absence of Ca^{2+} only 1% of the original activity was found; 3 mM Ca^{2+} was required for maximal activity. N2 (A_2/Japan) neuraminidase required 0.3 mM Ca^{2+} for maximal activity, a tenfold difference between N1 and N2 type neuraminidases. Much of the difficulty in determining a Ca^{2+} requirement can be attributed to the low quantity required, (particularly for N2) and the fact that most substrates as prepared contain divalent cations in sufficient quantity to meet the Ca^{2+} requirement for influenza viral neuraminidase (N2) (Wilson and Rafelson, 1967).

Heat stability studies by several investigators have shown the neuraminidases of N1 subtype to be heat labile and those of N2 subtype to be heat stable. Rafelson and co-workers (1963a) found the neuraminidase of PR8 (N1) to be completely inactivated by heat at 55°C for 30 minutes, whereas the Asian (N2) enzyme retained 67% of its activity after such treatment. Wide ranges in heat stability for the neuraminidases were found by Paniker (1968). The A_2 (N2) strains had the most stable enzymes with activity unaffected by heating at 45°C for 1 hour, NWS and WSE (N1) possessed the most heat-labile neuraminidases.

V. Neuraminidase Content of the Envelope

Neuraminidase has been estimated to be about 7% of the total protein of the influenza virion for such disparate strains as (A_0/Bel/42), bearing the N1 subtype (Skehel and Schild, 1971), X-7 bearing the N2 subtype (Laver and Kilbourne, 1966) and a B strain, B/Lee (Laver, 1963). In spite of the apparent consistency among these findings, it has been found that the amount of neuraminidase incorporated into the virion can be quite variable, depending on the host cell in which the virus is grown and on the strain of virus. Laver (1963) found the quantity of neuraminidase to vary depending on the cell line in which the virus was grown, representing 6% of the total protein when grown *in ovo,* 14% if the virus was grown in calf kidney cells. Laver and Kilbourne (1966) found twice as much neuraminidase in the X-7(F1)(H0N2) variant as in the X-7(H0N2) strain when both strains were grown *in ovo.* Palese and Schulman (1974) found a tenfold variation in the quantity of neuraminidase from two antigenically identical laboratory recombinants (H0N2) grown *in ovo.* Mowshowitz and Kilbourne (1975) observed a similar variation in neuraminidase activity between two wild-type Aichi (H3N2) virus isolates. Based on particle counts of virus, Seto (1964) found the incomplete virus of PR-8 (H0N1) and Japan 305 (H2N2) to have neuraminidase specific activities of one-half to one-fourth that of standard virus.

If the composition of neuraminidase is 7% of the total protein (and protein is 70% of the weight of the virion) (Frommhagen *et al.*, 1959) and the weight of the viral particle is assumed to be 4×10^{-16} gm (W) (Reimer *et al.*, 1966), then the number of molecules of neuraminidase can be determined per virion by the following equation (Skehel and Schild, 1971). A tetrameric neuraminidase of 240,000 daltons is assumed (Wrigley *et al.*, 1973) and N is Avogadro's number:

$$\frac{N \times W \times \% \text{ of total}}{\text{MW of NA} \times 100\%} = 49 \text{ neuraminidase molecules per virion}$$

Kendal and associates (1968) determined an absolute protein concentration of 4×10^{-16} gm per viral particle and made the estimate of 100 neuraminidase molecules per virion for A₂ Sing/1/57 (H2N2) based on a neuraminidase content of 10% of total viral protein and a molecular weight of 220,000. The total number of surface projections including hemagglutinin and neuraminidase was estimated to be 550–600 by Tiffany and Blough (1970); therefore, 50–100 would be those of neuraminidase, the approximately 500 remaining spikes would be those of hemagglutinin.

A. Solubilization of Neuraminidase

To investigate its properties, enzymatic and antigenic, it is helpful to deal with the enzyme as an entity separate from the other components of the envelope. Since the neuraminidase is situated in the envelope, one must find a means of solubilizing the neuraminidase and removing it from the envelope and other viral components. Techniques can be separated into (a) solubilization by proteolytic agents and (b) solubilization by surface active agents. A summary of purification by both types of techniques is presented in Table 4.2.

Solubilization of neuraminidase does not seem to alter its enzymatic properties. Neuraminidase which is biologically and antigenically active has been isolated by proteolysis or by surface active agents of an ionic or nonionic nature (Drzeniek *et al.*, 1966). The neuraminidase still possesses identical K_m, pH optima, and Ca^{2+} requirements (Drzeniek *et al.*, 1966). Neuraminidase which had been separated from the virion after detergent solubilization or by treatment with a proteolytic enzyme was neutralized by antisera to the same extent as neuraminidase of intact virions (Easterday *et al.*, 1969). However, it must be noted that Webster and Laver (1967) found the N2 detergent-solubilized neuraminidase to possess "poor" antigenicity when compared with the antigenicity of the neuraminidase *in situ*.

Table 4.2 Purification of Influenza Viral Neuraminidase Following Solubilization by Proteolytic Agents or Detergents

Agent	Strain	Yield (%)	Specific activity (μM/min/mg)[a]	Fold purification[d]	Reference
Proteolytic					
Trypsin	PR-8 (N1)	—	—	—	Mayron et al. (1961)
	Asian (N2)	50–80	386[b]	23	Noll et al. (1962)
	B/Lee	90	—	—	Wilson and Rafelson (1963)
Chymotrypsin	polyvalent vaccine	32	0.67	8	Rafelson et al. (1966)
	PR-8 (N1)	—	—	—	
Pronase	Jap 305 (N2)	70–90	23.4	12	Seto et al. (1966)
	A₂/Sing/57 (N2)	50–100	38–188[b]	3–15	Drzeniek et al. (1966)
	A₂/Sing/57 (N2)	11	173[b]	18	
	FPV (Rostock)	—	88–180[b]	9–40	
	A/Eng/939/69 (N2)	13	10.6[c]	32	Kendal and Kiley (1973)
B. subtilis protease	A₂/Sing/57 (N2)	120	9.9[c]	15	Biddle (1968)
Subtilisin BPN′	X-7/F1 (N2)	24	11.6[c]	16	Kendal and Eckert (1972)
	A₂/RI5⁺(W2)	15	11.0[c]	14	Kendal and Kiley (1973)
	A/AA/60 (N2)	19			
Detergents					
Sodium dodecyl sulfate	B/Lee	80–90	—	—	Laver (1963)
Sodium deoxycholate	X-7/F1 (N2)	20	—	—	Laver and Kilbourne (1966)
Sodium dodecyl sulfate	A₂/Sing/57 (N2)	—	—	—	Drzeniek et al. (1968)
Sodium dodecyl sulfate	B/Lee				
Sodium dodecyl sulfate with Triton X-100	X-7 (N2)	123	189	77	Bucher (1973, 1975)
	X-31 (N2)				
	B/Mass				
Tween 20	X-7 (N2) other strains bearing N1 or N2	50–100	—	—	Webster and Darlington (1969)
NP-40	WSN (N1)	20–40	—	13	Gregoriades (1972)

[a] μM, N-acetylneuraminic acid released per minute per mg protein. Different substrates and assay conditions make absolute comparisons difficult.
[b] Our calculations of specific activity based on 16% N content of protein.
[c] Our calculations based on units of Kendal and Eckert (1972).
[d] Fold purification is based on increase in specific activity of purified enzyme from the starting material.

B/Lee neuraminidase has proved to be the most stable and can be recovered in essentially 100% yield after SDS treatment or proteolysis by
trypsin (Laver, 1963). B/Lee neuraminidase is also unaffected by sodium
deoxycholate (Laver, 1963). Among the A strains the A_2 (N2) neuraminidases are the most readily recovered either by SDS treatment or proteolysis
and also are relatively heat stable. The use of neutral detergents has permitted the isolation of neuraminidases of the N2 subtype (Webster and
Darlington, 1969) as well as the neuraminidase of N1 subtype, which had
been especially difficult to obtain in pure form (Gregoriades, 1972). Hoyle
and Almeida (1971) found the neuraminidases of A_2 (N2) and B/Lee
to be almost completely resistant to pronase and trypsin, the neuraminidases
of PR-8 (N1) and swine (N1) to be partially resistant, and the neuraminidases of A_1 (N1) and A/DSP (N1) to be highly susceptible to pronase
and trypsin. The A_0 and A_1 neuraminidases which are sensitive to proteolytic
enzymes are also destroyed by SDS and urea (Hoyle and Almeida, 1971).

Techniques such as sonication, ether disruption, extraction with solvents,
solubilization by chaotropic agents (urea and guanidine hydrochloride) are
barely adequate for solubilization of the enzyme, perhaps because of the
great tendency of neuraminidase to aggregate. Ether disruption of virions
apparently liberates the hemagglutinin and neuraminidase as components
aggregated together (Hoyle, 1952; Davenport et al., 1960; Schäfer, 1963).
Ether disruption had been commonly used for disruption of viral particles
up to the time of Laver's isolation of neuraminidase (Hoyle, 1952; Lief
and Henle, 1956; Paucker et al., 1959; Hoyle et al., 1961).

Preferably one would wish to isolate an enzyme without the necessity for
cleavage of any covalent bonds. The use of detergent solubilization for the
isolation of neuraminidase permits the separation of other viral proteins
which have not been altered chemically from the same viral preparation,
although they may be biologically inactive (Bucher, 1975). It appears that
the peptide lost in proteolytic solubilization is necessary as an anchor for
holding the neuraminidase in the envelope and is not involved with the
functioning of the enzyme. Lazdins et al. (1972) found a loss of 7000 daltons
per neuraminidase subunit for proteolytically (trypsin) derived B/Lee neuraminidase versus that isolated with detergent (SDS); Wrigley et al. (1973)
found a loss of 12,000 daltons per subunit for B/Lee neuraminidase under
similar conditions.

A major distinction observed between the proteolytically derived and
detergent-solubilized neuraminidase(s) has been the lack of aggregation of
the proteolytically derived product. "Permanent" solubilization occurs for
the proteolytically derived product versus reaggregation of the detergent-
solubilized neuraminidase on removal of the solubilizing agent (Lazdins et

al., 1972). Any purification steps for detergent-solubilized neuraminidase must be performed in the presence of detergents, both for the maintenance of the dissociated state and the preservation of activity. Laver and Valentine (1969) and Rott *et al.* (1970) show aggregated structures on removal of detergent from N2 neuraminidases. Gregoriades (1972) found aggregation and loss of activity for WSN (N1) neuraminidase on removal of detergent. Webster (1970b) found considerable aggregation of detergent-solubilized neuraminidase even in the presence of 6 M guanidine HCl under reducing conditions.

1. USE OF PROTEOLYTIC AGENTS

The fact that proteolytic enzymes with different substrate specificities or mixtures of proteolytic enzymes (such as pronase) can be used to solubilize an active product tells us that (1) the neuraminidase active center is greatly resistant to proteolytic agents and (2) cleavage of the hydrophobic fiber will occur with practically any proteolytic agent. Several susceptible amino acids must be available for cleavage; hydrolysis at one site or another is a matter of no great consequence. These proteolytic agents are employed at high concentrations (1–2 mg/ml, or higher), which are nearly equivalent to the viral protein concentration, with short exposure times. Since the viral neuraminidase is in the "native" state, it is likely to be more resistant to proteolysis than a denatured enzyme. Carbohydrate residues on the enzyme may play a role in protecting the enzyme from proteolytic attack and also "direct" proteolytic enzymes to a specific area for cleavage.

Considering enzymes which have been employed for solubilization of the neuraminidase, trypsin has the most restricted specificity known of the endopeptidases with cleavage occurring on the carboxyl side of lysyl and arginyl residues (Walsh, 1970). Chymotrypsin favors cleavage of the protein at aromatic amino acid residues of the polypeptide chain (Wilcox, 1970). Nagarse protease (or subtilisin BPN′) is a serine protease which cleaves a variety of peptide and ester bonds (Ottesen and Svendsen, 1970). Pronase is a mixture of several proteolytic enzymes including endopeptidases and exopeptidases which are produced by a strain of *Streptomyces griseus* K-1 (Narahashi, 1970).

2. USE OF DETERGENTS

Detergents used for the isolation of viral neuraminidases can be divided into two major categories, ionic (primarily anionic) and nonionic. Among the first detergents to be used for solubilization of the enzyme with maintenance of enzymatic activity were sodium dodecyl sulfate and sodium deoxycholate, both strongly anionic-type detergents. The neuraminidase of the A_0 strains (N1) are sensitive to SDS (Gregoriades, 1972; Laver and Baker, 1972), and are inactivated by this agent; those of the A_2 strains (N2) can be isolated by SDS solubilization. A ratio of about 2:1 (w/w) protein/detergent has been found optimal for solubilization of N2 neuraminidase with maintenance of activity (Laver, 1963, Rott et al., 1970). The nonionic type detergents employed have been those of the nonionic Tween series, Tween 20 or Tween 80, often with ether, or more recently, NP40 (Gregoriades, 1972) and Triton X-100 (Bucher, 1973, 1975). The nonionic detergents generally have a much lower inactivating effect on enzymatic activity than the ionic detergents. As with the proteolytic enzymes the type of detergent does not seem to be of major importance in determining the properties of the solubilized enzyme, as long as activity is maintained.

Isolation of active neuraminidase by electrophoresis on cellulose acetate strips (Laver, 1963, 1964) with SDS is dependent on having an SDS-sensitive hemagglutinin coupled with an SDS-resistant neuraminidase. Thus, frequently the neuraminidase of the strain of interest must be genetically segregated into a recombinant with an SDS-sensitive hemagglutinin. After disruption of the viral particles with SDS, the neuraminidase, migrating by endosmotic flow, moves toward the cathode and is separated from the hemagglutinin component. With the A_2 strains, HA and NA migrate together (toward the cathode) and require genetic recombination with earlier strains to produce a hemagglutinin which is inactive in SDS (migrates toward the anode). The neuraminidase of NWS (N1) is denatured by SDS.

B. Purification of Neuraminidase

Following solubilization of the neuraminidase from purified virus, separation of the neuraminidase can be achieved by a combination of centrifugal, chromatographic, and/or electrophoretic steps. Since the active enzyme has a sedimentation rate of 8.0 S to 10.0 S and other viral components may have lower or higher sedimentation velocities, a frequent first step is that of ultracentrifugation, generally performed on either a sucrose or sodium glutamate gradient. The latter has the advantage of permitting a direct measurement of neuraminidase activity in a thiobarbituric acid assay without interference of the sucrose (Biddle, 1968). A relatively low speed spin will separate the neuraminidase from the viral particles, and a second higher speed centrifugation or use of a sharper sucrose gradient will separate the slowly sedimenting soluble proteins from the more rapidly sedimenting neuraminidase.

Later steps frequently involve chromatographic techniques separating macromolecules either by size, as with gel filtration utilizing a material such as Sephadex G-200 or Bio-Rad A-5 (Kendal *et al.*, 1968; Bucher and Kilbourne, 1972) or the use of an ion exchange resin, such as DEAE cellulose, to which N1 neuraminidase adsorbs rather strongly at neutral pH (Gregoriades, 1972). Cellulose acetate electrophoresis in the presence of SDS has been used with much success by Laver (1963, 1964). Electrophoresis in SDS on polyacrylamide gels has been shown to separate on the basis of size (Weber and Osborne, 1969) and has been used to isolate influenza viral neuraminidase (Bucher and Kilbourne, 1972). Electro-focusing has also been an aid in purifying detergent-solubilized neuraminidase (Gregoriades, 1972). Purification based on activity can be achieved with the use of affinity columns bearing a small molecular weight inhibitor, N-p-aminophenoloxamic acid (Cuatrecasas and Illiano, 1971; Bucher, 1973, 1975). Influenza viral neuraminidase has also been purified by exploiting its carbohydrate content, adsorbing the enzyme by lectin affinity chromatography (Hayman *et al.*, 1973).

C. Demonstration of Purity

Following isolation one can apply several criteria for purity of influenza viral neuraminidase. One criterion would be the increase in specific activity under defined conditions. If the neuraminidase represents 7% of the total protein, then one should see an increase in specific activity of about 14- to 15-fold. However, this parameter is difficult to use since generally there is an increase in neuraminidase activity on release of the neuraminidase from the envelope, accompanied simultaneously by a variable amount of denaturation depending on the strain and conditions of solubilization. Thus, it is difficult to judge purity based on specific activity.

A criterion for the purity of a neuraminidase preparation has been nonadsorption of product to red blood cells, but in spite of nonadsorption, antibodies to hemagglutinin may be produced (Wilson and Rafelson, 1963; Drzeniek and Rott, 1963). Thus, an additional criterion for purity has been that no antibodies be produced against any component other than neuraminidase when this enzyme is used as an immunogen.

Since we now know the position of the neuraminidase on polyacrylamide gels, another criterion may be the presence of one high molecular weight glycoprotein band under nonreducing conditions. After reduction, there should be total conversion to one or two glycoprotein bands of about 60,000 daltons with no other polypeptides present, when 5–10 μg of protein is applied to a polyacrylamide gel (Bucher, 1975).

VI. Characterization of the Isolated Product

A. Amino Acid Composition

The amino acid composition has been determined for neuraminidase isolated via detergent treatment for two A subtypes, N1 (Be1) and N2
(X-7/F1), and for a B strain (B/Lee) by Laver and Baker (1972). The
amino acid composition has also been determined for proteolytically derived
neuraminidase of an A subtype, N2 (X-7/F1) by Kendal and Eckert
(1972). The data from both groups of investigators are summarized in
Table 4.3.

In comparison with the amino acid composition of the other major polypeptides of influenza virus, neuraminidase is richer in total cysteine residues

Table 4.3 Amino Acid Composition for N2 (X-7/F1) Neuraminidase

Polar residues	SDS derived N2[a] (residues/monomer)	Proteolytically derived N2[b] (residues/monomer)
Lysine	24.1	20.3
Histidine	6.4	9.7
Arginine	32.6	29.8
Aspartate	77.6	74.3
Threonine	38.0	30.7
Serine	55.1	59.0
Glutamate	46.5	40.0
Residues of intermediate polarity		
Glycine	48.7	50.6
Alanine	20.3	15.3
Nonpolar residues		
Proline	26.2	23.3
Valine	39.1	36.1
Methionine	5.9	9.3
Isoleucine	45.5	34.1
Leucine	25.1	19.4
Tyrosine	12.8	12.6
Phenylalanine	17.7	14.8
Total cysteine	13.9	21.4

[a] Monomer 60,000 daltons (our estimate). (Laver and Baker, 1972.)

[b] Monomer, 54,000 daltons (our calculation based on a mean residue
weight per amino acid of 112. (Kendal and Eckert, 1972.)

(Laver and Baker, 1972). Assuming a molecular weight of 60,000 daltons per subunit and a mean residue weight per amino acid of 112, we calculate a chain length of 535 amino acids per neuraminidase polypeptide. For the neuraminidase of X-7/F1) (N2), Laver and Baker found the total cysteine to represent 2.6% or 13.9 residues. Kendal and Eckert (1972) found an even higher content of total cysteine, 21.4 residues.

Since aggregation occurs though the "fiber" of the SDS-derived neuraminidase on the removal of the detergent, persumably because of the hydrophobicity of this area (see Fig. 4.4, Laver and Valentine, 1969), and since it is known that this portion of the molecule is lost on proteolysis (Lazdins et al., 1972; Wrigley et al., 1973), it is interesting to make a comparison of the total number of polar and nonpolar residues for N2 (X-7/F1) neuraminidase derived by the detergent technique (Laver and Baker, 1972) and that derived by proteolysis (Kendal and Eckert, 1972). It would be more valid to make such comparisons using data obtained by the same group of investigators, but unfortunately such data is not presently available. If one considers the polar residues to be lysine, histidine, arginine, aspartic acid, threonine, serine, and glutamic acid, then one finds that out of 535 residues (see above) there are 280 polar residues for detergent-derived neuraminidase and 264 polar residues for proteolytically derived neuraminidase, a loss of 6% of the polar residues. If the nonpolar residues are considered to be proline, valine, methionine, isoleucine, leucine, tyrosine, phenylalanine, and total cysteine, one finds 186 nonpolar residues in detergent-derived neuraminidase and 171 nonpolar residues in proteolytically derived neuraminidase, a loss of 8% of nonpolar residues. Thus it appears that the amino acids in the area of the neuraminidase molecule cleaved by proteolysis are not significantly more hydrophobic than the remainder bearing the active sites. Conformation of the polypeptide chain must be more important in conferring a hydrophobic character to this region than the actual amino acid content.

The number of lysyl plus arginyl residues are of interest with respect to peptide mapping of a tryptic hydrolysate of this enzyme. Kendal and Eckert (1972) found a total of 50.1 lysine plus arginine residues per subunit, Laver and Baker found 57.0 such residues per subunit. The number of total cysteine residues found is also considerably different; Kendal and Eckert (1972) found 21 total cysteine residues; Laver and Baker (1972) found only 14 residues. The two groups of investigators also found different number of methionine residues; for the same subtype of neuraminidase, Kendal and Eckert (1972) found 9.3, and Laver and Baker (1972) found 5.9. The content of methionine is important for study of the substructure of neuraminidase using cyanogen bromide cleavage at methionine residues. From the work of Kendal and Eckert (1972) we would predict 9–10 fragments after such cleavage. Laver and Baker's data (1972) would suggest 6 or 7 fragments. Additional determinations of amino acid composition are necessary to resolve these discrepancies.

Little is known about the carbohydrate content of neuraminidase, a glycoprotein. Kendal and Eckert (1972) found 5.7 glucosamine residues per polypeptide chain. Lazdins et al. (1972) reported the loss of a glucosamine-rich fraction on preparation of proteolytically derived neuraminidase.

B. Amino Acids at the Active Site

Some investigators have attempted to determine the nature of the amino acid residues at the active site with less than definitive results. Hoyle (1969) found evidence for the presence of the residues tyrosine and histidine at the active site and could not find any suggestion for the presence of cysteine, methionine, tryptophan, arginine, or lysine. On the other hand, Bachmayer's (1972) investigation with N-bromosuccinimide modification strongly suggests that tryptophan is present at the active site. Complete loss of neuraminidase activity occurred on treatment of pronase derived neuraminidase A_2 (N2) with N-bromosuccinimide. Substrates such as sialyllactose and fetuin protected the enzyme against inactivation.

C. Isoelectric Point

The isoelectric point has been determined for neuraminidase which was proteolytically derived (Neurath et al., 1970; Kendal et al., 1973) or detergent derived (Neurath et al., 1970; Gregoriades, 1972). Neurath and associates (1970) and Kendal and associates (1973) found great heterogeneity of isoelectric points for N2 neuraminidase whether the enzyme was derived by proteolytic or detergent techniques. Gregoriades (1972) purified neuraminidase of the N1 subtype (WSN) with the aid of nonionic detergents and found the preparation to be homogeneous with an isoelectric point (pI) of 6.0. Kendal and associates (1973) found at least 6 peaks on isoelectric focusing for N2 neuraminidase ranging from pI = 5.2 to 6.5 with major peaks at pI = 5.5 to 5.8. In both cases the isoelectric point was slightly acidic. Denatured neuraminidase (Kendal et al., 1973) had an isoelectric point 1.5 to 2 pH units lower than native neuraminidase, suggesting that many side chain carboxyl groups may be conformationally masked in the native molecule. For A_2/Aichi/68 and B/Mass/66, Neurath et al. (1970) found a wide range of peaks of pI from 5 to 9, with viral neuraminidase possessing an isoelectric point closer to neutrality than Clostridrium per-

frigens (pI = 4.95) or *Vibrio cholerae* (pI = 4.80) neuraminidases, both of which possessed sharp isoelectric points. Neurath and associates (1970) did not include detergent in the electrofocusing experiments with detergent-derived neuraminidase, thus aggregation may have created the heterogeneity. Gregoriades (1972) obtained a homogeneous isoelectric point at pH 6.0 for detergent-derived neuraminidase and had included nonionic detergents in the media. One might expect proteolytically isolated neuraminidase to be heterogeneous, as cleavage might be expected to occur at more than one site on the polypeptide chain. However, Kendal and associates (1973) found heterogeneity of neuraminidase fractions even after taking individual isoelectric peak fractions and resubjecting them to electrofocusing.

VII. Structure of Neuraminidase

Neuraminidase evidently exists as a spikelike projection on the surface of the influenza virion. To date, however, no one has achieved the resolution under electron microscopy necessary to observe differences among spikes on the viral surface and definitely identify individual spikes as being neuraminidase and not those of hemagglutinin. Laver and Valentine (1969) were unable to identify specific neuraminidase spikes because of the close packing of the surface projections. Both Kendal and Madeley (1970) and Compans and associates (1969) noted the appearance of patches of flocculated antibody on the virion surface when antisera to the neuraminidase was incubated with whole virus particles, suggesting that the neuraminidase may exist in discrete areas. Their observations also demonstrated that neuraminidase is not confined to the base of spikes, since the antibodies clearly were attached to the tips of spikes.

Whether influenza viral neuraminidase is removed from viral particles by proteolytic or detergent techniques, a macromolecule sedimenting within the range of 8.0 S to 10.0 S is observed, and a molecular weight of 200,000 to 250,000 daltons has been calculated. Proteolytically derived neuraminidase has been found to have a lower sedimentation rate and molecular weight than neuraminidase isolated by detergent techniques. Noll and associates (1962) predicted a molecular weight of 190,000 based on a sedimentation rate of 9.0 S and a partial specific volume ($\bar{V}$) of 0.7 cm/gm for B/Lee neuraminidase solubilized with the aid of trypsin. Kendal and associates (1968) calculated a molecular weight of 220,000 based on a sedimentation rate of 8.0 S and a $\bar{V}$ of 0.733 cm/gm for N2 neuraminidase solubilized with nagarse protease. Wrigley and associates (1973) estimated a molecular weight of 207,400 by sedimentation equilibrium based on a $\bar{V}$ of 0.719 and had found a sedimentation rate of 9.0 S for B/Lee neuraminidase-solubilized with trypsin. Higher sedimentation rates were observed for detergent-solubilized neuraminidase. Webster and Darlington (1969) found a rate of 10.8 S for N2 (X-7) neuraminidase with Tween 20, and Bucher and Kilbourne (1972) found a rate of 11.0 S for N2 (X-7) neuraminidase with SDS. Rott and associates (1970) found a sedimentation rate of 10 S for SDS-solubilized influenza A neuraminidase, treatment with pronase reduced the sedimentation rate to 9 S.

The active unit of neuraminidase was predicted to be tetrameric based on its behavior under reducing conditions (Kendal and Eckert, 1972; Bucher and Kilbourne, 1972; Lazdins et al., 1972). Several investigators showed that the 10 S active unit can be dissociated into monomeric units with a molecular weight of 50,000 to 60,000 daltons when treated with reducing agents, such as mercaptoethanol or dithiothreitol (Webster, 1970a,b; Kendal and Eckert, 1972; Bucher and Kilbourne, 1972; Skehel and Schild, 1971; Lazdins et al., 1972). Proof of the tetrameric structure of the neuraminidase was provided with the publication of the fine electron micrographs of Wrigley and associates (1973).

Under the electron micrograph, proteolytically derived neuraminidase exists as planar tetrameric units which are about 40Å in cross section and are more cubical than round as shown in Fig. 10.4 in Chapter 10 and in the diagram in Fig. 4.3 (Wrigley et al., 1973). If the neuraminidase tetramers are detergent (SDS) derived, they retain "fibers" or "tails" of 100 Å in length with a "foot" of about 40 Å in diameter (Laver and Valentine, 1969; Wrigley et al., 1973). Viewed on a side, these neuraminidase tetramers particles have a club-shaped appearance. If the detergent is removed, the neuraminidase units have a great propensity for aggregation, and the aggregated tetramers exhibit the appearance of what has been colorfully described as "seeding dandelions" with a diameter of 320 Å (Laver and Valentine, 1969; Wrigley et al., 1973). If hemagglutinin subunits are present, the neuraminidase will form *mixed* aggregates with the hemagglutinin on the removal of detergent (Laver and Valentine, 1969).

The neuraminidase evidently must be tetrameric to possess enzymatic activity (Bucher and Kilbourne, 1972; Kendal and Eckert, 1972). Gregoriades (1972) reported activity with a smaller unit based on detergent gradient gel filtration, but the neuraminidase may have reassociated to tetrameric form after elution on gel filtration as has been observed by Bucher and Kilbourne (1972). These investigators found that although the neuraminidase was eluted at a point of 53,000 daltons after chromatography on Bio-Gel A-5 (Bio Rad), the enzyme had spontaneously reassociated to active tetrameric units, as measured by sucrose gradient centrifugation. A summary of level of monomeric association and activity is shown in Fig. 4.4.

Although disulfide bonds play an important role in the tetrameric struc-

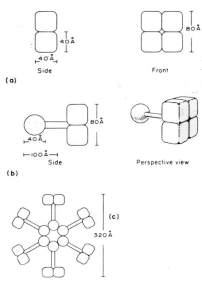

Fig. 4.3. Diagrammatic representation of neuraminidase structure as interpreted from the electron micrographs of Laver and Valentine (1969) and Wrigley and associates (1973). Proteolytically derived neuraminidase (a) possesses coplanar structure of the tetrameric unit, with side and front views shown. The tail fiber has been removed during proteolysis. Detergent-derived neuraminidase (b) shows the attached fiber with the club-shaped head as seen on a side view. On removal of detergent (c) the neuraminidase molecules (up to twelve units) aggregate to produce the appearance of a "seeding dandelion" of Laver and Valentine (1969), evidently through hydrophobic interaction of the tips of the fiber. Throughout the diagram, the subunits are visualized as more cubic than spherical (Wrigley and associates, 1973).

ture as noted above, this is apparently at the level of intrachain and/or between dimers rather than among all four subunits, as shown in Fig. 4.5 (Bucher and Kilbourne, 1972; Lazdins *et al.*, 1972). Bucher and Kilbourne (1972) noted diffusion on polyacrylamide gel electrophoresis beyond the extent predicted for a molecule of that size (200,000–250,000) without the addition of reducing agent. Under nonreducing conditions, Lazdins and associates (1972) found a polypeptide band at 120,000 for B/Lee neuraminidase, reduction was required to produce the monomeric unit. They suggested that the monomers are linked together by disulfides to form dimers, and the dimers in turn form a tetrameric structure by noncovalent interaction.

Although the tetrameric structure of neuraminidase has been resolved, the existence of four equivalent monomers (Kendal and Eckert, 1972; Wrigley *et al.*, 1973) or two types of nonequivalent monomers (Bucher and Kilbourne, 1972) still is a matter of debate. One suggestion has been that the finding of one or two types of subunits may be a function of strain. The rather exotic club-shaped structure may suggest more than one type of com-

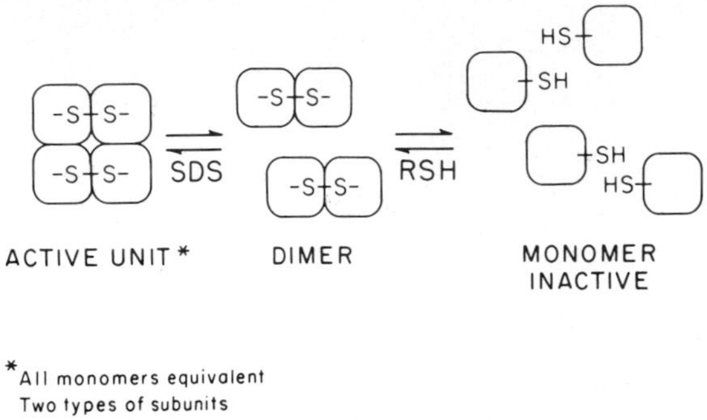

ACTIVE UNIT*   DIMER   MONOMER INACTIVE

*All monomers equivalent
Two types of subunits

Fig. 4.4. Structure of neuraminidase as related to activity. Neuraminidase evidently requires a tetrameric association for its enzymatically active unit (Kendal and Eckert, 1972; Bucher and Kilbourne, 1972). Dissociation to dimeric units can occur in the presence of detergent (Lazdins *et al.*, 1972). Dissociation to monomeric units requires sulfhydryl reagents (Webster, 1970 a,b; Kendal and Eckert, 1972; Bucher and Kilbourne, 1972). The dissociation is not irreversible, reassociation to an active tetrameric unit can occur under appropriate conditions (Bucher and Kilbourne, 1972).

PHENYLGLYOXAL   PHENYLOXAMIC ACID   β-PHENYL-α-MERCAPTO-ACRYLIC ACID

2-(O-AMINOPHENYL) BENZIMIDAZOLE

1-(O-AMINOPHENYL)-3,4-DIHYDROISOQUINOLINE   3-AZA-2,3,4-TRIDEOXY-4-OXO-D-ARABINO-OCTONIC ACID-δ-LACTONE   2-DEOXY-2,3-DEHYDRO-N-TRIFLUOROACETYL-NEURAMINIC ACID (FANA)

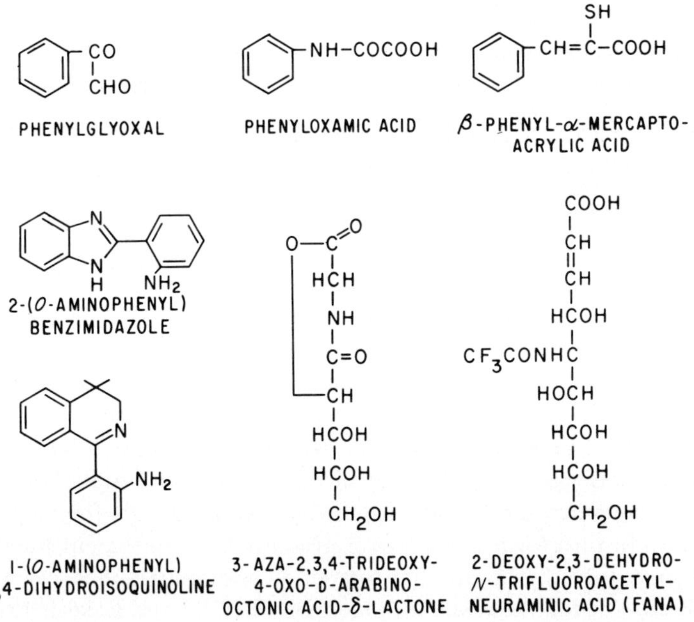

Fig. 4.5. Chemical structure of synthetic neuraminidase inhibitors. The different classes and their derivatives are described in the text.

ponent. Investigators studying neuraminidase (N2) isolated from the recombinant strains of X-7 or X-7(F1) by detergent techniques have found two components, although there has been disagreement as to the ratio of the monomeric units (Webster, 1970a; Bucher and Kilbourne, 1972; Skehel and Schild, 1971; Lazdins *et al.*, 1972). Bucher and Kilbourne (1972) have found the monomers to be present in equimolar concentrations; other investigators have found a smaller concentration of the more rapidly moving component (Skehel and Schild, 1971; Lazdins *et al.*, 1972). Kendal and Eckert (1972) found only one component for neuraminidase isolated from X-7(F1), but the enzyme was solubilized by proteolysis. Gregoriades (1972) found only one subunit for neuraminidase (N1) derived from WSN. Investigators who have examined the neuraminidase of B/Lee have found only one type of subunit (Lazdins *et al.*, 1972; Laver and Baker, 1972; Wrigley *et al.*, 1973).

Kendal and Kiley (1973) observed only one polypeptide band on electrophoresis after reduction for proteolytically derived neuraminidase from X-7(F1) (N2). Peptide maps of tryptic hydrolysates of proteolytically derived neuraminidase suggest the presence of only one type of subunit based on the number of radiolabeled sulfhydryl groups observed (Kendal and Kiley, 1973). After tryptic digestion of [^{14}C]carboxamidomethylated neuraminidase subunits, Kendal and Kiley (1973) observed about 20 spots on autoradiographs of their peptide maps; this strongly suggests the presence of only one type of subunit since they found 21 total cysteine residues. If there are two types of neuraminidase subunits, twice that number of spots (42) should have been observed. However, Laver and Baker (1972) found considerably fewer total cysteine residues, only 14; twice that number would be 28, perhaps within the experimental error for 20 peptides observed by Kendal and Kiley (1973) on peptide mapping. It had been predicted that the number of peptides observed might be dependent on the technique of isolation, that is whether the neuraminidase is detergent-derived or proteolytically derived. However, peptide maps of neuraminidase isolated by either technique showed no significant differences (A. P. Kendal and D. J. Bucher, unpublished).

Lazdins and associates (1972) have suggested that the component migrating more rapidly under electrophoresis could be proteolytically derived. Kendal and Kiley (1973) have offered a similar explanation for the existence of the second component. Another possible explanation might lie in differences in carbohydrate composition of the monomers. Confirmation of the nature of the differences between the two types of monomers, whether real or artifactual, awaits the separation and isolation of these components. The existence of two types of subunits would increase genetic encumbrance but would also increase the potential for genetic variation.

VIII. Neuraminidase as an Antigen

Neuraminidase has emerged as an antigenically significant component of the virion. Influenza viral neuraminidase is unique in that it is an enzyme which is also significant as an antigen in a disease. Antibodies to the neuraminidase can confer protection against disease or modify the course of influenza viral infection (see Chapter 12). Using recombinant viruses possessing common neuraminidases but serologically unrelated hemagglutinins, Schulman and associates (1968) found that antibodies to neuraminidase inhibited viral replication in the mouse lung, diminishing the viral titer and the extent of lung lesions.

As does the hemagglutinin, neuraminidase undergoes antigenic "shift" and "drift." The neuraminidase component shows antigenic variation independent of the hemagglutinin (Paniker, 1968; Schulman and Kilbourne, 1969). Although a new A_1 subtype of influenza virus was introduced in 1947, with a dramatic change in the hemagglutinin, the neuraminidase component was cross-reactive with the A_0 neuraminidase; the neuraminidases in both subtypes have been designated as N1 (Paniker, 1968; World Health Organization, 1972). In 1957–1958, the A_2 strain appeared with both novel hemagglutinin (H2) and neuraminidase (N2). No cross-reaction of antisera could be found between Asian (N2) and PR8(N1) or B as observed by Råfelson et al. (1963a,b). The strain appearing in 1968 possessed a novel hemagglutinin (H3) although the neuraminidase was highly cross-reactive with the A_2 strains, and thus was designated N2 (World Health Organization, 1972). Minor antigenic changes, "drift," had been occurring throughout the decades when no major shift occurred (Schulman and Kilbourne, 1969).

Interaction of the neuraminidase with antibodies can be measured by several techniques. These include such diverse procedures as inhibition of enzymatic activity (Fazekas de St. Groth, 1962, 1963; Aymard-Henry et al., 1973), immunoprecipitation (Easterday et al., 1969; Schild and Pereira, 1969; Palese et al., 1973), reduction in plaque size (Jahiel and Kilbourne, 1966), and mouse titration tests (Schulman et al., 1968). The immunoprecipitation band of neuraminidase can be directly visualized after immunodiffusion if the small chromogenic substrate, MPN, is employed (Palese et al., 1973).

One of the techniques most widely used for the determination of antineuraminidase antibodies is the inhibition of neuraminidase activity using a large substrate which is a neuraminic acid-containing glycoprotein. The level of inhibition by antibody has been found to be independent of substrate concentration (Fazekas de St. Groth, 1963; Rafelson et al., 1963a). The neuraminidase inhibition assay has been standardized with the use of fetuin as substrate, and the degree of inhibition is measured as that dilution of antibody producing 50% inhibition of neuraminidase activity (Aymard-Henry *et al.*, 1973). A straight line is obtained when the percentage inhibition is plotted versus the logarithm of the dilution of antisera. The final assay conditions are 1.2% fetuin in 0.1 M sodium phosphate buffer, pH 5.9, with 1.5 mM CaCl$_2$ in a 0.2 ml volume. Sensitivity of the test has been increased by lengthy incubation of the neuraminidase with antisera and substrate (17 hours at 37°C).

The inhibition of neuraminidase activity by antibodies was found to be dependent on the size of the substrate (Fazekas de St. Groth, 1963; Rafelson *et al.*, 1963b). Inhibition of the neuraminidase of *Vibrio cholerae* showed a similar dependence on substrate size (Mohr and Schramn, 1960). It was observed that neuraminidase activities of influenza virus could be inhibited with specific antibody if the substrate was large (orosomucoid, fetuin, or urinary glycoprotein), but little or no inhibition of activity could be observed if a small substrate, sialyllactose, were employed. This suggested that inhibition of enzymatic activity occurred by a steric process: antibody is not directed against the active site but against an adjacent site(s) and inhibition becomes greatest with the largest substrate employed (Fazekas de St. Groth, 1962).

Fazekas de St. Groth (1963) found in a comparison of A and B strains, that the A$_0$(Mel) strain had neuraminidase disposed so that it is more readily neutralized by antibody, and the maximum level of inhibition with the same substrate is higher for A$_0$(Mel) than for B(Lee). The A$_2$ strain shows steric inhibition with large substrates and some inhibition with sialyllactose, unlike the B strains which show no inhibition with sialyllactose, 80% inhibition with large substrates (such as fetuin, orosomucoid, and trypsin-treated urinary mucoid) and 100% inhibition with very large substrates (such as erythrocytes, urinary mucoid, and ovomucin). This may indicate greater distance between the antigenic and active sites in the B strains as compared to the A strains.

Fazekas de St. Groth (1963) also showed that after papain cleavage of antibodies, steric inhibition was greatly diminished, although the equilibrium binding constant was identical to that for intact antibodies. Fazekas de St. Groth (1963) found that the inhibition is by a noncompetitive mechanism and is dependent on (1) the distance between antigenic determinants and the enzyme active center, (2) the shape and size of substrate molecules, and (3) the size of the antibody molecule. An estimate was made of a 20 Å distance between the antigenic and active sites of neuraminidase (Fazekas de St. Groth, 1962). These experiments were performed with antisera to the intact virus particle, containing both anti-hemagglutinin and anti-neuraminidase antibodies. Monospecific antisera to the neuraminidase should be employed to verify this interpretation.

The property of nonantigenicity of the active site is not unique to neur-aminidase, but apparently is a phenomenon which is common to several enzymes and may be a reflection of the immutability of the active site among species (Cinader, 1967). One theory may be that since the host recognizes the influenza viral neuraminidase active site as identical to the active site of its own neuraminidase, it is unable to produce antibodies to this area.

Antibodies to hemagglutinin can inhibit neuraminidase activity to varying degrees for several strains (Paniker, 1968; Webster and Pereira, 1968). The neuraminidase inhibition mediated by hemagglutinin antibodies can be elim-inated if the neuraminidase (X-7) is solubilized by Tween 20 (Webster, 1970a), or SDS, or pronase (Easterday et al., 1969). Conversely, antibody to neuraminidase can inhibit hemagglutination for some viral strains (Kil-bourne, 1968; Schulman and Kilbourne, 1969); generally, antibodies to neuraminidase do not prevent hemagglutination, but strongly inhibit *elution* of virus (Brown and Laver, 1968). The hemagglutination inhibition test has been used to determine anti-neuraminidase antibodies using X-15 and the X-15(HK) recombinants (Kendal et al., 1972). The sensitivity of the test has been increased by the inclusion of anti-human IgG (Kendal et al., 1972) (see also Chapter 11).

IX. Lectins and Neuraminidase

Concanavalin A, a lectin or phytagglutinin, will inhibit influenza viral neuraminidase activity in a manner similar to that of antibodies specific to the enzyme, when a large molecular substrate such as fetuin is used (Palese et al., 1973; Zalan et al., 1974). Concanavalin A agglutinates com-pounds possessing α-D-glucopyranosyl, α-D-mannopyranosyl, and α-D-fructo-furanosyl residues (Goldstein et al., 1965; Goldstein and So, 1965). As with antibodies, a neuraminidase precipitation line can be visualized on immuno-diffusion using the small chromogenic substrate, MPN, when a solution of concanavalin A is used in place of antisera and diffused toward a prepara-tion of the disrupted virus, even though activity is inhibited by concanavalin A when a large substrate is employed (Palese et al., 1973). Thus concanava-lin A behaves similarly to anti-neuraminidase antibodies in that it blocks the active site sterically, not directly.

Rott and co-workers (1972) demonstrated the precipitation of neuramini-dase by concanavalin A and believed this to be the sole surface component reacting with the lectin; these workers had found that addition of con-canavalin A to fowl plague virus-infected chick embryo fibroblast cells prevented assembly or release of virus. If virus was disrupted with Triton X-100, hemagglutinin activity was found in the supernatant and neuraminidase was precipitated by concanavalin A. However, with proteolytically derived neuraminidase only one-third of the enzyme could be precipitated by concanavalin A, with two-thirds of the neuraminidase remaining in the supernatant. This suggests that a carbohydrate-rich fraction is eliminated from proteolytically derived neuraminidase, as has also been shown by Lazdins and associates (1972) utilizing very different techniques.

Zalan and coworkers (1974) had initially suggested that neuraminidase activity was blocked through the interaction of concanavalin A with the hemagglutinin component. However, isolated neuraminidase possessed an identical degree and pattern of blocking as the enzyme *in situ*. Sensitivity to inhibition by concanavalin A was found to vary according to strain. Evidently the carbohydrate residues of the neuraminidase are readily accessible on the envelope, and solubilization of the neuraminidase does not open up previously "hidden" areas. In addition, it was found that whereas isolated neuraminidase could be adsorbed to Sepharose Con A (Pharmacia), an agarose material substituted with concanavalin A, the hemagglutinin component did not adsorb (E. Zalan, personal communication). The work of Rott and associates (1972) and E. Zalan (personal communication) would suggest that the carbohydrate moieties on neuraminidase and hemagglutinin are significantly different.

Neuraminidase is also bound by lens culinaris phytohemagglutinin columns (Hayman *et al.*, 1973), as is the hemagglutinin. This lectin recognizes glucose, mannose, and sterically related sugar residues (Stein *et al.*, 1971). Studies with lectins should aid in localizing the active site of the neuraminidase molecule and help to provide information on the nature of the carbohydrate residues of neuraminidase.

X. Inhibitors to Neuraminidase Activity

Inhibition of neuraminidase activity can be mediated by antibodies or lectins, but blockage of neuraminidase activity can also occur with several other types of agents. Inhibitors to neuraminidase may be natural or synthetic in origin, large or small, and highly specific or relatively nonspecific. Interest in inhibitors to this enzyme has been heightened by the possibility that neuraminidase inhibitors might serve as chemotherapeutic agents specifically directed against viruses containing neuraminidase.

Inhibitors which will block neuraminidase activity frequently do not affect the hemagglutinin, even though both viral proteins interact with neuraminic acid. Neuraminyllactose is cleaved by neuraminidase but is not an inhibitor of hemagglutination (Bogoch, 1957). Orosomucoid is not a hemagglutination inhibitor but is cleaved by neuraminidase (Mayron *et al.*, 1961). Neuraminic acid will inhibit neuraminidase but is not an inhibitor of hemagglutination (Odin, 1952).

Drzeniek (1966, 1970) and Becht and Drzeniek (1967) observed that polyanions have a marked inhibitory effect on viral neuraminidase. Ribonucleic and deoxyribonucleic acids, dextran sulfate, pig submaxillary mucin, and heparin inhibit neuraminidases from influenza and parainfluenza viruses in concentrations in the range of 0.005 to 0.5 μg/ml. Synthetic and inorganic polyanions such as trypan red, congo red, and phosphotungstic and silicotungstic acids also inhibit FPV/Rostock and influenza A_2 viral neuraminidases in concentrations varying from 10^{-4} to 10^{-7} M. The activity of these compounds, however, is not specific because the inhibition can be reversed with albumin or small amounts of polycations such as poly-L-lysine.

Sulfhydryl reagents such as thioglycolate, glutathione, cysteine, merthiolate, and Hg^{2+} inhibit the neuraminidases of influenza A_2/Jap 305/57 (H2N2) virus and PR8 (H0N1) virus, although the concentrations required to achieve 50% inhibition are high and vary between 10^{-2} and 10^{-3} M (Rafelson *et al.*, 1963a). EDTA, also, at high concentrations (10^{-2} to 10^{-4} M) inhibits all influenza viral neuraminidases tested.

Many structurally unrelated compounds have been shown to inhibit neuraminidases (see Fig. 4.5). Edmond *et al.* (1966) found that phenyl-glyoxal derivatives and substituted oxamic acids inhibit the neuraminidase of influenza A/Engl/1/61 (H2N2) virus. The best inhibitor of this group, *N*-phenyloxamic acid, causes a 50% enzyme inhibition between 2×10^{-4} to 5×10^{-4} M. Despite the fact that oxamic acid derivatives are nonspecific neuraminidase inhibitors which interfere with enzyme reactions not related to neuraminic acid, such as lactate dehydrogenase, aminophenyloxamic acid coupled to a solid matrix has been successfully used for the purification of bacterial and viral neuraminidases (Cuatrecasas and Illiano, 1971; Bucher, 1973). Some of the compounds described by Edmond *et al.* (1966) have a weak antiviral effect on PR-8 (H0N1) influenza virus grown in allantoic membranes but are ineffective when tested in embryonated eggs. Haskell *et al.* (1970) describes another class of acidic neuraminidase inhibitors which are substituted β-aryl-α-mercaptoacrylic acids (Fig. 4.5). These inhibitors also cause a 50% inhibition of viral and bacterial neuraminidases at the relatively high concentration of 5×10^{-4} M. Another group of neuraminidase inhibitors, derivatives of aminophenyl-benzimidazoles, are interesting because they are basic in contrast to the inhibitors mentioned above which all possess a carboxyl group; however the benzimidazole derivatives are also relatively weak neuraminidase inhibitors (Haskell *et al.*, 1970).

Dihydro- and tetrahydroisoquinoline derivatives were reported to inhibit neuraminidase activity (Brammer *et al.*, 1968; Haskell *et al.*, 1970) and to be active against influenza virus infections in mice and humans (Brammer *et al.*, 1968). Recently Shinkai and Nishimura (1972) claimed that two isoquinoline derivatives tested did not inhibit neuraminidase activity but rather interfered with the thiobarbituric acid test. In the light of these data the experiments by Brammer *et al.* (1968), Tute *et al.* (1970), and Haskell *et al.* (1970) should be reexamined.

In an effort to provide specific inhibitors to neuraminidase, several investigators have synthesized compounds structurally related to *N*-acetylneuraminic acid. *N*-Acetylneuraminic acid itself was shown to be a weak inhibitor of influenza virus A/Sing/1/57 (H2N2) neuraminidase with a K_i of 5×10^{-3} M compared to a K_m of 6×10^{-4} M for sialyllactose. Khorlin *et al.* (1970) found that 2-deoxy-2-*p*-nitrophenylthio-*N*-acetyl-α-D-neuraminic acid, an α-ketoside of *N*-acetylneuraminic acid, is a competitive inhibitor of *Vibrio cholerae* neuraminidase with a K_i of 2.3×10^{-4} M versus a K_m of 1.67×10^{-3} M for *N*-acetylneuraminyllactose. Another neuraminic acid analog, 3-aza-2,3,4-trideoxy-4-oxo-D-arabinooctonic acid-δ-lactone, is even more effective with a K_i of 4×10^{-5} M for *V. cholerae* neuraminidase (Fig. 4.5). Both compounds show inhibitory activity against all viral neuraminidases tested.

Recently, derivatives of deoxyneuraminic acid with specific blocking activity against neuraminidases have been synthesized (Meindl and Tuppy, 1969a, 1973). 2-Deoxy-2,3-dehydro-*N*-acetylneuraminic acid is a competitive inhibitor of *V. cholerae* neuraminidase with a high affinity for the bacterial enzyme ($K_i = 1 \times 10^{-5}$ M) and a marked inhibitory activity on myxoviruses in tissue culture (Meindl and Tuppy, 1969b; Meindl *et al.*, 1971). 2-Deoxy-2,3-dehydro-*N*-acetylneuraminic acid differs from *N*-acetylneuraminic acid only because of a double bond between carbon atom 2 and 3. Derivatives of this compound obtained by substituting the *N*-acetyl group with a *N*-fluoro, *N*-difluoro, *N*-trifluoro, or *N*-chloroacetyl group are even more effective inhibitors (Meindl *et al.*, 1974). Eighteen derivatives were tested against a variety of influenza viral neuraminidases. The most active of these derivatives, 2-deoxy-2,3-dehydro-*N*-trifluoroacetylneuraminic acid (FANA), competitively inhibits enzyme activity with a K_i of 7.9×10^{-7} M for influenza A/Mel/35(H0N1) viral neuraminidase. So far, FANA is the most potent specific neuraminidase inhibitor known; the affinity of viral neuraminidase for small molecular weight, as well as large molecular weight, substrates is about 1000 times lower than that for FANA (Meindl *et al.*, 1974; Schulman and Palese, 1975). FANA causes a 50% enzyme inhibition at concentrations as low as 2×10^{-6} to 5×10^{-6} M at substrate concentrations of 10^{-3} M and seems to be specific for neuraminidases and reactions involving neuraminic acid. The hemagglutination of influenza A and B viruses is not inhibited, but FANA interferes with the hemagglutination by parainfluenza viruses, NDV and SV5, above concentrations of 10^{-7} and 10^{-6} M, respectively. Because hemagglutination by Sendai virus is not inhibited, hemagglutination inhibition by FANA does not seem to be a general characteristic of parainfluenza viruses (Meindl et al., 1974).

FANA was further shown to inhibit influenza virus replication in tissue culture. All influenza viruses tested were shown to be inhibited by FANA (Palese et al., 1974a; Schulman and Palese, 1975). Differences in susceptibility, however, were found. Viruses containing the N1 neuraminidase of WSN (H0N1) virus showed inhibition in a plaque size reduction test at a FANA concentration of 2×10^{-6} to 4×10^{-6} M; viruses with the N2 neuraminidase of the recombinant virus X-7 (H0N2) required 50–100 times higher FANA concentrations for the same degree of inhibition. The fact that influenza viruses with the same hemagglutinin but different neuraminidases show a different response to FANA strongly suggests that the antiviral effect of FANA is specifically mediated by inhibition of neuraminidase activity (Schulman and Palese, 1975). Furthermore, FANA has no effect on the replication of other enveloped viruses, such as measles and vesicular stomatitis virus, that do not possess neuraminidase (Kilbourne et al., 1974; Palese et al., 1974a).

XI. Role of Neuraminidase

Since the discovery of the neuraminidase more than 30 years ago several theories have been advanced to explain the function of this enzyme. In addition to the possible physiological role of *removing neuraminic acid from mucins,* which are hemagglutination inhibitors, it has been suggested that during the replicative cycle neuraminidase may function either in the *penetration* of virus into the cell or in the *release* of progeny virus. Recent evidence suggests a fourth potential role, that of *preventing aggregation* of newly formed virus.

It was originally suggested that neuraminidase may be responsible for the *penetration* of the virus into susceptible cells following attachment to neuraminic acid at the cell surface. The cleavage of neuraminic acid could be required for entry of the virion into the cell (Hirst, 1942). Several observations argue against such a role. Virus with heat-inactivated neuraminidase still penetrates into cells (Fazekas de St. Groth, 1948), interferes with the multiplication of active virus (Isaacs and Edney, 1950), and participates in genetic recombination with other viruses (Burnet and Lind, 1954). Proteolytic removal of the neuraminidase does not affect the infectivity of the WSN (H0N1) strain (Schulze, 1970). Inhibition of neuraminidase activity with the neuraminidase inhibitor FANA at 10^{-3} M, which assures virtually complete inhibition of neuraminidase activity, does not affect penetration (J. L. Schulman and P. Palese, unpublished results). Antibodies to neuraminidase do not affect the infectivity of influenza virus (Seto and Rott, 1966; Jahiel and Kilbourne, 1966; Webster and Laver, 1967; Kilbourne et al., 1968). All this evidence suggests that neuraminidase activity is not essential during the early steps of influenza virus replication. It could, however, be argued that inactivation or removal of the neuraminidase by heat, proteolytic enzymes, inhibitors, or antibody is not complete and that a remaining fraction of the enzyme activity is sufficient to facilitate the first step(s).

Hoyle (1950) proposed, that the neuraminidase acts on cellular substrates resulting in the *release* of virus from the cell surface. Padgett and Walker (1964) came to a similar conclusion by showing that a variant of influenza B/Lee virus with low neuraminidase activity is more slowly released from cells than the stock Lee virus with a higher neuraminidase activity, and the variant also has a slower growth rate in multicycle replication. In the light of recent experiments with variants of influenza A viruses differing in their neuraminidase content by a factor of eight- to tenfold, it seems that the correlation of neuraminidase activity and release or growth may depend on the host cell system employed. Although the high neuraminidase-containing variant replicates more rapidly in eggs and chorioallantoic membrane pieces, the variant with low neuraminidase content replicates to higher titer in clone 1-5C-4 cells (Palese and Schulman, 1974; J. L. Schulman, unpublished results).

Support for the *release* role of neuraminidase has come from experiments using anti-neuraminidase antibodies which do not interfere with adsorption of the virus but which prevent release of newly synthesized virions (Seto and Rott, 1966; Jahiel and Kilbourne, 1966; Webster and Laver, 1967; Kilbourne et al., 1968; Compans et al., 1969). It was believed that antibodies would inhibit the hydrolysis of terminal neuraminic acid molecules thereby blocking the release of viral particles attached to neuraminic acid molecules at the cell membrane. This role was supported by experiments demonstrating that inhibition of virus release in the presence of antibodies could be partially overcome by the addition of an excess of external bacterial neuraminidase (Compans et al., 1969; Webster, 1970a). Becht and accociates (1971) were not able to confirm these results and found that monovalent anti-neuraminidase antibodies present during a single cycle of replication would not block the release of virus, although they inhibited neuraminidase activity. Other experiments also cast doubt on the role of the

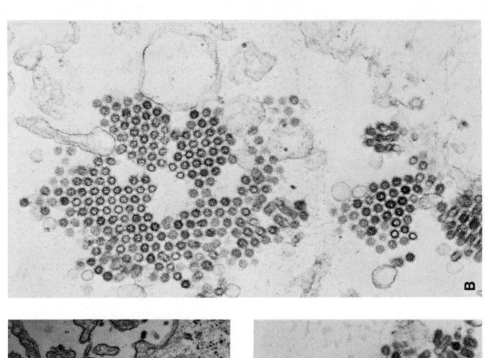

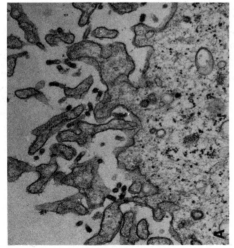

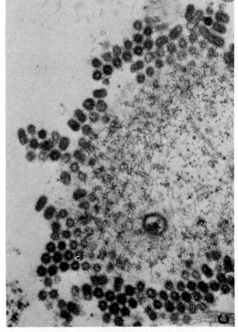

enzyme during *release* of virus. The same amount of cellular neuraminic acid is released from infected cells in the presence or absence of antibody (Dowdle *et al.*, 1974). The time of maximal neuraminidase production is long before the release of the virus (Schlesinger and Karr, 1956; Lipkind and Tsvetkova, 1973).

The effect of bivalent anti-neuraminidase antibodies has more recently been attributed to a bridging or clumping of virus by antibodies (originally proposed by Kilbourne and Schulman, 1965) and attachment of viral aggregates to the cell surface, rather than to their neuraminidase-inhibiting activity (Kendal and Madeley, 1970; Becht *et al.*, 1971; Dowdle *et al.*, 1974). The bridging effect of anti-neuraminidase antibodies may not be the only mechanism by which neuraminidase antibodies act to inhibit influenza virus production. In contrast to the findings of Becht and associates (1971), monovalent anti-neuraminidase antibodies have been shown to inhibit virus replication when assayed in the more sensitive plaque size reduction test which involves a multicycle growth of the virus (Kilbourne *et al.*, 1974). During multicycle replication even slight reductions in virus yield are magnified and repeated during each subsequent cycle. This would indicate that at least part of the inhibitory activity of anti-neuraminidase antibodies may be mediated by specific neuraminidase inhibition. Experiments described earlier with FANA, a small molecular weight neuraminidase inhibitor, support the idea that inhibition of neuraminidase activity influences virus replication of neuraminidase-containing viruses (Palese *et al.*, 1974a; Schulman and Palese, 1975) and suggests that an active neuraminidase is indeed essential for influenza virus replication.

A new role of the viral neuraminidase, that of *preventing virus aggregation,* has been proposed from studies with ts (temperature sensitive) mutants of influenza virus and provides further evidence for the essential role of the enzyme in the replicative cycle of influenza virus (Palese *et al.*, 1974b,c). Sugiura and associates (1972) have isolated ts mutants of influenza WSN (H0N1) virus, each of which falls into one of several complementation groups. Two of these mutants were shown to be neuraminidase-defective mutants (Palese *et al.*, 1974b). When grown at nonpermissive temperature

---

Fig. 4.6. Aggregation of ts3 influenza WSN (H0N1) virus grown at non-permissive temperature or in the presence of FANA. Thin sections were prepared according to Palese *et al.* (1974b). Ts3 grown at permissive temperature; virus particles are budding; no aggregation (A). Ts3 grown at nonpermissive temperature; particles possess no neuraminidase activity and contain neuraminic acid on the envelope; aggregation occurs (C). Ts3 grown at permissive temperature in the presence of the neuraminidase inhibitor FANA (6.0×10^{-1} *M*); particles contain neuraminic acid on the envelope; aggregation occurs (B). Electron micrograph by R. W. Compans, P. Palese, and M. Ueda.

the neuraminidase-defective mutants produce particles that contain neuraminic acid on their envelopes and form large aggregates. It had been previously shown that the envelope of influenza virus particles and the membrane patches at the site of virus budding are devoid of neuraminic acid, presumably due to the viral neuraminidase (Klenk *et al.*, 1970). It has been speculated that the removal of the neuraminic acid may be necessary to permit assembly of the virus (Klenk *et al.*, 1970). From the results obtained with the neuraminidase-defective mutant it is clear that morphologically intact virus particles with neuraminic acid on their envelope do bud from the cell but form aggregates rather than being released as individual virions (Fig. 4.6). Since the virions are sialylated, the hemagglutinin of neighboring virions may recognize the viral envelope as a receptor and attach particles to each other, creating large aggregates. The interesting results by Schulze (1975) on the effect of *in vitro* sialylation of influenza WSN virus might also suggest the formation of small aggregates (see Chapter 3). The observed increase of infectivity of *in vitro* sialylated virus may be caused by the aggregation of 2–4 noninfectious virus particles. This phenomenon has been described by Hirst and Pons (1973).

Thus the role of *prevention of aggregation* of virions by the action of neuraminidase can be summarized as follows. Neuraminidase is responsible for the removal of sialic acid from the envelope of the virion, thus eliminating receptors on the surface which would cause the virus to aggregate and form conglomerates of up to 500 particles (Fig. 4.6). The neuraminidase protects the virus from its own hemagglutinin which attaches to neuraminic acid-containing receptors (Palese *et al.*, 1974b).

The theory for this proposed role suggests that only those viruses which possess a hemagglutinin with neuraminic acid as receptor on the cell (i.e., orthomyxo- and paramyxoviruses) need a neuraminidase and provides an explanation for the observation that other budding viruses do not possess a neuraminidase. From the limited amount of data available it seems that budding viruses, such as RNA tumor viruses, VSV, Sindbis, and rabies virus, possess neuraminic acid on their envelope (Burge and Huang, 1970; Klenk and Choppin, 1971; Lai and Duesberg, 1972; Schlumberger *et al.*, 1973; Krantz *et al.*, 1974). Incorporation of neuraminic acid in the envelope of all budding viruses may be part of the maturation process; only orthomyxoviruses and paramyxoviruses must remove neuraminic acid from their envelope to avoid aggregation.

From the electron micrographic studies it can be seen that virus with temperature-sensitive neuraminidase appears to aggregate rather than attach to neuraminic acid receptors on the cell membrane. One possible explanation for this could be that during the budding process the virions are already in close contact at the membrane, and when leaving the cell they remain attached to each other instead of reattaching to the cell surface. Figure 4.6 shows the phenomenon of aggregation of a neuraminidase-deficient mutant when grown at nonpermissive temperature. A similar effect is seen when the mutant is grown at permissive temperature in the presence of FANA, a neuraminidase inhibitor. Under these conditions the viral neuraminidase is inhibited and the virions carry neuraminic acid receptors causing aggregation (P. Palese and R. W. Compans, 1975).

One must also consider the role that viral neuraminidases may have in removing neuraminic acid receptors from cell membranes and mucin layers to prevent virus from reattaching to these receptors. This might be particularly important in natural infections when virus could be trapped by mucin layers or other hemagglutination inhibitors, and the neuraminidase might serve not only to disaggregate the particles but also to free the virus from these glycoproteins to allow infection of other susceptible cells. Thus, there may not be a single function, but several functions which neuraminidase may serve in the replicative cycle.

Acknowledgments

The authors wish to express their appreciation to Dr. Vannie W. Wilson, Jr., for his helpful discussions and review of the manuscript. Part of the work carried out in the authors' laboratories was supported by Public Health Service Research Grants AI 09304, AI 10884, and AI 11823-01 and by Contract U-2076 from the Health Research Council of the City of New York.

References

Ada, G. L., and Lind, P. E. (1961). *Nature (London)* **190,** 1169.
Ada, G. L., Lind, P. E., and Laver, W. G. (1963). *J. Gen. Microbiol.* **32,** 225.
Aminoff, D. (1959). *Virology* **7,** 355.
Aminoff, D. (1961). *Biochem. J.* **81,** 384.
Aymard-Henry, M., Coleman, M. T., Dowdle, W. R., Laver, W. G., Schild, G. C., and Webster, R. G. (1973). *Bull. W.H.O.* **48,** 199.
Bachmayer, H. (1972). *FEBS (Fed. Eur. Biochem. Soc.) Lett.* **23,** 217.
Becht, H., and Drzeniek, R. (1967). *J. Gen. Virol.* **2,** 261.
Becht, H., Hammerling, U., and Rott, R. (1971). *Virology* **46,** 337.
Biddle, F. (1968). *J. Gen. Virol.* **2,** 19.
Blix, G., Gottschalk, A., and Klenk, E. (1957). *Nature (London)* **179,** 1088.
Bogoch, S. (1957). *Virology* **4,** 458.
Boschman, T. A. C., and Jacobs, J. (1965). *Biochem. Z.* **342,** 532.
Brammer, K. W., McDonald, C. R., and Tute, M. S. (1968). *Nature (London)* **219,** 515–517.
Brown, J., and Laver, W. G. (1968). *J. Gen. Virol.* **2,** 291.
Bucher, D. J. (1973). *Abstr. Amer. Soc. Microbiol.* p. 215.
Bucher, D. J. (1975). *In* "The Negative Strand Viruses" (R. Barry and B. Mahy, eds.). Academic Press. New York (in press).

Bucher, D. J., and Kilbourne, E. D. (1972). *J. Virol.* **10**, 60.
Burge, B., and Huang, A. S. (1970). *J. Virol.* **6**, 176.
Burnet, F. M. (1951). *Physiol. Rev.* **31**, 131.
Burnet, F. M., and Lind, P. E. (1954). *Aust. J. Exp. Biol. Med. Sci.* **32**, 133.
Burnet, F. M. and Stone, J. D. (1947). *Aust .J. Exp. Biol. Med. Sci.* **25**, 227.
Cinader, B. (1967). *In* "Antibodies to Biologically Active Molecules" (B. Cinader, ed.), Vol. 1, pp. 85–137. Pergamon, Oxford.
Compans, R. W., Dimmock, N. J., and Meier-Ewert, H. (1969). *J. Virol.* **4**, 528.
Cuatrecasas, P., and Illiano, G. (1971). *Biochem. Biophys. Res. Commun.* **44**, 178.
Davenport, F. M., Rott, R., and Schäfer, W. (1960). *J. Exp. Med.* **112**, 765.
Dimmock, N. J. (1971). *J. Gen. Virol.* **13**, 481.
Dowdle, W. R., Downie, J. C. and Laver, W. G. (1974). *J. Virol.* **13**, 269.
Drzeniek, R. (1966). *Nature (London)* **211**, 1205.
Drzeniek, R. (1967). *Biochem. Biophys. Res. Commun.* **26**, 631.
Drzeniek, R. (1970). *Z. Med. Mikrobiol. Immunol.* **156**, 1.
Drzeniek, R. (1972). *Curr. Top. Microbiol. Immunol.* **59**, 35.
Drzeniek, R. (1973). *Histochem. J.* **5**, 271.
Drzeniek, R., and Gauhe, A. (1970). *Biochem. Biophys. Res. Commun.* **38**, 651.
Drzeniek, R. and Rott, R. (1963). *Z. Naturforsch. B* **18**, 1127.
Drzeniek, R., Seto, J. T., and Rott, R. (1966). *Biochim. Biophys. Acta* **128**, 547.
Drzeniek, R., Frank, H., and Rott, R. (1968). *Virology* **36**, 703.
Easterday, B., Laver, W. G., Pereira, H. G., and Schild, G. C. (1969). *J. Gen. Virol.* **5**, 83.
Edmond, J. D., Johnston, R. G., Kidd, D., Rylance, H. J. and Sommerville, R. G. (1966). *Brit. J. Pharmacol.* **27**, 415.
Enzyme Nomenclature. (1965). *Compr. Biochem.* **13**, 138.
Faillard, H., Do Amaral, C. F. and Blohm, M. (1969). *Hoppe Seyler's Z. Physiol. Chem.* **350**, 798.
Fazekas de St. Groth, S. (1948). *Nature (London)* **162**, 294.
Fazekas de St. Groth, S. (1962). *Advan. Virus Res.* **9**, 1.
Fazekas de St. Groth, S. (1963). *Ann. N.Y. Acad. Sci.* **103**, 674.
Flockton, H. I., and Hobson, D. (1970). *In* "The Biology of Large RNA Viruses" (R. D. Barry and B. W. J. Mahy, eds.), pp. 535–541. Academic Press, New York.
Frommhagen, L. H., Knight, C. A., and Freeman, N. K. (1959). *Virology* **8**, 176.
Goldstein, I. J., and So, L. L. (1965). *Arch. Biochem. Biophys.* **3**, 404.
Goldstein, I. J., Hollerman, C. E., and Merrick, J. M. (1965). *Biochim. Biophys. Acta* **97**, 68.
Gottschalk, A. (1957). *Biochim. Biophys. Acta* **23**, 645.
Gottschalk, A. (1958). *Nature (London)* **181**, 377.
Gottschalk, A. (1960). "The Chemistry and Biology of Sialic Acids and Related Substances," pp. 1–115. Cambridge Univ. Press, London and New York.
Gottschalk, A., and Drzeniek, R. (1972). *In* "The Glycoproteins" (A. Gottschalk, ed.), pp. 381–402. Elsevier, Amsterdam.
Gottschalk, A., Belyavin, G., and Biddle, F. (1972). *In* "The Glycoproteins" (A. Gottschalk, ed.), pp. 1082–1096. Elsevier, Amsterdam.
Gregoriades, A. (1972). *Virology* **49**, 333.
Haskell, T. H., Peterson, F. E., Watson, D., Plessas, N. R., and Culbertson, T. (1970). *J. Med. Chem.* **13**, 697.
Hayman, M. J., Skehel, J. J., and Crumpton, M. J. (1973). *FEBS (Fed. Eur. Biochem. Soc.) Lett.* **29**, 185.

Heimer, R., and Meyer, K. (1956). *Proc. Nat. Acad. Sci. U.S.* **42**, 728.
Hirst, G. K. (1942). *J. Exp. Med.* **76**, 195.
Hirst, G. K., and Pons, M. W. (1973). *Virology* **56**, 620.
Howe, C., Lee, L. T., and Rose, H. M. (1961). *Arch. Biochem. Biophys.* **95**, 512.
Hoyle, L. (1950). *J. Hyg.* **48**, 277.
Hoyle, L. (1952). *J. Hyg.* **50**, 229.
Hoyle, L. (1969). *J. Hyg.* **67**, 289.
Hoyle, L., and Almeida, J. D. (1971). *J. Hyg.* **69**, 461.
Hoyle, L., Horne, R. W., and Waterson, A. P. (1961). *Virology* **13**, 448.
Huang, R. T. C., and Orlich, M. (1972). *Hoppe-Seyler's Z. Physiol. Chem.* **352**, 318.
Isaacs, A., and Edney, M. (1950). *Aust. J. Exp. Biol. Med. Sci.* **28**, 231.
Jahiel, R. I., and Kilbourne, E. D. (1966). *J. Bacteriol.* **92**, 1521.
Kathan, R. H., and Weeks, D. I. (1969). *Arch. Biochem. Biophys.* **134**, 572.
Kathan, R. H., and Winzler, R. J. (1963). *J. Biol. Chem.* **238**, 21.
Kendal, A. P., and Eckert, E. A. (1972). *Biochim. Biophys. Acta* **258**, 484.
Kendal, A. P., and Kiley, M. P. (1973). *J. Virol.* **12**, 1482.
Kendal, A. P., and Madeley, C. R. (1969). *Biochim. Biophys. Acta* **185**, 163.
Kendal, A. P., and Madeley, C. R. (1970). *Arch. Gesamte Virusforsch.* **31**, 219.
Kendal, A. P., Biddle, F., and Belyavin, G. (1968). *Biochim. Biophys. Acta* **165**, 419.
Kendal, A. P., Minuse, E., and Davenport, F. M. (1972). *Z. Naturforsch. B* **27**, 241.
Kendal, A. P., Kiley, M. P., and Eckert, E. A. (1973). *Biochim. Biophys. Acta* **317**, 28.
Khorlin, A. Ya., Privalova, I. M., Zakstelskaya, L. Ya., and Molibog, E. V. (1970). *FEBS (Fed. Eur. Biochem. Soc.) Lett.* **8**, 17.
Kilbourne, E. D. (1968). *Science* **160**, 74.
Kilbourne, E. D., and Schulman, J. L. (1965). *Trans. Ass. Amer. Physicians* **78**, 323.
Kilbourne, E. D., Laver, W. G., Schulman, J. L., and Webster, R. G. (1968). *J. Virol.* **2**, 281.
Kilbourne, E. D., Palese, P., and Schulman, J. L. (1974). *Perspect. Virol.* **9**, 99.
Klenk, H. D., and Choppin, P. W. (1971). *J. Virol.* **7**, 416.
Klenk, H. D., Compans, R. W., and Choppin, P. W. (1970). *Virology* **42**, 1158.
Krantz, M. J., Lee, Y. C., and Hung, P. P. (1974). *Nature (London)* **248**, 684.
Kuhn, R., and Brossmer, R. (1958). *Angew. Chem.* **70**, 25.
Lai, M. M. C., and Duesberg, P. H. (1972). *Virology* **50**, 359.
Laver, W. G. (1963). *Virology* **20**, 251.
Laver, W. G. (1964). *J. Mol. Biol.* **9**, 109.
Laver, W. G., and Baker, N. (1972). *J. Gen. Virol.* **17**, 61.
Laver, W. G., and Kilbourne, E. D. (1966). *Virology* **30**, 493.
Laver, W. G., and Valentine, R. C. (1969). *Virology* **38**, 105.
Lazdins, I., Haslam, E. A., and White, D. O. (1972). *Virology* **49**, 758.
Lief, F. S., and Henle, W. (1956). *Virology* **2**, 753.
Lipkind, M. A., and Tsvetkova, I. V. (1973). *Arch. Gesamte Virusforsch.* **42**, 125.
Mayron, L. W., Robert, B., and Winzler, R. J. (1961). *Arch. Biochem. Biophys.* **92**, 475.
Meindl, P., and Tuppy, H. (1966a). *Monatsh. Chem.* **97**, 990.
Meindl, P., and Tuppy, H. (1966b). *Monatsh. Chem.* **97**, 1628.

Meindl, P., and Tuppy, H. (1967). *Monatsh. Chem.* **98**, 53.

Meindl, P., and Tuppy, H. (1969a). *Monatsh. Chem.* **100**, 1295.

Meindl, P., and Tuppy, H. (1969b). *Hoppe-Seyler's Z. Physiol. Chem.* **350**, 1088.

Meindl, P., and Tuppy, H. (1973). *Monatsh. Chem.* **104**, 402.

Meindl, P., Bodo, G., Lindner, J., and Palese, P. (1971). *Z. Naturforsch. B* **26**, 792.

Meindl, P., Bodo, G., Palese, P., Schulman, J., and Tuppy, H. (1974). *Virology* **58**, 457.

Mohr, E., and Schramm, G. (1960). *Z. Naturforsch.* **25**, 568–575.

Mowshowitz, S., and Kilbourne, E. D. (1975). *In* "Negative Strand Viruses" (R. Barry and B. Mahy, eds.). Academic Press, New York (in press).

Narahashi, Y. (1970). *In* "Methods in Enzymology" (G. E. Perlman and L. Lorand, eds.), Vol. 19, pp. 651–664. Academic Press, New York.

Neurath, A. R., Hartzell, R. W., and Rubin, B. A. (1970). *Experientia* **26**, 1210.

Noll, H., Aoyagi, T., and Orlando, J. (1962). *Virology* **18**, 154.

Odin, L. (1952). *Nature (London)* **170**, 663.

Ohman, R., and Hygstedt, O. (1968). *Anal. Biochem.* **23**, 391.

Ottesen, M., and Svendsen, I. (1970). *In* "Methods in Enzymology" (G. E. Perlman and L. Lorand, eds.) Vol. 19, pp. 199–215. Academic Press, New York.

Padgett, B. L., and Walker, D. L. (1964). *J. Bacteriol.* **87**, 383.

Palese, P., and Schulman, J. L. (1974). *Virology* **57**, 227.

Palese, P., and Compans, R. W. (1975). *Nature (London)* in press.

Palese, P., Bodo, G., and Tuppy, H. (1970). *J. Virol.* **6**, 556.

Palese, P., Bucher, D., and Kilbourne, E. D. (1973). *Appl. Microbiol.* **25**, 195.

Palese, P., Schulman, J. L., Bodo, G., and Meindl, P. (1974a). *Virology* **59**, 490.

Palese, P., Tobita, K., Ueda, M., and Compans, R. W. (1974b). *Virology* **61**, 397.

Palese, P., Schulman, J. L., Tobita, K. (1974c). *Behring Werk Mitt.* **55**, 11.

Paniker, C. K. J. (1968). *J. Gen. Virol.* **2**, 385.

Paucker, K., Birch-Anderson, A., and von Magnus, P. (1959). *Virology* **8**, 1.

Priwalowa, I. M., and Khorlin, A. J. (1969). *Izv. Akad. Nauk. SSSR, Ser. Khim.* **12**, 1785.

Rafelson, M. E., Schneir, M., and Wilson, V. W. (1963a). *Arch. Biochem. Biophys.* **103**, 424.

Rafelson, M. E., Schneir, M., and Wilson, V. W. (1963b). *In* "The Amino Sugars" (R. W. Jeanolz and E. A. Balazs, eds.), Vol. II, pp. 171–179. Academic Press, New York.

Rafelson, M. E., Gold, S., and Priede, I. (1966). *In* "Methods in Enzymology" (E. F. Neufeld and V. Ginsburg, eds.), Vol. 8, pp. 677–679. Academic Press, New York.

Reimer, C. B., Baker, R. S., Newlin, J. E., and Havens, M. C. (1966). *Science* **152**, 1379.

Rott, R., Drzeniek, R., and Frank, H. (1970). *In* "The Biology of Large RNA Viruses" (R. D. Barry and B. W. J. Mahy, eds.), pp. 75–85. Academic Press, New York.

Rott, R., Becht, H., Klenk, H. D., and Scholtissek, C. (1972). *Z. Naturforsch. B* **27**, 227–233.

Schafer, W. (1963). *Bacteriol. Rev.* **27**, 1.

Schauer, R., and Faillard, H. (1968). *Hoppe-Seyler's Z. Physiol. Chem.* **349**, 961.

Schild, G. C., and Pereira, H. G. (1969). *J. Gen. Virol.* **4**, 355.

Schlesinger, R. W., and Karr, H. V. (1956). *J. Exp. Med.* **103**, 309.

Schlumberger, H. D., Schneider, L. G., Kulas, H. P., and Diringer, H. (1973). *Z. Naturforsch. C* **28**, 103.

Schneir, M. L., and Rafelson, M. E. (1966). *Biochim. Biophys. Acta* **130**, 1.

Schulman, J. L., and Kilbourne, E. D. (1969). *Proc. Nat. Acad. Sci. U.S.* **63**, 326.

Schulman, J. L., and Palese, P. (1975). *Virology* **63**, 98.

Schulman, J. L., Khakpour, M., and Kilbourne, E. D. (1968). *J. Virol.* **2**, 778.

Schulze, I. T. (1970). *Virology* **42**, 890.

Schulze, I. T. (1975). *In* "Negative Strand Viruses" (R. D. Barry and B. W. J. Mahy, eds.). Academic Press, New York (in press).

Sedmak, J. J., and Grossberg, S. E. (1973). *Virology* **56**, 658.

Seto, J. T. (1964). *Biochim. Biophys. Acta* **90**, 420.

Seto, J. T., and Rott, R. (1966). *Virology* **30**, 731.

Seto, J. T., Drezeniek, R., and Rott, R. (1966). *Biochim. Biophys. Acta* **113**, 402.

Shinkai, K., and Nishimura, T. (1972). *J. Gen. Virol.* **16**, 227.

Skehel, J. J., and Shild, G. C. (1971). *Virology* **44**, 396.

Spiro, R. G. (1960). *J. Biol. Chem.* **235**, 2860.

Stein, M. D., Howard, I. K., and Sage, H. J. (1971). *Arch. Biochem. Biophys.* **146**, 353.

Sugiura, A., Tobita, K., and Kilbourne, E. D. (1972). *J. Virol.* **10**, 639.

Suttajit, M., and Winzler, R. J. (1971). *J. Biol. Chem.* **246**, 3398.

Tiffany, J. M., and Blough, H. A. (1970). *Virology* **41**, 392.

Tuppy, H., and Gottschalk, A. (1972). *In* "The Glycoproteins" (A. Gottschalk, ed.), pp. 403–449. Elsevier, Amsterdam.

Tuppy, H., and Palese, P. (1969). *FEBS (Fed. Eur. Biochem. Soc.) Lett.* **3**, 72.

Tute, M. S., Brammer, K. W., Kaye, B., and Broadbent, R. W. (1970). *Med. Chem.* **13**, 44.

Walop, J. N., Boschman, T. A. C., and Jacobs, J. (1960). *Biochim. Biophys. Acta* **44**, 185.

Walsh, K. A. (1970). *In* "Methods in Enzymology" (G. E. Perlman and L. Lorand, eds.), Vol. 19, pp. 41–63. Academic Press, New York.

Warren, L. (1959). *J. Biol. Chem.* **234**, 1971.

Warren, L. (1963). *In* "Methods in Enzymology" (S. P. Colowick and N. O. Kaplan, eds.), Vol. 6, pp. 453–465. Academic Press, New York.

Weber, K., and Osborne, M. (1969). *J. Biol. Chem.* **244**, 4406.

Webster, R. G. (1970a). *In* "Biology of Large RNA Viruses" (R. Barry and B. Mahy, eds.), pp. 53–74. Academic Press, New York.

Webster, R. G. (1970b). *Virology* **40**, 643.

Webster, R. G., and Darlington, R. W. (1969). *J. Virol.* **4**, 182.

Webster, R. G., and Laver, W. G. (1967). *J. Immunol.* **99**, 49.

Webster, R. G., and Pereira, H. G. (1968). *J. Gen. Virol.* **3**, 201.

Wilcox, P. E. (1970). *In* "Methods in Enzymology" (G. E. Perlman and L. Lorand, eds.), Vol. 19, pp. 64–112. Academic Press, New York.

Wilson, V. W., and Rafelson, M. E. (1963). *Biochem. Prep.* **10**, 113.

Wilson, V. W., and Rafelson, M. E. (1967). *Biochim. Biophys. Acta* **146**, 160.

Winzler, R. J. (1972). *In* "Glycoproteins" (A. Gottschalk, ed.), pp. 1268–1293. Elsevier, Amsterdam.

World Health Organization. (1972). *Bull. W.H.O.* **45**, 119.

Wrigley, N. G., Skehel, J. J., Charlwood, P. A., and Brand, C. M. (1973). *Virology* **51**, 525.

Zalan, E., Wilson, C., Freitag, R., and Labzoffsky, N. A. (1974). *Abstr. Amer. Soc. Microbiol.* p. 221.

5

The Biologically Active
Proteins of Influenza Virus:
Influenza Transcriptase
Activity of Cells and Virions

Robert W. Simpson and William J. Bean, Jr.

I. Introduction

This chapter involves an area of influenza virus biology which is of recent inception and, as such, provides much information which is fragmentary in content, still leaving many questions unanswered. The basic premise upon which this chapter will be based is that myxoviruses are "negative" stranded viruses (Barry and Mahy, 1975) with an obligative need for a virion-bound RNA polymerase which transcribes the segmented viral genome into complementary RNA molecules endowed with messenger function for viral protein synthesis. The separation of the discussion into a consideration of an RNA polymerase associated with infected cells in one case and with purified virus particles in the other was dictated by convenience and should not be construed as an endorsement of the concept that distinct enzymes are operative in these two systems.

II. RNA Polymerase Activity of Infected Cells

The first observation of an RNA-dependent RNA polymerase activity in cells infected with influenza virus was made by Ho and Walters (1966), who detected such enzyme function in minced chorioallantoic membranes exposed to virus after removal from embryonated chicken eggs. Addition of actinomycin D but not guanidine hydrochloride was found to inhibit the appearance of this enzyme activity. Subsequent confirmation of this work came from several laboratories which focused on the various requirements of the system, the temporal aspects of enzyme appearance, and the nature of the products made (Ruck *et al.*, 1969; Page *et al.*, 1968; Skehel and Burke, 1968; Scholtissek and Rott, 1969a). In an early related study, the interesting finding was made that infection of cells with fowl plaque virus was accompanied by a measurable effect on host cell polymerases (Borland and Mahy, 1968). In this and a series of later investigations (Mahy, 1970; Mahy *et al.*, 1972, 1974), these workers examined the nucleolar activity (polymerase I) and the nucleoplasmic activity (polymerase II) assayed in fractions of purified nuclei from infected chick embryo fibroblast cells and differentiated both by their ionic requirements and their respective sensitivities to the drug α-amanitin. It was found that the α-amanitin-insensitive activity (polymerase I) decreased after infection, while the drug-sensitive polymerase II which is believed to synthesize cellular mRNA species (Roeder and Rutter, 1970; Zylber and Penman, 1971; Reeder and Roeder, 1972) showed increased activity to a level 70% greater than that seen in uninfected cells (Mahy *et al.*, 1974). The latter enhancement of polymerase II activity in isolated nuclei corresponded to the first of two distinct periods of increased RNA synthesis detected in infected cells at 90 minutes and 3 hours, respectively, by pulse labeling techniques. Only the first of these two peak activities was effected by α-amanitin introduced 1 hour before the pulse. Since this drug is known to block influenza replication (Rott and Scholtissek, 1970;

Mahy *et al.*, 1972) and since a requirement for functional DNA (see Chapter 8) is also recognized, these data lend support to the working hypothesis that one or more host mRNA species is needed for influenza replication early in the viral growth cycle.

A. Enzyme Activity of Different Cellular Fractions and Requirements of the *in Vitro* Assay System

The results of various investigations concerning the nature of viral-induced polymerase activity in influenza infected cells are in general agreement for several points. In most studies, the activity has been detected in microsomal fractions at 1 to 2 hours after infection (Ho and Walters, 1966; Scholtissek and Rott, 1969a; Skehel and Burke, 1969). Additionally, in all cases the enzyme function has shown to be RNA dependent, to possess an endogenous template (Schwarz and Scholtissek, 1973), and to be insensitive to the effects of exogenous RNA, deoxyribonuclease, or actinomycin D (Table 5.1) (Ho and Walters, 1966; Scholtissek and Rott, 1969a; Skehel and Burke, 1969). Virus-specific RNA polymerase activity associated with infected cells invariably has been detected in particulate cellular fractions inclusive of microsomal elements and nuclei, but not in the cell sap normally sequestered in the supernatant fraction of cell homogenates subjected to ultracentrifugation (Scholtissek and Rott, 1969a).

The common features of the *in vitro* polymerase reaction catalyzed by the cell-derived enzyme include a requirement for all four nucleoside triphosphates (Ruck *et al.*, 1969), a temperature optimum of about 28°C (Paffenholz and Scholtissek, 1973), and linear kinetics for at least the first 2 hours of incubation. It should be mentioned that while the *in vitro* reaction is best sustained for maximum periods at 28°C, incubation of these reaction mixtures at higher temperatures approaching the optimum for viral replication *in vivo* results in a higher initial rate of RNA synthesis but a concomitant and abrupt termination of the activity within 30 to 60 minutes (Paffenholz and Scholtissek, 1973). The latter effect may be related to the apparent instability of the enzyme–template complex at supraoptimal temperatures in *in vitro* reaction mixtures as discussed below for the virion-bound polymerase of influenza virus.

There is still considerable disagreement regarding the exact requirements of the *in vitro* reaction stimulated by either the cell- or virion-derived enzyme for various cations. The literature includes reports attesting to a need for both Mn^{2+} and Mg^{2+} ions or for only one of these cations. The disparity in this case has probably been accentuated by differences in the choice of

Table 5.1 The Effect of Various Inhibitors on Virus-Specific RNA Synthesis[a]

Drug	Inhibition of influenza replication	In vitro activity		In vivo activity	
		Cell-associated polymerase	Virion-associated polymerase	Total viral RNA synthesis	Primary transcription by the virion polymerase enzyme
Actinomycin D	+	−	−	+[b]	+
Cycloheximide	+	−	−	+[c]	−
α-Amanitin	+[d]	−	−	+[b]	−[e]

[a] +, inhibition; −, no inhibition.
[b] Preferential inhibition of complementary RNA synthesis (Scholtissek and Rott, 1970; Pons, 1973; Rott and Scholtissek, 1970).
[c] Preferential inhibition of virion RNA synthesis (Scholtissek and Rott, 1970; Pons, 1973).
[d] Inhibitory if added during the first 2 hours following infection (Rott and Scholtissek, 1970).
[e] Primary transcription inhibited only by pretreatment of cells with drug at high concentration (Bean, 1974).

cell–virus systems, the purification procedure employed, and the actual concentration of ions used in the final reaction mixture. Table 5.2 summarizes the various findings of investigations concerning ionic requirements of the cell-derived polymerase. Recently, a study conducted by Horrisberger and colleagues (Horrisberger and Guskey, 1974; Horrisberger and Schulze, 1975) demonstrated that an *in vitro* RNA polymerase function could be detected in the postmitochondrial supernatant fraction of lysates of cells infected with A_0/NWS virus using either Mn^{2+} or Mg^{2+} ions in the complete reaction mixture. The finding that addition of KCl to reaction mixtures stimulated the synthesis of RNA in the presence of Mn^{2+} but depressed this reaction when only Mg^{2+} ions were present has generated several interpretations, including the suggestion that two enzymes with different ionic requirements may function in this system (Horrisberger and Guskey, 1974). This conclusion was also bolstered by the observation that the activity in the presence of Mg^{2+} showed a higher initial rate, which became depressed within 20 minutes, whereas the reaction stimulated in the presence of Mn^{2+} alone was sustained for at least 2 hours. It is obvious that further work is required to substantiate the validity of a two-enzyme hypothesis.

B. Nature of the RNA Products Synthesized *in Vitro* by Polymerase-Containing Fractions of Infected Cells

As discussed in greater detail elsewhere (see Chapter 8), infection of permissive cells with myxoviruses results in the appearance of virion-specific RNA representing all of the genome size classes present in purified virus. Virion-type RNA is found associated with a major nucleoprotein (RNP) fraction in both the cytoplasm and the nucleoplasm, while viral complementary RNA is found in the cytoplasm as an RNP minor fraction (Pons, 1971; Krug, 1972) and appears to be at least the predominant species associated with polysomes (Pons, 1972; Nayak, 1970). A small amount of double-stranded RNA, also representing all size classes of the virion RNA, has been detected, but its exact role in influenza biosynthesis is uncertain (Pons, 1967; Pons and Hirst, 1968). By contrast with the *in vivo* system, the identity of RNA products generated *in vitro* by the cell-associated enzyme system is still open to question. Several laboratories (Ruck *et al.,* 1969; Skehel and Burke, 1969; Mahy and Bromley, 1969) have observed the appearance of a 10 S to 12 S ribonuclease-resistant RNA in reaction mixtures catalyzed by microsomal fractions of infected cells, which some workers contend does not represent a precursor of single-stranded species (Mahy and Bromley, 1969). Even less certainty surrounds the types of single-stranded RNA which may be made under these conditions. By base ratio analysis of the products

Table 5.2 Summary of Ionic Requirements for *in Vitro* RNA Synthesis of Influenza Virus

Original source of enzyme system	Material tested	Time of isolation (hours)	Assay temp. (°C)	Ions required for optimal activity	Reference
Infected cells[a]					
CAM infected with PR 8	Microsomes (P-78,000)[b]	3	37	Mg^{2+} (4 mM)	Ho and Walters, 1966
CAM from Inf. A2 infected eggs	Microsomes (P-78,000)	7	37	Mg^{2+} (8 mM)	Page et al., 1968; Ruck et al., 1969
CEF infected with FPV	Microsomes (P-100,000) and nuclei	3	37	Mg^{2+} (4 mM)	Scholtissek and Rott, 1969a
CEF infected with FPV	Cytoplasmic extract (S-600)[c]	6	37	Mn^{2+} (4.5 mM) or Mg^{2+} (3 mM)	Skehel and Burke, 1968, 1969
	Microsomes (P-130,000)	6	37	Mn^{2+} (3 mM) or Mg^{2+} (1.5 mM)	
	nuclei	6	37	Mn^{2+} or Mg^{2+}	
CEF infected with FPV	Microsomes (P-105,000)	6	28	Mg^{2+} (2.5 mM)	Mahy and Bromley, 1969, 1970
CEF infected with FPV	Microsomes (P-105,000) and nuclei	6	28	Mg^{2+} (10 mM)	Hastie and Mahy, 1973
MDBK or BHK cells infected with WSN	Purified ribonucleoprotein	4	33	Mn^{2+} (1 mM) and Mg^{2+} (10 mM)	Compans and Caliguri, 1973
Virions					
Purified WSN grown in CEF	Whole virus		37	Mn^{2+} (1.9 mM)	Chow and Simpson, 1971
Purified NWS grown in eggs	Whole virus		37	Mn^{2+} (4 mM)	Penhoet et al., 1971
Purified FPV grown in CEF	Whole virus		37	Mn^{2+} (3 mM) or Mg^{2+} (1.5 mM)	Skehel, 1971
Purified WSN grown in CEF	Whole virus		31	Mn^{2+} (1 mM) and Mg^{2+} (10 mM)	Bishop et al., 1971a
Purified WSN grown in CEF	Whole virus		31	Mn^{2+} (2 mM)	O. Rochovansky (personal communication)
	Isolated ribonucleoprotein		31	Mn^{2+} (2 mM) or Mg^{2+} (10 mM)	

[a] CAM, chorioallantoic membrane; CEF, chick embryo fibroblast; FPV, fowl plague virus.
[b] P-78,000, pellet produced by centrifugation of postmitochondrial supernatant at 78,000 g.
[c] S-600, supernatant obtained following centrifugation at 600 g.

made using microsomes of chorioallantoic membranes from infected eggs (A_2/Leningrad/62 [H2N2] virus), Ruck *et al.* (1969) showed that the RNA made *in vitro* had a base composition similar to that of the virion RNA. However, Scholtissek (1969) demonstrated that 85 to 100% of *in vitro* product made in a system utilizing microsomal fractions obtained at 6 hours from fowl plague infected chick embryo cells would specifically hybridize with the homologous virion RNA. By monitoring the same virus–host cell system at both early and late times during infection, Hastie and Mahy (1973) were able to demonstrate an *in vitro* microsomal RNA polymerase product consisting of 67 to 93% complementary RNA depending on the time of cell extraction. These workers have also clearly shown by appropriate hybridization techniques that purified nuclei from these cells synthesize both viral RNA and its complement *in vitro* in approximately equal amounts. This nuclear polymerase activity appeared earlier than that seen in cytoplasmic fractions. Such findings suggest that the reported inconsistencies concerning the various classes of single-stranded RNA species made *in vitro* by enzyme produced in cells in response to infection with influenza virus may relate to both the time that cells were monitored for this activity and the type of cellular fraction examined.

III. Virion-Associated RNA Polymerase Activity

The report of an RNA-dependent RNA polymerase activity in purified particles of reovirus (Shatkin and Sipe, 1968; Borsa and Graham, 1968) was followed by the demonstration of virion-bound transcriptase in rhabdoviruses (Baltimore *et al.*, 1970), RNA tumor viruses (Temin and Mitzutani, 1970; Baltimore, 1970), and paramyxoviruses (Huang *et al.*, 1971). Initial efforts to find such enzyme activity in particles of WSN influenza virus in our own laboratory met with failure owing to the special ionic requirements of the *in vitro* assay system. With the introduction of Mn^{2+} ions in reaction mixtures, it was possible for us to demonstrate positive RNA polymerase activity in several influenza strains (Chow and Simpson, 1971), an observation which was soon confirmed in other laboratories (Penhoet *et al.*, 1971; Skehel, 1971). By comparison with other viruses possessing a virion RNA polymerase, the transcriptase of influenza virus is about 750 times less active than the enzyme found in reovirus and about $\frac{1}{25}$ as active as vesicular stomatitis virus (VSV) (see Table 5.3). However, influenza A_0/WS strain is about four times more active than Newcastle disease virus and at least 20-fold more active than the reported values for Sendai virus. Reovirus remains the most active of all animal viruses with virion-bound transcriptases

Table 5.3 Comparison of Influenza Virus with Other Animal Viruses for *in Vitro* RNA-Dependent RNA Polymerase Activity of Free Virions

Virus	Approximate rate of *in vitro* RNA synthesis[a]	Requirements and special features	Reference
Myxoviruses			
Strain WS	1,000	Essential requirement	Chow and Simpson, 1971;
Strain WSN	500	for Mn^{2+}; activity unstable at 37°C	Bishop *et al.*, 1971a, 1972; Bean, 1974
Rhabdoviruses			
VSV	25,000	Requires Mg^{2+}; inhibited by Mn^{2+}; repetitive initiation	Baltimore *et al.*, 1970; Roy and Bishop, 1972; Chow and Simpson, 1971; Aaslestad *et al.*, 1971
Kern Canyon virus	1,000	Like VSV	
Paramyxoviruses			
Newcastle disease virus	250	Requires Mg^{2+}	Huang *et al.*, 1971; Robinson, 1971; Stone *et al.*, 1971; Stone and Kingsbury, 1973
Sendai virus	50[b]	Requires Mg^{2+}; activity increases with time of incubation; stimulated by polyanions	
Reovirus			
Type 3	750,000	Requires removal of outer capsid or heat shock; very stable activity; all genome segments transcribed	Shatkin and Sipe, 1968; Borsa and Graham, 1968; Skehel and Joklik, 1968

[a] Rate of reaction expressed in picomoles of labeled nucleotide incorporated per mg viral protein per hour.
[b] Rate reported by Stone *et al.* (1971) after 3 hours of incubation.

with respect both to the rate of its RNA polymerase activity and its capacity for sustained transcription in an *in vitro* system (Skehel and Joklik, 1968).

A. Characterization of the *in Vitro* System

The composition of the complete reaction mixture necessary for the detection of *in vitro* RNA polymerase activity in influenza virions is basically similar to that used for transcriptase assay of other enveloped animal viruses and includes purified virions, all four nucleoside triphosphates, an appropriate detergent presumably needed to render the polymerase-ribonucleoprotein complex accessible, monovalent ions, and divalent cations under the conditions discussed below. Unlike the optimum temperature for growth of virus in cells (Scholtissek and Rott, 1969b), the influenza polymerase functions most efficiently for sustained RNA synthesis in *in vitro* reaction mixtures incubated at 31°–33°C (Bishop *et al.*, 1971a), a phenomenon which is probably related to the inherent instability of the polymerase–template complex at higher temperatures in the *in vitro* system.

The effect of cations on the *in vitro* synthesis of RNA products by the influenza virion transcriptase has been of special interest to several investigators. In the initial studies of this enzyme activity, an obligate requirement for Mn^{2+} ions was reported by two groups (Chow and Simpson, 1971; Penhoet *et al.*, 1971), who described a minimal need of 1.9 and 4 mM, respectively. In reaction mixtures in which Mn^{2+} ions are replaced by Mg^{2+}, RNA synthesis proceeds at a greatly reduced level (Chow and Simpson, 1971; Skehel, 1971), while Mg^{2+} ions can serve to augment enzyme activity in reactions containing suboptimal concentrations of Mn^{2+} (Bishop *et al.*, 1971a). It appears, therefore, that Mn^{2+} is an essential divalent cation for *in vitro* function of the influenza virion polymerase.

In addition to the effect of omission of essential ingredients from reaction mixtures, *in vitro* transcriptase activity of influenza particles is inhibited by ribonuclease and polyanions (Chow and Simpson, 1971). No inhibition is observed in this system in the presence of actinomycin D, rifamipicin, α-amanitin, or deoxyribonuclease (Chow and Simpson, 1971; Penhoet *et al.*, 1971; Skehel, 1971). As will be noted below, however, actinomycin D does appear to block early transcription in infected cells mediated by the virion-bound enzyme (see Table 5.1). Oxford and colleagues have demonstrated an inhibition of the influenza transcriptase in *in vitro* reactions by selenocystamine, phenenthrolene derivatives, and thiosemicarbazones, all compounds which are strong chealators of "soft" heavy metals such as zinc (Oxford, 1973a; Oxford and Perrin, 1974). The inhibition of the cell-associated viral enzyme by selenocystine had been previously described (Ho *et al.*, 1968; Ho and Walters, 1971). That the virion-associated enzyme may actually be a zinc metalloenzyme as are the cellular RNA or DNA polymerases of *Escherichia coli* (Scrutton *et al.*, 1971; Slater *et al.*, 1971) is suggested by the finding of zinc in purified influenza particles using atomic absorption and atomic mass spectrometry (Oxford and Perrin, 1975). It also is significant to note in this connection that zinc has recently been reported to be present in the virion RNA-dependent DNA polymerase of oncornaviruses (Auld *et al.*, 1974). Stimulation of the *in vitro* RNA synthesis catalyzed by the virion polymerase has recently been found to occur in the presence of cell-derived host factors (O. Rochovansky, personal communication). One of these factors has tentatively been identified as inorganic pyrophosphatase, since the purified enzyme gives about a twofold stimulation of RNA influenza polymerase activity as do extracts of normal chick embryo cells and can negate the inhibitory effect of exogenous pyrophosphate added to reaction mixtures. The identity of another host factor which appears to enhance *in vitro* transcription is still under study.

B. Reaction Products of the Virion RNA Polymerase

The *in vitro* reaction catalyzed by influenza particles is initially linear and is proportional to the amount of viral protein used in test mixtures. When the RNA synthesized under these conditions is phenol extracted and tested for degradation by a mixture of ribonuclease A and T_1, 60–80% of the product exhibits ribonuclease resistance (Bishop *et al.*, 1971b). Most of the remaining ribonuclease-sensitive product made can be converted into a nuclease-resistant form by annealing the RNA in the complete test mixture. Analysis of this product by polyacrylamide gel electrophoresis using differentially radiolabeled template and product precursor reveals the early appearance of RNA molecules comigrating with the virion template RNA inclusive of all its size classes as well as a somewhat larger species (Bishop *et al.*, 1971b.) These reaction products can be converted to a more rapidly migrating form with a molecular weight ranging between 5×10^4 to 3×10^5 daltons when the product RNA is melted at 100°C. The general conclusion that can be drawn from these studies regarding the RNA synthesized by the influenza virion transcriptase is that the bulk of the product made *in vitro* is complementary RNA, apparently linked by hydrogen bonds to the template RNA to form multistranded complexes of an obscure nature. There is no evidence for the rapid displacement of low molecular weight complementary strands from these complexes during the transcription process as is the case with rhabdoviruses such as VSV (Bishop and Roy, 1971).

The initiation sequence of the *in vitro* RNA polymerase product has been determined by Hefti *et al.* (1975). These workers isolated the ribonucleoprotein component from WSN influenza virions and labeled the 5′-termini of the transcriptase product generated *in vitro* with γ-labeled nucleoside triphosphates. Only one major initiation sequence, pppGpCp, was found. While the authors concluded that transcription may be initiated by this one unique sequence, they were unable to ascertain whether every segment of the fragmented influenza genome is actually transcribed in this system. Recently, McGeoch and Kitron (1975) reported that the addition of guanosine to influenza polymerase reactions stimulated the synthesis of viral complementary RNA. Under their test conditions, guanosine was incorporated at the 5′-terminus in the sequence GpCp. Stimulation of the virion transcriptase was also obtained with guanosine 5′–monophosphate and the dinucleotides GpC and GpG.

C. Virion Transcriptase Activity of Different Virus Strains

The first report of an RNA polymerase associated with influenza virus particles included observations for strain variation for *in vitro* transcriptase activity among human and nonhuman myxoviruses (Chow and Simpson, 1971). Subsequent work carried out in this laboratory (Bean, 1974) on this particular problem has revealed that the apparent difference in transcriptase activity of certain influenza prototypes is strongly influenced by the relative sensitivity of the reaction to the incubation temperature employed. Figure 5.1 illustrates the kinetics for the *in vitro* reaction of influenza WS and its derivative strain, WSN, showing that these viruses can be differentiated for their initial reaction rates at either optimal (32°C) or supraoptimal (37°C) temperatures. With WS virus, the initial rate of synthesis is always higher at 37°C than at 32°C while the opposite is true for WSN. When specific recombinants of the WS and WSN strains are examined for their virion RNA polymerase activity, it is observed that the overall rate of reaction and the relative rates at the two assay temperatures assort as independent

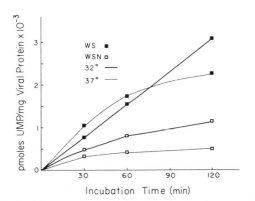

Fig. 5.1. *In vitro* RNA synthesis by the virion transcriptase of influenza WS and WSN in reaction mixtures incubated at 32° and 37°C. Standard influenza polymerase reaction mixtures (Bishop *et al.*, 1971a) containing either purified WS or WSN virus were incubated at the temperatures indicated and assayed for acid-precipitable radioactivity at different times.

properties among progeny found to be hybrid for other genetic markers. It is not known whether these *in vitro* reaction properties reflect the relative physical stability of the transcribing complex or one of its specific components such as the RNA polymerase.

Conditional lethal temperature-sensitive (ts) mutants of the WSN strain representing members of seven distinct recombination–complementation groups (Hirst, 1973) were recently examined in this laboratory for their virion polymerase activity *in vitro*. All of these viruses showed a diminished enzyme function by comparison with the wild-type while one of these mutants (WSN ts 24) showed only 5% or less of WSN activity. We have been unable to correlate aberrant transcriptase activity of such mutants with their specific temperature-sensitive defect(s). When five complementation tester strains of fowl plague virus were analyzed for their virion-associated transcriptase activity in reaction mixtures maintained at the permissive and nonpermissive viral growth temperatures of 36° and 42°C, respectively, one mutant exhibited a 71% reduction of enzyme activity while the other viruses and their wild-type progenitor were reduced in their activity by 8–20% at the higher temperature employed (Ghendon *et al.*, 1973). None of these fowl plague mutants was found to possess a virion-bound polymerase, which was nonfunctional in cells incubated at temperatures restrictive for viral replication (but see Chapter 7). However, Scholtissek *et al.* (1974) have recently described a ts mutant of fowl plague virus which fails to induce detectable virus-specific RNA synthesis in cells incubated at nonpermissive temperature, despite the fact that a microsomal RNA polymerase activity could be demonstrated in extracts of these cells in *in vitro* reaction mixtures held at the restrictive viral growth temperature of 40°C. These workers were unable to explain the reason for this apparent discrepancy concerning the functional efficiency of the influenza RNA polymerase in the two systems.

Evidence for the distinctiveness of the influenza RNA-dependent RNA polymerases of heterologous influenza serotypes is found in the report of Scholtissek and colleagues (1971), which indicated that convalescent serum from chickens infected with fowl plague virus would inhibit the *in vitro* function of the microsomal RNA polymerase activity from cells infected with either homologous virus or heterologous type A myxoviruses but not type B influenza or the paramyxovirus NDV. These data were offered as further evidence that the influenza RNA polymerase enzyme is at least partially coded for by the viral genome. While most of the studies conducted thus far on the influenza virion transcriptase have concerned type A prototypes, Oxford (1973b) has recently conducted an investigation of two influenza B strains which has shown that these viruses can also be distinguished according to reproducible differences in their respective *in vitro* RNA polymerase activity.

D. *In Vitro* RNA Polymerase Activity of Incomplete Virus and Subviral Components

Previous studies in other laboratories have demonstrated that incomplete or defective particles of influenza virus (von Magnus type) generated by serial high multiplicity passage in an appropriate host are deficient for their content of virion RNA and their infectivity (von Magnus, 1954; Ada and Perry, 1956; Pons and Hirst, 1969; Duesberg, 1968). We have recently examined the RNA polymerase activity of von Magnus preparations of influenza virus (Bean, 1974; Bean and Simpson, 1975) considering the fact that incomplete T particles of certain rhabdoviruses were previously shown to be devoid of normal transcriptase activity (Roy and Bishop, 1972; Reichman *et al.*, 1974). We have found that incomplete preparations of influenza A virus (WS or WSN strains), which exhibited a 10,000-fold reduction of normal infectivity levels and which are deficient for the high molecular weight class of virion RNA as described earlier (Pons and Hirst, 1969; Duesberg, 1968), showed at most about a twofold reduction in their *in vitro* transcriptase activity. Since it has been previously reported that each size class of virion-derived nucleoprotein has a detectable RNA polymerase activity (Bishop *et al.*, 1972), one would expect that incomplete particles of influenza virus would still be capable of catalyzing *in vitro* transcriptase reactions despite their other deficiencies. It is interesting to note, in this respect, that one can obtain defective preparations of influenza virus which show an apparently normal RNA complement but a 20-fold reduction of infectivity (Pons and Hirst, 1969). In this laboratory, we have found that neither the maximum reduction of the largest virion RNA species (i.e., about two-thirds) nor the moderate loss of virion-associated RNA polymerase activity appear to account sufficiently for the much greater decrease in infectivity of these incomplete virus populations. Collectively, these observations suggest that other unrecognized factors are responsible for the impaired infectivity of such influenza preparations.

E. Identity of Viral Polypeptide Responsible for Transcriptase Activity

Two basic questions that remain unanswered at this time concern the identification of the structural polypeptide(s) responsible for the virion transcriptase activity of influenza virus and the exact relationship of such polypeptide(s) to the cell-associated enzyme. The protein composition of transcriptase-positive ribonucleoprotein fractions obtained from dissociated influenza WS particles has included predominantly the NP protein (MW, about 55,000) and a trace of the large P polypeptides (MW about 90,000)

(Bishop *et al.*, 1972). Recent examination of ribonucleoprotein derived from the WSN strain has confirmed this initial observation and further shown that both the P1 and P2 components of the large molecular weight structural proteins are associated with transcriptase active material (O. Rochovansky, personal communication). The recent finding that polymerase-active nucleocapsid components of identical morphological appearance and buoyant density can be isolated from either purified influenza particles or the microsomal fraction of infected cells provides strong suggestive evidence that the latter cell-associated structures physically correspond to the transcribing complex found in intact virions (Compans and Caliguiri, 1973). Although it was initially reported that viral nucleocapsid components with transcriptase activity from influenza-infected cells contain only NP protein (Compans and Caliguiri, 1973), the same investigators have since found P polypeptide in these fractions by use of appropriate radiolabeling techniques necessary for detecting this protein, which appears to be made very early in the infectious cycle (Caliguiri and Compans, 1974). Thus far, all attempts to separate the microsomal polymerase from its internal template and to obtain an enzyme functionally dependent upon the addition of exogenous RNA have failed (Schwarz and Scholtissek, 1973). The failure of such attempts, thus far, to isolate a free enzymatically active polymerase could result from irreversible damage to the viral enzyme itself or an absolute requirement for the presence of an intact ribonucleoprotein as the functional template. Similarly, methods which have been successfully applied to dissociate and reconstitute the virion transcriptase activity from the nucleoprotein of rhabdoviruses (Bishop *et al.*, 1974) have not been successful when tested with purified influenza virus (D. H. L. Bishop, personal communication). In the final analysis, the identification of the virion- and cell-associated RNA polymerases of influenza virus and their attendant template requirements must await the successful outcome of further efforts to isolate these enzymes in a functionally active form.

F. Kinetics of Influenza Transcription in Infected Cells

Both the noninfectious nature of the influenza genome and the presence of a virion-associated RNA polymerase in myxoviruses are the same findings in keeping with the concept that the initial event in influenza infected cells involves transcription of the viral template RNA into a complementary form (Baltimore, 1971). In our laboratory we studied these early events in infected cells to determine whether *in vivo* transcription of the virion RNA resembles that observed in the *in vitro* systems discussed above for such things as reaction kinetics and sensitivity to various inhibitors.

As reported recently (Bean and Simpson, 1973), it is possible to follow the conversion of ^{32}P-labeled viral template RNA into ribonuclease-resistant complexes formed by hybridization with newly synthesized complementary RNA strands present in annealing mixtures of the total RNA extracted at different times from cells infected with radiolabeled influenza virus. This technique is useful for monitoring the production of complementary RNA in cells until such time during infection that sufficient amounts of newly synthesized virion RNA are made to compete with the labeled input RNA in annealing mixtures. Figure 5.2 illustrates the kinetics of *in vivo* complementary RNA synthesis as measured by this method. The principal feature of *in vivo* transcription is its biphasic nature. Transcription, first detectable at 40–60 minutes, proceeds linearly until about 90 minutes, after which it becomes greatly amplified. The effect of the drugs actinomycin D and cycloheximide on *in vivo* transcription are of interest in light of their differential inhibition of complementary RNA and viral RNA synthesis, respectively (Scholtissek and Rott, 1970; Pons, 1973). Actinomycin added at the time of infection completely blocks *in vivo* transcription, while cycloheximide does not prevent initial (primary) transcription from occurring but prevents its subsequent amplification (Fig. 5.2). When the *in vivo* transcription process is followed over a longer time course as illustrated in Fig. 5.3, the level

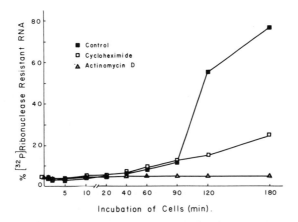

Fig. 5.2. Measurement of *in vivo* transcription of the influenza genome in chick embryo cells by a template labeling technique. Cell-associated RNA synthesis of WSN influenza was monitored by following the conversion of ^{32}P-labeled virion RNA into a ribonuclease-resistant form after annealing total RNA extracted from infected cells after incubation at 37°C (see Bean and Simpson, 1973). In two of the groups represented, cells were pretreated with either actinomycin D (5 μg/ml) or cycloheximide (20 μg/ml) 20 minutes before infection with radiolabeled virus.

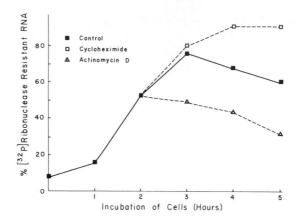

Fig. 5.3. Effect of delayed addition of actinomycin D or cycloheximide on *in vivo* RNA synthesis induced in cells by influenza virus. Primary CEF cultures were infected with ^{32}P-labeled WSN virus and incubated over a 5 hour period at 37°C. Either actinomycin D (5 μg/ml) or cycloheximide (100 μg/ml) were added to infected cultures at 2 hours and incubation was continued. The ribonuclease-resistant fraction of the labeled RNA extracted from cells at the times indicated was determined after annealing as shown for Fig. 5.2.

of detectable ribonuclease-resistant RNA is seen to decline after 3 hours, an event which we have ascribed to the appearance of competing virion-type RNA in the infected cell (Bean and Simpson, 1973). If, however, cycloheximide is added to cells after the onset of amplified transcription, this decline does not occur, presumably because of the selective inhibition of virion RNA synthesis by this drug (Scholtissek and Rott, 1970; Pons, 1973). Conversely, the delayed addition of actinomycin D 2 hours after infection results in an abrupt drop in the level of ribonuclease-resistant RNA detectable after annealing of total cell RNA. A reasonable explanation for this effect is that actinomycin D preferentially inhibits complementary RNA synthesis but allows additional viral RNA to be made which competes with labeled template RNA during annealing, a conclusion previously offered by other workers (Scholtissek and Rott, 1970; Pons, 1973). Additional studies recently cordycepin, α-amanitin, mitomycin C, interferon, or ultraviolet light (Bean on the *in vivo* transcription process. We can also report that influenza virus transcription is inhibited *in vivo* by pretreatment of chick embryo cells with cordycepin, α-amanitin, mitomycin C, interferon, or ultraviolet light (Bean and Simpson, 1973; Bean, 1974). The apparent need for an endogenous functional host DNA for initiation of influenza transcription in permissive cells is reflected by the dose-dependent inhibition of *in vivo* transcription in cells exposed to ultraviolet radiation prior to infection.

IV. Conclusions and Remarks

The studies cited in this chapter provide a useful foundation for future work on the RNA-dependent RNA polymerases of myxoviruses and their role in the infectious process. Whether the complementary RNA species synthesized by these enzymes play a direct role in viral protein synthesis is still open to question (Seigert *et al.,* 1973; Kingsbury and Webster, 1973) and needs clarification. Similarly, the chemical identity of the influenza transcriptase is unknown at this time, and valiant efforts should be made to isolate this enzyme in a functional form in order to allow its full characterization. Perhaps the most perplexing question that remains to be answered concerns the role of the host cell in the initiation and maintenance of viral RNA synthesis. Although actinomycin D has no apparent effect on the *in vitro* activities of the virion- or cell-associated polymerases, this drug, as well as ultraviolet light and other inhibitors of cell DNA function, block transcription *in vivo*. These findings, and the failure to detect any viral products in infected enucleated cells (Follet *et al.,* 1974; Kelley *et al.,* 1974), indicate that influenza transcription requires a nuclear function. However, the detection of *in vivo* primary transcription in the presence of cycloheximide further indicates that transcription does not require the translation of a newly synthesized mRNA. At present, no entirely satisfactory hypothesis has been proposed that will help to reconcile these puzzling data. With more investigators pursuing such intriguing problems, hopefully, we may gain clearer understanding of how influenza transcription is regulated by host and viral factors. Such knowledge may better equip us for devising effective chemotherapeutic approaches to the control of human and animal myxovirus infections.

Acknowledgments

Work described in this chapter which was conducted in the authors' laboratory was supported by funds from Research Grant AI-09124 from the National Institute of Allergy and Infectious Diseases, United States Public Health Service.

References

Aaslestad, H. G., Clark, H. F., Bishop, D. H. L., and Koprowski, H. (1971). *J. Virol.* **7,** 726.
Ada, G. L., and Perry, B. T. (1956). *J. Gen. Microbiol.* **14,** 623.
Auld, D. S., Kawaguchi, D. M., Livingston, D. M., and Vallee, B. L. (1974). *Proc. Nat. Acad. Sci. U.S.* **71,** 2091.
Baltimore, D. (1970). *Nature (London)* **226,** 1209.

Baltimore, D. (1971). *Bacteriol. Rev.* **35**, 235.

Baltimore, D., Huang, A. S., and Stampfer, M. (1970). *Proc. Nat. Acad. Sci. U.S.* **66**, 572.

Barry, R. D., and Mahy, B. W. J., eds. (1975). "Negative Strand Viruses." Academic Press, New York.

Bean, W. J., Jr. (1974). Doctoral Dissertation, Rutgers, The State University of New Jersey, New Brunswick.

Bean, W. J., Jr., and Simpson, R. W. (1973). *Virology* **56**, 646.

Bean, W. J., Jr., and Simpson, R. W. (1975). *J. Virol.* Submitted for publication.

Bishop, D. H. L., and Roy, P. (1971). *J. Mol. Biol.* **57**, 513.

Bishop, D. H. L., Obijeski, J. F., and Simpson, R. W. (1971a). *J. Virol.* **8**, 66.

Bishop, D. H. L., Obijeski, J. F., and Simpson, R. W. (1971b). *J. Virol.* **8**, 74.

Bishop, D. H. L., Roy, P., Bean, W. J., Jr., and Simpson, R. W. (1972). *J. Virol.* **10**, 689.

Bishop, D. H. L., Emerson, S. U. and Flamand, A. (1974). *J. Virol.* **14**, 139.

Borland, R., and Mahy, B. W. J. (1968). *J. Virol.* **2**, 33.

Borsa, J., and Graham, A. F. (1968). *Biochem. Biophys. Res. Commun.* **33**, 895.

Caliguiri, L. A., and Compans, R. W. (1974). *J. Virol.* **14**, 191.

Chow, N.-L., and Simpson, R. W. (1971). *Proc. Nat. Acad. Sci. U.S.* **68**, 752.

Compans, R. W., and Caliguiri, L. A. (1973). *J. Virol.* **11**, 441.

Duesberg, P. H. (1968). *Proc. Nat. Acad. Sci. U.S.* **59**, 930.

Follett, E. A. C., Pringle, C. R., Wunner, W. H., and Skehel, J. J. (1974). *J. Virol.* **13**, 394.

Ghendon, Y. Z., Markushin, S. G., Marchenko, A. T., Sitnikov, B. S., and Ginsburg, V. P. (1973). *Virology* **55**, 305.

Hastie, N. D., and Mahy, B. W. J. (1973). *J. Virol.* **12**, 951.

Hefti, E., Roy, P., and Bishop, D. H. L. (1975). *In* "The Negative Strand Viruses" (R. D. Barry and B. W. J. Mahy, eds.), pp. 307–326. Academic Press, New York.

Hirst, G. K. (1973). *Virology* **55**, 81.

Ho, P. P. K., and Walters, C. P. (1966). *Biochemistry* **5**, 231.

Ho, P. P. K., and Walters, C. P. (1971). *Ann. N.Y. Acad. Sci.* **173**, 438.

Ho, P. P. K., Walters, C. P., Streightoff, F. Baker, L. A., and De Long, D. C. (1968). *Antimicrob. Ag. Chemother.* pp. 636–641.

Horrisberger, M., and Guskey, L. E. (1974). *J. Virol.* **13**, 230.

Horrisberger, M., and Schulze, C. (1974). *Arch. Gesamte Virsuforsch.* **46**, 148.

Huang, A. S., Baltimore, D., and Bratt, M. A. (1971). *J. Virol.* **7**, 389.

Kelley, D. C., Avery, R. J., and Dimmock, N. J. (1974). *J. Virol.* **13**, 1155.

Kingsbury, D. W., and Webster, R. G. (1973). *Virology* **56**, 654.

Krug, R. M. (1972). *Virology* **50**, 125.

McGeoch, D., and Kitron, N. (1975). *J. Virol.* **15**, 686.

Mahy, B. W. J. (1970). *In* "The Biology of Large RNA Viruses" (R. D. Barry and B. W. J. Mahy, eds.), pp. 392–415. Academic Press, New York.

Mahy, B. W. J., and Bromley, P. A. (1969). *Biochem. J.* **114**, 64P.

Mahy, B. W. J., and Bromley, P. A. (1970). *J. Virol.* **6**, 259.

Mahy, B. W. J., Hastie, N. D., and Armstrong, S. J. (1972). *Proc. Nat. Acad. Sci. U.S.* **69**, 1421.

Mahy, B. W. J., Brownson, J. M. T., Carroll, A. R., Hastie, N. D., and Raper, R. H. (1974). *In* "Negative Strand Viruses" (R. D. Barry and B. W. J. Mahy, eds.), pp. 445–467. Academic Press, New York.

Nayak, D. P. (1970). *In* "The Biology of Large RNA Viruses (R. D. Barry and B. W. J. Mahy, eds.), pp. 371–391. Academic Press, New York.

Oxford, J. S. (1973a). *J. Gen. Virol.* **18,** 11.

Oxford, J. S. (1973b). *J. Virol.* **12,** 827.

Oxford, J. S., and Perrin, D. D. (1974). *J. Gen. Virol.* **23,** 59.

Oxford, J. S., and Perrin, D. D. (1975). *In* "Negative Strand Viruses" (R. D. Barry and B. W. J. Mahy, eds.). Academic Press, New York.

Paffenholz, V., and Scholtissek, C. (1973). *Z. Naturforsch. B* **28,** 208.

Page, M. G., Ruck, B. J., and Brammer, K. W. (1968). *Biochem. J.* **109,** 43P.

Penhoet, E., Miller, H., Doyle, H., and Blatti, S. (1971). *Proc. Nat. Acad. Sci. U.S.* **68,** 1369.

Pons, M. W. (1967). *Arch. Gesamte Virusforsch.* **22,** 203.

Pons, M. W. (1971). *Virology* **46,** 149.

Pons, M. W. (1972). *Virology* **47,** 823.

Pons, M. W. (1973). *Virology* **51,** 120.

Pons, M. W., and Hirst, G. K. (1968). *Virology* **35,** 182.

Pons, M. W., and Hirst, G. K. (1969). *Virology* **38,** 68.

Reeder, R. H., and Roeder, R. G. (1972). *J. Mol. Biol.* **67,** 433.

Reichmann, M. E., Villarreal, L. P., Kohne, D., Lesnaw, J., and Holland, J. J. (1974). *Virology* **58,** 240.

Robinson, W. D. (1971). *J. Virol.* **8,** 81.

Roeder, R. G., and Rutter, W. J. (1970). *Proc. Nat. Acad. Sci. U.S.* **65,** 675.

Rott, R., and Scholtissek, C. (1970). *Nature (London)* **228,** 56.

Roy, P., and Bishop, D. H. L. (1972). *J. Virol.* **9,** 946.

Ruck, B. J., Brammer, K. W., Page, M. G., and Coombes, J. D. (1969). *Virology* **39,** 31.

Scholtissek, C. (1969). *Biochim. Biophys. Acta* **179,** 389.

Scholtissek, C., and Rott, R. (1969a). *J. Gen. Virol.* **4,** 125.

Scholtissek, C., and Rott, R. (1969b). *J. Gen. Virol.* **5,** 283.

Scholtissek, C., and Rott, R. (1970). *Virology* **40,** 989.

Scholtissek, C., Becht, H., and Rott, R. (1971). *Virology* **43,** 137.

Scholtissek, C., Kruczinna, R., Rott, R., and Klenk, H. D. (1974). *Virology* **58,** 317.

Schwarz, R. T., and Scholtissek, C. (1973). *Z. Naturforsch. B* **28,** 202.

Scrutton, M. C., Wu, C. W., and Goldthwait, D. A. (1971). *Proc. Nat. Acad. Sci. U.S.* **68,** 2497.

Seigert, W., Bauer, G., and Hofschneider, P. H. (1973). *Proc. Nat. Acad. Sci. U.S.* **70,** 2960.

Shatkin, A. J., and Sipe, J. P. (1968). *Proc. Nat. Acad. Sci. U.S.* **61,** 1462.

Skehel, J. J. (1971). *Virology* **45,** 793.

Skehel, J. J., and Burke, D. C. (1968). *Biochem. J.* **110,** 41P.

Skehel, J. J., and Burke, D. C. (1969). *J. Virol.* **3,** 429.

Skehel, J. J., and Joklik, W. K. (1968). *Virology* **39,** 822.

Slater, J. P., Mildvan, A. S., and Loeb, L. A. (1971). *Biochem. Biophys. Res. Commun.* **44,** 37.

Stone, H. O., and Kingsbury, D. W. (1973). *J. Virol.* **11,** 243.

Stone, H. O., Portner, A., and Kingsbury, D. W. (1971). *J. Virol.* **8,** 174.

Temin, H. M., and Mitzutani, S. (1970). *Nature (London)* **226,** 1211.

von Magnus, P. (1954). *Advan. Virus Res.* **2,** 59.

Zylber, E. A., and Penman, S. (1971). *Proc. Nat. Acad. Sci. U.S.* **68,** 2861.

6

Influenza Virus RNA(s)

Marcel W. Pons

I. Introduction

Influenza virus has a unique spectrum of biological activities among animal viruses, such as multiplicity reactivation (Henle and Liu, 1951), incomplete virus formation (von Magnus, 1954), sensitivity to actinomycin D (Barry *et al.*, 1962), a noninfectious nucleic acid, and high rates of genetic recombination (Simpson and Hirst, 1961; Hirst, 1962). This last property led to the proposal that the influenza genome consisted of two or more single-stranded ribonucleic acid (RNA) segments rather than one continuous chain of covalently linked nucleotides (Burnet, 1956; Hirst, 1962). The hypothesis was subsequently confirmed by biochemical analysis of RNA extracted from virions (Duesberg, 1968; Pons and Hirst, 1968a), and its biological validity was reinforced by the subsequent finding that the intracellular replicative form of the virion RNA also existed in similar segments (Pons and Hirst, 1968b).

The RNA of influenza virus comprises 0.8–1.1% of the dry weight of the particle (Ada and Perry, 1954; Frisch-Niggemeyer and Hoyle, 1956; Frommhagen *et al.,* 1959). Chemical analysis of RNA obtained from purified virions led to an estimate of 2×10^6 to 3×10^6 daltons of RNA per virion (Ada and Perry, 1954; Frisch-Niggemeyer and Hoyle, 1956), but these values were undoubtedly too low. Although reasonably close to the currently accepted values of 4.5×10^6 to 5×10^6 daltons RNA per virion, the small amount of RNA in each virion and/or the presence of incomplete virus in the preparations may have led to underestimates of the amount of RNA present per virion (see Section III,B).

II. Methods

A. Growth and Purification of Influenza Virus

There exist several different methods for the purification of influenza virus. Presented here is the one currently in use in our laboratory and, with minor modifications, in several other laboratories. This procedure has the advantage of serving equally well for purifying virus grown in embryonated eggs or in tissue cultures of chick embryo fibroblast (CEF) monolayers. In addition, this method yields virus of high purity, a 40% recovery of the starting virus, and very little loss in infectivity or hemagglutinating activity (HA). There are other methods of purification, such as those which utilize an ammonium sulfate precipitation step which also yields virus of high purity, although the high salt concentration has an adverse effect on the infectivity of the virus. It should be pointed out here that, in general, all manipulations of the virus are conducted in such a way as to minimize inactivation of virus infectivity.

The majority of the biochemical work done on influenza virus in the United States has been done with the WSN strain. In Europe, much of the work has been done with fowl plague virus, another type A influenza strain. The differences between these two strains, as far as their nucleic acid and its replication are concerned, are probably minimal.

The WSN strain of influenza virus is usually grown in primary chick embryo fibroblast (CEF) monolayers. In order to prepare large amounts of virus [of the order of 5×10^{10} to 10×10^{10} plaque forming units (PFU)], 40 to 80 confluent CEF monolayers are inoculated with virus at a multiplicity of infection of approximately 5×10^{-5} PFU/cell. The monolayers are incubated at 37°C for 40 hours in a 5% CO_2 atmosphere (Simpson and Hirst, 1961) and the virus purified from the supernatant fluids, as described below. In order to prepare radioactively labeled virus, the appropriate isotopes, usually [^{3}H]5-uridine (2–5 μCi/ml) or [^{3}H]- or [^{14}C] amino acids (2–5 μCi/ml) are added just prior to incubation at 37°C.

To purify the virus, the supernatant fluids are first centrifuged at low speed to remove cells and large particles of cellular debris, and then at 53,700 g for 130 minutes to pellet the virus. These, and all subsequent operations, are performed at 0°–4°C. The virus pellet is resuspended in a small volume of STE buffer (0.1 M NaCl, 1 mM EDTA, in 0.01 M Tris-HCl, pH 7.2), homogenized, and centrifuged at 10,000 g for 10 minutes. At this point we frequently treat the supernatant fluid with 1.0 μg/ml RNase A for 10 minutes at 37°C. Extraneous free RNA's of viral and host cell origin are commonly found absorbed to the virus envelope, and this brief RNase treatment removes the contaminating RNA's. Care must be taken to remove all the added RNase, particularly if the viral RNA is to be examined by polyacrylamide gel electrophoresis (PAGE). When such analyses are to be performed, the enzyme treatment is frequently omitted, resulting in the appearance of extra RNA segments in the 4 S to 7 S regions of the gels.

After RNase treatment the virus is layered over 4.0 ml 30% sucrose in STE and centrifuged for 1 hour at 145,000 g. STE buffer is added, the pellet homogenized to resuspend it, and centrifuged at low speed to remove debris. The supernatant fluid is layered over linear sucrose gradients, 10 ml each of 30% and 60% sucrose in STE buffer through 10 ml of mineral oil and centrifuged to equilibrium for 17 hours at 96,000 g. The visible virus band appears at a density of 1.18–1.19 gm/cm^3 and is collected from the bottom of the tube in fractions of approximately 1 ml. Sucrose is removed from virus solutions either by chromatography through Sephadex G-50 or by pelleting the virus by centrifugation for 60 minutes at 145,000 g and resuspending the pellet in STE buffer.

B. Extraction of Viral RNA's

1. EXTRACTION OF RNA FROM VIRIONS

Virus, purified as described above and pelleted to free it of sucrose, is resuspended in a small volume of STE buffer (usually 0.2 to 0.4 ml). After complete dispersal of the pellet, 1.0 to 2.0 ml of SLA buffer is added (0.5% SDS, 0.14 M LiCl, in 0.01 M acetate buffer, pH 4.9) and an equal volume of freshly distilled water saturated phenol : chloroform (1 : 1) added. The mixture is shaken by hand for 4 minutes, the phases separated by centrifugation at low speed, and the upper aqueous phase removed carefully without disturbing the interphase. After the addition of 2 volumes of 95% ethanol, the RNA is precipitated overnight at −20°C, collected by centrifugation, redissolved in the appropriate buffer, and reprecipitated with alcohol. When PAGE analyses are to be done, it is particularly important that the RNA from the first alcohol precipitation be redissolved in RNA electrophoresis buffer (5 mM EDTA, 10 mM NaCl, 0.05% SDS, 5 mM Tris-HCl, pH 7.4). If the NaCl concentration exceeds 10 mM by a small amount, much of the viral RNA tends to stay at the top of the gels resulting in poor electropherograms.

2. EXTRACTION OF VIRAL RNA FROM INFECTED CELLS

Three types of viral specific RNA may be extracted from infected cells: (1) virion-type RNA (vRNA), (2) RNA complementary to virion RNA (vcRNA), and (3) double-stranded (ds) RNA. The extraction of relatively pure vRNA may be accomplished by first isolating the viral RNA as an RNA–protein complex, the ribonucleoprotein (RNP). This will be described in Section V,A,1. The isolation of vcRNA can best be accomplished by isolating this species of RNA from polysomes, since most, if not all, of the viral messenger RNA (mRNA) is vcRNA (Section V,B,1).

The isolation of virus-specific double-stranded RNA (dsRNA) from infected cells has been described in detail elsewhere (Pons, 1967b; Pons and Hirst, 1968b). Briefly restated, the procedure involved phenol–SDS extraction of infected cells and repeated chromatography of the isolated RNA on CF 11 cellulose columns (Franklin, 1966) until a product with a RNase resistance of greater than 90% is achieved. RNA, isolated by these techniques and analyzed by PAGE, reveals six distinct species of ds virus-specific RNA (Fig. 6.1). Denaturation of the dsRNA by dimethyl sulfoxide yields single-stranded RNA's (ssRNA) with electrophoretic mobilities identical to those of vRNA's (Pons and Hirst, 1968b).

C. Analysis of Extracted RNA

There are many techniques available for extraction of viral RNA from infected cells and virions. The selection of a method is dictated, to a large extent, by the method to be used to analyze the product and the use to

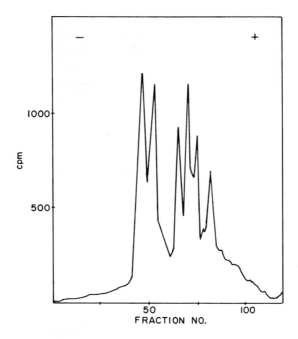

Fig. 6.1. Polyacrylamide gel electrophoresis of [³H]uridine labeled double-stranded RNA obtained from chick embryo fibroblasts infected with influenza virus.

which the extracted material is to be put. That is, if one were interested in examining the extracted material for biological activity it would be desirable to have a small amount of Mg^{2+} present during the extraction. However, the presence of Mg^{2+} causes influenza virus RNA to aggregate and, unless removed (by the addition of EDTA, for example) prior to analyses, would give spurious results if the RNA were examined by velocity sedimentation analyses. In most instances, virus-specific RNA is extracted using SDS and 1:1 phenol:chloroform (Penman, 1969) in SLA buffer.

1. ANALYSIS OF EXTRACTED RNA BY GRADIENT CENTRIFUGATION

Velocity gradient centrifugation analysis is the simplest method for determining sedimentation values and obtaining general information of virion and intracellular virus-specific RNA's. RNA obtained from phenol:chloroform-SDS extracted virions is redissolved from an alcohol precipitation in STE buffer. The RNA is layered over linear 10–35% glycerol gradients (17 ml each) in STE buffer containing 1 M urea (STEU buffer). We have

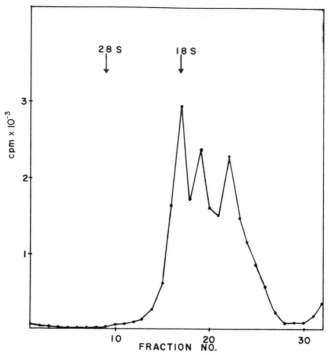

Fig. 6.2. Glycerol gradient velocity sedimentation analysis of purified [³H]-uridine labeled influenza virus RNA. The gradients are linear 10–35% glycerol solutions (w/w) in STEU buffer (0.1 *M* NaCl, 1 m*M* EDTA, 10 m*M* Tris-HCl, pH 7.2, 1 *M* urea).

found that coating the centrifuge tubes with a thin layer of silicone grease improves the resolution and reduces wall effects during centrifugation. Glycerol is used for most analyses (but not for polysome analyses) since it has a lower density than sucrose; it can be autoclaved to sterilize it and destroy any contaminating RNase while sucrose cannot; it will not freeze at −20°C, and this avoids some of the problems encountered when freezing biological material, and, lastly, glycerol quenches very little (compared to sucrose) in most liquid scintillation counting solutions.

After centrifuging the viral RNA through glycerol gradients at 120,000 *g* for 17 hours, 1 ml fractions are collected from the bottom of the tubes and radioactivity of each fraction determined. As seen in Fig. 6.2, these procedures will resolve the RNA into three size classes with sedimentation values of approximately 18 S, 14 S, and 11 S. If the virus is not treated with RNase during its purification a fourth peak at 4 S to 7 S is usually seen. This latter material most likely represents host and free virion RNA absorbed on the coat of the virion.

2. Analysis of Extracted RNA by Polyacrylamide Gel Electrophoresis (PAGE)

Analysis of influenza virus RNA by PAGE is more difficult than sedimentation analysis but yields much more information. Basically, two types of gel systems have been used, an agarose–acrylamide gel system using bisacrylamide as the cross-linking agent (Pons and Hirst, 1968a), and an acrylamide system using ethylene diacrylate as the cross-linker without agarose (Duesberg, 1968). Both systems have certain advantages and disadvantages, however, we shall describe only the former system in detail. Our experience with the agarose–acrylamide–bisacrylamide system has shown several pitfalls which must be avoided in order to get successful results. The details of the method are given in Pons and Hirst (1968a) and Pons (1972). Some of the essential details alluded to above but not described in those reports are the necessity for casting and running gels in glass tubes coated with a siliconizing agent such as dimethyldichlorosilane, the need to overlay gels with water immediately after casting and before polymerization occurs and, lastly, not mixing the marker dye with the RNA to be analyzed. The dye is run in parallel with the unknown RNAs on a separate gel.

Figure 6.3 depicts a typical gel electrophoresis pattern obtained with $[^3H]5$-uridine labeled vRNA obtained from virions. Clearly, there are five distinct classes of vRNA present. Gel electrophoresis of dsRNA obtained from infected cells indicates there are six different-sized RNA molecules present (Fig. 6.1) (Pons and Hirst, 1968b). Skehel (1971) has reported that six different ssRNA molecules are observed when virus is disrupted with lithium dodecyl sulfate and subjected to PAGE. On the other hand, Lewandowski et al. (1971), using other methods, have estimated the minimum number of RNA molecules per virion, based on the number of 3'-termini, as seven. At the moment it appears that the influenza genome consists of 6 or 7 individual RNA molecules. The uncertainty as to the exact number of segments per virion makes it impossible to determine the molecular weight of the virus genome. However, estimates based on the coding requirements for virus-specific polypeptides make it appear that a genome must have a minimum molecular weight of 3.5×10^6 to 4×10^6 daltons. Lewandowski et al. (1971) have estimated that the seven segments they described would have a minimum molecular weight of 4.7×10^6 daltons of RNA.

Recently, we have developed a new gel electrophoresis system using slab gels rather than cylindrical gels. These methods show that the influenza genome consists of 8 separate pieces of single-stranded (ss) RNA. Isolation of double-stranded (ds) RNA from infected cells also yields 8 pieces of ds RNA. In both cases the RNA's are grouped as follows: 3 closely grouped large RNA's, 3 more widely separated intermediate size pieces, and 2 small

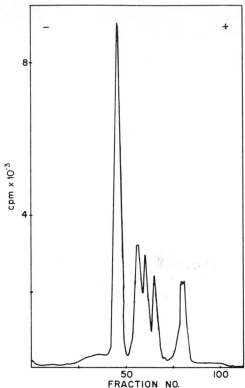

Fig. 6.3. PAGE of [³H]uridine labeled single-stranded RNA obtained from purified influenza virus (WSN strain) by phenol–SDS extraction. Electrophoresis was for 110 minutes at 10 mA/gel at 0°C.

pieces. Dr. Peter Palese, using a similar method for analyzing ssRNA finds 9 pieces of RNA (P. Palese, personal communication). The extra or ninth RNA piece has a low molecular weight and its presence seems to be related to the multiplicity of infection.

3. Analysis of Extracted RNA by Chromatography on
   Methylated Albumin Kieselguhr (MAK) Columns

Influenza virus RNA may be analyzed on MAK columns as described by Mandell and Hershey (1960). Under gradient elution conditions the vRNA's elute from such columns at 1.00 M NaCl (Pons, 1967a) as a single peak. Subsequent velocity sedimentation analysis of this RNA shows that the RNA sediments as a broad area with an average sedimentation value of 18 S. The usefulness of MAK analysis is limited when examining vRNA obtained from purified virions, but is quite useful for examining RNA obtained from infected cells. Phenol–SDS extracted infected cell RNA chromatographed on MAK separates the viral single-stranded and double-stranded RNA's. The ssRNA's elute with host 28 S ribosomal RNA. If this mixture of host and vRNA's is subjected to velocity sedimentation, the viral RNA's (which have a mean sedimentation constant of 18 S) and 28 S host ribosomal RNA separate leaving a relatively pure product, as viral RNA's, obtained from the cell.

III. Physical and Chemical Characteristics of Influenza Viral RNA's

A. RNA from Infectious Virus

In the preceding sections we have described the various methods employed in the isolation and analysis of RNA from virus. With the possible exception of the studies of Li and Seto (1970), who claimed that RNA from virus particles could be extracted as single long chain RNA molecules, which could be visualized by electron microscopy, all of the data obtained by many workers indicate that the viral RNA is segmented. As indicated above, there is uncertainty about the exact number of segments per virion, which makes it impossible to determine the molecular weight of the whole genome with any degree of certainty.

The base composition of vRNA isolated from the PR 8 strain was determined by Duesberg and Robinson (1967) to be uracil 33%, cytosine 24%, adenine 23%, and guanine 19.5%. Earlier, Ada and Perry (1956) found the base composition of vRNA varied slightly but significantly from strain to strain. The base composition of the vRNA and its sensitivity to RNase digestion indicate that it is single-stranded. Since there is no annealing between RNA molecules extracted from virions the ssRNA in virions is of one strand sense (Scholtissek and Becht, 1971; Pons, 1971).

The essential point regarding influenza virus RNA is its segmented nature. Apparently many of the biological properties of the virus which set it apart from most of the other animal viruses can be explained by this fact. Although several plant viruses seem to have segmented genomes, the only other animal viruses that are known (to date) to have a segmented RNA are reovirus and RNA tumor viruses. There is physical, chemical, and biological evidence establishing the segmented nature of the influenza genome.

Sedimentation analysis of labeled RNA extracted from purified virus particles led many different workers to the conclusion that the extracted RNA had a molecular weight too low to account for the information necessary to synthesize virus-specific polypeptides (Davies and Barry, 1966; Duesberg and Robinson, 1967; Nayak, 1969; Pons, 1967a). In these last two reports the isolation of a high molecular weight RNA was demonstrated (see also Agrawal and Bruening, 1966), but it now appears that this may have been aggregated RNA segments or incompletely deproteinized RNP molecules. PAGE analysis of vRNA by Duesberg (1968) and Pons and Hirst (1968a) shows that the genome consisted of at least five segments of RNA. Subsequently, it was shown that viral-specific dsRNA extracted from infected cells was also in pieces which, when separated into ssRNA segments by melting, had electrophoretic mobilities similar to virion RNA (Pons and Hirst, 1968b). This observation indicated that the segments had biological significance and were not simply degradation products of the extraction procedures.

The above biochemical work suggested that the virus genome was segmented. Several bits of biological data also indicated a segmented genome in this virus. The high recombination frequency obtained with genetic crosses of influenza virus suggested a mechanism similar to random assortment of segments rather than true genetic recombination with crossing-over within pieces of RNA (Simpson and Hirst, 1961; Hirst, 1962). Scholtissek and Rott (1964) found that Bayer 139 inactivated virus functions in a stepwise fashion, which suggested to them a multicomponent genome. Multiplicity reactivation (Henle and Liu, 1951; Barry, 1961) and ultraviolet light inactivation studies (Joss *et al.,* 1969; Gandi and Burke, 1970) also were interpreted as showing the possible existence of a multicomponent genome.

Although the biochemical and biological data were very suggestive, the most conclusive data establishing the segmented nature of the genome was from the following: Young and Content (1971) separated the virion RNA into three size classes by velocity sedimentation. Each of the three classes of RNA had as its 5'-terminal nucleotide, pppAp. Lewandowski *et al.* (1971) showed that the 3'-termini were unphosphorylated uridine (U-OH). In addition, Content and Duesberg (1971) showed base sequence differences between the three size classes of virion RNA, while Horst *et al.* (1972) found different oligonucleotides in each of these size classes. These data, taken with the previous work, make it highly unlikely, if not impossible, that RNA segments arise from cleavage of a covalently linked single-stranded RNA molecule.

It is clear that the genome is segmented, and there is no evidence to suggest any type of linkage between segments such as overlapping complementary base pairing. Since virus-specific RNA obtained from infected cells is also segmented, it is unclear how virus maturation with the inclusion of the proper number and type of pieces takes place. This will be discussed in Section V.

B. RNA from von Magnus or Incomplete Virus

One of the peculiarities of this virus is that when serially passaged at high multiplicities in eggs or tissue culture a diminishing amount of infectious virus is produced although the hemagglutination (HA) titer remains high. This virus, with low infectivity and high HA activity, is incomplete or von Magnus virus (von Magnus, 1954). Duesberg (1968) showed by PAGE that incomplete virus had diminished amounts of the larger RNA segments. Pons and Hirst (1969) showed that it was only the largest RNA segment which was greatly diminished in incomplete virus after two high multiplicity passages, while the polypeptide composition of incomplete virus was affected only quantitatively. It should be noted that although we refer to this largest piece as being "missing" it might still be present in a cleaved form. That is, if the RNA were cleaved at one or more points along the chain, the RNA would still be present in the virion but would migrate in gels to a different location and thus appear to be missing. There is no evidence for this, however.

Choppin (1969) found that serial high multiplicity passage of the WSN strain of influenza virus in MDBK cells did not lead to the formation of substantial amounts of incomplete virus until several such passages were made. On the other hand, a single passage of virus in HeLa cells led to the production of noninfective HA particles (Henle *et al.,* 1955; Hillis *et al.,* 1960; White *et al.,* 1965; TerMeulen and Love, 1967). Choppin and Pons (1970) examined the RNA's of virus grown in MDBK and HeLa cells and found the largest RNA segment was decreased in MDBK-grown virus but only slowly, and not until the fourth successive high multiplicity passage was it greatly reduced (as opposed to two passages in eggs and CEF monolayers). In HeLa cells, a single passage of egg-grown virus was sufficient to show the loss of the largest RNA segment. Lerner and Hodge (1969) found that HeLa cells infected with PR 8 strain of influenza virus produced all seven pieces of dsRNA, but the ssRNA in incomplete particles was not examined.

These results with incomplete virus show that the host cell plays a significant role in the replication of virus RNA, although the nature of this influence is uncertain. The mechanism by which a single RNA segment is excluded from virions is also uncertain, although the following explanation has been suggested (Choppin and Pons, 1970): Since the replication of a smaller RNA segment would be completed more rapidly than that of a larger segment (Mills *et al.,* 1967; Spiegelman *et al.,* 1968), overloading a cell with influenza virus might cause a depletion in available pools of nucleotides or some other material(s) required for the synthesis of the larger RNA molecules. This hypothesis, that small RNA segments have a competitive advantage in replication, assumes that replication of each piece is independent of the others, and that packaging of the RNA is random (Compans *et al.,* 1970). Since this hypothesis was put forth, Bishop *et al.* (1972) have shown that each piece of RNA carries its own polymerase molecules, a fact which strengthens the above argument.

IV. Protein-Associated RNA (The RNP)

A. Physical and Chemical Characteristics

When influenza virions are disrupted with ether (Hoyle, 1952; Lief and Henle, 1956; Davenport *et al.,* 1959), sodium deoxycholate (Duesberg, 1969; Kingsbury and Webster, 1969), or Nonidet P-40 (NP40) (Pons *et al.,* 1969), a stable complex consisting of RNA and protein is released. This ribonucleoprotein (RNP) consists of 10% RNA and 90% protein. The protein moiety of the RNP has a molecular weight of approximately 55,000 to 65,000 daltons and is designated the NP (Pons *et al.,* 1969). Velocity gradient centrifugation of RNP on 10–35% glycerol gradients in STEU buffer resolves the RNP into three classes with mean sedimentation coefficients of 48 S, 40 S, and 34 S (Pons, 1971). Duesberg (1969) and Kingsbury and Webster (1969) also isolated three size classes of RNP but reported higher S values of approximately 70 S, 60 S, and 50 S. The discrepancy probably arises from differences in the methods of extraction and analysis of the isolated RNP, the material having a tendency to aggregate in the absence of urea or in low salt solutions. After gluteraldehyde fixation RNP has a buoyant density of 1.34 gm/cm^3 in CsCl (Krug, 1971).

Pons (1971), using PAGE analysis of isolated RNP, confirmed the earlier suppositions of Duesberg (1969) and Kingsbury and Webster (1969) that each of the three size classes of RNP isolated on velocity gradients consisted of different RNA segments associated with the NP. There is no evidence to date for the existence of a continuous strand of RNP (i.e., RNA segments held together on a continuous backbone of NP) either within the virion or in the infected cell.

In contrast to the RNP's of paramyxoviruses (Compans and Choppin, 1967), the RNP's of influenza virus are sensitive to RNase digestion (Duesberg, 1969; Pons *et al.,* 1969). The influenza virus RNP's are, however, less sensitive to RNase digestion than free RNA (Pons *et al.,* 1969). Pronase treatment of isolated RNP's digested the NP and left free viral RNA (Pons *et al.,* 1969). Mild pronase treatment did not digest the NP (Duesberg, 1969). These data suggest that both the RNA and NP are exposed in the

RNP complex, although each component does offer some protection to the other against degradation.

Pons *et al.* (1969) examined isolated RNP by electron microscopy after staining with uranyl acetate or negative staining with potassium phosphotungstate. The structures appeared to have helical or twisted midsections with alternate deep and shallow grooves and with loops at either end. These structures varied in length from 500 to 1500 Å with a constant thickness of 150 Å (75 Å at the terminal loops) (Schulze *et al.*, 1970) (Fig. 6.4A). Compans *et al.* (1972) obtained similar results and showed that the length of each RNP piece reflects the size of the RNA molecule associated with it. The morphology of the RNP suggests a helical structure consisting of RNA and protein, neither of which encases the other, which is coiled back on itself to form a highly twisted structure.

Scholtissek and Becht (1971) showed that the NP has an equal affinity for vRNA and vcRNA. It also binds to AMP-rich cellular RNA and to other single-stranded viral RNA's but not dsRNA. As indicated above, once formed the RNP complex is stable in 1 M urea and also in 0.8 M NaCl or 1 M KCl. Under *in vitro* assay conditions, there does not appear to be a great deal of specificity in the association of NP and RNA molecules. Another indication of this lack of specificity was demonstrated by the following work: Pons *et al.* (1969) and Goldstein and Pons (1970) showed that polyvinyl sulfate (PVS) displaced the RNA from the protein backbone leaving a PVS–NP complex which had sedimentation properties and the morphological appearance of the original RNP (Fig. 6.4B). The free viral RNA sedimented at 18 S, was as susceptible to RNase digestion as phenol-extracted RNA, while the PVS-NP complex was not destroyed by RNase. These results were important since they showed that the morphology of RNP is largely determined by interactions between NP molecules, since two such widely different molecules as PVS and RNA, when associated with NP, had a similar appearance. Furthermore, the PSV–NP complex, which was identical physically and morphologically to RNP, could only be obtained when PVS was added to intact RNP. Addition of PVS to free NP subunits gave a heterogeneous mixture of PVS–protein molecules, none of which sedimented or looked like RNP. The interaction of PVS with RNP also indicates, as pointed out by Schulze (1973), that charge interactions between protein molecules and the phosphodiester backbone of the RNA seem to be involved in the formation of RNP, since the RNA can be substituted for by a polymer containing charged phosphate groups.

Several different methods have been developed for isolating RNP's from infected cells (Pons, 1971, 1972). Each of these methods yields RNP's with buoyant density, sedimentation, and morphological characteristics identical to those of virion RNP's. There is one difference between RNP's isolated

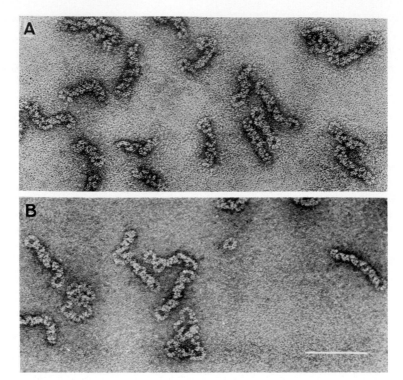

Fig. 6.4. Electron micrographs of isolated, purified ribonucleoprotein. (A) RNP negatively stained with uranyl acetate, pH 5.0. (B) RNP in which the RNA has been replaced by polyvinyl sulfate. Negatively stained with uranyl acetate, pH 5.0. ×180,000; marker, 1000 Å. (From Pons *et al.*, 1969.)

from virions and those found free in infected cells: Virion RNP's consist of protein complexed to vRNA, while 90% of the cellular RNP's contain vRNA and 10% vcRNA. Although Krug (1972) has reported the presence of free vcRNA in infected cells, we have found no free viral-specific RNA intracellularly (other than dsRNA). Our techniques enable us to isolate all the intracellular virus-specific RNA as RNP's. The reasons for this discrepancy are not yet clear.

B. Biological Properties of RNP

As yet, there is no evidence that the protein portion of RNP serves any function other than to protect the RNA. It is conceivable that RNA segments might be joined into a single unit on a continuous backbone of NP.

Although such a structure has not been demonstrated, a model for the replication of viral RNA based on such a structure has been proposed (Pons, 1970). Also, the NP or RNP might serve some regulatory function in transcription, translation, or replication processes. Answers to these questions may be forthcoming from studies on *in vitro* transcription and translation.

Hirst and Pons (1972) reported that virus extracts containing RNP isolated from wild-type WSN strain influenza virus had marker rescue activity when tested against temperature-sensitive mutants. The nature and complexity of the material active in rescue was not determined, but free viral RNA, prepared by phenol–SDS extraction of RNP or virions or by treatment of RNP with polyvinyl sulfate, was totally inactive in such tests. Whether NP alone, or NP plus polymerase, is sufficient for rescue activity must be determined.

V. Intracellular Virus-Specific RNA's

A. Virion-Type RNA (vRNA)

1. SYNTHESIS OF THE vRNA

Although much work has been done on the intracellular synthesis of influenza virus RNA, studies have been impeded by the virus' sensitivity to actinomycin D (AD) inhibition. Several workers presented evidence which was interpreted as showing that viral RNA synthesis became resistant to AD inhibition at 2 to $2\frac{1}{2}$ hours after infection (Barry *et al.*, 1962; Barry, 1964; Granoff and Kingsbury, 1964; see reviews by Kingsbury, 1970; Blair and Duesberg, 1970). Still other evidence can be interpreted as showing inhibition by AD irrespective of the time of drug addition (Scholtissek and Rott, 1970; Gregoriades, 1970; Pons, 1973). Regardless of when the drug is added it inhibits viral dsRNA synthesis (Pons, 1967b), specifically the synthesis of strands complementary to virion RNA, i.e., vcRNA (Scholtissek and Rott, 1970; Pons, 1973). This work will be discussed in detail in Section VI,A. We have raised the point here to emphasize the fact that the work to be discussed below was, for the most part, done without using any inhibitors of viral RNA synthesis, and, as a consequence, a great deal of effort was directed toward separating viral and host cell products during viral maturation.

As mentioned in Section II,C,1 virus-specific RNA's have a mean sedimentation value of 18 S. Mammalian host ribosomal RNA's sediment at

28 S and 18 S. Therefore, when no inhibitors are used to halt host ribosomal RNA synthesis, viral RNA synthesis is partially obscured by the host 18 S RNA. To avoid this problem, a technique was devised for isolating viral RNA's from infected cells as the RNP. The RNP has a mean sedimentation constant of 30 S to 50 S, is stable to EDTA, high salt, and urea treatments which break down host ribosomes, and can be concentrated by isoelectric point precipitation (Schäfer and Munk, 1952). Taking advantage of these properties, infected cells were disrupted with NP 40, the RNP removed and concentrated by precipitation with 0.1 M acetate buffer pH 4.5, and purified by velocity sedimentation through one or two glycerol gradients (Pons, 1971). The isolated and purified product RNP's have a buoyant density, sedimentation properties, and morphological characteristics of RNP's isolated from virions. However, whereas RNA isolated from virions does not self-anneal, RNA isolated from intracellularly obtained RNP's self-anneal to a maximum of about 20%. These data, in addition to data obtained by annealing competition experiments, indicate that intracellular RNP's consist of 90% vRNA and 10% vcRNA (Pons, 1971).

Scholtissek *et al.* (1969) reported that viral RNA synthesis was linked to the synthesis of the NP polypeptide. These data made it feasible to study the kinetics of viral RNA synthesis by following the intracellular appearance of RNP. In addition, the methods developed for studying intracellular events during virus replication have led to the view that there are no free viral-specific RNA's within the infected cell (Pons, 1971, 1972). That is, as soon as an RNA chain is synthesized, or perhaps while being synthesized, it rapidly becomes associated with NP. Krug (1971) has interpreted his data to mean that vcRNA synthesis occurs much earlier than the formation of vcRNP's. Regardless of this discrepancy, it still appears valid to use RNP synthesis as a gauge of viral RNA synthesis. Pons (1971) showed that RNP could be detected as early as 1 hour after infection. Earlier, it was shown that viral-specific dsRNA could be detected at $\frac{1}{2}$ hour after infection (Pons, 1967b). The difference is merely one of methodology and sensitivity for the curve showing the kinetics of RNP production can be extrapolated back to zero time. The kinetics of RNP production have all the characteristics expected for the synthesis of a self-replicating molecule (Pons, 1971).

In summary, the data obtained to date indicate that viral RNA synthesis, as reflected in the appearance of RNP, begins almost immediately after infection. The asymptotic appearance of the curve of the kinetics of RNP production indicates a self-duplicating molecule is involved. In CEF monolayers, RNP production is at a maximum 4–5 hours after infection, at which time new virus accumulates in the extracellular fluid and some cell disintegration occurs. Another aspect of intracellular viral RNA synthesis is the site of synthesis, which will be dealt with in Chapter 8.

2. Maturation and Packaging of RNA into Virions

The mechanisms involved in packaging RNA (or RNP) into virions are unknown. Clearly, there is a selective process involved since only RNP's containing vRNA are packaged in new virions, while vcRNA containing RNP's are excluded. Although there are no data concerning this, we may speculate that the initial maturation steps involve the association of some polypeptide (perhaps the M polypeptide) with a recognition site on the vRNP's. Once this initial event occurs, other polypeptides or more subunits of the same polypeptide condense around the RNP and self-assembly begins and finally ends with the maturation of new particles at specific locations on the cell membranes, which have been altered at these locations to contain viral components.

How a complete array of virus RNA segments (as RNP) is packaged into a single virion is a large problem especially in view of the segmented nature of the viral genome. Although we have not excluded the possibility that various RNA segments are aligned or linked in some orderly array on a continuous protein backbone, there is no evidence for this. Compans *et al.* (1970) calculated that if five segments of RNA are required for a complete genome and if seven segments were actually packaged randomly, approximately 22% of the resulting particles would have the total complement of five different pieces. The data now indicate at least six or seven different segments are carried in each virion and so one must assume that, if their scheme was operative in this system, nine to ten pieces would have to be packaged. Although this seems to be a bit high based on the chemical estimates on the amount of RNA per virion, it is still possible and connot be excluded. Such a system of maturation, coupled with the virions' tendency to aggregate and enhance their infectivity (Hirst and Pons, 1973), would give the virus a distinct competitive survival advantage in nature.

One experimental approach to this question is quite straightforward but in practice it has proved very difficult technically. If we assume replication of RNP pieces is random, we can make the following prediction. Random or unregulated synthesis of RNP segments would produce an overabundance of the smaller RNP segments. This prediction assumes that the polymerase molecule on each segment of RNP (Bishop *et al.*, 1972) replicates at the same rate. Thus, since the smallest RNP segment is $\frac{1}{3}$ the length of the largest segment, there might be three times as much of the former as the latter. Our data do not show this but instead agree with those of Bishop *et al.* (1972) that the segments are in the ratio of $2:1:1:1:2$ (heaviest to lightest) (M. W. Pons, unpublished results). It is conceivable that maturation involves random packaging, but replication or transcription of virus-specific RNA's are regulated or controlled somehow. If packaging of RNP segments is random, then the distribution of RNP pieces, relative to one another, should be the same in virions as in the intracellular pool from which they are withdrawn. Preliminary data are equivocal, the experiments being technically very difficult because of the presence of incomplete virus in the population and the lack of synchrony in infection.

B. Complementary or Messenger RNA (vcRNA)

1. Intracellular Location of vcRNA

It has been shown that the RNA complementary to that found in virions was associated with polysomes in infected cells (Pons, 1972). As stated (Section V,A,1), 10% of the intracellular virus-specific RNA isolated as RNP was vcRNA. When cells were fractionated, however, it was found that most of the virus-specific RNA found associated with polysomes was vcRNA (Pons, 1972). Recently, Etkind and Krug (1974) reported that all of this RNA is vcRNA. This differs from our results, since we had to apply a correction factor to eliminate the contribution of the host cell RNA. Etkind and Krug (1974) have effectively removed all of the contaminating host RNA. It would appear that influenza is like other viruses which carry RNA-dependent RNA polymerases associated with the particle (vesicular stomatitis virus, for example) and, consequently, is able to generate functional messenger RNA shortly after infection.

Evidence from another kind of experimental approach gives some results which might lead to a different conclusion about the nature of the mRNA. These results are highly contradictory and, at the moment, must be considered as inconclusive. Siegert *et al.* (1973) have reported synthesis of NP polypeptide in an *E. coli* cell-free protein-synthesizing system using vRNA as messenger. In direct contrast, Kingsbury and Webster (1973) found that vRNA could not function as mRNA in a rabbit reticulocyte cell-free system, but RNA obtained from infected cells (a mixture of vRNA and vcRNA) could function as messenger and direct the synthesis of the M polypeptide. These opposing reports are difficult to reconcile but, given the preliminary nature of these findings and until confirmatory data have appeared, we can tentatively suggest that one of the segments of RNA found in virions may have the capacity to function as mRNA. The annealing data to date of Etkind and Krug (1974) and Pons (1972) make it unlikely that more than one piece of vRNA is doubling as a template for both transcription and translation.

2. KINETICS OF vcRNA SYNTHESIS

The work discussed above, concerning RNP and dsRNA synthesis, show that vcRNA synthesis begins very shortly after infection. A more critical study of only this type of RNA synthesis can be made by following the appearance of vcRNA on polysomes. Cells are pulse-labeled with [³H]uridine for short intervals at various times after infection and polysomes isolated and analyzed after phenol : chloroform-SDS extraction. The data show that after an initial depression of host polysome formation vcRNA synthesis increases steadily. The majority of the vcRNA is synthesized $2\frac{1}{2}$ to 3 hours postinfection, after which time its synthesis declines (M. W. Pons, in preparation). Similarly, Krug and Etkind (1973), studying RNA synthesis in the cytoplasm and nucleus of infected cells, found vcRNA synthesis is completed by 4 hours after infection. Thus, these data indicate vcRNA synthesis begins very shortly after infection and is completed by 4 hours, at which time new virus particles begin to appear extracellularly. The nature of the shutoff mechanism is unknown.

3. THE PHYSICAL STATE OF THE mRNA

A study of the vcRNA associated with polysomes (mRNA) has led to the finding that most, if not all, of the mRNA is in the form of RNP. Polysomes were isolated, disrupted with high salt, EDTA, and puromycin (Blobel, 1971) and the mRNA examined. Less than 2% of the vcRNA was found as free RNA, the remainder was in the form of RNP. Great care was taken to ensure that the NP polypeptide (the only polypetide found associated with the isolated mRNP) was not nonspecifically being absorbed to free mRNA during its isolation. It is difficult to be sure that the mRNP is a complete RNP, i.e., without areas free of proteins, but, based on the sedimentation characteristics of the isolated mRNP and its buoyant density in CsCl, it appears to be physically identical to RNP isolated from virions.

Many workers have suggested that mammalian mRNA's can exist and function as messengers when in the form of RNP's (Spirin and Nemer, 1965; Spirin, 1966; Perry and Kelley, 1968; Henshaw, 1968; Kumar and Lindberg, 1972; Bryan and Hayashi, 1973; for reviews, see Gross, 1968; Spirin, 1969). Clearly, a mRNP, being more resistant to RNase digestion, would have greater stability than free mRNA. Just how such a molecule would be translated is unclear, but presumably it might involve a dissociation of the polypeptide subunit and RNA at the point of contact between ribosomes and mRNA. It is also possible that the polypeptide portion of the complex plays a regulatory role in translational processes. A clearer understanding of these problems will come from studies using *in vitro* protein synthesizing systems.

VI. Effect of Inhibitors on RNA Synthesis

A. Actinomycin D

We have already stated (Section V,A,1) that AD inhibits the synthesis of vcRNA completely, no matter when it is added in the replicative cycle, while it inhibits vRNA synthesis only slightly (Scholtissek and Rott, 1970; Pons, 1973). Gregoriades (1970) showed that the vcRNA synthesized prior to inhibition continued to function as mRNA as long as 17 hours after drug addition. It seems clear now that the interpretation of the data by the workers who claimed the drug was not inhibitory when applied 2 to 3 hours after infection (Barry *et al.*, 1962; Barry, 1964; Granoff and Kingsbury, 1964) and those who said the drug was inhibitory at all times (Scholtissek and Rott, 1970; Pons, 1967c) was extreme, and the actual effect lies somewhere between. The drug is inhibitory at all times after infection to vcRNA synthesis, and this causes a decrease in viral polypeptide synthesis, particularly when added before much mRNA has been synthesized. If the drug is added after a sufficient amount of vcRNA has been produced to give enough vcRNA to make the required polypeptides and to serve as template for vRNA synthesis, virus will be produced. Thus, after that time the drug appears to be noninhibitory. It must be emphasized that the drug *is* inhibitory for vcRNA synthesis and must be used with caution when studying intracellular events.

The nature of the inhibition of vcRNA synthesis is unclear. It would appear that actinomycin D is inhibiting a cellular function necessary for vcRNA synthesis, since the drug is effective if given prior to infection of cells. That is, functional host DNA is required [but not host DNA synthesis (Barry, 1964)] for virus multiplication. The drug does not inhibit the *in vitro* synthesis of vcRNA (Chow and Simpson, 1971), but unexpectedly does inhibit intracellular primary transcription (Bean and Simpson, 1973). It is conceivable that the drug inhibits the synthesis of a host cell factor(s) required for transcription. This factor is lacking in the *in vitro* system, and, although some synthesis of vcRNA occurs, it can be substantially stimulated by the addition of a host cell factor(s) (O. Rochovansky, personal communication).

Work on influenza RNA synthesis has been hampered by the inability to conduct pulse-chase experiments in CEF monolayers; the cells continue to incorporate labeled uridine even in the presence of large excesses of unlabeled uridine. Recently, AD has been used to halt incorporation of labeled uridine into vcRNA associated with polysomes. Although not a "chase" in the true sense of the word, the treatment does enable one to follow the fate of preexisting vcRNA. It was found that when vcRNA was isolated from infected cells after a brief (30 minute) pulse the majority of the RNA sedimented with an average value of 14 S. As the pulse interval was increased, the sedimentation value increased until, with a $1\frac{1}{2}$ hour pulse, the RNA had an average sedimentation value of 18 S and a distribution similar to vRNA.

When cells were pulse-labeled for 30 minutes and then exposed to AD for various times in the absence of label, it was found that there was a shift in the distribution of labeled RNA examined by velocity sedimentation analysis. Immediately after this labeling interval, approximately 70% of the labeled vcRNA was in the 9 S to 15 S region and 30% in the 15 S to 22 S region. (RNA extracted from virions is distributed as 20% 9 S to 15 S and 80% 15 S to 22 S.) At the end of the 30 minute labeling period the isotope was removed, AD added, and aliquots of cells withdrawn at 30 minute intervals. After 60 minutes exposure to AD (there was no further change beyond this time), the label was distributed 40% in 9 S to 15 S and 60% in 15 S to 22 S RNA; these values are intermediate between those found with vRNA and vcRNA at the end of a 30 minute pulse label. Significantly, the apparent increase in 15 S to 22 S RNA was not due to an increase in the amount of this RNA but to a decrease in 9 S to 15 S RNA. These results may be interpreted as showing that AD stops vcRNA synthesis, as was expected. However, the decrease in smaller vcRNA segments may mean that these RNA's were not excessive amounts of small vcRNA's but rather incomplete larger RNA molecules. When their synthesis was halted by the drug these growing molecules were dissociated from polysomes, leaving only complete vcRNA molecules associated with polysomes which had approximately the same distribution of RNA segments, relative to one another, as vRNA from virions.

These experiments have been given in some detail for they reveal several significant facts about vcRNA synthesis. (1) The uneven distribution of vcRNA molecules after a relatively short pulse labeling interval was due to the presence of incomplete RNA strands rather than an overabundance of smaller strands. As discussed in Section V,A,2, if duplication of vcRNA was random and uncontrolled, one would expect to find many more small than large RNA segments. Since this does not appear to be the case, there must be a control over RNA synthesis which determines the amount of each piece made. (2) Since incomplete RNA molecules (in the form of RNP's) were found associated with polysomes, it suggests that as vcRNA transcription is going on the NP polypeptide is added to the uncompleted strand. This is in distinction to the synthesis of a complete strand of RNA which is then proteinized. Furthermore, since these incomplete molecules are isolated from polysomes it suggests that translation of vcRNA occurs while the strand is still being synthesized. Such is the case in most bacterial systems which have been examined.

B. Cycloheximide

Cycloheximide inhibits protein synthesis by inhibiting polypeptide chain elongation (Wettstein et al., 1964; Stanners, 1966; Watanabe et al., 1967). Treatment of influenza virus infected cells with cycloheximide decreases the synthesis of vcRNA but completely abolished the synthesis of vRNA (Pons, 1973). These results were similar to those of Scholtissek and Rott (1970) who examined whole cell extracts using annealing techniques.

The nature of the inhibitory effect with cycloheximide is unclear. The different responses of vRNA and vcRNA synthesis to cycloheximide and AD treatment indicate that two different enzymes may be involved in their synthesis (or if not two enzymes, a single "core" enzyme with different subunits, which may be either host-or virus-specified polypeptides), the synthesis of which are being affected by the drugs.

C. Cordycepin

Cordycepin is an inhibitor of poly(A) synthesis (Penman et al., 1970; Darnell et al., 1971), a substance which has been shown to be important for the production of functional messenger RNA's in a variety of viral and host cell systems. Cells (both CEF and BHK-21 cells) were infected with influenza virus, treated with cordycepin for 45 minutes sometime between 2 and 4 hours after infection, and then labeled with [^{3}H]uridine for 30 minutes. Polysomes and RNP were extracted from these cells and compared with untreated infected and control cells. In infected cells, the drug caused a 70% inhibition of uptake of label into both polysomes and RNP and a 60% inhibition of HA and infectious virus production. Polysome labeling of uninfected CEF cells was inhibited about 80%. In BHK-21 cells, however, the drug had no effect on HA or infectious virus production, inhibited polysome and RNP synthesis only slightly but inhibited polysome labeling of uninfected cells 86% (Rochovansky and Pons, 1975).

Etkind and Krug (1974) have shown that poly(A) is present on influenza mRNA's. Since the vRNA does not contain poly(U) segments (Marshall and Gillespie, 1972; Rochovansky and Pons, 1975) the poly(A) found on vcRNA must be added after transcription. It is conceivable that CEF cells, which are, relatively speaking, metabolically inactive under our experimental conditions [but more active in the system of Mahy *et al.* (1973) where cordycepin had little effect on fowl plague virus production in CEF cells], may have to synthesize some cellular component, such as poly(A), before virus replication can proceed. BHK-21 cells, however, are much more metabolically active and presumably there would be larger pools of virus-required host factor available. The suggestion that some host synthesis is required for virus production is supported by the results of Mahy *et al.* (1972) who showed a stimulation of cellular DNA-dependent RNA polymerase II of CEF cells infected with fowl plague virus. RNA polymerase II is the enzyme involved in the production of host mRNA's.

VIII. Conclusions

This discussion of the chemical, biological, and morphological characteristics of influenza virus RNA and RNP make it clear that the genome consists of several single-stranded RNA segments. End-group analyses of the various RNA segments and the presence of polymerase molecules on each segment make it highly likely that each piece is replicated separately. Less clear, however, is how the proper number and type of segments are packaged to produce an infectious virus particle. Is the selection of pieces under some regulatory mechanism or is it a random process? By what means are vcRNA segments excluded from this process? The answers to these questions are being sought in several laboratories.

Related to these questions are the questions of regulation of RNA transcription, translation, and replication in virus-infected cells. Very little is known about these processes although they are the subject of much current work. The use of *in vitro* RNA- and protein-synthesizing systems should provide some of the answers to the questions raised here.

References

Ada, G. L., and Perry, B. T. (1954). *Aust. J. Exp. Biol. Med. Sci.* **32**, 453.
Ada, G. L., and Perry, B. T. (1956). *J. Gen. Microbiol.* **14**, 623.
Agrawal, H. O., and Bruening, G. (1966). *Proc. Nat. Acad. Sci. U.S.* **55**, 818.
Barry, R. D. (1961). *Virology* **14**, 398.
Barry, R. D. (1964). *Cell. Biol. Myxovirus Infect., Ciba Found. Symp., 1964* pp. 51–75.

Barry, R. D., Ives, D. R., and Cruickshank, J. G. (1962). *Nature (London)* **194,** 1139.

Bean, W. J., and Simpson, R. W. (1973). *Virology* **56,** 646.

Bishop, D. H., Roy, P., Bean, W. J., Jr., and Simpson, R. W. (1972). *J. Virol.* **10,** 689.

Blair, C. D., and Duesberg, P. H. (1970). *Annu. Rev. Microbiol.* **24,** 539.

Blobel, G. (1971). *Proc. Nat. Acad. Sci. U.S.* **68,** 832.

Bryan, R. N., and Hayashi, M. (1973). *Nature (London) New Biol.* **244,** 271.

Burnet, F. M. (1956). *Science* **123,** 1101.

Choppin, P. W. (1969). *Virology* **39,** 130.

Choppin, P. W., and Pons, M. W. (1970). *Virology* **42,** 603.

Chow, N., and Simpson, R. W. (1971). *Proc. Nat. Acad. Sci. U.S.* **68,** 752.

Compans, R. W., and Choppin, P. W. (1967). *Proc. Nat. Acad. Sci. U.S.* **57,** 949.

Compans, R. W., Dimmock, N. J., and Meier-Ewert, H. (1970). *In* "The Biology of Large RNA Viruses" (R. D. Barry and B. W. J. Mahy, eds.), pp. 87–108. Academic Press, New York.

Compans, R. W., Content, J., and Duesberg, P. H. (1972). *J. Virol.* **10,** 795.

Content, J., and Duesberg, P. H. (1971). *J. Mol. Biol.* **62,** 273.

Darnell, J. E., Philipson, L., Wall, R., and Adesnik, M. (1971). *Science* **174,** 507.

Davenport, F. M., Rott, R., and Schaefer, W. (1959). *Fed. Proc., Fed. Amer. Soc. Exp. Biol.* **18,** 563.

Davies, P., and Barry, R. D. (1966). *Nature (London)* **211,** 384.

Duesberg, P. H. (1968). *Proc. Nat. Acad. Sci. U.S.* **59,** 930.

Duesberg, P. H. (1969). *J. Mol. Biol.* **42,** 485.

Duesberg, P. H., and Robinson, W. S. (1967). *J. Mol. Biol.* **25,** 383.

Etkind, P. R., and Krug, R. M. (1974). *Virology* (in press).

Franklin, R. M. (1966). *Proc. Nat. Acad. Sci. U.S.* **55,** 1504.

Frisch-Niggemeyer, W., and Hoyle, L. (1956). *J. Hyg.* **54,** 201.

Frommhagen, L. H., Knight, C. A., and Freeman, N. K. (1959). *Virology* **8,** 176.

Gandi, S. S., and Burke, D. C. (1970). *In* "The Biology of Large RNA Viruses" (R. D. Barry and B. W. J. Mahy, eds.), pp. 675–383. Academic Press, New York.

Goldstein, E. A., and Pons, M. W. (1970). *Virology* **41,** 382.

Granoff, A., and Kingsbury, D. W. (1964). *Cell. Biol. Myxovirus Infect., Ciba Found. Symp., 1964* pp. 96–119.

Gregoriades, A. (1970). *Virology* **42,** 905.

Gross, P. R. (1968). *Annu. Rev. Biochem.* **37,** 631.

Henle, G., Girardi, A., and Henle, W. (1955). *J. Exp. Med.* **101,** 25.

Henle, W., and Liu, O. C. (1951). *J. Exp. Med.* **94,** 305.

Henshaw, E. S. (1968). *J. Mol. Biol.* **36,** 401.

Hillis, W. D., Moffat, M. A. J., and Holtermann, O. A. (1960). *Acta Pathol. Microbiol. Scand.* **50,** 419 and 429.

Hirst, G. K. (1962). *Cold Spring Harbor Symp. Quant. Biol.* **27,** 303.

Hirst, G. K., and Pons, M. W. (1972). *Virology* **47,** 546.

Hirst, G. K., and Pons, M. W. (1973). *Virology* **56,** 620.

Horst, J., Content, J., Mandeles, S., Frankel-Conrat, H., and Duesberg, P. H. (1972). *J. Mol. Biol.* **69,** 209.

Hoyle, L. (1952). *J. Hyg.* **50,** 229.

Joss, A., Gandhi, S. S., Hay, A. J., and Burke, D. C. (1969). *J. Virol.* **4,** 816.

Kingsbury, D. W. (1970). *Progr. Med. Virol.* **12,** 49.

Kingsbury, D. W., and Webster, R. G. (1969). *J. Virol.* **4,** 219.

Kingsbury, D. W., and Webster, R. G. (1973). *Virology* **56,** 654.

Krug, R. M. (1971). *Virology* **44,** 125.

Krug, R. M. (1972). *Virology* **50,** 103.

Krug, R. M., and Etkind, P. M. (1973). *Virology* **56,** 334.

Kumar, A., and Lindberg, V. (1972). *Proc. Nat. Acad. Sci. U.S.* **69,** 681.

Lerner, R. A., and Hodge, L. D. (1969). *Proc. Nat. Acad. Sci. U.S.* **64,** 544.

Lewandowski, L. J., Content, J., and Leppla, S. H. (1971). *J. Virol.* **8,** 701.

Li, K. K., and Seto, J. T. (1970). *J. Virol.* **7,** 524.

Lief, F. S., and Henle, W. (1956). *Virology* **2,** 753.

Mahy, B. W. J., Hastie, N. D., and Armstrong, S. J. (1972). *Proc. Nat. Acad. Sci. U.S.* **69,** 1421.

Mahy, B. W. J., Cox, N. J., Armstrong, S. J., and Barry, R. D. (1973). *Nature (London) New Biol.* **243,** 172.

Mandell, J. D., and Hershey, A. D. (1960). *Anal. Biochem.* **1,** 66.

Mills, D. R., Peterson, R. L., and Spiegelman, S. (1967) *Proc. Nat. Acad. Sci. U.S.* **58,** 217.

Nayak, D. P. (1969). *Fed. Proc., Fed. Amer. Soc. Exp. Biol.* **28,** 1858.

Penman, S. (1969). *In* "Fundamental Techniques in Virology" (K. Habel and N. P. Salzman, eds.), Vol. 1, pp. 35–48. Academic Press, New York.

Penman, S., Rosbash, M., and Penman, M. (1970). *Proc. Nat. Acad. Sci. U.S.* **67,** 1878.

Penman, S. (1969). *In* "Fundamental Techniques in Virology" (K. Habel and N. P. Salzman, eds.), Vol. 1, pp. 35–48. Academic Press, New York.

Penman, S., Rosbash, M., and Penman, M. (1970). *Proc. Nat. Acad. Sci. U.S.* **67,** 1878.

Perry, R. P., and Kelley, D. E. (1968). *J. Mol. Biol.* **35,** 37.

Pons, M. W. (1967a). *Virology* **31,** 523.

Pons, M. W. (1967b). *Arch. Gesamte Virusforsch.* **22,** 203.

Pons, M. W. (1967c). *Virology* **33,** 150.

Pons, M. W. (1970). *Curr. Top. Microbiol. Immunol.* p. 142.

Pons, M. W. (1971). *Virology* **46,** 149.

Pons, M. W. (1972). *Virology* **47,** 823.

Pons, M. W. (1973). *Virology* **51,** 120.

Pons, M. W., and Hirst, G. K. (1968a). *Virology* **34,** 386.

Pons, M. W., and Hirst, G. K. (1968b). *Virology* **35,** 182.

Pons, M. W., and Hirst, G. K. (1969). *Virology* **38,** 68.

Pons, M. W., Schulze, I. T., Hirst, G. K., and Hauser, R. (1969). *Virology* **39,** 250.

Rochovansky, O., and Pons, M. W. (1975). *In* "Negative-Strand Viruses" (R. D. Barry and B. W. J. Mahy, eds.). Academic Press, New York (in press).

Schäfer, W., and Munk, K. (1952). *Z. Naturforsch. B* **7,** 573.

Scholtissek, C., and Becht, H. (1971). *J. Gen. Virol.* **10,** 11.

Scholtissek, C., and Rott, R. (1964). *Virology* **22,** 169.

Scholtissek, C., and Rott, R. (1970). *Virology* **40,** 989.

Scholtissek, C., Drzeniek, R., and Rott, R. (1969). *In* "The Biochemistry of Viruses" (H. Levy, eds.). Dekker, New York.

Schulze, I. T. (1973). *Advan. Virus Res.* **18,** 1.

Schulze, I. T., Pons, M. W., Hirst, G. K., and Hauser, R. (1970). *In* "The Biology of Large RNA Viruses" (R. D. Barry and B. W. J. Mahy, eds.), pp. 324–346. Academic Press, New York.

Siegert, W., Bauer, G., and Hofschneider, P. H. (1973). *Proc. Nat. Acad. Sci. U.S.* **70**, 2960.

Simpson, R. W., and Hirst, G. K. (1961). *Virology* **15**, 436.

Skehel, J. J. (1971). *J. Gen. Virol.* **11**, 103.

Spiegelman, S. Pace, N. R., Mills, D. R., Levisohn, R. Eikhom, T. S., Taylor, M. M., Peterson, R. L., and Bishop, D. H. L. (1968). *Cold Spring Harbor Symp. Quant. Biol.* **33**, 101.

Spirin, A. S. (1966). *Curr. Top. Develop. Biol.* **1**, 1.

Spirin, A. S. (1969). *Eur. J. Biochem.* **10**, 20.

Spirin, A. S., and Nemer, M. (1965). *Science* **150**, 214.

Stanners, C. P. (1966). *Biochem. Biophys. Res. Commun.* **24**, 758.

TerMeulen, V., and Love, R. (1967). *J. Virol.* **1**, 626.

von Magnus, P. (1954). *Advan. Virus Res.* **2**, 59.

Watanabe, Y., Kudo, H., and Graham, A. F. (1967). *J. Virol.* **1**, 36.

Wettstein, F. O., Noll, H., and Penman, S. (1964). *Biochim. Biophys. Acta* **87.** 525.

White, D. O., Day, H. M., Batchelder, E. J., Cheyne, I. M., and Wansbrough, A. J. (1965). *Virology* **25**, 289.

Young, R. J., and Content, J. (1971). *Nature (London) New Biol.* **230.** 140.

7

Influenza Virus Genetics

Akira Sugiura

I. Introduction—Historical Review

This section was written without the intention of reviewing all literature relevant to the genetic studies of influenza virus. This has been done in greater detail by Kilbourne (1963) and by Hoyle (1968). I have tried to follow, in roughly chronological order, only those findings which directly evolved into important concepts and theories in this field. I have also tried to attach new interpretations to some older experimental findings using the

171

current terminology and to modify some former interpretations which are no longer relevant in the light of present knowledge. The history of genetic studies of influenza viruses is divided into two periods. The first phase encompasses roughly the entire 1950's, while the developments from the early 1960's through the present will be dealt as the second period, the beginning of which was marked by the wider use of cell cultures and the adoption of plaquing technique.

A. Genetic Studies in the First Period

The first evidence of genetic interaction with influenza viruses was obtained by Burnet and Lind (1949) during the study of the interference phenomenon in the mouse brain. From mouse brains infected simultaneously with the neurotropic variant of the WS strain (NWS) and other non-neurotropic strains, WSM or SW-15, they isolated virus strains which apparently combined the characters of the two inoculum viruses, i.e., neurovirulence from NWS, and either heat-stable hemagglutinin from WSM, or serological type from SW-15. For the ensuing 10 years, Burnet and his co-workers were the main students of the genetics of influenza virus.

In 1951, Henle and Liu found that multiple infection of allantoic cells with either PR8(A) or Lee(B) viruses that had been inactivated by ultraviolet radiation or heating led to a partial restoration of lost infectivity. They interpreted the phenomenon as analogous to multiplicity reaction in T-even bacteriophage, a form of genetic interaction between different viral genomes within the same strain.

In 1952, Appleby reported the isolation of a new strain of virus from embryonated eggs which had received a mixture of NWS and Kunz strains, both inactivated by ultraviolet radiation. The new virus was serologically Kunz but behaved like NWS parent in tissue tropism, i.e., in neurovirulence and pathogenicity on intranasal inoculation in mice. Its origin was attributed to recombination.

In 1953, Hirst and Gotlieb (1953a) started to work on influenza genetics, and their group, along with Burnet's, constituted two main schools in this field in 1950's. Among other combination forms of WSN and Mel strains, they obtained X_3 virus which appeared to have inherited antigens from both parent viruses and had been stable in repeated passages in limiting dilution.

In 1955, Baron and Jensen observed that genetic traits of NWS or Wright strains, rendered noninfectious by ultraviolet radiation, could be rescued in mixed infection with active virus. The progeny virus had the genetic traits of the inactive parent and the serotype of the active parent.

Thus, the existence of genetic interaction or genetic recombination was

firmly established during this period by several groups of investigators working independently.

1. GENETIC STUDIES CONDUCTED BY BURNET AND CO-WORKERS

At the beginning of genetic studies, NWS, a neurotropic variant of WS
strain, was almost exclusively employed as a donor of genetic character because of its unique property, the ability to multiply in the mouse brain causing incoordination, paralysis, and death after intracerebral inoculation. In
the experiments of Burnet and Lind (1951a), WSM, a non-neurotropic derivative of WS, served as the other parent. Besides neurovirulence, NWS
and WSM differed in the stability of hemagglutinin. The hemagglutinating
activity of NWS was completely destroyed by heating at 54°C for 30 minutes, while the hemagglutinin of WSM withstood heating at 62°C. When
mixtures of the two viruses in suitable proportions were inoculated into
mouse brain, virus strains referred to as WS-NM were isolated, which were
neurovirulent in mice, although to a variable extent, but had hemagglutinin
as resistant to heating as that of WSM. These characters were stable for
at least two limiting dilution passages in eggs.

In the next series of experiments (Burnet and Lind, 1951b; Burnet and
Edney, 1951), a variety of genetic markers were employed in recombination
between NWS and Mel, a non-neurotropic strain belonging to a different
serological subtype from NWS. Neurotropic recombinants with the serological character of Mel, ("NM" strains) were isolated from mixedly infected
mouse brains. NM's possessed characters of the Mel parent, such as thermo-
stability of the hemagglutinin and agglutination of RDE-treated erythrocytes, properties attributable to the hemagglutinin of Mel strain. NM recombinants had, on the other hand, diminished enzymic action on ovomucin
inhibitor and did not readily elute from erythrocytes. In these characters,
they were like the NWS parent. However, they were readily converted to
the "indicator state,"* unlike either of the parent. These properties of NM
recombinants can be explained by the relatively weak and thermolabile neuraminidase activity characteristic of the NWS strain. The conversion to the
indicator state by heating requires preservation of hemagglutinating activity,
while inactivating the viral neuraminidase. Mel could not be converted to
the indicator state due to its thermostable neuraminidase. Nor could NWS
be converted, but because of its heat-labile hemagglutinin. Only when thermostable hemagglutinin of Mel and the thermolabile neuraminidase of NWS

---

* When some influenza virus strains are heated, usually at 56°C for 30 minutes,
hemagglutination becomes inhibitable by some mucoproteins to which unheated
virus is not sensitive. This state is called the "indicator state." Conversion to indicator
state is believed to be a result of inactivation of neuraminidase activity.

were combined in the NM recombinant, was it convertible to the indicator state by differential inactivation. One sees in the NM recombinant the association of genetic characters which was later to be developed into the concept of "linkage groups." Mel [HA(Mel-serotype, thermostable), NA(active, thermostable), non-neurovirulent] × NWS [HA(NWS-serotype, thermolabile), NA(weak, thermolabile), neurovirulent] → NM [HA(Mel-serotype, thermostable), NA(weak, thermolabile), neurovirulent].

From 1952 on, the WSE strain came to be used as one of the participants in genetic experiments more frequently than NWS because of its better growth in the allantoic cavity in chick embryo. The pair of WSE and Mel was probably the most intensively studied combination in the genetic studies of influenza virus. Important findings obtained from this series of experiments can be summarily listed below.

a. Phenotypic Mixing. The progeny virus from the mixed infection, particularly when the neurotropic recombinants NM were found among them, was neutralizable by both anti-Mel and anti-NWS antisera (Fraser, 1953). The anomalous hemagglutinin, as referred to by Fraser, was different from simple mixtures of Mel and NWS and indicated that a majority of virus particles has an antigenic mosaic on their surface.

b. Capability of Inactivated Virus to Participate in Genetic Interactions. Heat inactivation of one component at 56°C for 30 minutes did not prevent the appearance of recombinants of the same serological type as the heated component (Burnet and Lind, 1954b). An appropriate degree of inactivation of one parent by mild thermal inactivation at 37°C for 7 days actually facilitated the detection of recombinants. The virus inactivated by ether treatment, however, was incompetent in recombination (Fraser, 1959a).

c. Linkage Groups. Mel and either WSE or NWS differed in a number of easily recognizable characters as shown in Table 7.1. Mel was represented as *ABCDEFG*, WSE as *abcdef*, and NWS as *ab(c)(d)efg*. *c* and *d* were parenthesized for NWS, because its convertibility to the indicator state could not be tested due to its extremely heat-labile hemagglutinin. In the cross of Mel and WSE, the progeny virus fell into the patterns shown in the tabulation (Burnet and Lind, 1952).

ABDF-CE	Mel parent type
abdf-ce	WSE parent type
ABDF-ce	Recombinant M⁺
abdf-CE	Recombinant WS⁻

Table 7.1   Genetic Markers of Mel and WSE or NWS

Serological character	*A* Mel	*a* WS
Thermostability of hemagglutinin	*B* stable	*b* labile
Inhibition of heated virus by mucoids, ovomucin, or meconium inhibitor;	*C* not inhibited	*c* inhibited
sheep salivary mucin	*D* not inhibited	*d* inhibited
Pathogenicity for chick embryo[b] inoculated on chorioallantois	*E* no lesions	*e* hemorrhagic lesions
Pathogenicity for mouse lung[b]	*F* nonfatal lesions	*f* fatal consolidation
Pathogenicity for mouse brain[a]	*G* nil	*g* fatal

[a] From Burnet (1960). Reproduced by permission of the author.
[b] In the tests for pathogenicity, fluids were diluted to give one hemagglutinating dose.

When NWS was used instead of WSE with the inclusion of *Gg* marker (Lind and Burnet, 1954), the recombination took the form of

$$ABDF\text{-}CEG + ab(d)f\text{-}(c)eg \rightarrow ABDF\text{-}ceg$$
$$\text{Mel} \qquad \text{NWS} \qquad \text{NM}$$

In this case the reciprocal form of recombinant was not isolated because of the selective procedures employed. Characters *ABDF, abdf* were always linked and thus constituted one linkage group, so did the characters, *CE, ce* or *CEG, ceg,* the other. From the currently prevailing theory in influenza virus genetics that each RNA segment codes for a single polypeptide, the existence of a linkage group is inexplicable unless one assumes that all linked markers are different phenotypic expressions of one virus-coded protein. The above findings might be interpreted in the following manner. *ABD* and *abd* are clearly the phenotypes of the hemagglutinin, and *C* and *c* are those of the neuraminidase of Mel and NWS, respectively. The reason that the hemagglutination of heated Mel was not inhibited by sheep salivary mucin could be that the Mel hemagglutinin lacked the affinity for it. On the other hand, the Mel hemagglutinin might have had affinity for ovomucin or meconium inhibitor, but because its neuraminidase was heat stable and able to destroy these inhibitors even after heating, hemagglutination was not inhibited in the hemagglutination inhibition tests employed. The situation was the opposite for NWS. The character *C, c* represents the heat stability of neuraminidase, as discussed already. If this interpretation is correct, the capacity to grow in the mouse lung was determined by the NWS hemagglutinin. It should be pointed out, however, that a particular linkage of markers is only relevant to the particular combination of parent virus strains, for in the recombination between WSE and CAM, the character *F* and *f* was transferable independently from characters of the hemagglutinin (Burnet and Lind, 1955). For neurovirulence, the presence of NWS neuraminidase appeared to be indispensable, at least for the combination of NWS and other H0N1 or $H_{sw}1N1$ strains. All neurotropic recombinants obtained by Burnet and his co-workers from NWS as one parent and WSM, SW-15, Mel, or Ocean Island strains as the other possessed phenotypes attributable to NWS neuraminidase (Burnet and Lind, 1951a,b). A neurotropic recombinant, obtained independently by Appleby from the cross between NWS and Kunz strains also conformed to this pattern (Appleby, 1952). The recombinant NK was definitely of Kunz serotype in hemagglutination inhibition test as well as in neutralization *in ovo,* but was also neutralized by NWS antiserum to a very slight extent. In tissue tropism, it was as neurovirulent as the NWS parent. It also resembled NWS in its sensitivity to sputum inhibitor and low enzymic (neuraminidase) activity. NK had probably received the hemagglutinin from Kunz and the neuraminidase from NWS. The low degree of neutralization by anti-NWS antiserum could have been the suppression of multi-cycle growth in the continued presence of antibody directed to the neuraminidase (Chapter 12).

Invasiveness for the chick embryo upon chorioallantoic inoculation (character *e*) was tightly linked to mouse neurovirulence (*g*) and thermolabile NWS neuraminidase (*c*), as interpreted. The two virulence characters are likely to be different expressions of the same genotype. Fraser (1959d) compared the virulence for the above two hosts of various NM recombinant strains isolated from either mouse brain or chick embryo brain. All strains which were weakly pathogenic for chick embroys were nonpathogenic on intracerebral inoculation of mice. He concluded that the two pathogenicities were different degrees of the same inherited quality, and mouse neurovirulence could be manifested only when a certain degree of chick embryo pathogenicity had been exceeded.

d. High Frequency of Recombination.   At the time of these studies, viral clones were isolated solely from embryonated eggs infected at the limiting dilution. Minority types in the progeny could not usually be obtained, unless very large number of eggs were used. In most cases, recombinants were isolated by selective methods, such as the use of antiserum, or the restrictive host systems, or frequently both. Therefore, the recombination frequency or the proportion of recombinants among the progeny could not be determined. Only in the cross between Mel and WSE, in which both types of virus grew at nearly equal rates, was recombination looked at quantitatively (Burnet and Lind, 1952). After infection of deembryonated eggs with a high concentration of both viruses, sufficient to infect all cells simultaneously, inoculum virus was removed by the use of receptor destroying enzyme

(RDE). The first-cycle yield harvested at 6–6.5 hours was analyzed by isolating viral clones at limiting dilution and by testing markers of individual clones. Forty-one clones tested were classified as 22 Mel, 6 M^+, 9 WS^-, and 4 WSE. The recombination frequency was thus $15/41$ or 37%.

e. Redistribution of Virulence. When recombination took place between NWS and Mel in the mouse brain or in the chorioallantois of the chick embryo, selective hosts for neurotropic virus strains, neurotropic Mel (*ABDF-ceg*) was easily obtained. When the mixed infection was carried out in the allantoic cavity and progeny virus clones were isolated without a selective process, strains with combined characters *A-ce* exhibited a whole range of neuropathogenicity from virtually no virulence to the full virulence comparable to the NWS parent, but recombinants with low or equivocal neuropathogenicity predominated. These recombinants of low or intermediate pathogenicity, however, although incapable of killing adult mice on intracerebral inoculation, did multiply to a certain extent in the brain and did cause a fatal infection when inoculated into 2- to 4-day-old baby mice (Lind and Burnet, 1957b). They were at least partially neurotropic. Similar variability of expression was observed by Fraser (1959d) in the pathogenicity of NM recombinants on chorioallantoic inoculation, ranging from full virulence, i.e., invasion of the embryo with hemorrhagic lesions and eventual death, to production of well-defined foci on the chorioallantois but without invasion of the embryo. As described before, the pathogenicity for chick embryos and neurovirulence for mice were correlated.

When virulence is used as a marker, one almost inevitably encounters such variable expression, a phenomenon referred to as "redistribution of virulence" by Burnet and co-workers, and it was probably the phenomenon most difficult to explain in genetic terms. As the word "redistribution" implies, they postulated that the degree of virulence was determined by the number of copies of a putative "virulence gene" (Burnet and Lind, 1954a), independently replicating and reassorting during genetic interaction, contained in the individual viral genome, or by the number of copies of equally putative "suppressor gene" in the case of avirulent mutants (Lind and Burnet, 1958). Later workers tended rather to regard virulence as multigenic without specifying whether this meant multiple copies of the same virulence gene or that virulence was a composite character determined by more than one different genes. In interpreting genetic studies dealing with virulence as a marker, one should take the following two facts into consideration. First, the variable expression of virulence is by no means characteristic to recombinants descended from a virulent parent. Even NWS itself is more or less subject to variation, unless it is propagated in the mouse brain (which ensures that virulent forms are constantly selected against less virulent forms) or is passaged at limiting infective dilution in the allantoic cavity (so that the original characters are maintained). On low dilution passages in the latter hosts, a gradual shift toward lesser neurovirulence invariably takes place (Burnet, 1951), indicating that neurovirulence offers no advantage for the virus in this host system and that the mutation toward lesser neurovirulence is relatively frequent. Second, virulence, unlike other *in vitro* markers (such as serotype or heat stability of the hemagglutinin), is a character that can be recognized only after extensive viral multiplication and is, therefore, likely to be influenced by an alteration in any step in multi-cycle growth. For virulence to become manifest, each step must proceed with maximal efficiency. The slightest incompatibility between different genes within a genome or the introduction of an inappropriate gene, unrelated to the putative virulence gene, might derange the efficient process, leading to diminished virulence. An example can be seen in the mutation of recombinant M^+ (*ABDF-ce*) to M^+d (*AbdF'-cE*),* in which the change in the first linkage group from *ABDF* to *AbdF'*, i.e., the loss of heat-stability of the hemagglutinin, acquisition of affinity to sheep mucoid receptor, and further attenuation of mouse lung pathogenicity, was accompanied by the loss of pathogenicity for the chick embryo on chorioallantoic inoculation, the change involving the second linkage group (Burnet and Lind, 1957b). In addition, M^+d grew more slowly in the allantoic cavity than M^+. Since M^+d mutant reverted readily to the original M^+ form, double mutation affecting both linkage groups was unlikely. It is conceivable that the mutation had taken place in the gene coding for the hemagglutinin, resulting in its phenotypic modification (*ABDF→AbdF'*) and slower growth rate at the same time. Even though the gene related to the second linkage group, normally related to the virulence (and presumably coding for the neuraminidase) was unchanged and M^+d still remained potentially or genotypically virulent, the retarded growth rate of the virus deterred its expression.

2. Genetic Studies Conducted by Hirst and Gotlieb

Hirst and Gotlieb (1953) used only Mel and WSN in their studies. The latter was a neurotropic variant of NWS, equivalent to NWS, but of different derivation. Mixed infections were performed in the allantoic cavity of chick embryos. Significant findings obtained in their studies will be summarized.

a. Combination Forms with Respect to Antigenic Specificity. Double infection of the allantoic sac of chick embryos with Mel and WSN resulted in the formation of progeny virus which combined some of the antigenic prop-

---

* *F*, No killing of mouse but partial consolidation in the lung; *F'*, no consolidation.

erties of both parents. Three kinds of combination form were distinguished (Hirst and Gotlieb, 1953b).

X_1: The hemagglutinin of this form was doubly neutralizable in the same way as was discussed in Section I,A,1,a. Hemagglutinin titration of the mixed yield, carried out in the presence of antiserum to either Mel or WSN revealed that the doubly neutralizable fraction, i.e., X_1, constituted as high as 95% of the total hemagglutinin (Table 7.2). Each antiserum inhibited the hemagglutination of X_1 as efficiently as it inhibited its homologous virus. X_1 was produced only when the majority of cells were simultaneously infected with both parent viruses. It did not breed true, i.e., it reverted to either Mel or WSN and not both, when propagated at the limiting dilutions. The X_1 form arose as a result of phenotypic mixing.

X_2: This form was also doubly neutralizable in the same way as X_1. But it was distinguished from X_1 in that X_2 at the limiting infective dilution, i.e., its single infective particle, gave rise to progeny containing both Mel and WSN and occasionally X_2 in addition. X_2 could, therefore, be propagated at least for a few generations at the limiting dilution without changing its character, but it eventually segregated. It was considered to be formed by heterozygosis or diploidy.

X_3: Only one strain of this form was obtained in the entire series of experiments encompassing more than 20 passages of X_2 form. X_3 appeared to be a true and stable recombinant which bred true at least for five passages at the limiting infective dilution without giving rise to Mel or WSN. X_3 was strongly inhibited in hemagglutination by anti-WSN antiserum but, unlike X_1 or X_2, weakly inhibited (i.e., inhibited only at very high concentrations) by anti-Mel antiserum (Table 7.3). It was concluded, therefore, that X_3 possessed two antigenic specificities, the major antigen derived from WSN and the minor antigen from Mel parents. In retrospect, it is probable that X_3 was a recombinant containing the WSN hemagglutinin and Mel

Table 7.2 Double Neutralization of the Fluid from the Mixedly Infected Eggs by Mel and WSN $(P_1)^{a,b}$

	Total titer	Mel titer	WSN titer	Discrepancy (%)
P_1	1024	48	16	94
Mel	2000	2000	<32	—
WSN	2000	<32	2000	—

[a] From Hirst and Gotlieb (1953b).

[b] Mel titer was determined by hemagglutination in the presence of anti-WSN antiserum, and WSN titer in the presence of anti-Mel antiserum.

Table 7.3 Inhibition of X_3 Hemagglutinin by
Anti-Mel or Anti-WSN Antiserum[a]

	Anti-Mel	Anti-WSN
X_3	64	500
Mel	32,000	16
WSN	16	1500

[a] From Hirst and Gotlieb (1953b).

neuraminidase, weak inhibition by anti-Mel antiserum being mediated through a steric hindrance effect (Chapter 12). Neutralization of X_3 *in ovo* by anti-Mel antiserum to a greater extent than expected from its hemagglutinin-inhibition titer also argues for the above presumption, because the continued presence of antibody directed to the neuraminidase could suppress the virus yield below its detectability by hemagglutination, making the extent of neutralization appear greater than it actually is (Chapter 12).

b. Behavior of the Neurovirulence Marker. In their studies of recombination between WSN and Mel, only two markers, i.e., the presence or absence of neurovirulence for mice and the serological type, were employed. Recombinants found were very asymmetrical. While WS-type recombinants lacking neurovirulence (W⁻)* were obtained readily, the reciprocal type, i.e., neurovirulent Mel (M⁺) was not encountered (Hirst and Gotlieb, 1955). Only when Mel which had been inactivated by ultraviolet radiation was reactivated by infective WSN, was the existence of M⁺ demonstrated, although the neurovirulence of some recombinants was unstable and variable from passage to passage (Gotlieb and Hirst, 1956). However, some Mel-type progeny virus strains, non-neurovirulent on direct intracerebral inoculation into mice, were shown to be potentially or genotypically neurovirulent, because their cross with W⁻, non-neurovirulent recombinant, yielded unequivocally neurotropic WSN. This is a phenomenon analogous to redistribution of virulence observed by Burnet and co-workers (Section I,A,1,e). The virulence of M⁺ ranges from its apparent absence to that nearly equivalent to WSN, and the nonvirulent forms predominated. In phenotypically non-neurovirulent M⁺, the gene for neurovirulence appeared to be prevented from expression when it was combined with Mel serotype. Only when it was recombined with WS serotype was virulence restored to the latter.

* Note that the terms W⁺, W⁻, M⁺, and M⁻ were used under quite different denotation from those used by Burnet's group. W and M denote WS and Mel serotypes [of the hemagglutinin], while + and − denote the presence and absence of neurovirulence for mice, respectively.

c. The Role of Heterozygotes in Recombination. In a series of experiments, the mixture of Mel (M⁻) and WSN (W⁺), each at high concentration, was inoculated into either the allantoic sac of whole chick embryos or deembryonated eggs (Hirst and Gotlieb, 1955). Clones were isolated at the limiting infective dilution (the dilution at which 25% or less of eggs became infected) from mixed yields without a selective process using antiserum. Out of 220 clones isolated, 85 yielded only M type progeny and 58 only W type progeny on further passage. The remaining 77 clones gave rise to both M and W types in the next generation. These clones were, therefore, serotypic heterozygotes, or more precisely diploids, since so-called heterozygotes were often heterozygous for several factors. W progeny derived from such heterozygotes contained a strikingly high proportion of non-neurovirulent WSN (W⁻), a recombinant with respect to serotype and neurovirulence, i.e., 41 out of 77 clones. In contrast, only 2 of 58 homozygous W type clones were W⁻. Hirst and Gotlieb (1955) suggested that heterozygotes were the preliminary step leading to the formation of recombinants. Since heterozygotes were also phenotypically mixed, i.e., doubly neutralizable, the use of antiserum for the purpose of selecting a particular type of progeny greatly diminished the chance of detecting recombinants. In the studies of these authors, the proportion of heterozygotes were generally very high (in the experiment cited above, $^{77}/_{220}$ or 35% were heterozygotes). On the other hand, Lind and Burnet (1957a) found heterozygotes in lower proportion, 3 serotypic heterozygotes in 24 clones isolated from the cross between NWSE and Mel. Furthermore, they found a high proportion of recombinants, unassociated with the heterozygotes, and they did not consider that heterozygotes played any significant role in generating recombinants. Why there was such a discrepancy between the two groups cannot be explained. The existence of heterozygotes itself appears to be questionable, particularly in the light of a recent finding, the universal occurrence of aggregates of virus particles (Hirst, 1973). It seems that the role played by either heterozygotes or aggregates in the formation of recombinants is still an unsettled question.

During this first period of study, the lack of precise methods of quantitating infectious virus and reliable techniques for obtaining pure clones were the chief limitations to progress. Infectivity had to be measured by end-point titrations in the allantoic cavity of chick embryos and the only practical way of obtaining pure clones was repeated passages at limiting infective dilution also in the allantoic cavity. Any meaningful experiments required an enormous number of eggs. The situation was described by Burnet himself.

> After 10 years' study of recombination in influenza viruses and many attempts to bring the phenomena into a satisfying pattern, some of which achieved publication, the author has been forced to retreat to an almost nihilistic attitude. In all quantitative experiments the variability of the re-

sults is such that for data which would allow, for example, the recognition of a linear sequence of the genetic determinants of certain characters, experiments would be needed of a magnitude beyond the resources of any laboratory interested in the problem. It is perhaps significant that all the groups interested in influenza virus genetics have now ceased publishing reports on this topic. There is no doubt at all about the facts but no theoretical framework in which to present them (Burnet, 1960).

Despite limitations, however, it is remarkable that these earlier studies had strong influence upon subsequent studies. Nearly all important concepts still valid today, such as phenotypic mixing, heterozygosis, linkage groups, high frequency of recombination, genetic competence of inactivated virus, had already been formulated during this period.

B. Genetic Studies in the Second Period

The second period was initiated by the study conducted by Simpson and Hirst (1971), who, for the first time, applied the plaquing technique to the genetic study of influenza viruses. Despite their fruitful application of cell cultures and the plaque method and substantial technical improvements thereafter, the fastidious behavior of most influenza virus strains in cell cultures limited progress in comparison with that made with other animal viruses, which could be handled more easily in cell cultures. This problem, which still plagues us today, is the reason for the predilection of investigators for WSN, NWS, and fowl plague virus (FPV), which are good plaque-formers in many cell culture systems, in the genetic studies. Because the contemporary nature of studies during this period hardly requires description and reinterpretation in detail, the major progress will be summarized only briefly.

Simpson and Hirst (1961) employed WSN as a donor of plaque-forming character to other influenza A virus strains which did not form plaques at all or formed only faint plaques at a very low efficiency on chick embryo cells. WSN grew to high titer and formed large and clear plaques with efficiency nearly equal to that found in infection of the chick embryo in the allantoic cavity. Mixed infection of chick embryo cells with WSN, inactivated by ultraviolet radiation, and infective non-plaque-forming or poorly plaque-forming strains led to the appearance of plaques far exceeding in number those of residual infective WSN. Most of the plaques which resulted from cross-reactivation were easily distinguishable from those of WSN by their difference in plaque size and/or morphology. Virus strains isolated from such plaques usually possessed markers inherited from reactivating non-plaque-forming parents. Cross-reactivation proved a very efficient way of

obtaining recombinants, and plaque-forming recombinants of many serotypes, such as WS, Mel, PR8, FM-1, S-1, Jap305, and swine, were isolated.

In 1962, Hirst proposed the hypothesis which was to have a profound
impact on subsequent studies of influenza virus. The hypothesis consisted
of essentially two separate, although interrelated, postulates. First, he speculated that the amount of RNA contained in the influenza viral genome
varied from particle to particle. This was inferred from the physical and
morphological heterogeneity observed with virus particles in standard preparations, the imperfect manner of virus maturation, and the frequent occurrence of heterozygosis. Except for von Magnus incomplete virus, the validity
of this postulate is still far from decided today, as will be discussed in Section
V,A,3. The second proposal stated that influenza RNA occurs in subgenomic
pieces, presumably capable of semiautonomous replication and random reassortment during the process of assembly. The frequency of recombination
would not be expected to be higher than 1% considering the size of influenza
virus RNA, based on experience with DNA bacteriophages and poliovirus,
if recombination took place by a similar mechanism. The far higher rate
observed can only be explained by genetic interaction by some unusual mechanism, as postulated. The prototype of this hypothesis could be found already
in 1952 in the postulation of linkage groups (Section I,A,1,c), and a similar
mechanism of recombination was less precisely defined by Burnet (1956).
But distinction between different subgenomic pieces and multiple copies of
the same piece was not made at the time. In this hypothesis only, an extraordinary mechanism of genetic interaction was proposed explicitly. Four
years later, "the divided genome" hypothesis was partly corroborated by the
discovery of small and heterogeneous species of RNA extracted from influenza virus (Davies and Barry, 1966), which was followed by an abundance
of biophysical and chemical evidence (reviewed by Shatkin, 1971; Young
and Content, 1971; Lewandowski et al., 1971; Bishop et al., 1971; Skehel,
1971; Horst et al., 1972; Bromley and Barry, 1973) all leading to the same
conclusion.

Tumova and Pereira (1965) followed the method of Simpson and Hirst
(1961), but they chose FPV for a plaque-forming virus to be reactivated
and A2 virus as a reactivant. All of more than 50 clones derived from reactivated plaque-formers contained the hemagglutinin of FPV. However, the
strain-specific complement fixation tests revealed the presence of A2 antigen,
in addition to FPV antigen, in about half of them. The A2 antigen contained
by one of these antigenic hybrids FPV-A2(R4) was later identified as the
neuraminidase of A2 virus (Easterday et al., 1969).

Independent and contemporaneous experiments by Kilbourne and his associates (Kilbourne and Schulman, 1965; Jahiel and Kilbourne, 1966; Kilbourne et al., 1967) of recombinants of NSW (H0N1) and RI/5+ (H2N2)

viruses conclusively established with a variety of serological techniques that "antigenic hybrids" could be readily produced. These experiments were greatly facilitated by the development of a new influenza virus plaquing system in aneuploid human cells, clone 1-5C-4 (Sugiura and Kilbourne, 1965). Because many strains, including NWS, formed plaques on this cell line, all progeny virus types produced in the mixed infection could be scored, which permitted the determination of the recombination frequency. Using a two-factor cross involving serotype and plaque type, the recombination frequency was demonstrated to be as high as 34% after one-cycle growth of NWS and CAM, confirming the earlier figure obtained by Burnet and Lind (1952) (Section I,A,1,d) (Sugiura and Kilbourne, 1966).

In this system, the existence of two kinds of antigens on the viral surface was recognized by the phenomenon of plaque size reduction (Kilbourne and Schulman, 1965; Jahiel and Kilbourne, 1966) during the characterization of X-7, an antigenic hybrid virus derived from the cross between NWS and A2/RI/5+/57. Antiserum to either NWS or RI/5, incorporated in the agar overlay, exerted a markedly different effect on the formation of plaques by X-7 on clone 1-5C-4 cells. While anti-NWS antiserum either prevented the appearance of plaques completely or reduced both the number and the size of plaques concomitantly at the end point (plaque inhibition), the anti-RI/5 antiserum greatly reduced only plaque size without affecting the number over a wide range of serum concentration (plaque size reduction). Anti-RI/5 antiserum had virtually no effect on X-7 in preinoculation neutralization tests, nor inhibited the hemagglutination by X-7. Anti-NWS antiserum, on the other hand, neutralized the infectivity and inhibited hemagglutination. X-7, in addition to the hemagglutinin of, undoubtedly, NWS, contained the antigenic determinant derived from the A2 parent. Earlier, it had been found that immunization of mice with X-7 virus, then known as "X" (Kilbourne and Schulman, 1965), provided protection against challenge with either parent virus. That the A2 antigen was in fact neuraminidase was proved by Laver and Kilbourne (1966) by electrophoretic analysis of the viral structural proteins.

After X-7, Kilbourne (1968) obtained several recombinants containing the hemagglutinin of equine influenza virus and neuraminidase of human influenza viruses by a similar method. These findings, together with those of Tumova and Pereira (1965) cited already, led to the conclusion that the potential for recombination was universal for all influenza A viruses, irrespective of the host species from which they were isolated.

The demonstration of neuraminidase as a component that is antigenically distinct from the hemagglutinin and the occurrence of recombination with respect to the two components are probably the major contributions of genetic studies not only to the elucidation of virion structure but, when coupled with the recognition of genetic compatibility between human and animal viruses, also to the understanding of ecological features of influenza virus (see Chapters 9 and 15).

For many years, almost all genetic studies made use of naturally occurring virus strains differing in a number of biological properties. Whether a recognizable difference originated in a single gene or was polygenic in nature was not known. Furthermore, although an abundance of markers are apparently available for influenza viruses, most of them were probably manifestations of only few genes, particularly the ones related to the virion surface proteins. Changes in proteins situated inside the envelope could not be recognized. Fenner and Sambrook (1964) had pointed out shortcomings of this approach and stressed the importance of employing conditional lethal mutants, which had been successfully utilized in bacteriophage genetics. These are mutants which fail to yield infectious progeny under certain, easily reproducible condition, but which replicate normally or nearly normally under other conditions. Theoretically it should be possible to obtain mutants only a single step away from a parent strain or wild-type virus. Due to the absence of suppressor-sensitive mechanisms in animal cells (Fenner, 1970), most conditional lethal mutants from animal viruses are temperature-sensitive mutants.

The first isolation of temperature-sensitive conditional lethal (ts) mutants of influenza virus was reported by Simpson and Hirst (1968). Both recombination and complementation were observed between certain pairs of these mutants, and they were classified into five complementation groups. This was another turning point in the genetic study of influenza virus. Since then, many ts mutants have been isolated by various groups of workers, but these will be described in a later section.

II. The Influenza Viral Genome

Since the RNA of influenza virus and its replication are discussed in greater detail in Chapters 6 and 8, only those aspects minimally required for the understanding of genetics will be summarized below. Genetic information for producing infectious progeny virus are encoded in the virion single-stranded RNA. Polypeptides which are at present known to be synthesized in the cell infected by influenza A virus are shown in Table 7.4 (reviewed by White, 1974) (see also Chapter 2). The presence of P_2 and NS_2 has yet to be confirmed. HA and NA are glycosylated after translation. HA may then be separated to HA_1 and HA_2 by proteolytic cleavage before being incorporated into the virion, depending upon the host cells or the environ-

Table 7.4 Polypeptides Known to Be
Synthesized in Influenza
Virus A-Infected Cells[a]

Viral polypeptides	Molecular weight (10^3 daltons)
P_1	94
P_2	81
HA	75–85
NP	50–65
NA	45–65
M	21–30
NS_1	23–30
NS_2	11

[a] From White (1974).

mental condition (Cahpter 3). Enzymatically active neuraminidase is known to be a tetramer, but evidence so far obtained is conflicting as to whether it is made up of four identical subunits (NA), or two molecules each of two different subunits (NA_1 and NA_2) (Chapter 4). Therefore, the minimum number of polypeptides coded for by the viral genome would be six (P, HA, NP, NA, M, and NS), and the maximum would be nine (P_1, P_2, HA, NP, NA_1, NA_2, M, NS_1, and NS_2). Coding for these 6 to 9 gene products requires single-stranded RNA of the size range of 4×10^6 to 5×10^6 daltons. Electrophoretic analysis of RNA extracted from the virion revealed, in good agreement with the prediction, that there existed at least five, and as many as ten species, ranging from 2×10^5 to 10^6 daltons. The total amount contained in a virion was estimated to be between 4×10^6 and 5×10^6 daltons (reviewed by Shatkin, 1971; Lewandowski *et al.*, 1971; Young and Content, 1971; Bishop *et al.*, 1971; Skehel, 1971; Horst *et al.*, 1972; Bromley and Barry, 1973; see also Chapter 6). It is believed that the virion RNA's are transcribed by virion-associated RNA-dependent RNA polymerase into complementary RNA's which also occur as heterogeneous species of similar size range as virion RNA segments. Most available evidence suggests that complementary RNA's are mRNA (Pons, 1972; Kingsbury and Webster, 1973; Etkind and Krug, 1974). From approximate correspondence between RNA's and polypeptides not only in number but also in size range (maximum coding capacity of single-stranded RNA of 2×10^5 to 10^6 daltons is polypeptides of 22×10^3 to 110×10^3 daltons), it is tempting to speculate that each RNA segment is a monocistronic message (Skehel, 1972). Hybridization study of virion RNA's and double-stranded RNA present in infected cells indicates that most RNA segments have unique base sequences and replicate independently (Content and Duesberg, 1971; Bromley and Barry, 1973). Synthesis of virion RNA's presumably proceeds on complementary RNA's as template. The RNA-dependent RNA polymerase catalyzing this reaction has not been characterized, but it is apparently distinct from the virion-associated transcriptase, because the transcriptase was blocked by actinomycin D in infected cells (Bean and Simpson, 1973), while the replication of virion RNA continued unaffected by the presence of the drug (Scholtissek and Rott, 1970; Pons, 1973). A probable candidate is the RNA-dependent RNA polymerase synthesized in the infected cell, which is different from virion-associated transcriptase in ionic requirement in *in vitro* reactions (Horisberger and Guskey, 1974). Close association of NP subunits with both virion RNA and complementary RNA indicates that the ribonucleoprotein, rather than free RNA plays an important role as the replicating and functional form of the viral genome (Duesberg, 1969; Pons, 1971, 1972). Persistence of reactivable genome in the cells for as long as 16–17 hours (Gotlieb and Hirst, 1956; Kilbourne, 1960) without being inactivated intracellularly by ribonuclease can also be explained by its existence as RNP, which is more resistant to the enzyme than free RNA (Pons *et al.,* 1969). It had been postulated that influenza viral genome is a continuous structure in which RNA segments are held together by the protein backbone formed by NP subunits (Pons, 1970). Such a mechanism would impose a certain degree of orderliness on the replication and assembly of RNA, ensuring that all RNA segments are assembled for maturation.

Influenza virus B has not been studied as intensively as influenza virus A. Virtually no work has been done on its RNA. However, in view of its morphological and functional resemblance, similar structural components (Laver and Baker, 1972; Oxford, 1973), and comparable efficiency of recombination (Tobita and Kilbourne, 1974), the genome of influenza virus B is unlikely to be significantly different from that of influenza virus A.

III. Mutation, Variation, Adaptation, and Host-Controlled Modification

A. Mutation and Variation

The terms "mutation" and "variation" are sometimes employed interchangeably, but more often with different connotations. Mutation might be defined as a change in inheritable character caused by alteration of the genome. Variation, on the other hand, usually implies the change resulting from a complex series of mutations and ensuing process of selection, but it sometimes includes changes not necessarily attributable to mutation, as

in the case of antigenic variation involving antigenic shift. Antigenic variation or antigenic change of mainly surface glycoproteins occurring in nature
will be fully discussed in Chapter 10 and therefore will not be dealt here.

There is no experimental evidence which substantiates the generally held
notion that influenza virus is notoriously labile or unusually mutable among
animal viruses. On this point, however, the scarcity of data relevant to mutation in influenza virus is rather surprising. In one of few studies focused
on mutation, the mutation rate from sensitivity to resistance to β inhibitor
in the bovine serum has been calculated to be 0.7×10^{-8} to 3.3×10^{-8} per
particle per duplication for different strains of influenza virus (Medill-Brown
and Briody, 1955). This is about $\frac{1}{1000}$ of the rate of mutation yielding d^+
character in poliovirus (Dulbecco and Vogt, 1958), or slightly lower than
the rate of acquisition of guanidine resistance in poliovirus (Carp, 1963).
Wild-type fowl plague virus gave rise to small plaque mutant k with an
unusually high frequency (Staiger, 1964). Unfortunately, however, this phenomenon has not been studied since, and whether it was truly caused by
mutation is not known. Certain chemicals which modify the structure of
RNA or interfere with correct base pairing during its replication significantly
raise mutational frequency and are used as mutagens. The frequency of isolation of ts mutants of influenza virus with or without the use of mutagens
is not very different from that in other viruses. The impression of high mutability probably originated in the unique epidemiological features of influenza
virus involving frequent antigenic variation (Chapters 10 and 15).

B. Adaptation

Adaptation means to obtain spontaneous mutants, often, but not necessarily, multi-step, that have survival advantage in a particular host or under
a particular environmental condition, namely, an attempt to bring about
variation in a direction which an experimenter desires. A classical and probably best-studied example of the change associated with adaptation is O–D
variation (reviewed by Burnet, 1955). Certain strains of influenza A virus
(H0N1 and H1N1), on primary isolation from human materials, grow only
in the amniotic cavity of chick embryo. Infected amniotic fluid agglutinates
human or guinea pig red blood cells but not chicken cells. The virus of
such characters was said to be in the "O" or original phase. During passages in the amniotic cavity, virus acquires the capacity to agglutinate
chicken, as well as human or guinea pig erythrocytes. This change is accompanied by the capacity to multiply also in the allantoic cavity. This character
of the virus was referred to as "D" or derivative phase. Passages of the
O virus at the limiting dilution maintain its character, but passages at the

low dilution inevitably lead to the change from O to D phase. Burnet and Bull's interpretation was that O virus constantly gave rise to mutant D form at an estimated rate of about 10^{-5} per particle per duplication, which was better fitted to the growth in and multiplied faster in the avian host than O virus. If a dilute inoculum containing only O particles initiates infection in the amniotic cavity, it would reach the final titer before the emergence of significant number of D form, and the resultant amniotic fluid would still retain the character of O virus. On the other hand, however, if a large inoculum containing even a small number of D particles is employed, the D form would gradually overgrow O virus. The rule that limiting dilution passages perpetuate original characters while low dilution passages favor the change (namely, the emergence and predominance of mutant forms with survival advantage in the given condition) was shown to hold for a number of other instances, such as morphological change of virus particles from filamentous to spherical forms (Burnet and Lind, 1957a) and diminution of neurovirulence of NWS on egg passages (Burnet, 1951).

C. Host-Controlled Modification

Host-controlled modification is the change in a viral phenotype determined by the host cell in which the virus has been grown. Because all viral polypeptides are coded for by the viral genome, they are the same regardless of the host cells. However, all carbohydrates and lipids contained in the virus and the way they are incorporated are under the genetic control of the host cell.

1. MODIFICATION OF VIRAL GLYCOPROTEINS

Glycoproteins, the hemagglutinin and neuraminidase, are partly determined by the host cell which provides enzymes necessary for the synthesis of carbohydrates and the glycosylation of virus-coded polypeptides. Therefore, glycoproteins of viruses from different cells may show different electrophoretic mobilities when analyzed in polyacrylamide gel and different stabilities to various dissociating conditions (Haslam et al., 1970; Schulze, 1970). Furthermore, the total amount of glycoprotein contained by virions may vary with the host cell (Lazarowitz et al., 1973). Highly purified virus grown in the allantoic cavity contains an antigen present in normal allantoic fluid (Knight, 1944). This host antigen was shown to be a high molecular weight carbohydrate attached covalently to protein, probably to the hemagglutinin (Harboe, 1963a,b; Haukenes et al., 1965; Laver and Webster, 1966). A recent report suggests the presence of host antigen also in the neuraminidase (Haheim and Haukenes, 1973).

2. MODIFICATION OF THE VIRAL ENVELOPE

Because the envelope of influenza virus and related viruses is derived from host cell plasma membrane during budding, the chemical composition of lipids and glycolipids of the envelope (and hence of virus particles) closely resembles that of the plasma membrane (Frommhagen *et al.*, 1959; Klenk and Choppin, 1969, 1970). Varying sensitivity of viral infectivity to phospholipase C is probably based on the difference in lipid composition. Virus grown in the allantoic cavity was resistant to phospholipase C, while virus of the same strain grown in chick embryo fibroblast cells in culture is highly sensitive (Simpson and Hauser, 1966). The blood group and Forssman antigens present in the virus are glycolipids derived from host cells (Rott *et al.*, 1966; Klenk *et al.*, 1972; Haheim and Haukenes, 1973).

3. MODIFICATON BY PROTEOLYTIC ENZYMES

The extent to which the HA polypeptide is cleaved into HA_1 and HA_2 before incorporation into virions is often determined by host cells. WSN and $RI/5^-$ strains, when grown in the allantoic cavity, contain more extensively cleaved HA than when grown in primary monkey kidney cells (Lazarowitz *et al.*, 1973; see Chapter 3). In Sendai virus, the cleavage of one glycopeptide by proteolytic enzymes of the host cell is apparently an essential step for the acquisition of hemolytic and cell fusion activity and infectivity (Homma and Ohuchi, 1973; Scheid and Choppin, 1974). No similar mechanism is known for influenza virus. But in view of the fact that the addition of proteolytic enzymes into cultures infected with influenza virus greatly facilitates multi-cycle growth of some virus strains (Came *et al.*, 1968; Tobita and Kilbourne, 1974; Appleyard and Maber, 1974), a similar situation might exist also for influenza virus.

IV. Genetic Markers

Because of the large number of genetic studies carried out with influenza virus, many markers have been described. Some are still useful, but many of them will be of little practical value for future studies. Regardless of their usefulness, markers frequently used in the past will be reviewed here with an attempt to clarify, wherever possible, the genetic basis of these markers from present knowledge.

A. Markers Based on the Phenotype of the Virus

1. PHENOTYPES ATTRIBUTABLE TO THE HEMAGGLUTININ

a. Serotype.   The serotype of the hemagglutinin is the most well-characterized marker of the hemagglutinin. It can be identified by a variety of immunological methods, (hemagglutination inhibition, neutralization, plaque inhibition (Jahiel and Kilbourne, 1966), or immunodiffusion, with the reservation that the antibody to the neuraminidase sometimes causes hemagglutination inhibition or neutralization (Chapter 10). An antigenic hybrid within the hemagglutinin itself has not been obtained. Antigenic hybrids so far described, containing unequal proportions of both parent antigens, demonstrable by hemagglutination inhibition or neutralization (Appleby, 1952; Hirst and Gotlieb, 1953b), were probably antigenic hybrids that had received the hemagglutinin from one parent and the neuraminidase from the other.

b. Heat Stability of Hemagglutinating Activity.   In recombination between WSE and Mel, the difference in heat stability was attributable to the hemagglutinin, because the heat stability was linked to the serotype of the hemagglutinin (Section I,A,1,c). With some *ts* mutants in which the hemagglutinin was affected, hemagglutinating activity was markedly heat labile (M. Ueda, K. Tobita, and A. Sugiura, unpublished). There have been other instances, however, where heat stability was segregated from the serotype of the hemagglutinin during recombination (Simpson and Hirst, 1961; Tumova and Pereira, 1965; McCahon and Schild, 1971), suggesting that the heat stability of hemagglutinating activity could be determined also by some other virus-coded structural component(s).

c. Stability of Hemagglutinating Activity to Chemicals or Enzymes.   Stability to sodium dodecyl sulfate (Simpson, 1964) or guanidine hydrochloride (David-West, 1973) is probably the property of the hemagglutinin. But stability to trypsin treatment, i.e., to the proteolytic cleavage of the hemagglutinin spikes from the envelope, does not appear to be determined exclusively by the hemagglutinin, since this character can be segregated from the hemagglutinin serotype (Kilbourne, 1963; Kilbourne, *et al.,* 1972).

d. Affinity for Receptor.   The capacity of virus to agglutinate erythrocytes of different animal species or those treated with RDE is determined primarily by the affinity of the hemagglutinin for the receptor substance. However, visible hemagglutination, being the combined result of viral attachment to the receptor and the subsequent elution through the enzymatic destruction of the receptor substance, can also be influenced by the neuraminidase. The example is seen in X-7 (H0N2), a recombinant between NWS (H0N1) and A/RI/5$^+$/57 (H2N2). Despite the inability of both parental viruses to elute from chicken erythrocytes, X-7 eluted rapidly. The "new" phenotype conferred during genetic interaction apparently resulted from a combination of low affinity of HO, compared to H2, for the erythrocyte receptor and the high neuraminidase activity of N2 (Laver and Kilbourne, 1966). Affinity of the hemagglutinin for certain receptor substances is sometimes manifested by the sensitivity to hemagglutination inhibition by these substances. Heated preparations of WSE were sensitive to sheep salivary gland mucin, while heated Mel were not. These properties were linked to the hemagglutinin serotype of the respective viruses (Section I,A,1,c). There are two contrasting types of H2N2 virus strains isolated in 1957 which differ strikingly in sensitivity to inhibitor contained in the normal horse serum (Choppin and Tamm, 1960). Circumstantial evidence indicates that the difference resides in the hemagglutinin, probably in the different affinity of the hemagglutinin for the inhibitor, rather than in the neuraminidase (Choppin and Tamm, 1960; Sugiura *et al.,* 1961; McCahon and Schild, 1971). Intensive effort to segregate inhibitor sensitivity from hemagglutinin serotype through genetic recombination has been unrewarding (E. D. Kilbourne, unpublished data).

Because the hemagglutinin is a single gene product, a covariation may be observed in the above markers (*a, b, c,* and *d*) when mutation takes place, as exemplified by the mutation of M$^+$ to M$^+$d (Section I,A,1,c).

2. Phenotypes Attributable to the Neuraminidase

Although, it has not been resolved whether the neuraminidase is composed of one or two kinds of polypeptides, no genetic finding so far suggests its dual genetic control. Obvious difference in quantity of neuraminidase per virion will be described below (Section IV,A,2,d).

a. Serotype. The serotype can be identified by neuraminidase inhibition, plaque size reduction, or by immunodiffusion tests. It can sometimes be identified also by hemagglutination inhibition.

b. Stability. Heat stability of the neuraminidase can be tested directly *in vitro* (Drzeniek *et al.,* 1966; Palese *et al.,* 1974). A marker often employed before the introduction of *in vitro* neuraminidase assay, the convertibility to "indicator" state to a certain inhibitor is essentially a test of the heat stability of the neuraminidase, on the condition that the hemagglutinating activity is not destroyed by the heating and that the hemagglutinin does have affinity for the inhibitor in question. Stability to guanidine hydrochloride was reported to be correlated with serotypes of the neuraminidase (David-West, 1973).

c. Enzyme Activity.   Low neuraminidase activity of NWS and WSN as contrasted with high activity of other virus strains has often been utilized as a marker (Appleby, 1952; Burnet and Lind, 1951a,b; Burnet and Edney, 1951; Hobson *et al.*, 1968). However, the enzyme activity is also determined by substrates. The neuraminidase of WSN, the activity of which was low on fetuin as a substrate, was as active as that of N2-containing virus strains when tested on a low molecular synthetic substrate, methoxyphenylacetyl-α-neuraminic acid (Palese *et al.*, 1973). The rate of elution of the virus from red blood cells is partly determined by neuraminidase activity, but again the affinity of the hemagglutinin for the erythrocyte receptor is another factor involved. Biochemical parameters of the neuraminidase, such as pH optima, K_m, and substrate specificity may also serve as genetic markers. NWS neuraminidase, compared with WS neuraminidase, showed a restricted range of substrate specificity. NWS enzyme was active on human α-glycoprotein or ovomucin, but was unable to cleave sialic acid from porcine submaxillary gland mucin. WS was active on all three substrates. Because porcine submaxillary gland mucin contained predominantly *N*-glycolylneuraminic acid, it was suggested that WS could liberate both *N*-acetyl- and *N*-glycolylneuraminic acid, while NWS could liberate only the *N*-acetyl form (Jameson and Levine, 1965).

d. Amount of Neuraminidase Contained by a Virion.   There have been a number of observations indicating that there is a severalfold difference in the amount of neuraminidase synthesized in infected cells and incorporated into a virion (Webster *et al.*, 1968; Webster and Campbell, 1972; Palese and Schulman, 1974; Mowshowitz and Kilbourne, 1974). It is clearly a genetically determined character of a virus strain. No satisfactory explanation is available at present for this puzzling phenomenon from a genetic standpoint.

3. MORPHOLOGY OF THE VIRION

Allantoic fluid preparations of virus strains which have not been adapted to the allantoic cavity often contain mainly filamentous virions. Adaptation to growth in the allantoic cavity is accompanied by a change from filamentous to spherical forms. The original filamentous morphology, however, can be maintained if the passage is done at the limiting dilution (Burnet and Lind, 1957a). These findings suggest that morphology is a genetically determined trait, subject to frequent mutation from filamentous to spherical forms, and that the latter form has a survival advantage over the former in the allantoic cavity. Definitive evidence for morphology as a genetically determined character came from the recombination between spherical PR8 and filamentous A2 virus strains which gave rise to spherical A2 and filamentous PR8 serotypes in the progeny (Kilbourne and Murphy, 1960). Morphology was linked to neither serotype of the hemagglutinin nor to that of the neuraminidase, but the change from filamentous to spherical form was associated with increased growth capacity in the allantoic cavity and higher mouse lung pathogenicity (Kilbourne and Murphy, 1960; Kilbourne *et al.,* 1971). It is unknown which viral structural protein(s) determines morphology. Virion morphology, besides being a genetic trait, is also modified by environmental condition. The addition of vitamin A alcohol to the allantoic cavity resulted in the formation of large number of filamentous PR8 virions, which were predominantly spherical in the absence of vitamin A (Blough, 1964).

B. Markers Demonstrable as a Consequence of Virus Multiplication

Such markers as host range, pathogenicity, or plaque-type have been extensively employed for influenza virus, but they are less well characterized than markers based on phenotypes of the virion. This is partly because of the still incomplete understanding of biochemical steps in viral replication and partly because of the inevitably polygenic nature of these markers, in the sense that multi-cycle growth of virus requires participation and coordination of all gene products as discussed in Section I,A,1,e.

1. HOST RANGE

Influenza virus can attach to, penetrate, and initiate infection in a uniquely wide range of cells, both in terms of animal species and kinds of tissues or organs. In most cases, however, it results in abortive infection, i.e., RNA's of both complementary and virion type and proteins are synthesized but very little infectious virus is produced (Schlesinger, 1950; Isaacs and Fulton, 1953; Henle *et al.,* 1955; Lerner and Hodge, 1969; Haslam *et al.,* 1970; Choppin and Pons, 1970; Sugiura, 1972). The cause of abortive infection apparently resides in a relatively late stage of viral replication. It is not known whether the same step is blocked in all virus–cell systems leading to abortive infection. The abortive infection in which migration of RNP antigen from the nucleus to the cytoplasm is prevented (Franklin and Breitenfeld, 1959; Hillis *et al.,* 1960; Löffler *et al.,* 1962; Ter Meulen and

Love, 1967; Ghandi *et al.,* 1971) and the abortive infection in which the migration occurs normally (Sugiura *et al.,* 1962; Fraser, 1967; Pristasova *et al.,* 1967; Zavadova *et al.,* 1968; Fedova and Tumova, 1968) may have defects at different steps (see also Chapter 8).

The distinction between productive and abortive infections is not absolute, for even in abortive infection, a small amount of infectious virus, although insufficient for continued multi-cycle growth, is sometimes produced (Choppin and Pons, 1970; Sugiura and Ueda, 1971).

Host range markers are usually tested by plaque formation on given cells. Plaque formation, requiring the production of infectious virus exceeding a certain limit in each cycle of multi-step growth, may be a too rigorous criterion for a host range marker. Virus clones which have received the gene(s) necessary for productive infection during recombination would produce varying amounts of infectious progeny, but usually less than the productive parent. This is probably the reason why the plaque-forming character was significantly less frequent among the progeny from a cross between plaque-forming and non-plaque-forming viruses (Tobita, 1971). Comparison of virus yield per cell would have provided a more appropriate criterion for the host range marker.

In crosses between FPV and either A2 virus strains of 1957 (H2N2) or the Hong Kong strain (H3N2), the hemagglutinin (but not the neuraminidase) of FPV appeared to be essential for plaque formation on chick embryo cells and for virulence for the chick embryo (Tumova and Pereira, 1965; McCahon and Schild, 1971). FPV, inactivated by ultraviolet light or ethylene iminoquinone, was reactivated by live H2N2 or H3N2 viruses. In the absence of selection, markers of a live parent usually predominate the progeny. Nevertheless, all clones isolated from plaques on chick embryo cells had FPV hemagglutinin. In contrast, many of these clones contained neuraminidase of N2 type, indicating that the FPV neuraminidase could be replaced by N2 without impairing the plaque-forming property (McCahon and Schild, 1971).

2. PATHOGENICITY

Whether a virus is pathogenic by a particular route of inoculation depends on the capability of the virus to produce infectious progeny virus in the cells at or around the site of inoculation. Host range and pathogenicity are considered as essentially the same phenomenon at different levels. For the same reason, therefore, a criterion for pathogenicity, as judged by cumulative virus growth, might be as stringent as plaque formation for a host range marker. This might also partially explain the redistribution of virulence (Section I,A,1,e). The possible association of neurovirulence with NWS neuraminidase, and mouse lung pathogenicity with the hemagglutinin of either NWS or WSE, in recombination between Mel and NWS or WSE has been already mentioned (Section I,A,1,c). Mayer *et al.* (1972) examined NWS, A2/Jap/305, and recombinants of them (H0N2 and H2N1) by a sensitive test for neurovirulence—virus multiplication in the brain of immunosuppressed mice. Neither H0N2 nor H2H1 was as fully virulent as NWS, but both of them, unlike the A2 parent, multiplied to a limited extent in the brain. Their conclusion was that the neurovirulence was linked to neither the hemagglutinin or neuraminidase exclusively. The finding, in addition to the above conclusion, suggests the distinction of H2 and H3 from H0 and H1 in terms of potentiality for neurovirulence. It might be postulated that H0 and H1 hemagglutinins are associated with incomplete but cryptic neurovirulence, i.e., a limited multiplication in the brain, the combination with NWS neuraminidase permitting the full expression of virulence. On the other hand, H2 and H3 hemagglutinins are not associated with the growth. The introduction of NWS neuraminidase results only in a slight increase in the virus growth. The above postulate will explain why the neurovirulence was linked to NWS neuraminidase in the cross between Mel and NWS, while it was under dual genetic control in the cross between A2 and NWS. Supporting evidence is the growth capability of CAM (H1N1) in the mouse brain, although to a limited extent, found by the same authors, and a similarly limited but definite growth of Mel in the brain of very young mice (Fraser, 1959b).

Mouse lung pathogenicity after intranasal inoculation is more complex. Most influenza virus strains are probably endowed with potential pathogenicity, since they can be more readily adapted to mouse lung than to mouse brain. There have been instances in which mouse lung virulence was apparently linked to the hemagglutinin (Mel × WSE or NWS, Burnet and Lind, 1952), to the neuraminidase (WSE × CAM, Burnet and Lind, 1955; WSE × SW, Burnet and Lind, 1956) or to neither(A2 × PR8, Kilbourne and Murphy, 1960; Hong Kong × PR8, Kilbourne *et al.*, 1971; A/England/939/69 × PR8, McCahon and Schild, 1972). Which gene product further promotes the growth of a particular virus strain in the mouse lung might vary depending on the combination of virus strains.

Linkage of chick embryo lethality with the FPV hemagglutinin in the cross between FPV and the Hong Kong virus strain has been mentioned in Section IV,B,1.

3. GROWTH CAPACITY IN THE ALLANTOIC CAVITY OF
   CHICK EMBRYOS

Association of growth capacity with the spherical morphology of the virion has been described (Section IV,A,3). Lack of linkage of the growth capacity to either of the hemagglutinin or neuraminidase has been shown in a number of combinations (A2 × PR8, Kilbourne and Murphy, 1960; Hong Kong × PR9, Kilbourne *et al.*, 1971; A/England/939/69 × PR8, McCahon and Schild, 1972).

4. PLAQUE TYPE

The size and morphology of plaques are seemingly convenient markers but they are poorly characterized. The mechanism and genetic basis of their manifestation are completely obscure. Increased uptake of neutral red by cells infected with certain virus strains, producing red bordered plaques, *r* character (Sugiura and Kilbourne, 1966), is believed to be related to the activation of lysosomal enzymes and therefore to the mode of the initiation of cytopathic effect (Allison and Mallucci, 1965).

C. Conditional Lethal Mutants

1. TEMPERATURE-SENSITIVE (*ts*) MUTANTS

The *ts* mutants provide the most useful markers in the genetic studies of animal viruses. So much space is devoted to the discussion of *ts* mutants in other sections that only contrasting features of *ts* mutants to other markers will be pointed out below.

1. The genome of *ts* mutants may be identical to that of the wild-type virus except in a single locus. With such mutants, the question of compatibility of genes or polygenic control of a marker would not arise.

2. The mutation can take place, at least theoretically, in all genes. Therefore, the use of *ts* mutants may greatly broaden the scope of genetic analysis, possibly to the entire genome.

3. The *ts* mutants, if they are sufficiently low reverting and nonleaky, can provide a powerful resolution. While the difference in the virus yield is of the order of only 100-fold between productive and abortive infections (Sugiura *et al.*, 1969; Choppin and Pons, 1970), some *ts* mutants exhibit over 10^6-fold difference between permissive and nonpermissive temperatures.

2. HOST RANGE MUTANTS

Host range mutants of influenza virus have not been obtained. They have been isolated from vesicular stomatitis virus, which in many respects resembles influenza virus (Simpson and Obijeski, 1974). In view of the possible participation of the host cell genome in viral replication (Borland and Mahy, 1968; Mahy *et al.*, 1972) and a marked dependence of successful maturation on host cells, a similar effort to look for host range mutants of influenza virus seems to be worthwhile.

V. Genetic Interactions

A. Genetic Recombination

1. Recombination in Influenza A Virus

In order for genetic recombination to be studied from the quantitative viewpoint, the following requirements should be fulfilled in experimental design.

1. Mixed infection should be carried out under conditions that permit nearly balanced replication of two virus strains.
2. All cells present in the system should be infected simultaneously with both virus strains. The inoculum virus should be removed as completely as possible before the emergence of progeny virus.
3. The progeny virus should be assayed in a host cell system in which all infective progeny virus particles can be registered.
4. Markers should be well characterized and identifiable without ambiguity.

Inoculation of high concentration of virus, as required by the simultaneous infection of all cells with both types of virus, inescapably leads more or less to the occurrence of the von Magnus phenomenon. One should, therefore, interpret the results always on the assumption that infective virus is genotypically representative, at least for the markers employed, of the total progeny virus, consisting predominantly of incomplete virus.

Among recombination studies using naturally existing virus strains, the experiments reported by Tobita (1971, 1972) were conducted approximately in conformity with the above requirements. Mixed infection was carried out in the human conjunctival cell line, clone 1-5C-4 (Kilbourne, 1969) with NWS (H0N1) and Hong Kong (H3N2) strains, both of which formed plaques with comparable efficiency on the above cells. Progeny virus clones were isolated randomly from plaques formed on the same cells in the absence of selective pressure and were tested for the serotype of the hemagglutinin and neuraminidase. The frequency of four possible genotypes among 191 progeny clones, obtained from four separate experiments is presented in

Table 7.5 Genotypes of Progeny Virus Obtained from Mixed Yields of NWS (H0N1) and Hong Kong (H3N2) Viruses[a]

Genotypes	Expt. 1	Expt. 2	Expt. 3	Expt. 4	Totals
H0N1	15[b]	4	7	7	33
H3N2	14	30	30	28	102
H0N2	7	8	7	9	31
H3N1	3	8	6	8	25
Totals	39	50	50	52	191
No. of recombinants	10	16	13	17	56
Recombinants (%)	25.6	32.0	26.0	32.8	29.3

[a] From Tobita (1971, 1972).
[b] Number of clones.

Table 7.5. The proportion of recombinants was fairly constant from experiment to experiment. The average recombination frequency was 29.3%, which confirmed the values given by previous workers [Burnet and Lind, 1952 (Section I,A,1,d) ; Sugiura and Kilbourne, 1966 (Section I,B)].

With the use of *ts* mutants, similar experiments have been done on a larger scale and with more ease. Illustrative examples of mixed infection between certain *ts* mutants of WSN showing the presence and absence of recombination are presented in Tables 7.6 and 7.7, respectively. Recombination frequency (%) is calculated by the following formula.

$$\frac{[AB_{33}]_{39.5} - ([A_{33}]_{39.5} + [B_{33}]_{39.5})}{[AB_{33}]_{33}} \times 100 \times 2$$

$[X_{33}]_{39.5}$ is the titer of the virus grown at 33°C but assayed at 39.5°C. A and B denote single yields, and AB the mixed yield. The degree of complementation is expressed by the complementation level defined as

$$\frac{[AB_{39.5}]_{33} - [AB_{39.5}]_{39.5}}{[A_{39.5}]_{33} + [B_{39.5}]_{33}}$$

Recombination frequency is derived from the proportion of ts^+ (wild-type) recombinants among the progeny produced at the permissive temperature after subtraction of appropriate controls. This value is multiplied by 2 on the assumption that the same number of reciprocal ts^{--} recombinants are present in the progeny. On the other hand, the complementation level represents the amount of virus which has managed to replicate at the nonpermissive temperature, despite its *ts* character, in comparison with the single infection controls.

Table 7.6　Virus Yields after Single and Mixed Infections with ts-3 and ts-8[a,b]

Inoculum viruses	Incubation temp (°C)	10 hour yield (PFU/ml) assayed at	
		33°C	39.5°C
ts-3	33	9,200,000	78,000
	39.5	34,000	20
ts-8	33	5,300,000	<3
	39.5	720	<3
ts-3 × ts-8	33	23,000,000	1,600,000
	39.5	18,000,000	500,000

[a] From Sugiura et al. (1972).

[b] ts-3 (8.8 PFU/cell), ts-8 (6.7 PFU/cell), or the mixture thereof (the same multiplicity as in single infection for each mutant) were inoculated into cultures of MDBK cells in duplicate. One set of cultures were incubated at the permissive temperature (33°C), the other at the nonpermissive temperature (39.5°C). Titration of progeny virus was done by plaque assay on MDBK cells at the two temperatures.

Recombination frequency:

$$\frac{1,600,000 - (7800 + 0)}{23,000,000} \times 100 \times 2 = 14.0\%$$

Complementation level

$$\frac{18,000,000 - 500,000}{34,000 + 720} = 504$$

Results so far obtained clearly show the "occurrence or nonoccurrence" pattern of recombinational event among mutants. Between mutants with a relatively low reversion rate and a low degree of leakiness, recombination either occurred at a frequency ranging from 2 to 33% or was not detectable at the level of 0.02%. Mutants could be divided into groups or clusters within which no recombination occurs. Such a pattern of recombination implies that it takes place primarily as an exchange of gene segments. The results obtained by Mackenzie (1970), which he considered to indicate a linear map for the viral genome, are also compatible with the above scheme. They show that mutants are divided into five clusters within which recombination does not occur, with some exceptions, but between which a frequency of over 2% is recorded.

The presence of intragenic recombination by a mechanism such as crossing-over cannot be definitely ruled out at present. But if it does exist, as in poliovirus (Cooper, 1969; Cooper et al., 1971), a frequency up to 0.3% may be expected from the comparison of the size of poliovirus genome and

Table 7.7 Virus Yields after Single and Mixed Infections with *ts*-1 and *ts*-6[a,b]

Inoculum viruses[c]	Incubation temp (°C)	10 hour yield (PFU/ml) assayed at	
		33°C	39.5°C
ts-1	33	11,000,000	200
	39.5	900	27
ts-6	33	25,000,000	110
	39.5	210	13
ts-1 × *ts*-6	33	28,000,000	120
	39.5	1,500	27

[a] From Sugiura *et al.* (1972).
[b] Methods were the same as described in Table 7.6.
[c] Multiplicity: *ts*-1, 4.8 PFU/cell; *ts*-6, 6.7 PFU/cell.

Recombination frequency

$$\frac{120 - (200 + 110)}{28,000,000} \times 100 \times 2 = <7.2 \times 10^{-6}\%$$

Complementation level

$$\frac{1,500 - 27}{900 + 210} = 1.3$$

influenza virus RNA segments. A frequency of this order would be easily detectable with a suitable combination of *ts* mutants. There has so far been no finding suggestive of intragenic recombination.

Sugiura *et al.* (1972) did not find a discrepancy between the occurrence of recombination and complementation. This supports the presumption that each subgenomic segment is a monocistronic message (Skehel, 1972). On the other hand, Simpson and Hirst (1968) and Markushin and Ghendon (1973) described certain complementing pairs of mutants in which recombination was absent. The discrepancy between recombination and complementation, suggesting either intragenic complementation or the presence of two genes in one piece of RNA segment, must be resolved by further study.

Recombination frequency is often quite variable from experiment to experiment. Up to 30-fold (Mackenzie, 1970; Hirst, 1973) or severalfold (Sugiura *et al.*, 1972) fluctuation has been encountered with the same pair of mutants in supposedly identical experimental condition. According to Mackenzie (1970), the addition of RDE to the culture fluid after virus adsorption stabilized the frequency. He also included the same standard cross in all experiments and, with the use of RDE and by relating the observed recombination frequency between a certain pair to the value obtained in the standard cross, could minimize the variability. The reproducibility thus achieved, it was claimed, enabled him to demonstrate additivity of recombination frequency between a number of mutants and to construct a linearly arranged map. The same technique, however, was not successful in the system used by Hirst (1973). At present, whether or not genes are arranged in order cannot be answered conclusively.

Another outstanding feature of recombination invariably observed is that the input multiplicity can be lowered without significantly reducing the recombination frequency over a wide range (Simpson and Hirst, 1968; Mackenzie, 1970; Sugiura et al., 1972; Hirst, 1973). At the multiplicity of $\frac{1}{10}$ PFU/cell of each virus, where only 5% of total infected cells receive both viruses, recombination frequency is expected to drop to $\frac{1}{20}$ of the maximum level. The reduction is, however, actually less than twofold (Sugiura et al., 1972). This would be explicable only by assuming the presence of particles that are noninfective in an ordinary sense but capable of giving rise to infective recombinants as a consequence of genetic interaction with other virus (Section V,A,3).

2. RECOMBINATION WITH INFLUENZA B VIRUSES

Recombination between Lee and Mil strains of influenza virus B was demonstrated by Perry and Burnet (1953) and Perry et al. (1954). They obtained recombinants which contained the hemagglutinin of Mil type in serological specificity, heat stability, and receptor affinity, but inherited mouse lung pathogenicity from the Lee parent, and reciprocal recombinants, avirulent Lee.

Tobita and Kilbourne (1974) infected chick embryo cells with Lee and B/Massachusetts/1/71, antigenically distinguishable from Lee both in the hemagglutinin and neuraminidase, and isolated plaques randomly which developed in the absence of selective pressure. Clones were tested for markers, the serotype of the hemagglutinin and the neuraminidase. Thirty-one clones examined were divided into the following types

$$H_{Lee} - N_{Lee} \qquad 3 \text{ clones}$$
$$H_{Mass} - N_{Mass} \qquad 8 \text{ clones}$$
$$H_{Lee} - N_{Mass} \qquad 2 \text{ clones}$$
$$H_{Mass} - N_{Lee} \qquad 18 \text{ clones}$$

Twenty out of 31 clones (64%) were recombinants with respect to two surface antigens. Influenza virus B is, thus, not different from influenza virus A in terms of high recombination frequency.

Despite the efficient recombination both within type A and type B influenza viruses, intertypic recombinant has not been obtained.

3. Mechanism of Recombination

Features of recombination so far known for influenza virus bear a striking resemblance to those in reovirus. Statistical analysis of recombination frequency between reovirus *ts* mutants favored random assortment as a mechanism of recombination (Fields, 1971). For influenza virus, convincing evidence for a similar conclusion is still lacking.

The question of how recombination occurs is essentially to ask how the assembly of RNA segments takes place, and whether there is any orderly process to ensure collection of all RNA segments or not. One hypothesis is that assembly is a purely random process (Hirst, 1962, 1973). Inevitably a large number of randomly defective particles would be produced along with particles containing complete set of RNA segments. Such randomly defective particles, entering the same cell, would complement each other leading to the production of infective progeny virus. According to Hirst (1973) and Hirst and Pons (1973), when a mixture of two virus strains at relatively high concentration is kept for a certain period and then diluted and inoculated, a significantly higher proportion of cells are doubly infected than when the mixture is immediately diluted after mixing or when two viruses are diluted before mixing. After a sufficiently extended period of incubation at 4°C, the proportion of doubly infected cells among the total infected cells becomes constant, regardless of concentration of the inoculum, as though doubly infected cells are generated as a result of one-hit process instead of a two-hit process as would be expected when cells receive two independently infecting particles. Hirst suggested that double infection characterized by a one-hit process was initiated by preformed mixed aggregates. If an aggregate comprising virus particles missing different RNA segments enter the cell, it would materially increase the chance of successfully initiating infection due to its topographical proximity. Such a mechanism would enhance the chance of recombination in mixed infection experiments as well as in nature. If formation of mixed aggregates is a universal phenomenon, recombination frequency would not be as meaningful as was originally thought, because of difficulty to distinguish mixed aggregates from true recombinants. Furthermore, an extensive reactivation of randomly defective virus particles through the formation of mixedly aggregates would make the role of infective influenza virion questionable.

Random assembly of RNA segments might offer an advantage to the virus by greatly increasing the chance of genetic interaction, but it might be, on the other hand, uneconomical, since the probability of assemblying a complete set would be very small. Formation of mixed aggregates by defective virus particles as postulated above is a plausible explanation. Compans *et al.* (1970) also proposed a model which postulates the packaging of more than the basic number of RNA segments in a virion. Incorporation of an excess of two to three RNA segments per particle substantially increases the proportion of complete particles. It would be expected from both the above hypotheses that most virus particles constituting a mixed yield are, or behave like, partial heterozygotes. As discussed in Sections I,A,2,c and VI, however, there is still a disagreement among investigators over the frequency of heterozygotes among mixed yields and their significance in recombination. It will be necessary to resolve the discrepancy in order to determine the validity of these hypotheses.

On the other hand, Pons has proposed that the RNA segments are held together by a protein backbone consisting of RNP subunits and that the newly synthesized RNA is incorporated into RNP by displacing the template RNA from the backbone, (Pons, 1970). The biological function of RNP but not of RNA (Hirst and Pons, 1972) and the close association of RNP with RNA synthesizing activity (Compans and Caliguiri, 1973) indicate the importance of RNP rather than free RNA in RNA replication. The hypothesis would envisage, however, a linear arrangement of gene segments, for which, with the exception of the work of Mackenzie (1970), genetic studies are still unable to provide evidence.

B. Multiplicity Reactivation and Cross-Reactivation

Both multiplicity reactivation and cross-reactivation are genetic recombinations involving virus which has lost infectivity due to the damage to its RNA. Multiplicity reactivation occurs between inactivated virus of the same genotype when at least one complete set of intact gene segments are present within a multiply infected cell. Barry (1961), in the study of multiplicity reactivation with UV-irradiated influenza viruses, compared experimentally obtained dose–response curves between multiplicity of infection and the virus yield with curves theoretically constructed assuming different number of radiation sensitive units according to Luria and Dulbecco's recombinational model (1949). The closest fit was observed with the curve made on the assumption that the genome consists of six radiation sensitive units. It is tempting to equate radiation sensitive units with the RNA segments. However, because the virus yield can be affected by von Magnus phenomenon or by interference, unavoidable in such experiments, it may not accurately reflect the number of virus-producing cells. It is desirable that multiplicity reactivation be reinvestigated quantitatively with more refined techniques, such as the use of infective center assay or immunofluorescent counting of infected cells.

Failure to demonstrate multiplicity reactivation between von Magnus incomplete viruses can be interpreted as the deletion of a common portion of the genome (Rott and Scholtissek, 1963). Electrophoretic analysis of RNA revealed the absence of the largest piece of RNA in von Magnus virus preparations (Pons and Hirst, 1969; Choppin and Pons, 1970). It still seems premature, however, to conclude that this particlar piece of RNA represents the deleted portion of the genome in von Magnus virus because of the lack of quantitative correlation between the disappearance of the RNA piece and the degree of incompleteness. The RNA profile remains unchanged until PFU/HA ratio drops to $\frac{1}{30}$ or less.

Cross-reactivation is recombination between inactivated virus and live virus of a different genotype. It has been utilized extensively for the isolation of recombinants, because it offers a convenient way of selecting out desired types of recombinant by virtue of greatly depressed yield of inactivated parent (Kilbourne and Murphy, 1960), particularly when coupled with the use of selective host cells to suppress live parent type. There is no evidence that inactivation per se fundamentally alters the mechanism of recombination or enhances the recombination rate. The types of recombinants obtained are the same, regardless of whether one of the parents is inactivated or not (McCahon and Schild, 1971).

Cross-reactivation has been utilized for estimating the proportion of the genome involved in a particular function. By comparing the inactivation rate of infectivity and that of plaque-forming ability, after reactivation by a live non-plaque-forming virus, Sugiura and Ueda (1971) suggested that about $\frac{1}{3}$ of the genome was required for plaque formation of NWS on FL cells. Similar experiments by McCahon and Schild (1971) led to the conclusion that 50% of the genome was involved in FPV for forming plaques on chick embryo cells. These values are probably overestimates, in view of the possibility that plaque formation is too rigorous a criterion for the growth capacity in particular host cells, as discussed in Section IV,B,1.

C. Complementation

Table 7.6 shows a typical example of complementation between *ts* mutants, while Table 7.7 shows the lack of complementation in the other pair of mutants. Mutants belonging to different groups complement each other with a complementation level ranging from 21 to 17,900 in mixed infection (Sugiura *et al.*, 1972). Virus yield at the nonpermissive temperature resulting from complementation usually exceeds 10% of that at the permissive temperature. In some pairs, however, a much lower yield is obtained even in the presence of complementation as well as recombination, apparently because of mutual interference of mutants at the nonpermissive temperature.

An important feature of complementation, as opposed to recombination, is that most of the progeny virus produced at the nonpermissive temperature still retains the original *ts* character (Table 7.6). Along with complementation, recombination does occur at the nonpermissive temperature, but when mutants that are defective at the early stage of viral replication are involved, complementation is obviously a prerequisite to the formation of recombinants at the nonpermissive temperature.

Complementation between naturally existing virus strains has not been intensively looked for. A recovery of non-neurotropic Mel from the mouse brain mixedly infected with NWS and Mel could have represented an example of complementation (Fraser, 1959c).

VI. Phenotypic Mixing and Heterozygosis

Phenotypic mixing occurs in any combination of influenza viruses, irrespective of whether there is genetic compatibility, for example, between influenza viruses A and B (Gotlieb and Hirst, 1954) and even between influenza virus and a paramyxovirus (Granoff and Hirst, 1954). All instances in which phenotypic mixing was demonstrated dealt with the mixing of hemagglutinin, but there is no reason to doubt the phenotypic mixing with regard to the neuraminidase. Few new findings or interpretation have been added to what was described in Section I. Only a brief comment will be made on technical problems related to phenotypic mixing. Nearly all progeny virus issued by a mixedly infected cell is phenotypically mixed, or doubly neutralizable when the cross involves two antigenically different virus strains. Accordingly, the use of antiserum for the purpose of selecting a particular serotype eliminates a majority of the recombinants. It is preferable that the addition of antiserum be delayed until all phenotypically mixed virus particles enter the cells in the next passage, particularly when efficient isolation of recombinants is intended or when recombination is being studied quantitatively.

Despite the importance claimed for heterozygotes as a source of recombinants in the early stage of genetic studies (Hirst and Gotlieb, 1955) (Section I,A,2,c), convincing evidence for their existence is lacking. It is conceivable that "heterozygotes," as recognized at that time, were mostly mixed aggregates, comprising virus particles of two different genotypes. First, most of heterozygotes were probably diploids, since they were heterozygous for several factors (Hirst and Gotlieb, 1955). Second, a substantial proportion of particles in a virus preparation are in the form of aggregates (Hirst, 1973; Hirst and Pons, 1973). If a heterozygote exists as a separate entity from a mixed aggregate, it could not be proved at present, for there is no reliable method to distinguish the two forms experimentally, one containing two different genomes internally and the other consisting of two externally separate, but firmly bound virus particles. Either heterozygotes or mixed aggregates may be the predominant source of recombination under certain experimental conditions, but they do not seem to be responsible for the generation of recombinants in ordinary mixed infections, nor is their proportion high among the mixed yields. Assay of individual clones isolated from mixed yields of NWS and Hong Kong, which has been cited also in Section V,A,1 (Tobita, 1971, 1972), showed that only 3 clones out of 194 gave rise to two different genotypes in the next passage. Because all these clones were directly assayed for serotype of hemagglutinin and neuraminidase by the plaque method without intervening passages, the presence of double-yielders was easily detected in this study.

VII. Study of Gene Function by Characterization of *ts* Mutants

Conditional lethal mutants of bacteriophage were elegantly utilized to elucidate biochemical steps involved in virus replication (Epstein *et al.*, 1963). Similar studies have been initiated for influenza virus only recently.

Thirty-four *ts* mutants of WSN which were collected by Sugiura *et al.* (1972, 1975) were divided into seven nonoverlapping recombination–complementation groups (groups I–VII) based on the presence or absence of recombination and complementation in mixed infections carried out in pairwise fashion. Mutants belonging to groups I, II, III, and V failed to synthesize RNA at the nonpermissive temperature in the presence of actinomycin D, and are most probably defective in the early functions related to either transcription or RNA replication. Group IV, VI, and VII mutants did synthesize appreciable amounts of RNA in the same condition, exceeding 10% of that of *ts*[+]. They probably represent mutants defective in late functions (Sugiura *et al.*, 1975). Two of the group IV mutants so far examined produced neither functional hemagglutinin nor neuraminidase, although all polypeptides, as identified electrophoretically, were synthesized and, futhermore, electron microscopic study revealed the budding of virus particles at the nonpermissive temperature. Heat lability of the neuraminidase of the virion grown at the permissive temperature suggested that the cause of defectiveness for this group of mutants was in the neuraminidase (Palese *et al.*, 1974). With group VI mutants, on the other hand, heat lability of its hemagglutinin and its failure to give rise to HO-containing ts^+ recombinants in the cross with an H3-containing virus suggested the defectiveness of the hemagglutinin (M. Ueda, K. Tobita, A. Sugiura, unpublished).

The greatest difficulty in characterization is the extreme variability of such phenotypic expression as the synthesis of RNA or polypeptides and the production of RNP, hemagglutinin, or neuraminidase from mutant to mutant within the same group. This is particularly marked for early stage mutants. The current explanation is that phenotypic expressions as mentioned above are markedly influenced by the leakiness of a mutant, and, sometimes, a small amount of mRNA synthesized through a leak allows nearly normal expression of certain physiological functions. Conclusions were drawn, therefore, from characterization of the least leaky mutants of each group when it was possible.

Fourteen FPV *ts* mutants isolated by Ghendon *et al.* (1973b) were divided into four recombination or five complementation groups. Recombination was said to be absent between complementation groups A and B. Complementation group D is apparently defective in an early stage of viral replication. One mutant of this group was RNA$^-$ in the presence of actinomycin D and was unable to synthesize appreciable amount of gene products. Its virion-associated transcriptase was significantly less active at the nonpermissive temperature than at the permissive temperature. A mutant in group E was the opposite, i.e., capable of synthesizing RNA as well as polypeptides, including functional hemagglutinin and neuraminidase, and RNP in comparable amounts to ts^+.

WSN *ts* mutants isolated by Mackenzie (1970; Mackenzie and Dimmock, 1973) fell into five or possible six groups, when their less well-characterized *ts*-3 and *ts*-8 mutants are considered to constitute another group.

Nearly 80 WSN *ts* mutants studied by Hirst's group (Simpson and Hirst, 1968; Hirst and Pons, 1972; Hirst, 1973) were said to be classified into eight complementation–recombination groups.

The number of groups defined is thus coming closer to the presumed number of genes. Detailed characterization of these mutants will disclose hitherto unknown function of each gene and the complex interaction of their products. Then the genetics of influenza virus will be discussed undoubtedly from quite a different viewpoint.

Apart from their usefulness for genetic analysis, *ts* mutants can serve as candidates for attenuated live virus vaccine because of their significantly reduced pathogenicity in both animals and in man (Mackenzie, 1969; Mills and Chanock, 1971; Murphy *et al.*, 1972; Ghendon *et al.*, 1973a). A mutant which is known to possess a mutation in the part of the genome other than coding for either hemagglutinin or neuraminidase would be valuable for the potential donor of temperature sensitivity to any future epidemic strain.

VIII. Conclusions

At present, most of experimental findings are compatible with the postulate that the genome consists of subgenomic segments, transcripts of which function as monocistronic messages, and they are reassorted for formation of a mature virion during assembly. But the exact mechanism of assembly has yet to be clarified with respect to whether reassortment is a purely random process or whether some kind of mechanism is operative to ensure efficient maturation. Among other poorly understood phenomena is the apparently genetically controlled graded expression of the neuraminidase gene, as observed for X-7 versus X-7(F1) and many other instances.

Although the start of the genetic study of influenza virus and its development during the first several years were dramatic, subsequent progress has not been as rapid as expected, and we are still dominated by concepts and postulates formulated before the early 1960's. However, provided with more refined methodology, well-defined markers, and a clearer understanding of genetic mechanisms in animal viruses as a whole, influenza virus genetics appears to be in a better position for an accelerated advance now than at any time in its history.

Acknowledgments

I thank Dr. E. D. Kilbourne for permitting use of unpublished observations, and Drs. F. M. Burnet, G. K. Hirst, K. Tobita, and D. O. White for the permission of reproducing published materials.

References

Allison, A. C., and Mallucci, L. (1965). *J. Exp. Med.* **121**, 463.
Appleby, J. C. (1952). *Brit. J. Exp. Pathol.* **33**, 280.
Appleyard, G., and Maber, H. B. (1974). *J. Gen. Virol.* **25**, 351.
Barry, R. D. (1961). *Virology* **14**, 398.
Baron, S., and Jensen, K. E. (1955). *J. Exp. Med.* **102**, 677.
Bean, W. J. Jr., and Simpson, R. W. (1973). *Virology* **56**, 646.
Bishop, D. H. L., Obijeski, J. F., and Simpson, R. W. (1971). *J. Virol.* **8**, 74.
Blough, H. A. (1964). *Cell. Biol. Myxovirus Infec., Ciba Found. Symp., 1964* pp. 120–143.
Borland, R., and Mahy, B. W. J. (1968). *J. Virol.* **2**, 33.
Bromley, P. A., and Barry, R. D. (1973). *Arch. Gesamte Virusforsch.* **42**, 182.
Burnet, F. M. (1951). *J. Gen. Microbiol.* **5**, 54.
Burnet, F. M. (1955). "Principles of Animal Virology," 1st ed. Academic Press, New York.
Burnet, F. M. (1956). *Science* **123**, 1101.

Burnet, F. M. (1960). "Principles of Animal Virology," 2nd ed. Academic Press, New York.

Burnet, F. M., and Edney, M. (1951). *Aust. J. Exp. Biol. Med. Sci.* **29**, 353.

Burnet, F. M., and Lind, P. E. (1949). *Aust. J. Sci.* **12**, 109.

Burnet, F. M., and Lind, P. E. (1951a). *J. Gen. Microbiol.* **5**, 59.

Burnet, F. M., and Lind, P. E. (1951b). *J. Gen. Microbiol.* **5**, 67.

Burnet, F. M., and Lind, P. E. (1952). *Aust. J. Exp. Biol. Med. Sci.* **30**, 469.

Burnet, F. M., and Lind, P. E. (1954a). *Nature (London)* **173**, 627.

Burnet, F. M., and Lind, P. E. (1954b). *Aust. J. Exp. Biol. Med. Sci.* **32**, 133.

Burnet, F. M., and Lind, P. E. (1955). *Aust. J. Exp. Biol. Med. Sci.* **33**, 281.

Burnet, F. M., and Lind, P. E. (1956). *Aust. J. Exp. Biol. Med. Sci.* **34**, 1.

Burnet, F. M., and Lind, P. E. (1957a). *Arch. Gesamte Virusforsch.* **7**, 413.

Burnet, F. M., and Lind, P. E. (1957b). *Aust. J. Exp. Biol. Med. Sci.* **35**, 225.

Came, P. E., Pascale, A., and Shimonaski, G. (1968). *Arch. Gesamet Virusforsch.* **23**, 346.

Carp, R. I. (1963). *Virology* **21**, 373.

Choppin, P. W., and Pons, M. W. (1970). *Virology* **42**, 603.

Choppin, P. W., and Tamm, I. (1960). *J. Exp. Med.* **112**, 895.

Compans, R. W., and Caliguiri, L. A. (1973). *J. Virol.* **11**, 441.

Compans, R. W., Dimmock, N. J., and Meier-Ewert, H. (1970). *In* "The Biology of Large RNA Viruses" (R. D. Barry and B. W. J. Mahy, eds.), pp. 87–108. Academic Press, New York.

Content, J., and Duesberg, P. H. (1971). *J. Mol. Biol.* **62**, 273.

Cooper, P. D. (1969). *In* "The Biochemistry of Viruses" (H. B. Levy, ed.), pp. 177–218. Dekker, New York.

Cooper, P. D., Geissler, E., Scotti, P. D., and Tannock, G. A. (1971). *Strategy Viral Genome, Ciba Found. Symp.* pp. 75–95.

David-West, T. S. (1973). *Arch. Gesamet Virusforsch.* **41**, 143.

Davies, P., and Barry, R. D. (1966). *Nature (London)* **211**, 384.

Drzeniek, R., Seto, J. T., and Rott, R. (1966). *Biochim. Biophys. Acta* **128**, 547.

Duesberg, P. H. (1969). *J. Mol. Biol.* **42**, 485.

Dulbecco, R., and Vogt, M. (1958). *Virology* **5**, 220.

Easterday, B., Laver, W. G., Pereira, H. G., and Schild, G. C. (1969). *J. Gen. Virol.* **5**, 83.

Epstein, R. H., Bolle, A., Steinberg, C. M., Kellenberger, E., Boy de la Tour, E., Chevalley, R., Edger, R. S., Susman, M., Denhardt, G. H., and Lielausis, A. (1963). *Cold Spring Harbor Symp. Quant. Biol.* **28**, 375.

Etkind, P. R., and Krug, R. M. (1974). *Virology* **62**, 38.

Fedova, D., and Tumova, B. (1968). *Acta Virol. (Prague)* **12**, 331.

Fenner, F. (1970). *Annu. Rev. Microbiol.* **24**, 297.

Fenner, F., and Sambrook, J. F. (1964). *Annu. Rev. Microbiol.* **18**, 47.

Fields, B. N. (1971). *Virology* **46**, 142.

Franklin, R. M., and Breitenfeld, P. M. (1959). *Virology* **8**, 293.

Fraser, K. B. (1953). *Brit. J. Exp. Pathol.* **34**, 319.

Fraser, K. B. (1959a). *Virology* **8**, 544.

Fraser, K. B. (1959b). *Virology* **9**, 168.

Fraser, K. B. (1959c). *Virology* **9**, 178.

Fraser, K. B. (1959d). *Virology* **9**, 191.

Fraser, K. B. (1967). *J. Gen. Virol.* **1**, 1.

Frommhagen, L. H., Knight, C. A., and Freeman, N. K. (1959). *Virology* **8**, 176.

Ghandi, S. S., Bell, H. B., and Burke, D. C. (1971). *J. Gen. Virol.* **13**, 423.

Ghendon, Y. Z., Marchenko, A. T., Markushin, S. G., Ghenkina, D. B., Mikhejeva, A. V., and Rozina, E. E. (1973a). *Arch. Gesmate Virusforsch.* **42**, 154.

Ghendon, Y. Z., Markushin, S. G., Marchenko, A. T., Sitnikov, B. S., and Ginzburg, V. P. (1973b). *Virology* **55**, 305.

Gotlieb, T., and Hirst, G. K. (1954). *J. Exp. Med.* **99**, 307.

Gotlieb, T., and Hirst, G. K. (1956). *Virology* **2**, 235.

Granoff, A., and Hirst, G. K. (1954). *Proc. Soc. Exp. Biol. Med.* **86**, 84.

Haheim, L. R., and Haukenes, G. (1973). *Acta Pathol. Microbiol. Scand, Sect B* **81**, 657.

Harboe, A. (1963a). *Acta Pathol. Microbiol. Scand.* **57**, 317.

Harboe, A. (1963b). *Acta Pathol. Microbiol. Scand.* **57**, 448.

Haslam, E. A., Hampson, A. W., Egan, J. A., and White, D. O. (1970). *Virology* **42**, 555.

Haukenes, G., Harboe, A., and Mortensson-Egnund, K. (1965). *Acta Pathol. Microbiol. Scand.* **65**, 534.

Henle, G., Girardi, A., and Henle, W. (1955). *J. Exp. Med.* **101**, 25.

Henle, W., and Liu, O. C. (1951). *J. Exp. Med.* **94**, 305.

Hillis, W. D., Moffat, M. A. J., and Holtermann, O. A. (1960). *Acta Pathol. Microbiol. Scand.* **50**, 419.

Hirst, G. K. (1962). *Cold Spring Harbor Symp. Quant. Biol.* **27**, 303.

Hirst, G. K. (1973). *Virology* **55**, 81.

Hirst, G. K., and Gotlieb, T. (1953a). *J. Exp. Med.* **98**, 41.

Hirst, G. K., and Gotlieb, T. (1953b). *J. Exp. Med.* **98**, 53.

Hirst, G. K., and Gotlieb, T. (1955). *Virology* **1**, 221.

Hirst, G. K., and Pons, M. W. (1972). *Virology* **47**, 546.

Hirst, G. K., and Pons, M. W. (1973). *Virology* **56**, 620.

Hobson, D., Flockton, H. I., and Gould, E. A. (1968). *J. Gen. Virol.* **3**, 445.

Homma, M., and Ohuchi, M. (1973). *J. Virol.* **12**, 1457.

Horisberger, M., and Guskey, L. E. (1974). *J. Virol.* **13**, 230.

Horst, J., Content, J., Mandeles, S., Fraenkel-Conrat, H., and Duesberg, P. H. (1972). *J. Mol. Biol.* **69**, 209.

Hoyle, L. (1968). *In* "The Influenza Viruses," pp. 159–168. Springer-Verlag, Berlin and New York.

Isaacs, A., and Fulton, F. (1953). *Nature (London)* **171**, 90.

Jahiel, R. I., and Kilbourne, E. D. (1966). *J. Bacteriol.* **92**, 1521.

Jameson, P., and Levine, A. S. (1965). *J. Bacteriol.* **90**, 563.

Kilbourne, E. D. (1960). *Virology* **11**, 291.

Kilbourne, E. D. (1963). *Progr. Med. Virol.* **5**, 79.

Kilbourne, E. D. (1968). *Science* **160**, 74.

Kilbourne, E. D. (1969). *In* "Fundamental Techniques in Virology" (K. Habel and N. P. Salzman, eds.), Vol. 1, pp. 146–160. Academic Press, New York.

Kilbourne, E. D., and Murphy, J. S. (1960). *J. Exp. Med.* **111**, 387.

Kilbourne, E. D., and Schulman, J. L. (1965). *Trans. Ass. Amer. Physicians* **78**, 323.

Kilbourne, E. D., Lief, F. S., Schulman, J. L., Jahiel, R. I., and Laver, W. G. (1967). *Perspect. Virol.* **5**, 87.

Kilbourne, E. D., Schulman, J. L., Schild, G. C., Schloer, G., Swanson, J., and Bucher, D. (1971). *J. Infect. Dis.* **124**, 449.

Kilbourne, E. D., Choppin, P. W., Schulze, I. T., Scholtissek, C., and Bucher, D. J. (1972). *J. Infect. Dis.* **125**, 447.

Kingsbury, D. W., and Webster, R. G. (1973). *Virology* **56**, 654.
Klenk, H.-D., and Choppin, P. W. (1969). *Virology* **38**, 255.
Klenk, H.-D., and Choppin, P. W. (1970). *Proc. Nat. Acad. Sci. U.S.* **66**, 57.
Klenk, H.-D., Rott, R., and Becht, H., (1972). *Virology* **47**, 579.
Knight, C. A. (1944). *J. Exp. Med.* **80**, 83.
Laver, W. G., and Baker, N. (1972). *J. Gen. Virol.* **17**, 61.
Laver, W. G., and Kilbourne, E. D. (1966). *Virology* **30**, 493.
Laver, W. G., and Webster, R. G. (1966). *Virology* **30**, 104.
Lazarowitz, S. G., Compans, R. W., and Choppin, P. W. (1973). *Virology* **52**, 199.
Lerner, R. A., and Hodge, L. D. (1969). *Proc. Nat. Acad. Sci. U.S.* **64**, 544.
Lewandowski, L. J., Content, J., and Leppla, S. H. (1971). *J. Virol.* **8**, 701.
Lind, P. E., and Burnet, F. M. (1954). *Aust. J. Exp. Biol. Med. Sci.* **32**, 437.
Lind, P. E., and Burnet, F. M. (1957a). *Aust. J. Exp. Biol. Med. Sci.* **35**, 57.
Lind, P. E., and Burnet, F. M. (1957b). *Aust. J. Exp. Biol. Med. Sci.* **35**, 67.
Lind, P. E., and Burnet, F. M. (1958). *Aust. J. Exp. Biol. Med. Sci.* **36**, 159.
Löffler, H., Henle, G., and Henle, W. (1962). *J. Immunol.* **88**, 763.
Luria, S. E., and Dulbecco, R. (1949). *Genetics* **34**, 93.
McCahon, D., and Schild, G. C. (1971). *J. Gen. Virol.* **12**, 207.
McCahon, D., and Schild, G. C. (1972). *J. Gen. Virol.* **15**, 73.
Mackenzie, J. S. (1969). *Brit. Med. J.* **3**, 757.
Mackenzie, J. S. (1970). *J. Gen. Virol.* **6**, 63.
Mackenzie, J. S., and Dimmock, N. J. (1973). *J. Gen. Virol.* **19**, 51.
Mahy, B. W. J., Hastie, N. D., and Armstrong, S. J. (1972). *Proc. Nat. Acad. Sci. U.S.* **69**, 1421.
Markushin, S. G., and Ghendon, Y. Z. (1973). *Acta Virol. (Prague)* **17**, 369.
Mayer, V., Schulman, J. L., and Kilbourne, E. D. (1972). *J. Virol.* **11**, 272.
Medill-Brown, M., and Briody, B. A. (1955). *Virology* **1**, 310.
Mills, V. J., and Chanock, R. M. (1971). *J. Infect. Dis.* **123**, 145.
Mowshowitz, S., and Kilbourne, E. D. (1975). *In* "Biology of Negative Stranded RNA Viruses" (in press).
Murphy, B. R., Chalhub, E. G., Nusinoff, S. R., and Chanock, R. M. (1972). *J. Infec. Dis.* **126**, 170.
Oxford, J. S. (1973). *J. Virol.* **12**, 827.
Palese, P., and Schulman, J. (1974). *Virology* **57**, 227.
Palese, P., Bucher, D., and Kilbourne, E. D. (1973). *Appl. Microbiol.* **25**, 195.
Palese, P., Tobita, K., Ueda, M., and Compans, R. W. (1974). *Virology* **61**, 397.
Perry, B. T., and Burnet, F. M. (1953). *Aust. J. Exp. Biol. Med. Sci.* **31**, 519.
Perry, B. T., Van den Ende, M., and Burnet, F. M. (1954). *Aust. J. Exp. Biol. Med. Sci.* **32**, 469.
Pons, M. W. (1970). *Curr. Top. Microbiol. Immunol.* **52**, 142.
Pons, M. W. (1971). *Virology* **46**, 149.
Pons, M. W. (1972). *Virology* **47**, 823.
Pons, M. W. (1973). *Virology* **51**, 120.
Pons, M. W., and Hirst, G. K. (1969). *Virology* **38**, 68.
Pons, M. W., Schulze, I. T., and Hirst, G. K. (1969). *Virology* **38**, 250.
Pristasova, S., Lesso, J., and Szanto, J. (1967). *Acta Virol. (Prague)* **11**, 177.
Rott, R., and Scholtissek, C. (1963). *J. Gen. Microbiol.* **33**, 303.
Rott, R., Drzeniek, R., Saber, M. S., and Reichert, E. (1966). *Arch. Gesamte Virusforsch.* **19**, 273.

Scheid, A., and Choppin, P. W. (1974). *Virology* **57**, 475.

Schlesinger, R. W. (1950). *Proc. Soc. Exp. Biol. Med.* **74**, 541.

Scholtissek, C., and Rott, R. (1970). *Virology* **40**, 989.

Schulze, I. T. (1970). *Virology* **42**, 890.

Shatkin, A. J. (1971). *Bacteriol. Rev.* **35**, 250.

Simpson, R. W. (1964). *Cell Biol. Myxovirus Infect., Ciba Found. Symp., 1964* pp. 187–206.

Simpson, R. W., and Hauser, R. E. (1966). *Virology* **30**, 684.

Simpson, R. W., and Hirst, G. K. (1961). *Virology* **15**, 436.

Simpson, R. W., and Hirst, G. K. (1968). *Virology* **35**, 41.

Simpson, R. W., and Obijeski, J. F. (1974). *Virology* **57**, 357.

Skehel, J. J. (1971). *J. Gen. Virol.* **11**, 103.

Skehel, J. J. (1972). *Virology* **49**, 23.

Staiger, H. R. (1964). *Virology* **22**, 419.

Sugiura, A. (1972). *Virology* **47**, 517.

Sugiura, A., and Kilbourne, E. D. (1965). *Virology* **26**, 478.

Sugiura, A., and Kilbourne, E. D. (1966). *Virology* **29**, 84.

Sugiura, A., and Ueda, M. (1971). *J. Virol.* **7**, 499.

Sugiura, A., Shimojo, H., and Enomoto, C. (1961). *Jap. J. Exp. Med.* **31**, 169.

Sugiura, A., Enomoto, C., and Ayai, M. (1962). *Jap. J. Exp. Med.* **32**, 415.

Sugiura, A., Ueda, M., and Enomoto, C. (1969). *Arch. Gesamte Virusforsch.* **26**, 105.

Sugiura, A., Tobita, K., and Kilbourne, E. D. (1972). *J. Virol.* **10**, 639.

Sugiura, A., Ueda, M., Tobita, K., and Enomoto, C. (1975). *Virology* **65**, 363.

Ter Meulen, V., and Love, R. (1967). *J. Virol.* **1**, 626.

Tobita, K. (1971). *Arch. Gesamte Virusforsch.* **34**, 119.

Tobita, K. (1972). *Arch. Gesamte Virusforsch.* **38**, 100.

Tobita, K., and Kilbourne, E. D. (1974). *J. Virol.* **13**, 347.

Tumova, B., and Pereira, H. G. (1965). *Virology* **27**, 253.

Webster, R. G., and Campbell, V. H. (1972). *Virology* **48**, 528.

Webster, R. G., Laver, W. G., and Kilbourne, E. D. (1968). *J. Gen. Virol.* **3**, 315.

White, D. O. (1974). *Curr. Top. Microbiol. Immunol.* **63**, 1.

Young, R. J., and Content, J. (1971). *Nature (London) New Biol.* **230**, 140.

Zavadova, H., Vonka, V., Kutinova, L., and Tuckova, E. (1968). *J. Gen. Virol.* **2**, 341.

8

Influenza Virus Replication

Christoph Scholtissek and Hans-Dieter Klenk

I. Introduction

A series of previous reviews exist on influenza virus replication. The literature up to 1968 is covered in articles by Hoyle (1968) and Scholtissek (1969); more recent publications are those of White (1973) and Compans and Choppin (1974).

Most of the data on replication have been obtained from studies with

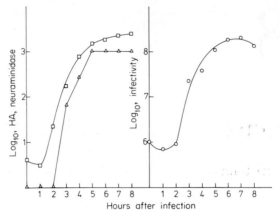

Fig. 8.1.   Multiplication of fowl plague virus in chick embryo cells. The various virus activities were determined in the cell extracts prepared at the times after infection as listed on the abscissa by three repeated cycles of freezing and thawing. Hemagglutination titer (HA), △; neuraminidase units, □; plaque forming units (infectivity), ○.

influenza A viruses. Major differences in the replication mechanisms of the other influenza virus types have not been found thus far.

Several cell culture systems have been developed which are very valuable for replication studies, e.g., the multiplication of the WSN strain in MDBK cells (Choppin, 1969) or of fowl plague virus in chick embryo fibroblasts. An example of a single cycle growth curve of the latter virus is shown in Fig. 8.1. The length of the latent period is about 3 hours and virus production reaches a plateau between 8 and 12 hours. In these systems in general high yields of infectious virus are produced and synthesis of host cell proteins is very efficiently shut off after infection. They are, therefore, very suitable for biochemical studies.

II. Adsorption, Penetration, Uncoating

Infection of a cell by a virus is initiated by adsorption, i.e., the attachment of the virus particle to the cell surface. Attachment requires two complementary structures, namely, the receptor sites on the host cell surface and the viral component responsible for recognition of the receptor sites. The ability of influenza virus to combine with and agglutinate a wide spectrum of erythrocytes has been known for many years (Hirst, 1941; McClelland and Hare, 1941). Hemagglutination has been used as a model reaction for the interaction of influenza viruses with the cell surface, and most of our knowledge on this subject has been derived from such studies. They should be generalized, however, only with caution, because the structure of the surface of erythrocytes and of permissive cells might be quite different (see also Chapter 3).

A. Role of Hemagglutinin in Adsorption

The component of the virion involved in binding is the hemagglutinin spike. The role of viral proteins in initiation of infection has been studied using antibody specific for the two surface proteins, hemagglutinin and neuraminidase, which can be prepared with the use of recombinant viruses. For example, a cross between an A_0 and an A_2 virus yielded a recombinant X-7F1, which possessed the A_0 hemagglutinin and the A_2 neuraminidase (Kilbourne *et al.*, 1968). Antiserum to X-7F1 does not inhibit the neuraminidase of A_0 viruses, but inhibits hemagglutination and neutralizes the infectivity of the virus. Interaction of the same serum with A_2 viruses does not inhibit hemagglutination or infectivity, although neutralization of the neuraminidase activity is complete. Thus, the neuraminidase is not involved in initiation of infection, and only the hemagglutinin appears to be responsible for adsorption. This concept is supported by the finding that virus particles from which only the neuraminidase spikes had been removed by proteolytic enzymes were still infective (Schulze, 1970).

There is evidence that the hemagglutinating principle is located on the carbohydrate-rich outer part of the hemagglutinin spikes (Chapter 3). Carbohydrate seems to be necessary for the function of the hemagglutinin, because unglycosylated hemagglutinin proteins are not able to bind to erythrocytes (Klenk *et al.*, 1972b).

B. Influenza Virus Receptor

Carbohydrates are essential constituents not only of the hemagglutinin, but also of the virus receptor on the cell surface. Hirst (1942) observed that the virus–red cell complex was unstable and that the receptor on the red cell surface were destroyed by a viral enzyme. This enzyme was later shown to be a neuraminidase which split neuraminic acid from glycoproteins (Klenk *et al.*, 1955; Klenk and Stoffel, 1956; Gottschalk, 1957). This represented the first demonstration of an enzyme as an integral part of a virus particle. Bacterial neuraminidases are also capable of destroying influenza virus receptors (Brunet and Stone, 1947). Thus it had been established that the receptor for influenza virus is a neuraminic acid-containing glycoprotein.

Since then much information on the nature of the myxovirus receptor has accumulated which recently has been reviewed by Hughes (1973). In essence, the receptor sites contain neuraminic acid residues which are present in the carbohydrate chains of glycoproteins. Nonreducing terminal neuraminosyl residues are necessary for the interaction of glycoproteins with influenza virus. Treatment with neuraminidase completely abolishes binding activity. Degradation studies with periodate suggest that an intact neuraminic acid molecule is required for activity (Suttajit and Winzler, 1971). Presumably the carboxyl group also plays an important function because electrostatic forces seem to be necessary, too (Huang, 1974). There appears to be little specificity as far as the structure is concerned to which neuraminic acid is linked because a whole series of different neuraminic acid-containing glycoproteins have been shown to bind to myxoviruses. Moreover, gangliosides (neuraminic acid-containing glycolipids) are also active (Haywood, 1975).

It can be expected that more light will be thrown on the binding of influenza viruses when the molecular structure of the receptor is elucidated. This has already been accomplished to a certain degree in the case of erythrocytes (Marchesi *et al.*, 1973). Attachment of myxoviruses to artificial membranes (Tiffany and Blough, 1971) also might provide valuable information.

C. Possible Mechanisms for Penetration and Uncoating

Two different mechanisms have been proposed for penetration and uncoating not only of influenza virus but of enveloped viruses in general. Both points of view are supported mainly by electron microscopic studies. One of them is *viropexis,* which has been postulated to be a pinocytotic process whereby whole virus particles are incorporated into a pinosome that subsequently fuses with lysosomes, the lysosomal enzymes causing uncoating of the virus (Fazekas de St. Groth, 1948). Electron microscopic support for this view was obtained by Dales and Choppin (1962) and by Dourmashkin and Tyrrell (1970). Virus particles were observed in direct contact with the cell surface 10 minutes after inoculation, and at 20 minutes particles were observed within cytoplasmic vacuoles. In contrast, the studies of Morgan and Rose (1968) suggest that penetration may result from the fusion of the viral envelope with the host cell membrane. Thus, at this time there is no general agreement on the mechanism of penetration of influenza virus.

As described in Chapter 5, influenza virions contain an RNA polymerase associated with their ribonucleoprotein components. Therefore the process

of uncoating is not likely to proceed beyond the release of the ribonucleoprotein. This step occurs at the cell surface according to the membrane fusion
mechanism of penetration and in phagocytotic vesicles according to the
viropexis mechanism.

III. Transcription

A. Time Course of RNA Synthesis

After uncoating, the single-stranded virion RNA has to be transcribed
into the complementary RNA. The RNA polymerase introduced by the infecting virus particle is supposed to function in the first step of viral RNA
multiplication (see Chapter 5). The influenza genome can be isolated from
the virion only in pieces (see Chapter 6). Furthermore it functions in pieces
as shown by genetic analysis (see Chapter 7) and by the stepwise inactivation of infectious virus (Scholtissek and Rott, 1964). Therefore it has to
be assumed that the polymerase initiates RNA synthesis on each individual
piece. Since RNA does not exist in cells as a free molecule but is always
bound to protein, the question arises to what protein viral RNA is bound
during its replication.

Experiments conducted to study the synthesis of influenza virus RNA are
rendered more difficult because actinomycin D cannot be utilized to unravel
the production of influenza RNA by specifically suppressing cellular RNA
synthesis, since this antibiotic interferes with the multiplication of influenza
viruses (Barry *et al.*, 1962; Rott and Scholtissek, 1964; Barry, 1964; White
et al., 1965; Pons, 1967). Therefore, specific hybridization of pulse-labeled
RNA at different times after infection with a surplus of either nonlabeled
virion RNA or complementary RNA and digestion with RNase has been
applied to follow the time course of viral RNA synthesis (Scholtissek and
Rott, 1970). It was found that early in the infectious cycle the synthesis
of complementary RNA prevails with a maximum at about 2 hours after
infection, while later most of the virus-specific RNA produced is virion
RNA. Krug (1972) using a different method also could show that 4 hours
after infection synthesis of complementary RNA almost had ceased. Relatively little double-stranded RNA after phenol extraction is found
(Scholtissek and Rott, 1970).

Since the one or the other type of viral RNA functions as messenger and
is used as template for viral protein synthesis (see Section IV,A), some translational control could occur on the level of a differential catabolism of viral
RNA. Therefore, pulse-chase experiments have been conducted to study the
stability of influenza RNA *in vivo*. It was found that in contrast to cellular

RNA both types of viral RNA are completely stable during a 90 minute chase period (Scholtissek *et al.*, 1972).

Earlier studies on the synthesis of viral RNA *in vivo,* in which actinomycin D was added later in the infectious cycle (Duesberg and Robinson, 1967; Nayak, 1970; Mahy, 1970) did not take into account that actinomycin D specifically inhibits synthesis of complementary RNA *in vivo* (Scholtissek and Rott, 1970; Pons, 1973). Since the double-stranded RNA has been isolated in at least 5 distinct pieces from infected cells, it is concluded that the viral RNA is also synthesized in pieces (Pons and Hirst, 1968).

B. Localization of Viral RNA Synthesis within the Host Cell

It has been claimed by using the technique of autoradiography that the site of viral RNA synthesis would be the cell nucleus (Scholtissek *et al.*, 1962; Barry *et al.*, 1974). Since the pulse lengths investigated in these studies are still too long, it cannot be ruled out that the viral RNA is synthesized within the cell cytoplasm and thereafter is transported to the nucleus, where it might accumulate. Furthermore virion RNA and complementary RNA could be synthesized at different sites within the cells.

C. Inhibition of Viral RNA Synthesis

1. ACTINOMYCIN D, MITHRAMYCIN, AND α-AMANITINE

When actinomycin D, or mithramycin, which both interfere with the template function of DNA, is added to infected cells at a time when viral RNA-dependent RNA polymerase is already present (e.g., 2 hours after infection), virion RNA is still subsequently synthesized for about 2 hours. Production of complementary RNA, however, ceases immediately. Later, virion RNA synthesis also is abolished, indicating that continuous production of complementary RNA is necessary for its synthesis (Rott *et al.*, 1965; Scholtissek and Rott, 1970; Scholtissek *et al.*, 1970; Pons, 1973). Gregoriades (1970) reported that actinomycin D also had a severe effect on the synthesis of virion RNA when added later in the infectious cycle. In these studies viral RNA synthesis was measured by the increased incorporation of labeled uridine into total RNA of infected cells. This increase could be abolished by addition of actinomycin D. It should be kept in mind, however, that infection with influenza virus causes an increased uptake of labeled uridine into the host cell after infection (Scholtissek *et al.,* 1967) and that actinomycin D has an inhibitory effect on this uptake (Scholtissek *et al.*, 1969). α-Amanitine, which has no affinity for DNA but which interferes with the activity of one of the cellular RNA polymerases (RNA polymerase II), also inhibits the synthesis of complementary RNA when added to the culture medium immediately after infection (Rott and Scholtissek, 1970; Mahy *et al.*, 1972).

The mechanism of the specific inhibition of the synthesis of complementary RNA by these antibiotics is not at all understood, since they have no effect on the production of complementary RNA *in vitro*. Thus the antibiotics act only *in vivo*, although the enzyme synthesizing the complementary RNA can be isolated from cells to which actinomycin D had been added 2 hours after infection (Scholtissek and Rott, 1969a).

The multiplication of influenza viruses can be inhibited also by other treatments of the host cell DNA, such as administration of mitomycin C, pretreatment with UV light, or removal of the cell nucleus prior to infection (Barry, 1964; Rott *et al.*, 1965; Nayak and Rasmussen, 1966; Follett *et al.*, 1974; Kelly *et al.*, 1974). The mechanism by which these treatments interfere with influenza multiplication might be the same as that of the other antibiotics. The only assumption which can be made from these studies is that we need a functional cell nucleus and/or a DNA-dependent host function for the multiplication of influenza viruses. What this function is cannot be said.

2. CYCLOHEXIMIDE

When cycloheximide, which specifically inhibits protein synthesis in animal cells, is added to cells 2 hours after infection with influenza virus, the production of virion RNA ceases immediately, while that of complementary RNA still proceeds at least for 2 hours (Scholtissek and Rott, 1970; Pons, 1973). It is not yet known whether one needs the continuous synthesis of viral or cellular protein used as a cofactor for the polymerase synthesizing virion RNA, or a protein (e.g., NP protein) to stabilize the newly synthesized virion RNA, or whether the inhibition of the synthesis of a certain virus protein causes a continuous production of complementary RNA normally switched off at about 3 hours after infection. This switch might be necessary to start virion RNA synthesis. Studies with temperature-sensitive mutants should answer some of these questions.

Recent experiments by Bean and Simpson (1973) have shown that the primary transcription *in vivo* (synthesis of complementary RNA on the virion RNA with the aid of the polymerase of the infecting particle) is not inhibited by cycloheximide, while actinomycin D inhibits it completely. Thus cycloheximide does not interfere *in vivo* with the polymerase activity introduced by the infecting particle synthesizing complementary RNA. It inhibits, however, the synthesis of new polymerase necessary for the production of complementary RNA.

3. GLUCOSAMINE

Glucosamine is known to deplete the UTP pool of chick embryo cells by forming UDP-N-acetylglucosamine (Scholtissek, 1971). When Earle's medium containing glucose is used as culture medium its effect is only on viral glycoprotein synthesis (see Section V). If, however, glucose is replaced either by pyruvate or fructose as energy source, the amino sugar is about 10 times more active with regard to the depletion of the UTP pool. Under these conditions the UTP pool of the host cells becomes specifically rate limiting for virion RNA synthesis, while cellular RNA synthesis is not yet affected (Scholtissek *et al.*, 1975). As a result of inhibition of viral RNA synthesis, none of the viral proteins is synthesized.

This observation might be interpreted in two ways: Either the viral RNA-dependent RNA polymerase has a lower affinity for UTP compared with the cellular DNA-dependent RNA polymerases, or there exist two more or less independent UTP pools within the cell, one of which might be used for viral RNA synthesis and is altered more severely by glucosamine than the other which might be used as substrate by cellular RNA polymerases.

D. Synthesis of Viral RNA *in Vitro*

An RNA-dependent RNA polymerase has been detected in influenza virus-infected cells by several investigators (Ho and Walters, 1966; Scholtissek and Rott, 1969a; Skehel and Burke, 1969; Ruck *et al.*, 1969; Mahy and Bromley, 1970; Compans and Caliguiri, 1973). Most of the enzyme activity was found with the microsomal fraction of the infected cells. In the *in vitro* test its activity is abolished by RNase but not by DNase. This means that the internal template is RNA. It is dependent on all four nucleoside triphosphates, and it is sensitive against polyanions, such as dextran sulfate and polyvinyl sulfate, but not against actinomycin D. Most of the *in vitro* product is of rather low molecular weight. Recent results by Horisberger and Guskey (1973) suggest that there might be two different enzyme activities present in the cytoplasm: One is Mg^{2+} dependent and is inhibited by relatively high salt concentrations; the other is Mn^{2+} dependent and is rather resistant to high salt. The latter enzyme activity is found also with virus particles (see Chapter 5).

Concerning the *in vitro* product of the cytoplasmic enzyme, conflicting results have been published. Ruck *et al.* (1969) reported that in their hands the enzyme synthesizes at least some virion type RNA (14 S to 19 S). They came to this conclusion by determining the base composition of the *in vitro* product after incubation of a microsomal fraction with all four ^{3}H-labeled nucleoside triphosphates of known specific radioactivity. The data obtained with [α-^{32}P]ATP on the nearest neighbor to adenylic acid published in the same paper, however, are in good agreement with the nearest neighbor analysis of Scholtissek (1969), from which the structure of the *in vitro* product was deduced to be complementary RNA. Mahy and Bromley (1970) in their original publication also claimed that some of the in vitro product obtained with the cytoplasmic enzyme would be virion RNA. Recently Hastie and Mahy (1973) confirmed, as originally shown by Scholtissek (1969), the production of complementary RNA almost exclusively by the cytoplasmic enzyme by nearest neighbor analysis and specific hybridization. Caliguiri and Compans (1974) also isolated an RNA polymerase from the cytoplasm of influenza-infected cells which synthesized *in vitro* an RNA at least 90% of which has a base sequence complementary to virion RNA. Hastie and Mahy (1973) found that a significant percentage of the *in vitro* product synthesized by the nuclear enzyme in the presence of actinomycin D was not hybridizable with nonlabeled virion RNA. It is not yet clear what kind of RNA this nonhybridizable portion is. Very little of the RNA synthesized under these conditions hybridizes with nonlabeled complementary RNA (C. Scholtissek, unpublished).

The kinetics of incorporation as labeled GTP into viral RNA can be interpreted as demonstrating that there is no reinitiation of RNA synthesis *in vitro*. If the crude enzyme preparation is incubated at low salt concentration almost all of the newly synthesized RNA originally is single stranded. After phenol extraction, however, a large percentage of the RNA becomes RNase resistant. Phenol converts a replicative intermediate structure composed of single-stranded template and newly synthesized complementary RNA held together at the site of replication by the polymerase molecule into a partially double-stranded structure (Feix *et al.,* 1967; Öberg and Philipson, 1971). The result on the *in vitro* product of the influenza enzyme has been interpreted as showing that the polymerase not only initiates and continues polymerization but it also separates the newly synthesized strand from its template. Otherwise a double-stranded RNA structure is formed which has no biological function (Paffenholz and Scholtissek, 1973). If the incubation is done at high salt concentration or with a purified enzyme a high percentage of the product is already double-stranded RNA prior to the phenol extraction (Schwarz and Scholtissek, 1973).

The property of the influenza virus RNA polymerase to synthesize exclusively complementary RNA *in vitro* has been used for establishing the genetic relatedness of different influenza strands by determination of the base sequence homology between them (Scholtissek and Rott, 1969b; Hobson and Scholtissek, 1970; Anschütz *et al.*, 1972).

IV. Synthesis of Viral Proteins

A. *In Vitro* Translation

The problem of whether virion or complementary RNA serves as messenger for viral protein synthesis is still unsolved. Conflicting results have been reported concerning the kind of virus-specific RNA bound to polysomes. Nayak (1970) found mainly virion RNA in the polysome region of sucrose gradients, while Pons (1972) isolated exclusively complementary RNA from polysomes. The latter result was confirmed by the observation that after addition at 2 hours after infection of actinomycin D, which preferentially interferes with the synthesis of complementary RNA (see Section III,C,1), no complementary RNA was found in the polysomes of infected cells (Pons, 1973).

Using a protein-synthesizing system from *E. coli* and influenza virion RNA as template, Siegert *et al.* (1973) found production of viral NP protein *in vitro*. The *in vitro* labeled NP protein was characterized by gel precipitation in the Ouchterlony test. In contrast to these results, Kingsbury and Webster (1973) did not observe any viral protein synthesis with virion RNA investigating a protein-synthesizing system isolated from rabbit reticulocytes. In this latter system, however, they found synthesis of the viral M protein (Chapter 2) with RNA isolated from infected cells as template. Thus the question of whether exclusively virion or complementary RNA is located on the polysomes, or some pieces of one type and other pieces of the other type are used as template for protein synthesis cannot be answered at the moment. Therefore it is still difficult to apply the new definition of "negative" or "positive" strand virus to influenza viruses as proposed by Baltimore (1971).

B. Synthesis of Viral Proteins *in Vivo*

Studies of influenza virus protein synthesis are facilitated by the finding that in infected cells virus-specific replaces host-specific polypeptide synthesis. In fowl plague virus-infected chick embryo fibroblasts (Joss *et al.*, 1969; Skehel, 1972; Klenk and Rott, 1973) and in BHK21-F cells infected with the WSN strain (Lazarowitz *et al.*, 1971) at 4 hours after infection viral proteins are synthesized almost exclusively (Fig. 8.2). In several early studies, three or four polypeptides were observed in infected cells (Taylor *et al.,* 1969; Joss *et al.,* 1969; Holland and Kiehn, 1970; White *et al.,* 1970). Subsequently additional polypeptides could be detected (Lazarowitz *et al.,* 1971; Skehel, 1972; Klenk *et al.,* 1972b; Krug and Etkind, 1973). In general, all structural proteins have been found in infected cells: one or two P proteins, the nucleocapsid subunit NP, the membrane protein M, the hemagglutinin glycoprotein in the uncleaved (HA) and the cleaved form (HA$_1$ and HA$_2$), and the neuraminidase subunit NA.

In addition to the virion proteins one or two nonstructural proteins (NS) have been described.

There are marked differences in the rates of synthesis of the different viral polypeptides. The NP and NS polypeptides are generally the first to be detected in infected cells. Skehel (1973) has suggested that the polypeptides P$_2$, NP, and NS, which were the first to be detected in fowl plague

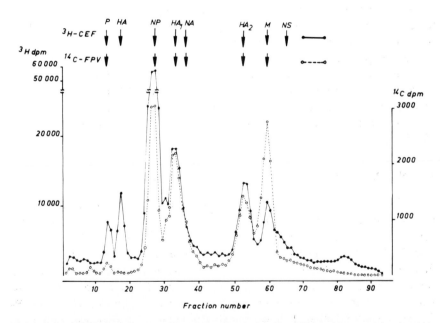

Fig. 8.2. Polyacrylamide gel electrophoresis of polypeptides synthesized in chick embryo fibroblasts 4 hours after infection with fowl plague virus (solid line). Polypeptides of purified virions were included as internal markers (dashed line). Migration is from the left to the right. (From Klenk *et al.,* 1972b). As indicated here previous results suggested that the neuraminidase glycoprotein NA is localized on the front slope of the HA$_1$ peak (Klenk *et al.,* 1972a). This position, however, appears not to be correct. Recent observations indicate that NA has a slightly lower electrophoretic mobility and is located between NP and HA$_1$ (H.-D. Klenk, unpublished results).

virus-infected cells, are products of RNA species produced by selective transcription of three of the viral genome segments by the virion polymerase. When cells were infected in the presence of cycloheximide and pulse-labeled after removal of the drug, only these three polypeptides were detected, suggesting that the messenger RNA's for these components were produced by primary transcription by the input virion transcriptase. From 4 to 6 hours after infection of chick fibroblasts by fowl plague virus, the rate of synthesis of M increased and that of NS decreased (Skehel, 1972, 1973). Thus the rates of synthesis of polypeptides may be controlled individually and may vary during the growth cycle.

Apart from the cleavage of HA into HA_1 and HA_2 there is no evidence that influenza virus-specific polypeptides are generated by cleavage of large precursors (Taylor et al., 1969; Lazarowitz et al., 1971; Skehel, 1972; Klenk and Rott, 1973).

New information on the location of viral components in infected cells has been obtained recently using autoradiography (Becht, 1971) or cell fractionation procedures and gel electrophoresis (Taylor et al., 1969, 1970). According to these studies the synthesis of all viral polypeptides appears to be cytoplasmic. Early immunofluorescence studies on the location of the nucleoprotein antigen have been interpreted as indicating nuclear synthesis followed by transport to the cytoplasm (Liu, 1955; Breitenfeld and Schäfer, 1957; Holtermann et al., 1960). However, it is clear that immunofluorescence detects antigen accumulation rather than synthesis (see Section IV, B,2).

1. RNA POLYMERASE

The virus-specific RNA-dependent RNA polymerase activity can be detected in influenza virus-infected cells between $1\frac{3}{4}$ to 3 hours after infection depending on the host system used (Scholtissek and Rott, 1969a; Skehel and Burke, 1969; Ruck et al., 1969; Mahy and Bromley, 1970). It is the first detectable virus-specific activity after infection. Most of the viral polymerase activity is isolated with the microsomal fraction; some of it stays with the nuclei and cannot be released from them by extensive washing. There is no fundamental difference in the kinetics of appearance or in cofactor requirements between the nuclear and microsomal enzyme (Scholtissek and Rott, 1969a; Mahy et al., 1975).

When the cytoplasm was further fractionated according to the method of Caliguiri and Tamm (1970) using a discontinuous sucrose gradient, the polymerase activity was found with the rough membranes (Compans and Caliguiri, 1973; Klenk et al., 1974a).

Since viral polymerase activity was found also with purified virus particles (see Chapter 5) the question arose as to which viral protein the polymerase activity might be associated with. The polymerase isolated from virus-infected cells has been purified about 200-fold. The only virus-specific product associated with polymerase activity was the RNP antigen (NP plus viral RNA determined by the complement-fixation test). All attempts to remove the latter led to a complete loss of enzyme activity (Schwarz and Scholtissek, 1973). The P protein has been suggested as a candidate for the viral polymerase (Kilbourne *et al.*, 1972). When the enzyme complex labeled *in vivo* with amino acids was isolated from influenza-infected cells and purified about 35-fold, electrophoretic analysis first revealed only the NP protein in this complex (Compans and Caliguiri, 1973). Subsequently, however, under different labeling conditions the P protein also could be detected (Caliguiri and Compans, 1974). On the other hand, Klenk *et al.* (1974) detected the P protein in the cytosol, which is almost free of polymerase activity (Scholtissek and Rott, 1969a; Skehel and Burke, 1969). This observation could mean that the P protein exerts its putative polymerase activity only when it is bound to the RNP antigen.

That the RNP antigen itself has polymerase activity is not very likely because hyperimmune serum against RNP antigen does not inhibit polymerase activity, while convalescent serum, which should contain antibodies against polymerase does inhibit the polymerase (Scholtissek *et al.*, 1971). This convalescent serum (which was obtained from an animal recovered from influenza A infection) inhibited the polymerase activities of all influenza A viruses tested but not that of an influenza B virus. All these observations are compatible with the idea that the RNP antigen (virion RNA plus NP protein) might be the template for the synthesis of complementary RNA.

2. NUCLEOCAPSID PROTEIN (NP)

The NP protein is bound to viral RNA forming the RNP antigen. This is true not only for the NP protein isolated from the virion but also for that isolated from infected cells (Schäfer, 1957). It can be detected by serological means first at about 3 hours after infection, which is 1 hour ahead of the appearance of hemagglutinin (Breitenfeld and Schäfer, 1957). Its titer does not increase significantly after this time. This might be due to an equilibrium reached between new synthesis and incorporation into mature particles. By labeling techniques the NP protein can be detected in the infected cells as early as 2 hours after infection (Scholtissek and Rott, 1961; Krug, 1972).

By fluorescent antibodies the RNP antigen is detected first in the cell nucleus. Later it appears also in the cytoplasm (Breitenfeld and Schäfer, 1957). Under certain conditions, such as abortive infection (Franklin and

Breitenfeld, 1959), in the presence of p-fluorophenylalanine (Zimmermann and Schäfer, 1960), or under von Magnus conditions (Rott and Scholtissek, 1963), the RNP antigen is retained within the nucleus.

The early accumulation of RNP antigen in infected cells does not mean that the NP protein is also synthesized within the nucleus. Autoradiographic and cell fractionation studies point to a cytoplasmic synthesis of this and another arginine-rich protein and a rapid transport from the cytoplasm into the nucleus (Taylor *et al.*, 1969, 1970; Becht, 1971).

In extracts of infected cells it has been found that a certain fraction of the RNP antigen contains complementary RNA (Pons, 1971; Krug, 1972; Krug and Etkind, 1973), although in virus particles only one type of RNA is found as shown by the absence of any self-annealing of virion RNA (Scholtissek and Becht, 1971; Pons, 1971). It cannot be decided whether the RNP antigen containing complementary RNA has a specific significance during virus multiplication, or whether it is only an artifact produced during cell fractionation. It has been shown that both RNA strands bind equally well to the NP protein *in vitro* (Scholtissek and Becht, 1971). Thus if there is any free NP protein and free complementary RNA, the corresponding RNP antigen is formed immediately during homogenization. Viral RNA can be replaced in the RNP antigen by polyvinyl sulfate (Pons *et al.*, 1969). Therefore it should be tested whether replacement of different viral RNA's in the RNP antigen in cell homogenates is possible. From the shifts of base composition of viral RNA, labeled for different lengths of time by ^{32}P and isolated from the cytoplasmic RNP antigen, Krug (1972) concludes that some of the complementary RNA exists free of NP protein before it is incorporated into the RNP antigen. The incorporation of ^{32}P into RNA of animal cells occurs with a considerable lag phase due to the rather slow labeling of the phosphorus in the α-position of the nucleoside triphosphates (Scholtissek, 1965). Unless corresponding corrections were made for the calculations of the shifts the data by Krug (1972) should be interpreted with caution.

A kinetic analysis of the appearance of RNP antigen in the nucleus and in the cytoplasm by Krug (1972) suggests that the RNP antigen accumulating in the nucleus is not the precursor of that found in the cytoplasm.

3. Nonstructural Proteins

Several nonstructural virus-specific proteins of unknown function have been described in infected cells. The most abundant one has a molecular weight of about 25,000 and has been designated NS (Lazarowitz *et al.*, 1971). On polyacrylamide gels it has a migration rate similar to that of the M protein. Both proteins, however, appear to be unrelated as indicated by different peptide maps. Large amounts of the NS protein are found in the nucleus (Lazarowitz *et al.*, 1971; Krug and Etkind, 1973). These findings are in agreement with previous immunofluorescence studies of Dimmock (1969) who observed bright nucleolar staining with antiserum specific for nonstructural viral antigens, which probably represented the NS protein. This protein is also found as a major virus-specific protein on free and membrane-bound ribosome fractions of infected cells (Pons, 1972; Compans, 1973a; Klenk *et al.*, 1974a). The association of NS with ribosomes appears to depend on the ionic strength (Krug and Etkind, 1973). In low ionic strength buffers, the polypeptide was found to be absorbed to both ribosomal subunits, whereas it was removed by higher salt.

A recent study (Gregoriades, 1973) raised some question about the identity of NS as a nonstructural polypeptide distinct from virion polypeptide M. It was possible to extract the M polypeptide from virions with acidic chloroform–methanol, and a protein of identical electrophoretic mobility could also be extracted from whole infected cells, nuclei, or polysomes. Analysis of tryptic digests of the M protein and the nuclear and polysome-associated proteins extracted by chloroform–methanol revealed many similarities, suggesting that the M and the NS protein were identical. Further information is, however, needed to conclusively explain these results.

In addition to NS, other nonstructural virus-specific polypeptides may exist, although none has been well characterized. Using antiserum directed against nonstructural viral antigens, Dimmock and Watson (1969) precipitated radioactively labeled polypeptides from infected cells. Analysis by polyacrylamide gel electrophoresis suggested the presence of several nonstructural polypeptides, with the major component corresponding to NS. One of the remaining nonstructural components migrated more rapidly, and may correspond to a 10,000 to 15,000 MW component described by Skehel (1972) and Krug and Etkind (1973).

4. Membrane Protein (M)

The M protein which lines the inner surface of the lipid bilayer of the envelope and is the most plentiful protein in the virion is found in relatively small amounts in infected cells. This suggested not only that synthesis of the M protein is controlled, but also that it might be a rate-limiting step in virus production (Lazarowitz *et al.*, 1971). This concept is supported by the finding that at 25°C, a temperature at which virus formation is inhibited, M protein is the only virus-specific protein which cannot be detected in infected cells (Klenk and Rott, 1973).

The M protein can be detected on smooth membranes and plasma membranes of infected cells (Lazarowitz *et al.*, 1971; Compans, 1973a; Klenk *et al.*, 1974a). These findings illustrate the membrane affinity of this protein.

5. HEMAGGLUTININ (HA)

The hemagglutinin is synthesized as a larger precursor glycoprotein HA which subsequently is cleaved into 2 smaller glycoproteins HA$_1$ and HA$_2$ (Lazarowitz *et al.*, 1971). Cleavage which can be inhibited by protease inhibitors (Klenk and Rott, 1973) appears to be carried out by host-specific proteolytic enzymes (Lazarowitz *et al.*, 1973a). The extent of cleavage depends on the virus strain, the host cell, the extent of cytopathic effect, and the presence or absence of serum in the medium (Lazarowitz *et al.*, 1971, 1973a,b; Klenk and Rott, 1973; Stanley *et al.*, 1973). Thus, fowl plague virions grown in chick embryo fibroblasts contain only cleaved hemagglutinin glycoproteins, whereas there is virtually no cleavage if WSN virions are grown in MDBK cells in the absence of serum. In the presence of serum, however, WSN hemagglutinin is cleaved, too. Cleavage takes place in this system at the plasma membrane (Lazarowitz *et al.*, 1971), and the enzyme responsible for cleavage is serum plasminogen activated by an activator produced by the host cell (Lazarowitz *et al.*, 1973b). In the fowl plague system the mechanism of cleavage appears to be different. Cleavage occurs on intracellular membranes and plasminogen is not required (Klenk *et al.*, 1974a). The rate of cleavage is drastically reduced at 25°C (Klenk and Rott, 1973).

Cleavage of HA is not a precondition for hemagglutinating activity and assembly of the virion (Lazarowitz *et al.*, 1973a; Stanley *et al.*, 1973), but recent studies have revealed that it is necessary for infectivity (Klenk *et al.*, 1975b). These findings are compatible with the hypothesis that, in addition to its role in adsorption, the hemagglutinin has another function in the infection process and that cleavage is required for this function. The observations, that cleavage of HA is a host-dependent phenomenon and that particles containing uncleaved HA have a low infectivity, suggest that host range and spread of infection of an influenza virus might depend on the presence of a host protease as an activating enzyme.

Cell fractionation studies of influenza virus-infected cells have revealed that the hemagglutinin glycoproteins are always associated with membranes (Compans, 1973a; Klenk *et al.*, 1974a). The intracellular location of these proteins and their migration from the rough to the smooth endoplasmic reticulum and the plasma membrane will be described in detail in Section VII, B.

6. Neuraminidase (NA)

Viral neuraminidase has been detected as active enzyme 3 hours after infection in chorioallantoic membranes, and, by extrapolation, its synthesis has been estimated to start as early as 1 to 2 hours after infection (Noll *et al.*, 1961). The intracellular location of the neuraminidase has been investigated by cell fractionation and appears to be similar to that of the hemagglutinin (Compans, 1973a; Klenk *et al.*, 1974a). The neuraminidase has been found in association with membranes derived from the smooth endoplasmic reticulum as detected by biological activity and polyacrylamide gel electrophoresis. Enzymatic activity has also been found in fractions containing rough membranes. These data are in agreement with immunofluorescence studies (Maeno and Kilbourne, 1970). Four hours after infection neuraminidase could be detected in the cytoplasm; later it appeared to be concentrated at the cell periphery.

V. Carbohydrate Synthesis

Carbohydrate is present in the influenza virus envelope in the formation of glycoproteins and glycolipids (Klenk *et al.*, 1972a). The glycolipids of myxoviruses are derived from the plasma membrane of the host cell (Klenk and Choppin, 1970b), but it has not been determined whether preformed or newly synthesized glycolipid is preferentially incorporated into the virion.

The use of radioactive precursors, such as glucosamine, mannose, galactose, and fucose, which are incorporated specifically into viral glycoproteins, has demonstrated that the carbohydrate side chains of these glycoproteins are newly synthesized during infection (Haslam *et al.*, 1970; Compans *et al.*, 1970a; Schwarz and Klenk, 1974). Cell fractionation studies have provided further information on the sites of glycosylation of the viral glycoproteins. Glucosamine is associated with the HA polypeptide in both the smooth and rough cytoplasmic membrane fractions; however, fucose is associated with HA in the smooth but not in the rough membranes (Compans, 1973b). Inhibition of protein synthesis by puromycin stops the incorporation of glucosamine almost immediately, whereas fucose continues to be incorporated for approximately 10–15 minutes (Stanley *et al.*, 1973). Finally, with fowl plague virus the precursor glycoprotein HA and the cleavage products HA_1 and HA_2 appear to contain the full mannose and glucosamine complement, whereas the fucose and galactose content is significantly higher in the cleavage products (Klenk *et al.*, 1975a; Schwarz and Klenk, 1974). These observations suggest that biosynthesis of the carbohydrate side chains of the hemagglutinin glycoproteins occurs in a stepwise manner, with different saccharide residues added in distinct cellular compartments. Glucosamine and mannose appear to be attached to HA polypeptides in rough membranes very soon after or even during polypeptide synthesis, whereas fucose appears to be attached later by transferases present in smooth membranes.

These glycosyl transferases are presumably host-specific enzymes. The carbohydrate moiety of the glycoproteins appears to be determined, therefore, by the host cell. There is evidence, however, that in addition to these host enzymes the viral neuraminidase plays an essential role in the formation of the carbohydrate side chains. It has been found that the surface of myxovirus envelopes is devoid of neuraminic acid (Klenk and Choppin, 1970b; Klenk et al., 1970), whereas in viral envelopes, which do not contain the enzyme, this carbohydrate is a common constituent (Klenk and Choppin, 1971; McSharry and Wagner, 1971; Renkonen et al., 1971). These findings suggest that the lack of neuraminic acid is an essential feature of myxoviruses. Recently it could indeed be shown that neuraminidase is responsible for removing neuraminic acid from the influenza virus envelope, thereby preventing the formation of receptors on the viral envelope, which otherwise would lead to formation of large aggregates of virus particles (Palese et al., 1974). These observations support the concept that the carbohydrate moiety of the hemagglutinin as the major envelope glycoprotein is the product of the combined action of host cell transferases and viral neuraminidase. By the action of the neuraminidase the virus is able to introduce a virus-specific modification into a primarily host-specific complex carbohydrate structure, a modification which appears to be essential for the biological activity of the virus.

D-Glucosamine and 2-deoxy-D-glucose inhibit the formation of biologically active hemagglutinin, neuraminidase, and infectious virus (Kilbourne, 1959; Kaluza et al., 1972), and biochemical studies have revealed that the sugars interfere with the biosynthesis of viral glycoproteins (Gandhi et al., 1972; Klenk et al., 1972b). In the presence of the inhibitors the size of the hemagglutinin glycoproteins decreases. The extent of the decrease is dose dependent. Thus, as the sugar concentration increases glycoprotein HA with a molecular weight of 76,000 is gradually converted into a compound of the molecular weight of 64,000, which has been designated HA_0 (Klenk et al., 1972b; Schwarz and Klenk, 1974). The shift in molecular weight is paralleled by a decrease of the carbohydrate content, and protein HA_0 has been shown to be almost free of carbohydrate (Schwarz and Klenk, 1974). These findings indicate that HA_0 is the incompletely glycosylated or unglycosylated polypeptide chain of glycoprotein HA and that the inhibitory effect of D-glucosamine and 2-deoxy-D-glucose is due to an impairment of glycosylation. Polypeptide HA_0 is associated with membranes as is the normal HA. It migrates also from rough to smooth endoplasmic reticulum, where it is cleaved into polypeptides HA_{01} and HA_{02}. Therefore the carbohydrates do not appear to be essential for the membrane affinity of the polypeptide. However, the lack of hemagglutinating activity in infected cells suggests that the unglycosylated protein is unable to bind to receptors.

VI. Lipid Synthesis

As enveloped viruses in general, influenza virus acquires its lipids by utilization of host cell lipids. This concept is supported by the following observations. The lipid composition of influenza virus was found to be similar to that of the host cell (Ambruster and Beiss, 1958; Frommhagen et al., 1959). Host cell lipids, labeled radioactively before infection, are incorporated into virus particles (Wecker, 1957). When virus was grown in different host cells, modifications of the viral lipids were detected (Kates et al., 1961, 1962). In general, lipids of viruses which bud at the cell surface closely reflect the lipid composition of the host cell plasma membrane (Klenk and Choppin, 1969, 1970a,b; Renkonen et al., 1971). The rate of de novo synthesis of phospholipids in chick embryo fibroblasts was unchanged up to 7 hours after infection with influenza virus; thereafter all lipid synthesis was depressed (Blough et al., 1973). This depression is probably not a primary effect, but may be secondary to inhibition of RNA or protein synthesis or other cytopathic effects. Thus, the results obtained to date suggest that synthesis of viral lipids occurs by the normal cellular process of lipid biosynthesis, and the viral envelope is formed by incorporation of lipids from the host cell plasma membrane.

VII. Assembly (see also Chapter 2)

A. Nucleocapsid Formation

As has been described above, the nucleocapsid protein is most likely synthesized in the cytoplasm. It appears that it is present there for a short period in a free form and that it then associates with viral RNA to form nucleocapsids (Klenk et al., 1974a; Compans and Caliguiri, 1973). Whereas the NP protein is rapidly incorporated into nucleocapsids, the RNA may be derived from a preformed pool (Krug, 1972). Because of the small size of the influenza nucleocapsids, they cannot be identified with certainty by electron microscopy in infected cells. Clusters of strands or fibers about

50 Å in diameter, observed in the cytoplasm, may represent viral ribonucleo-proteins (Apostolov *et al.*, 1970; Compans *et al.*, 1970b).

The available evidence indicates that the RNA genome of influenza virions consists of 5–7 segments (Chapter 6). An infective particle, therefore, requires one copy of each segment. Hirst (1962) has proposed that nucleo-capsids could be incorporated randomly into virions from the intracellular pool. The proportion of infective virions in a population may be increased by incorporation of extra pieces of RNA into the average virion (Compans *et al.*, 1970b). For example, if five different pieces of RNA were needed for infectivity, but each virion contained a total of seven pieces incorporated at random, then $\sim 22\%$ of the virions would be infective. Evidence in favor of random incorporation of RNA segments has been provided by the recent observations of Hirst (1973) that recombination occurs between non-plaque-forming particles in virus populations. The ability of non-plaque-forming particles to undergo recombination can be explained by the absence of one or more pieces from the particles, with the missing pieces varying from one particle to another; thus suitable pairs of defective virus can form recombinants.

B. Budding Process

As most enveloped viruses, influenza virus is assembled on preformed cellular membranes; assembly takes place by budding from the plasma membrane. The first demonstration of virus release from cells by a process not involving lysis was provided by Murphy and Bang (1952) in early electron microscopic studies of influenza virus-infected cells. Filaments and spheres were observed to project from the cell surface into the extracellular space. No virus particles were observed in the interior of cells at times when infective virus was produced, and it therefore appeared that the virus particles were formed at the cell surface. Using ferritin-labeled antibody, Morgan *et al.* (1961) observed that the cell surface contained viral antigen in areas where virus was forming. More recent electron microscopic studies have demonstrated that the envelope of the merging virus contains a unit membrane such as that of the host cell, with a layer of projections, corresponding to the viral spikes, on the outer surface. On the inner surface of the viral membrane is an additional electron-dense layer which is not found on the cell surface, which probably consists of the M polypeptide (Bächi *et al.*, 1969; Compans and Dimmock, 1969; Apostolov *et al.*, 1970). Electron microscopic observations have provided suggestive evidence for the order in which viral components associate at the cell surface (Bächi *et al.*, 1969; Compans and Dimmock, 1969; Compans *et al.*, 1970b). Viral envelope proteins appear first to be incorporated into areas of the membrane which appear to be of normal morphology; however, specific adsorption of erythrocytes is observed to such regions of membrane indicating the presence of HA protein. The membrane (M) protein then presumably associates with the inner surface of such regions of membranes, forming an electron-dense layer. The ribonucleoprotein then binds specifically to the membrane in such regions, and the process of budding occurs by an outfolding and pinching off of a segment of the membrane, enclosing the associated nucleoprotein. Polyacrylamide gel electrophoresis studies also support the idea that the envelope proteins associate with the plasma membrane more rapidly than the RNP (Lazarowitz *et al.*, 1971). Host cell polypeptides are excluded from the membrane which is a precursor to the viral envelope, since such polypeptides are not detected in purified virions. As already mentioned, neuraminic acid residues are absent in the envelope of budding influenza virus particles but are present in the adjacent cell membrane (Klenk *et al.*, 1970). These observations establish that there is an abrupt transition in chemical composition between the envelope of a budding virus particle and the abjacent cell membrane.

On the other hand, however, it is an important feature of the budding process that the viral envelope is continuous with and morphologically similar to the plasma membrane of the host cell (Compans and Dimmock, 1969). As has been pointed out above, the lipids in these envelopes very closely resemble those of the host cell membrane. These observations suggest that the lipids in the unaltered plasma membrane are easily exchangeable by lateral diffusion with those in budding virus particles.

It therefore appears that the envelope of a budding virion is derived from a patch of cell membrane modified by the incorporation of viral envelope proteins. This concept does not, of course, necessarily imply that all envelope components are synthesized on the plasma membrane. In fact, it has been known for a long time that envelope constituents have to migrate considerable distances from one cell compartment to another in order to get from the site of their biosynthesis to the site of envelope assembly. Breitenfeld and Schäfter (1957) have shown that in cells infected with influenza virus the hemagglutinin can first be seen throughout the cell and is located in a higher concentration in a juxtanuclear locus. Later the hemagglutinin accumulates in the peripheral region of the cell and also may be demonstrated in fine filaments which protrude from the cell margin.

The concept that envelope components migrate from the interior of the cell to the surface has recently been confirmed and extended by a series of studies employing cell fractionation and analysis of the viral proteins in the various cell fractions. As has been outlined above these studies suggest that the hemagglutinin glycoprotein and possibly the other envelope proteins are synthesized on the rough endoplasmic reticulum (Compans, 1973a; Klenk *et al.*, 1974). As detected by pulse-chase experiments, a few minutes later the hemagglutinin is present in the membranes of the smooth endoplasmic reticulum (Compans, 1973a; Stanley *et al.*, 1973; Klenk *et al.*, 1974) and in the plasma membrane (Stanley *et al.*, 1973). Although chase experiments from the smooth endoplasmic reticulum into the plasma membrane have not been carried out, it appears likely that the hemagglutinin migrates from the rough through the smooth endoplasmic reticulum to the plasma membrane. It should be pointed out that throughout this migration the hemagglutinin and the other envelope proteins are constituents of the membranes along which they move; they are never detected as soluble proteins. In smooth membrane fractions believed to be derived primarily from the endoplasmic reticulum all major envelope proteins are found (Compans, 1973a; Klenk *et al.*, 1974). However, their proportions differ from those in the plasma membrane and in the virion (Stanley *et al.*, 1973; Klenk *et al.*, 1974). The ratio of protein M to the hemagglutinin glycoproteins is much higher in mature viral envelopes than in membranes of the endoplasmic reticulum. This finding suggests that only a small amount of the membranes carrying hemagglutinin glycoprotein is converted into viral envelopes, namely, that fraction which also contains the carbohydrate-free protein. As has been pointed out above, the synthesis of M protein might be rate limiting for virus assembly.

Different rates of synthesis of the various envelope proteins support the hypothesis that the assembly of the envelope is a multistep process. Compatible with this concept is the processing of the hemagglutinin involving sequential attachment of the carbohydrate moiety and proteolytic cleavage of the primary gene product in the course of migration.

VIII. Release

The problem of release of influenza virus from the host cell appears to be closely linked to that of the function of the viral neuraminidase which has already been discussed in detail (Section V and Chapter 4). That the enzyme plays an essential role in virus release has been suggested by the ability of antibody specific for neuraminidase to inhibit release (Seto and Rott, 1966; Webster *et al.*, 1968). In addition such antibody prevents elution of virus from erythrocytes (Brown and Laver, 1968). Bacterial neuraminidase, which is not inhibited by antibody to viral neuraminidase, is able to cause release of virus from antibody-treated cells (Compans *et al.*, 1969; Webster, 1970). On the other hand, bivalent antibody to neuraminidase also causes virus aggregation (Seto and Chang, 1969; Compans *et al.*, 1969; Webster, 1970), and monovalent antibody does not prevent virus release, although inhibiting over 90% of the neuraminidase activity (Becht *et al.*, 1971). All of these data taken together suggest that bivalent antibodies prevent virus release by cross-linking virus to antigens present on the cell surface *and* by inhibiting the enzyme activity. That the neuraminidase indeed plays an essential role in virus release is also suggested by the recent observations of Palese *et al.* (1974), who found that the enzyme is required to remove neuraminic acid from the viral envelope in order to avoid aggregation of the progeny virus on the cell surface.

IX. Abnormal Forms of Multiplication

A. Host-Dependent Abortive Multiplication

Influenza viruses can infect a wide variety of host cells. In many of these infected cells, however, the yield of infectious progeny is either extremely low or not measurable, although viral components can be found in normal titers. This type of host-dependent interruption of the infectious cycle is called an abortive infection. Such an abortive infectious cycle was observed originally in mice injected intracerebrally with non-neurotropic strains of influenza virus (Schlesinger, 1953). The higher the inoculated dose of the virus, the higher was the amount of newly synthesized hemagglutinin. Several other influenza virus A–host cell systems have been described in the meanwhile in which only RNP antigen and hemagglutinin but no significant amounts of infectious virus are produced. In all systems so far tested the RNP antigen accumulates in the nucleus and cannot be detected by fluorescent antibodies within the cytoplasm (Henle *et al.*, 1955; Franklin and Breitenfeld, 1959; Ter Meulen and Love, 1967; Fraser, 1967).

B. von Magnus Phenomenon

During serial passages of influenza viruses at a multiplicity higher than 1 (Barry, 1961) increasing amounts of incomplete virus are formed which are released from the host cells (von Magnus, 1951, 1952). These virus particles have a surface structure very similar to infectious virus, they are immunogenic and they cause homologous interference. They contain less RNA and RNP antigen, show a lower infectivity to hemagglutinin ratio, and contain more lipid than complete virus particles (von Magnus, 1954; Isaacs, 1959; Pauker *et al.,* 1959; Rott and Schäfer, 1961; Rott and Scholtissek, 1963).

An analysis of the RNA of incomplete virus has revealed that viral RNA of relatively high molecular weight is either missing or present in reduced amounts, while the amount of a low molecular weight RNA increases (Duesberg, 1968; Pons and Hirst, 1969; Nayak, 1969).

In cells infected with the second undiluted passage of influenza virus, the total information is present in so far as complementary RNA isolated from these cells is able to render labeled RNA isolated from infectious virus completely RNase-resistant after annealing (Scholtissek and Rott, 1969b). Thus the appearance of increased amounts of low molecular weight RNA in incomplete particles might be at the expense of high molecular weight RNA, which might be incorporated into these particles as broken and therefore nonfunctional molecules. This idea is strengthened by the observation that with each undiluted passage the capacity to produce infectious virus is lost first, followed by the loss to synthesize hemagglutinin, neuraminidase, and finally of RNP antigen (Scholtissek *et al.,* 1966).

Nayak (1972) found that during the first passage of high multiplicity the early yield of virus was fully infectious and showed the normal pattern of RNA pieces of infectious virus in a sucrose gradient, while the late virus yield had an RNA pattern typical for von Magnus incomplete virus.

Acknowledgments

We thank Drs. L. A. Caliguiri, P. W. Choppin, R. W. Compans, and P. Palese for preprints of manuscripts in press.

References

Anschütz, W., Scholtissek, C., and Rott, R. (1972). *Med. Microbiol. Immunol.* **158,** 26.

Apostolov, K., Flewett, T. H., and Kendall, A. P. (1970). *In* "The Biology of Large RNA Viruses" (R. D. Barry and B. W. J. Mahy, eds.), pp. 3–26. Academic Press, New York.

Armbruster, O., and Beiss, U. (1958). *Z. Naturforsch. B* **13,** 75.

Bächi, T., Gerhard, W., Lindenmann, J., and Mühlethaler, K. (1969). *J. Virol.* **4,** 769.

Baltimore, D. (1971). *Strategy Viral Genome, Ciba Found. Symp.* pp. 99–100.

Barry, R. D. (1961). *Virology* **14,** 389.

Barry, R. D. (1964). *Virology* **24,** 563.

Barry, R. D., Ives, D. R., and Cruickshank, J. G. (1962). *Nature (London)* **194,** 1139.

Barry, R. D., Cox, N. J., and Armstrong, S. J. (1975). *In* "Negative Strand Viruses" (R. D. Barry and B. W. J. Mahy, eds.). Academic Press, New York.

Bean, W. J., Jr., and Simpson, R. W. (1973). *Virology* 56, 646.

Becht, H. (1971). *J. Virol.* 7, 204.

Becht, H., Hämmerling, U., and Rott, R. (1971). *Virology* 46, 337.

Blough, H. A., Gallaher, W. R., and Weinstein, D. B. (1973). *In* "Membrane Mediated Information" (P. W. Kent, ed.), Vol. I, pp. 183–199. MTP, Lancaster, England.

Breitenfeld, P. M., and Schäfer, W. (1957). *Virology* 4, 328.

Brown, J., and Laver, W. G. (1968). *J. Gen. Virol.* 2, 291.

Burnet, F. M., and Stone, J. D. (1947). *Aust. J. Exp. Biol. Med.* 25, 227.

Caliguiri, L. A., and Compans, R. W. (1974). *J. Virol.* 14, 191.

Caliguiri, L. A., and Tamm, I. (1970). *Virology* 42, 100.

Choppin, P. W. (1969). *Virology* 38, 130.

Compans, R. W. (1973a). *Virology* 51, 56.

Compans, R. W. (1973b). *Virology* 55, 541.

Compans, R. W., and Caliguiri, L. A. (1973). *J. Virol.* 11, 441.

Compans, R. W., and Choppin, P. W. (1974). *Compr. Virol.* (in press).

Compans, R. W., and Dimmock, N. J. (1969). *Virology* 39, 499.

Compans, R. W. Dimmock, N. J., and Meier-Ewert H. (1969). *J. Virol.* 4, 528.

Compans, R. W., Klenk, H.-D., Caliguiri, L. A., and Choppin, P. W. (1970a). *Virology* 42, 880.

Compans, R. W., Dimmock, N. J., and Meier-Ewert, H. (1970b). *In* "The Biology of Large RNA Viruses" (R. D. Barry and B. W. J. Mahy, eds.), pp. 87–108. Academic Press, New York.

Dales, S., and Choppin, P. W. (1962). *Virology* 18, 489.

Dimmock, N. J. (1969). *Virology* 39, 224.

Dimmock, N. J., and Watson, D. H. (1969). *J. Gen. Virol.* 5, 499.

Dourmashkin, R. R., and Tyrrell, D. A. J. (1970). *J. Gen. Virol.* 9, 77.

Duesberg, P. H. (1968). *Proc. Nat. Acad. Sci. (U.S.)* 59, 930.

Duesberg, P. H., and Robinson, W. S. (1967). *J. Mol. Biol.* 25, 383.

Fazekas de St. Groth, S. (1948). *Nature (London)* 162, 294.

Feix, G., Slor, H., and Weissmann, C. (1967). *Proc. Nat. Acad. Sci. U.S.* 57, 1401.

Follett, E. A. C., Pringle, C. R., Wunner, W. H., and Skehel, J. J. (1974). *J Virol.* 13, 394.

Franklin, R. M., and Breitenfeld, P. M. (1959). *Virology* 8, 293.

Fraser, K. B. (1967). *J. Gen. Virol.* 1, 1.

Frommhagen, L. H., Knight, C. A., and Freeman, N. K. (1959). *Virology* 8, 176.

Gandhi, S. S., Stanley, P., Taylor, J. M., and White, D. O. (1972). *Microbios* 5, 41.

Gottschalk, A. (1957). *Biochim. Biophys. Acta* 23, 645.

Gregoriades, A. (1970). *Virology* 42, 905.

Gregoriades, A. (1973). *Virology* 54, 369.

Haslam, E. A., Hampson, A. W., Egan, J. A., and White, D. O. (1970). *Virology* 42, 555.

Hastie, N. D., and Mahy, B. W. J. (1973). *J. Virol.* 12, 951.

Haywood, A. (1975). *In* "Negative-Strand Viruses" (R. D. Barry and B. W. J. Mahy, eds.), pp. 923–928. Academic Press, New York.

Henle, G., Girardi, A., and Henle, W. (1955). *J. Exp. Med.* 101, 25.

Hirst, G. K. (1941). *Science* 94, 22.

Hirst, G. K. (1942). *J. Exp. Med.* **76**, 195.
Hirst, G. K. (1962). *Cold Spring Harbor Symp. Quant. Biol.* **27**, 303.
Hirst, G. K. (1973). *Virology* **55**, 81.
Ho, P. P. K., and Walters, C. P. (1966). *Biochemistry* **5**, 231.
Hobson, D., and Scholtissek, C. (1970). *J. Gen. Virol.* **9**, 151.
Holland, J. J., and Kiehn, E. D. (1970). *Science* **167**, 202.
Holtermann, O. A., Hillis, W. D., and Moffat, M. A. J. (1960). *Acta Pathol. Microbiol. Scand.* **50**, 398.
Horisberger, M., and Guskey, L. E. (1973). *J. Virol.* **13**, 230.
Hoyle, L. (1968). *In* "Virology Monographs" (S. Gard, C. Hallauer, and K. F. Meyer, eds.), Vol. 4, Springer-Verlag, Berlin and New York.
Huang, R. T. C. (1974). *Med. Microbiol. Immunol.* **159**, 129.
Hughes, R. C. (1973). *Prog. Biophys. Mol. Biol.* **26**, 191.
Isaacs, A. (1959). *In* "The Viruses" (F. M. Burnet and W. M. Stanley, eds.), Vol. 3, pp. 143–150. Academic Press, New York.
Joss, A., Gandhi, S. S., Hay, A. J., and Burke, D. C. (1969). *J. Virol.* **4**, 816.
Kaluza, G., Scholtissek, C., and Rott, R. (1972). *J. Gen. Virol.* **14**, 251.
Kates, M., Allison, A. C., Tyrrell, D. S., and James, A. T. (1961). *Biochim. Biophys. Acta* **52**, 455.
Kates, M., Allison, A. C., Tyrrell, D. A., and James, A. T. (1962). *Cold Spring Harbor Symp. Quant. Biol.* **27**, 293.
Kelly, D. C., Avery, R. J., and Dimmock, N. J. (1974). *J. Virol.* **13**, 1155.
Kilbourne, E. D. (1959). *Nature (London)* **183**, 271.
Kilbourne, E. D., Laver, W. G., Schulman, J. L., and Webster, R. G. (1968). *J. Virol.* **2**, 281.
Kilbourne, E. D., Choppin, P. W., Schulze, I. T., Scholtissek, C., and Bucher, D. L. (1972). *J. Infec. Dis.* **125**, 447.
Kingsbury, D. W., and Webster, R. G. (1973). *Virology* **56**, 654.
Klenk, E., and Stoffel, W. (1956). *Hoppe-Seyler's Z. Physiol. Chem.* **303**, 78.
Klenk, E., Faillard, H., and Lempfrid, H. (1955). *Hoppe-Seyler's Z. Physiol. Chem.* **301**, 235.
Klenk, H.-D., and Choppin, P. W. (1969). *Virology* **38**, 255.
Klenk, H.-D., and Choppin, P. W. (1970a). *Virology* **40**, 939.
Klenk, H.-D., and Choppin, P. W. (1970b). *Proc. Nat. Acad. Sci. U.S.* **66**, 57.
Klenk, H.-D., and Choppin, P. W. (1971). *J. Virol* **7**, 416.
Klenk, H.-D., and Rott, R. (1973). *J. Virol.* **11**, 823.
Klenk, H.-D., Compans, R. W., and Choppin, P. W. (1970). *Virology* **42**, 1158.
Klenk, H.-D., Rott, R., and Becht, H. (1972a). *Virology* **47**, 579.
Klenk, H.-D., Scholtissek, C., and Rott, R. (1972b). *Virology* **49**, 723.
Klenk, H.-D., Wöllert, W., Rott, R., and Scholtissek, C. (1974a). *Virology* **57**, 28.
Klenk, H.-D., Wöllert, W., Rott, R., and Scholtissek, C. (1975a). *In* "Negative-Strand Viruses" (R. D. Barry and B. W. J. Mahy, eds.), pp. 621–634. Academic Press, New York.
Klenk, H.-D., Rott, Orlich, M., and Blödor, J. (1975b). *Virology* (in press).
Krug, R. M. (1972). *Virology* **50**, 103.
Krug, R. M., and Etkind, P. R. (1973). *Virology* **56**, 334.
Lazarowitz, S. G., Compans, R. W., and Choppin, P. W. (1971). *Virology* **46**, 830.
Lazarowitz, S. G., Compans, R. W., and Choppin, P. W. (1973a). *Virology* **52**, 199.

Lazarowitz, S. G., Goldberg, A. R., and Choppin, P. W. (1973b). *Virology* **56,** 172.

Liu, C. (1955). *J. Exp. Med.* **101,** 677.

McClelland, L., and Hare, R. (1941). *Can. Pub. Health. J.* **32,** 530.

McSharry, J. J., and Wagner, R. R. (1971). *J. Virol.* **7,** 59.

Maeno, K., and Kilbourne, E. D. (1970). *J. Virol.* **5,** 153.

Mahy, B. W. J. (1970). *In* "The Biology of Large RNA Viruses" (R. D. Barry and B. W. J. Mahy, eds.), pp. 392–415. Academic Press, New York.

Mahy, B. W. J., and Bromley, P. A. (1970). *J. Virol.* **6,** 259.

Mahy, B. W. J., Hastie, H. D., and Armstrong, S. G. (1972). *Proc. Nat. Acad. Sci. U.S.* **69,** 1421.

Mahy, B. W. J., Brownson, J. M. T., Caroll, A. R., Hastie, N. D., and Raper, R. H. (1975). *In* "Negative-Strand Viruses" (R. D. Barry and B. W. J. Mahy, eds.). Academic Press, New York.

Marchesi, V. T., Jackson, R. L., Segrest, J. P., and Kahane, I. (1973). *Fed. Proc., Fed. Amer. Soc. Exp. Biol.* **32,** 1833.

Morgan, C., and Rose, H. P. (1968). *J. Virol.* **2,** 925.

Morgan, C., Hsu, K. C., Rifkind, R. A., Knox, A. W., and Rose, H. M. (1961). *J. Exp. Med.* **114,** 825.

Murphy, J. S., and Bang, F. B. (1952). *J. Exp. Med.* **95,** 259.

Nayak, D. P. (1969). *Fed. Proc., Fed. Amer. Soc. Exp. Biol.* **28,** 1858.

Nayak, D. P. (1970). *In* "The Biology of Large RNA Viruses" (R. D. Barry and B. W. J. Mahy, eds.), pp. 371–391. Academic Press, New York.

Nayak, D. P. (1972). *J. Gen. Virol.* **14,** 63.

Nayak, D. P., and Rasmussen, A. F., Jr. (1966). *Virology* **30,** 673.

Noll, H., Aoyagi, T., and Orlando, J. (1961). *Virology* **14,** 141.

Öberg, B., and Philipson, L. (1971). *J. Mol. Biol.* **58,** 725.

Paffenholz, V., and Scholtissek, C. (1973). *Z. Naturforsch. C* **28,** 208.

Palese, P., Tobita, K., Ueda, M., and Compans, R. W. (1974). *Virology* **6,** 397.

Pauker, K., Birch-Anderson, A., and von Magnus, P. (1959). *Virology* **8,** 1.

Pons, M. W. (1967). *Virology* **33,** 150.

Pons, M. W. (1971). *Virology* **46,** 149.

Pons, M. W. (1972). *Virology* **47,** 823.

Pons, M. W. (1973). *Virology* **51,** 120.

Pons, M. W., and Hirst, G. K. (1968). *Virology* **35,** 182.

Pons, M. W., and Hirst, G. K. (1969). *Virology* **38,** 68.

Pons, M. W., Schulze, I. T., Hirst, G. K., and Hauser, R. (1969). *Virology* **39,** 250.

Renkonen, O., Kääriäinen, L., Simons, K., and Gahmberg, C. C. (1971). *Virology* **46,** 318.

Rott, R., Schäfer, W. (1961). *Z. Naturforsch. B* **16,** 310.

Rott, R., and Scholtissek, C. (1963). *J. Gen. Microbiol.* **33,** 303.

Rott, R., and Scholtissek, C. (1964). *Z. Naturforsch. B* **19,** 316–323.

Rott, R., and Scholtissek, C. (1970). *Nature (London)* **228,** 56.

Rott, R., Saber, S., and Scholtissek, C. (1965). *Nature (London)* **205,** 1187.

Ruck, B. J., Brammer, K. W., Page, M. G., and Coombes, J. D. (1969). *Virology* **39,** 31.

Schäfer, W. (1957). *Nature Viruses, Ciba Found. Symp., 1956* pp. 91–103.

Schlesinger, R. W. (1953). *Cold Spring Harbor Symp. Quant. Biol.* **18,** 55.

Scholtissek, C. (1965). *Biochim. Biophys. Acta* **103,** 146.

Scholtissek, C. (1969). *Biochim. Biophys. Acta* **179,** 389.

Scholtissek, C. (1971). *Eur. J. Biochem.* **24**, 358.
Scholtissek, C., and Becht, H. (1971). *J. Gen. Virol.* **10**, 11.
Scholtissek, C., and Rott, R. (1961). *Z. Naturforsch. B* **16**, 663.
Scholtissek, C., and Rott, R. (1964). *Virology* **22**, 169.
Scholtissek, C., and Rott, R. (1969a). *J. Gen. Virol.* **4**, 125.
Scholtissek, C., and Rott, R. (1969b). *Virology* **39**, 400.
Scholtissek, C., and Rott, R. (1970). *Virology* **40**, 989.
Scholtissek, C., Rott, R., Hausen, P., Hausen, H. and Schäfer, W. (1962). *Cold Spring Harbor Symp. Quant. Biol.* **27**, 245.
Scholtissek, C., Drzeniek, R., and Rott, R. (1966). *Virology* **30**, 313.
Scholtissek, C., Becht, H., and Drzeniek, R. (1967). *J. Gen. Virol.* **1**, 219.
Scholtissek, C., Drzeniek, R., and Rott, R. (1969). *In* "The Biochemistry of Viruses" (H. B. Levy, ed.), pp. 219–258. Dekker, New York.
Scholtissek, C., Becht, H., and MacPherson, I. (1970). *J. Gen. Virol.* **8**, 11.
Scholtissek, C., Becht, H., and Rott, R. (1971). *Virology* **43**, 137.
Scholtissek, C., Kaluza, G., and Rott, R. (1972). *J. Gen. Virol.* **17**, 213.
Scholtissek, C., Rott, R., and Klenk, H.-D. (1975). *Virology* **63**, 191.
Schultze, I. T. (1970). *Virology* **42**, 890.
Schwarz, R. T., and Klenk, H.-D. (1974). *J. Virol.* **14**, 1023.
Schwarz, R. T., and Scholtissek, C. (1973). *Z. Naturforsch. C* **28**, 202.
Seto, J. T., and Chang, F. S. (1969). *J. Virol.* **4**, 58.
Seto, J. T., and Rott, R. (1966). *Virology* **30**, 731.
Siegert, W., Bauer, G., and Hofschneider, P. H. (1973). *Proc. Nat. Acad. Sci. U.S.* **70**, 2960.
Skehel, J. J. (1972). *Virology* **49**, 23.
Skehel, J. J. (1973). *Virology* **56**, 394.
Skehel, J. J., and Burke, D. C. (1969). *J. Virol.* **3**, 429.
Stanley, P., Gandhi, S. S., and White, D. O. (1973). *Virology* **53**, 92.
Suttajit, M., and Winzler, R. J. (1971). *J. Biol. Chem.* **246**, 3398.
Taylor, J. M., Hampson, A. W., and White, D. O. (1969). *Virology* **39**, 419.
Taylor, J. M., Hampson, A. W., Layton, J. E., and White, D. O. (1970). *Virology* **42**, 744.
Ter Meulen, V., and Love, R. (1967). *J. Virol.* **1**, 626.
Tiffany, J. M., and Blough, H. A. (1971). *Virology* **44**, 18.
von Magnus, P. (1951). *Acta Pathol. Microbiol. Scand.* **28**, 278.
von Magnus, P. (1952). *Acta Pathol. Microbiol. Scand.* **28**, 311.
von Magnus, P. (1954). *Advan. Virus Res.* **2**, 59.
Webster, R. G. (1970). *Virology* **40**, 643.
Webster, R. G., Laver, W. G., and Kilbourne, E. D. (1968). *J. Gen. Virol.* **3**, 315.
Wecker, E. (1957). *Z. Naturforsch. B* **12**, 208.
White, D. O. (1973). *In* "Comprehenserie Treatise in Microbiology," Vol. 63, p. 1. Springer-Verlag, Berlin and New York.
White, D. O., Day, H. M., Batchelder, E. J., Cheyne, I. M., and Wansbrough, A. J. (1965). *Virology* **25**, 289.
White, D. O., Taylor, J. M., Haslam, E. A., and Hampson, A. W. (1970). *In* "The Biology of Large RNA Viruses" (R. D. Barry and B. W. J. Mahy, eds.), pp. 602–618. Academic Press, New York.
Zimmermann, T., and Schäfer, W. (1960). *Virology* **11**, 676.

9

Laboratory Propagation of Human Influenza Viruses, Experimental Host Range, and Isolation from Clinical Material

W. R. Dowdle and G. C. Schild

I. Introduction

The first successful experimental transmission of influenza virus was achieved during the early years of this century with fowl plague virus, although this agent was not recognized as an influenza virus until 1955 (Schäfer, 1955). In 1931, Shope transmitted "classical" swine influenza from pig to pig by the intranasal inoculation of filtrates of respiratory secretions. The first evidence of transmission of human influenza to laboratory animals was obtained by Smith *et al.* (1933). They demonstrated that ferrets inoculated with human respiratory secretions from influenza cases developed febrile respiratory infections which were naturally transmitted among cagemates. The results of these studies were quickly confirmed by Francis (1934). Subsequently it was observed that mice inoculated under anesthesia with nasal turbinate material from infected ferrets developed pneumonia (Andrewes *et al.*, 1934). The above findings led to the use of experimental animals as assay systems for virus infectivity and produced rapid developments in knowledge of the properties of the influenza virus and of immunity to infection.

A further significant event was the finding of Burnet (1940) that the influenza virus could be propagated in cells lining the allantoic and amniotic cavities of the developing chick embryo. This finding was of obvious benefit in enabling workers to avoid the disadvantages associated with reliance on experimental animals and had the further advantage that relatively large amounts of influenza virus could be harvested in the form of infected allantoic fluids. Furthermore, influenza virus could be isolated directly in eggs without the need of prior adaptation in ferrets or mice, a procedure which could result in the accidental contamination of virus strains by extraneous agents. The discovery of the hemagglutinating properties of the influenza virus particle (Hirst, 1941) was also of fundamental importance in enabling the presence of virus to be detected without requiring demonstration of infectivity. A further significant landmark which has obvious implications to the study of influenza virus replication was the cultivation of the virus in cell cultures (Mogabgab *et al.*, 1954). The development of plaquing systems (Hotchin, 1955; Ledinko, 1955) in cell monolayer cultures for the assay of virus infectivity has also ultimately led to the potential for obtaining pure "clones" of influenza virus for use in genetic experiments.

II. Laboratory Propagation

A. Cell Cultures

Inoculation of influenza type A and type B viruses into cell cultures produces one of three effects: (1) virus may replicate with varying efficiency, forming infectious virus (productive infection); (2) virus may undergo an incomplete growth cycle, forming incomplete virus at the cell surface or noninfectious virus particles in the medium (abortive infection); or (3) virus may fail to infect. Some experimental evidence also suggests that a state of chronic infection may be induced in which small quantities of infective virus are released over a long time period (persistent infection).

1. PRODUCTIVE INFECTION

The replicative cycle of influenza viruses has been described in detail in Chapter 8. In brief, the inoculation of virus into a susceptible cell culture is followed by an "eclipse" period of approximately 2 hours during which no biological or serological evidence of virus protein synthesis is detected. During this early period virus-specific polypeptides are synthesized, including virus-specific components which are not incorporated into the virion. Approximately 2 hours after infection, nucleoprotein (NP) antigen may be detected intracellularly. The quantity of this component reaches maximal level 5–6 hours after infection. The presence of hemagglutinin or surface antigens in cell extracts is detectable 3 hours after infection. Budding virus may be detected in cell membranes approximately $5\frac{1}{2}$ hours after infection. Virus release commences shortly thereafter, at approximately 6 hours, and infective virus reaches maximum concentration in the medium 7–8 hours after infection.

Productive cycles of infection with human influenza virus strains occur in a variety of primary cell cultures from avian and mammalian species. A listing of these cultures may be found in Hoyle (1968). Rather than repeat this list an attempt is made here to summarize some of the more pertinent findings representing over 20 years of experience by a number of investigators.

Epithelioid cells provide the most sensitive *in vitro* system for propagation of the largest array of influenza A and B strains. The most common of these include human fetal kidney (Mogabgab *et al.*, 1954), rhesus or green monkey kidney (Mogabgab *et al.*, 1961), calf kidney (Haas and Wulff, 1957; Lehmann-Grube, 1965), pig kidney (Lehmann-Grube, 1964), and hamster kidney (Heath and Tyrrell, 1959). Of these, primary monkey, human, and calf kidney cells have been most widely used. Monkey kidney is usually preferred because of superior growth and handling characteristics.

Not all epithelioid cell cultures are permissive for influenza virus infection. Primary diploid or heteroploid human amnion cells, as well as other heteroploid epithelial cells, are usually refractory. Heteroploid cells include lines such as HeLa, KB, or conjunctival cells (Green *et al.*, 1957), as well as Maf, human heart, and intestine (Wong and Kilbourne, 1961).

Epithelioid cell cultures derived from fully developed organs provide more uniform sensitivity to influenza viruses than cultures derived from organs in the embryonic state. In our own experiencé, cell cultures prepared from kidneys removed from human stillbirths are equally as sensitive as monkey kidney for influenza viruses, whereas cell cultures from younger human embryos are not. One major problem with embryonic kidney cells is the lack of uniformity from lot to lot. The kidneys are usually obtained from fetuses of different ages and collected under such conditions that the percentages of viable cells may vary widely. These factors contribute to the wide variation in ratio of epithelial-like to fibroblast-like cells usually seen in human fetal kidney cultures. This in turn may contribute to the wide variation in virus susceptibility. Epithelial-like cells support virus replication; fibroblast-like cells do not. The same observations have been made with pig kidneys. Cultures from mature pig kidneys consist predominantly of epithelioid cells and support influenza virus multiplication. Cultures from embryonic kidneys consist almost entirely of fibroblastic cells and are virtually insusceptible (Lehmann-Grube, 1964). Experience suggests that this is a general observation for kidney cultures from most species.

Susceptibility of epithelioid cells to influenza infection decreases upon subpassage. In some instances, such as human embryonic kidney, subpassage of cell cultures favors proliferation of nonsusceptible fibroblasts. In other instances, such as monkey kidney (W. R. Dowdle, unpublished observations) and calf kidney (Lehmann-Grube, 1964), cell cultures retained their epithelioid characteristics after numerous passages, but patterns of virus susceptibility changed after the first subculture. The diploid state of epithelioid cells is not in itself indicative of virus susceptibility.

Some viruses may grow or be adapted to growth in fibroblasts, or heteroploid cell line, but such strains are rare. The influenza type A strain NWS (H0N1) is unique in its wide cell tropism and may propagate in heteroploid epithelial cells (Wong and Kilbourne, 1961), fibroblasts (Kilbourne *et al.*, 1964), or MBBK, a heteroploid bovine kidney line (Choppin, 1969). Influenza B virus has also been reported to grow in a heteroploid canine kidney cell line (Green, 1962).

Host specificity of infection is not always predictable. Swine viruses have been reported not to grow on human kidney cells (Hinz and Syverton, 1959), but human viruses readily grow on pig kidney cells (Lehmann-Grube, 1964). Monkey kidney cell cultures are refractory to equine (Heq2Neq2) viruses when inoculated directly from clinical specimens, but the same viruses grow well in monkey kidney after a single passage in eggs (Dowdle *et al.*, 1963).

Failure to adequately remove serum constituents before virus inoculation is one of the major reasons for poor isolation rates or lower infectivity assays in susceptible cell cultures. Components of the serum required as an essential ingredient for the growth phase of cell cultures may cause nonspecific neutralization of virus. This is particularly true for viruses prevalent since 1957.

The inhibitory effect of serum can be removed by two or more washings of the cells with serum-free medium.

2. ABORTIVE INFECTION

Henle *et al.* (1955) were the first to demonstrate that HeLa cells (from human cervical carcinoma) inoculated with high multiplicities of egg-grown virus produced noninfectious hemagglutinating particles. Abortive infections also were shown to occur with Earle's L cells infected with fowl plague virus (Franklin and Breitenfeld, 1959), a variety of cell lines infected with swine influenza virus (Wong and Kilbourne, 1961), Krebs 2 ascites tumor cells (Low *et al.*, 1962), BHK-21 cells (Fraser, 1967), and BSC-1 cells (Nikitin *et al.*, 1972). Abortive infections are not restricted to heteroploid cells, but have been shown for human diploid fibroblasts as well (Kilbourne *et al.*, 1964).

The mechanism of abortive infection is not completely clear; presumably, there is a block at some stage of the virus growth cycle. In studies of incomplete cycles of influenza replication in HeLa cells (Henle *et al.*, 1955) or L cells (Franklin and Breitenfeld, 1959), both NP antigen and hemagglutinating particles were produced in considerable quantities. Loffler *et al.* (1962) showed that in the course of abortive infection of HeLa cells, nucleoprotein tended to accumulate in the nucleus, and the released virus particles were deficient in total complement of ribonucleic acid (RNA). Choppin and Pons (1970) found that these noninfectious hemagglutinating particles produced by HeLa cells were deficient in the largest piece of RNA but possessed an increased amount of small RNA. They also found that HeLa cells could produce infective influenza virus if the inoculum was free of incomplete virus. In this respect the abortive infection of HeLa cells was similar to the classical von Magnus type of incomplete virus production in chick embryos (see Chapter 8).

3. PERSISTENT INFECTION

Some experimental evidence suggests the existence of low-grade chronic infection of cell cultures by influenza viruses. Tyrrell (1959) described chronic infection of cultured calf kidney cells with WS virus. Gavrilov *et al.* (1972) found that persistent infection of serially cultivated porcine kidney cells with WSN virus could be detected up to 105 days. Wilkinson and Borland (1972) found evidence of persistent infection with PR8 virus up to 50 days after infecting human lung cell cultures. The cells did not show cytopathogenic effects, and small amounts of infective virus could be detected in the culture medium. Such reports indicate that, at least with certain influenza virus strains, the establishment of short-term chronic infections may be possible, but a "true" persistent infection with influenza viruses has not yet been demonstrated.

4. PARAMETERS OF INFECTIONS

a. Intracellular Products of Infection. Fluorescent antibody (FA) techniques (Weller and Coons, 1954) have been employed extensively as immunological "probes" to identify and locate virus-specific antigens in infected cells. The parameters of the direct and indirect immunofluorescence techniques for viruses have been described in detail elsewhere (Liu, 1969). The earliest applications of this technique to influenza were by Watson and Coons (1954) and Liu (1955), who demonstrated the essentially intranuclear distribution of the fluorescence due to the NP antigen in influenza-infected cells. Subsequently the method has been extensively used in studies of the distribution of influenza antigens at various times in the virus replication cycle. Maeno and Kilbourne (1970) described the distribution of NP, hemagglutinin (HA), and neuraminidase (NA). Oxford and Schild (1974) studied the distribution of all four major antigens of the virus, including the matrix (M) protein.

Attempts to quantitate influenza infection in cell cultures by means of FA techniques have been made by Oxford and Schild (1968), who described an infective center counting technique for estimating the numbers of fluorescent cells.

Dimmock (1969) described an influenza-specific antigen which was present in the nucleoli of influenza-infected cells. The antigen could be demonstrated by FA techniques using sera from infected mice but not with sera prepared against virus particles. Nucleolar fluorescence appeared early in infection and was thought to be due to an influenza antigen induced in infected cells but not incorporated in virus particles.

FA techniques are extremely sensitive in detecting small quantities of antibody or antigen and are susceptible to nonspecific effects. Stringent controls are necessary. For detecting particular antigens it is essential to use highly specific antisera prepared against purified antigens.

Radioactive labeling techniques have been widely applied to the detection of intracellular virus proteins during influenza replication. Becht (1969) used radioactive-labeled precursors followed by autoradiography to show that NP was mainly found in the nucleus of the infected cell. Others (Joss et al., 1969; Taylor et al., 1969; Skehel, 1972) have employed the use of radioactive pulse-labeling techniques and polyacrylamide gel electrophoresis. Such studies will be described in detail elsewhere and need only brief mention in this chapter. One of the most successful techniques in this connection

antigen may be released into the culture medium. The release of virus and "soluble" antigen from infected cells may be followed by testing the culture fluids for virus products employing tests for biological activity or by assays of influenza-specific antigens. The most frequently used test to follow the course of virus release is the HA test (Hirst, 1941). Tests for neuraminidase activity are infrequently performed unless for some specific purpose. Both these tests detect essentially virus particles. Complement fixation (CF) tests for detection of virus antigen in culture fluids have been frequently employed using either antibody to NP or antibody to surface antigens ("V" antisera). Antisera to pure HA or NA also could be used. The latter test detects essentially virus particles or free envelope antigens, while in tests employing antibody to NP or M the "soluble" antigens rather than virus particles are detected. The parameters of these test systems for biological properties of the virus and assays for influenza antigens are described in Chapter 12.

The presence of infective virus particles is established by the use of one or other of the infectivity assay systems available. The most generally applicable and sensitive method for assays of infectivity is by the use of endpoint infectivity titrations in embryonated eggs. The use of embryonated eggs is described in Section II,D in this chapter. The egg infective dose 50% (EID_{50}) is calculated from the eggs infected with each dilution of virus using a standard calculation (Reed and Muench, 1938). Titers are expressed as EID_{50} per ml of fluid. Assays of infectivity may also be carried out using the allantois on shell technique of Fazekas de St. Groth and White (1958), also described later in this chapter, but in general this method is of lower sensitivity than titrations in eggs.

Virus titrations may also be carried out in cell cultures in an analogous way to egg infective titrations, but evidence of infection of cultures is estimated by the hemadsorption technique previously described.

Cytopathogenic effects have not often been used as evidence of influenza virus infection in cell cultures. These effects (reviewed by Pereira, 1961) are extremely variable for different virus strains and different cell cultures. Since they are essentially degenerative, consisting of cytoplasmic granulation, vacuolation, nuclear pyknosis, and cellular contraction and disintegration, titration endpoints cannot be determined with accuracy. Basophilic cytoplasmic inclusions in influenza A-infected cells have been described, but they also are variable (Soloviev and Alekseeva, 1960). Basophilic cytoplasmic inclusions are often regularly observed in cells infected with certain influenza B viruses (Porebska et al., 1968).

For some influenza virus strains, for example, fowl plague virus and the neurotropic variants of human strains NWS or WSN, assays of infectivity may be carried out by counting plaques on cell monolayer cultures using one of the plaquing techniques described in Section II,B. When employing a plaquing technique it is important to establish its efficiency in relationship to the egg infectivity titration. For the above strains, this ratio is approximately 1:1, but for most human influenza isolates and most plaquing systems the relative efficiency of plaquing is low.

B. Plaque Techniques

Plaque formation with influenza viruses has been extremely variable. Many viruses do not plaque and those that do frequently plaque at very low plating efficiencies. These observations are particularly true for influenza A viruses. Plaquing ability is a characteristic of individual strains without regard to subtype.

Plaque formation in primary cell cultures has been reported for chick embryo fibroblasts (Simpson and Hirst, 1961), lung (Granoff, 1955), and kidney (Wright and Sagik, 1958). Success with primary chick fibroblasts has been restricted largely to the neurotropic NWS strain and to a few high passage influenza A and B laboratory strains. Chick kidney cells, however, provide a reasonable plaquing system for many influenza A strains (Beare and Keast, 1974).

Plaque formation by some influenza A and B viruses in chick embryo monolayers may be permitted or enhanced by pretreatment of the monolayers with the enzymes, pancreatin (Came *et al.*, 1968) or trypsin (Tobita and Kilbourne, 1974). The mode of action of these proteolytic enzymes is uncertain. It appears that they may either modify the cell surface to make it more susceptible to virus adsorption and penetration, or they may destroy some virus inhibitory factor associated with the cell or remaining after removal of growth media-containing serum.

Syrian hamster kidney cells were described by Grossberg (1964) as being a highly effective system for plaquing influenza A viruses without prior adaptation, but little other experience with these cells has been reported.

The two systems which have been used most frequently for general influenza virus plaquing are primary monkey kidney and bovine kidney cells. Most influenza A or B strains isolated and passaged in other hosts do not readily plaque in monkey kidney, but many strains can be adapted to produce plaques after several serial passages (Henry and Younger, 1957; Choppin, 1962). Takemoto and Fabisch (1963) suggested that inefficient plaquing of influenza A viruses in many instances resulted from the inhibition of virus adsorption to cells by sulfated agar polysaccharides. With some strains, plaque numbers and size were enhanced considerably by adding DEAE-dextran to the agar to form an inactive complex with the inhibitor. This ingredient is now incorporated into the overlay agar far most systems.

Calf kidney cells were reported earlier by Lehmann-Grube (1963) and more recently by Beare and Keast (1974) to be a highly efficient system for plaquing influenza B viruses. The uniformity of results obtained with the B strains was in striking contrast to the highly variable results obtained with the type A strains. The requirements for adapting type A strains to efficient plaquing on bovine kidney cells have not been thoroughly evaluated.

Of these two primary cell systems, monkey kidney has the best laboratory growth and handling characteristics. Although bovine kidney may grow readily, cell sheets frequently become detached from the glass once confluent monolayers have formed.

All primary cell systems have the major disadvantages of heterogeneity of cellular constituents and variability of susceptibility of cell cultures derived from individual animals. Some cells, particularly monkey kidney and bovine kidney, have the added disadvantage of the frequent occurrence of adventitious agents. These probems can be avoided in theory by the use of a heteroploid cell line. The Wong–Kilbourne variant of the Chang human conjunctival cell line has been successfully used by Sugiura and Kilbourne (1965) for plaquing influenza A and B viruses. Plaque formation in this cell line also has been reported for influenza A (H3N2) strains from clinical material (Rytel and Sedmak, 1973). Although passage through a heteroploid cell line makes the virus unacceptable for use in human studies or as a candidate for live vaccines, this line has proved to be particularly valuable for genetic studies and serologic assays.

C. Organ Cultures

Cell monolayers or suspension cultures consist of undifferentiated cells and, therefore, rarely retain the spectrum of virus susceptibility characteristic of the host organ from which they were derived. Organ cultures consist of fragments of embryonic or adult organs maintained in vitro without cell proliferation and, therefore, retain many of their in vivo characteristics of virus susceptibility. Because of this, organ cultures provide useful systems for in vitro studies of interactions between virus and the host target cells.

The most extensive studies of organ cultures derived from one species are described in a series of reports on the ferret by Basarab and Smith (1969, 1970), Gould et al. (1972), and Toms et al. (1974). Organ cultures of nasal turbinates, bladder, uterus, trachea, lung, conjunctiva, oviduct, and esophagus (in this order) were found to be susceptible to infection with egg-grown influenza A (H2N2) virus. Alimentary tract tissues were insusceptible, with the exception of the esophagus and pharynx which could be infected only after high virus inoculum. Also insusceptible were muscle, reticuloendothelial tissue, blood vessels, and kidney. In comparative *in vivo* studies conducted after intranasal inoculation of the same strain, only the nasal turbinates, lung, trachea, and esophagus were found to be infected. Of these, the nasal turbinates contained the majority of the virus detected. Bladder and uterus were not infected despite earlier findings that organ cultures of these tissues were as susceptible to infection as respiratory tissues. Both of these organs could also be infected by direct urogenital inoculation (Basarab and Smith, 1970). Infection of urogenital tissue by influenza viruses is not unique for the ferret. Rosztoczy *et al.* (1973) found that influenza A also would replicate in human embryonic endometrium organ culture as well.

Because tissues of the respiratory tract represent the major sites of *in vivo* virus replication, organ cultures derived from the respiratory tract have received greatest attention. Fragments of ciliated epithelial cells from the trachea and nasal mucosa from a variety of animals have proved to be highly useful for influenza virus replication; lung tissue fragments have been less so. A discussion of the use of organ cultures for virus propagation and the tissues examined for this purpose is found in the review by Hoorn and Tyrrell (1969). Methods for preparation of organ cultures are described by Hoorn and Tyrrell (1969) and Cherry and Taylor-Robinson (1970).

Little has been done to evaluate the efficacy of ciliated epithelial cells specifically for recovery of influenza viruses. In limited studies of respiratory disease, human embryo tracheal organ cultures were not found to offer any advantage over primary rhesus kidney cultures for isolation of influenza A (Roome *et al.,* 1971) or influenza B viruses (Votava and Tyrrell, 1970). Besides, human tracheal cultures are difficult to obtain and are more cumbersome to use than conventional cell cultures.

Chick embryo tracheal organ cultures were compared with primary African green monkey kidney cell cultures for isolation of influenza A by Blaskovic *et al.* (1972b). Approximately the same number of strains grew on each system as on both systems. They suggested that use of organ cultures and cell cultures might be combined to achieve the maximum isolation of viruses. Chick embryo tracheal organ cultures were not compared with embryonated eggs, which is an infinitely simpler system.

Because tissues in organ culture and in the intact host are similar in susceptibility and response to virus infection, it has been assumed that their response to antiviral drugs would also be similar. If this assumption is correct, organ culture can be useful for drug evaluation. However, there are both negative and positive aspects. On the negative side, an organ fragment removed from the whole animal is not subject to normal physiological functions which may influence drug efficacy. On the positive side, the concentration of drugs and duration of contact can be better controlled than in the live animal. Tyrrell *et al.* (1965) were the first to use human ciliated epithelial organ cultures for *in vitro* evaluations of an anti-influenza drug (amantadine). Herbst-Laier (1970) investigated a wide variety of organ culture systems, including tracheal explants from mice, hamsters, ferrets, rats, dogs, monkeys, pigs, and calves, and turbinates from dogs and ferrets. Of these, ferret and dog tracheae were found to be the most suitable systems for evaluating growth (or inhibition) of the reference influenza A and B strains. Dog trachea showed specific histological changes which were thought to be more useful criteria for evaluation than virus titers alone. The finding of Blaskovic *et al.* (1972a) of consistent cytopathic changes in chick embryonic tracheal organ cultures inoculated with influenza type A (Hong Kong/68) strains suggests that the chick tracheal system might also prove to be useful.

The use of ciliated epithelial organ cultures has been suggested for defining the host range of newly isolated influenza A viruses. Schmidt *et al.* (1974) have reported that the sensitivity of ciliated epithelial organ cultures from chickens, horses, ferrets, and pigs to infection with virus from humans, pigs, horses, and avian species correlated well with the natural passage history of the virus strains.

Organ culture also shows potential for screening virus strains for live vaccine candidates. Mostow and Tyrrell (1973) reported an apparent correlation between the ability of a virus to reduce ciliary activity and damage cells of human embryonic tracheal cultures and its ability to produce disease in man. However, this correlation did not extend to ferret organ cultures nor to all influenza viruses (Hara *et al.*, 1974). Influenza B viruses demonstrated uniform pathogeneity for human tracheal organ cultures despite differing virulence for man. It appears clear, therefore, that although organ cultures offer many advantages for virus studies, an organ cut into fragments and maintained apart from the host in a totally artificial environment does not react to infection precisely in the same manner as it would in the intact animal.

D. The Embryonated Chicken Egg

The chick embryo has been used extensively for the isolation and propagation of influenza viruses since the original description of the amniotic technique by Burnet in 1940. The classic report by Beveridge and Burnet on the cultivation of viruses and rickettsia in the chick embryo was published in 1946. Little new information of major importance has been added since that time.

Some of the early recommendations now seem outdated, however, because of the biological variability of the influenza viruses. In the 1940's, amniotic inoculation of the 13- to 14-day-old embryo was recommended for isolation of influenza A and B strains, and laboratory-adapted strains were inoculated via the allantoic cavity of the 10- to 12-day-old embryo. As late as 1967 most influenza A and some B strains could be isolated only by amniotic cavity inoculation, and they frequently required multiple passages before successful adaptation. Isolation in the allantoic cavity was a rare event. Since 1968, human influenza type A viruses have been isolated equally as well by inoculation of the embryo by either route; amniotic inoculation has offered no advantage. Experience with influenza B over the years has also been variable. Because it has been difficult to predict predilection of either virus, inoculation of 11-day-old embryos both intraamniotically and intra-allantoically is now recommended as standard procedure.

Unadapted viruses inoculated into the amnion of 13-day-old embryos replicate primarily in the trachea and lungs. They may or may not cause death. Viruses which have undergone multiple passages by this route may replicate in the amniotic membrane and the epithelial surfaces of the embryo, as well as in the respiratory tract, and cause multiple hemorrhages and rapid death. After several passages the isolates may grow readily in the allantoic cavity.

Isolates unadapted to the chick embryo (O or original phase) frequently demonstrate higher hemagglutination titers with guinea pig or human erythrocytes than with chicken erythrocytes. Once adapted to the allantoic cavity (D or derived phase), the virus will usually agglutinate chicken erythrocytes to titers equal to or higher than those obtained with mammalian erythrocytes. This progression from the O to D phase (Burnet and Bull, 1943) is not a consistent event. Most of the influenza A and B strains isolated since 1968 agglutinated chick and guinea pig cells to equal titers.

Adapted viruses inoculated intraallantoically into 11-day-old embryos replicate primarily in the endodermal cells of the chorioallantoic membrane, although virus may also be found in the amniotic membranes and the respiratory tract. Growth in the allantoic cavity has the obvious advantage of ease of harvest and high volumes of fluid. Well-adapted strains may yield 10^9 to 10^{11} virus particles per ml. The virus may grow equally as well in embryos ranging from 10 to 13 days old, but the volume of allantoic fluid decreases rapidly in embryos older than 13 days. The younger egg is also preferred because of lower urate content in the allantoic fluid. As the embryo develops the urate content increases. Eggs inoculated at 12 or 13 days yield allantoic fluids which become cloudy immediately upon chilling and form heavy precipitates after a few days. Urate precipitates contain virus and may greatly reduce the titer of the fluid.

The size of inoculum may have a considerable effect on virus yield. Recommended inocula range from 10^4 to 10^5 EID_{50} per ml. Below this level the virus yield may be low and the pattern of replication spotty. Above this, the titers may be considerably reduced (Miller, 1944). The higher inoculum also may produce the von Magnus effect, that is, an increased ratio of noninfective to infective virus particles (von Magnus, 1952). This phenomenon is discussed in Chapter 1.

For certain special studies it may be advantageous to cultivate the virus in the cells of the allantoic membrane without interference from virus replication in other tissues of the embryo. For such studies deembryonated eggs may be used (Bernkoff, 1949). Virus yield in the deembryonated egg is much lower than in the intact egg, and this method is not recomended for routine use.

E. Allantois on Eggshell

Because of the considerable expense and labor involved in performing experiments requiring inoculation of multiple embryonated eggs, the advantage of a technique which permits the same experiment to be conducted with fragments from a single egg is obvious. Such a procedure has the additional advantage of tissue homogeneity, thereby avoiding the major problem of variable susceptibility of different eggs.

Fulton and Armitage (1951) were the first to propose a technique for cutting the chorioallantoic membrane (CAM) into small pieces and maintaining the tissue in cups in plastic trays, but virus titers were found to be considerably lower than in the intact egg. Fazekas de St. Groth and White (1958) improved the technique by modifying the medium and using fragments attached to the eggshell. In this way, the eggshell served to buffer the medium and anchor the tissue, thereby exposing maximum tissue surface and presenting only that side of the CAM which is susceptible to virus infection. Infectivity titers with most influenza type A strains in the allantois on eggshell system are similar to those obtained after inoculation of the intact egg. Growth of influenza B strains has generally been less successful. This procedure has been particularly useful for virus infectivity assays and neutralization tests with influenza type A and, more recently, for rapid isolation and purification of type A recombinants (Webster, 1970).

III. Experimental Host Range

A. Ferrets

The influenza A virus of man was first isolated in ferrets (Smith *et al.*, 1933). Since that time the ferret has received considerable attention, initially as a means for virus isolation and later as a model for pathogenicity and immunology of influenza.

Ferrets are highly susceptible to infection with influenza A viruses. Intranasal inoculation of infectious virus produces within 48 hours a febrile (100° to 107°F) response which may last from 24 to 72 hours. Animals during this period show mild symptoms of influenza, commonly rhinitis, sneezing, dyspena, loss of appetite, and malaise. The virus is actively shed during the first few days of disease and may be readily transmitted to uninoculated ferrets and to man (Smith and Stuart-Harris, 1936). Uninoculated ferrets may also become naturally infected from human contacts; therefore, it is essential that prior to inoculation all experimental animals be examined for preexisting antibody to current human influenza viruses.

The ferret was reported to have been highly susceptible to the type A viruses prevalent in the mid-1930's, but less susceptible to the late H0 strains, H1, and influenza B strains (Hirst, 1947b; Sugg and Nagaki, 1955). This may well have been so, but there has been no systematic study of the use of ferrets for isolation of A and B viruses after the early 1940's. By that time the embryonated egg technique had been widely accepted, and the use of the ferret for virus isolation had declined for obvious reasons.

The ferret, however, still remains a popular animal model for studies of human influenza. Influenza in ferrets closely resembles that seen in humans (Shope, 1934; Francis and Stuart-Harris, 1938; Liu, 1955; Sugg and Nagaki, 1955; Haff et al., 1966). Different strains of influenza viruses may produce a wide spectrum of disease. Response to infection ranges from a mild nonfebrile upper respiratory infection with only focal histological changes in the anterior nares (Haff et al., 1966), to a sharp febrile reaction with rapid necrobiosis and desquamation of the ciliated epithelial cells (Shope, 1934; Francis and Stuart-Harris, 1938), and, finally, to a virus pneumonia with destruction of alveolar cell lining (Hers, 1963; Mulder and Hers, 1972). The early findings by light microscopy of virus-specific pathogenic changes in the respiratory epithelium have been confirmed and extended by electron microscopy (Hotz and Bang, 1957) and FA studies (Liu, 1955).

Sites of virus multiplication after intranasal inoculation are nasal turbinates, lungs, trachea, and esophagus (Basarab and Smith, 1969; Haff et al., 1966). The virus was restricted to those sites even though other tissues (bladder, uterus, and conjunctiva) were also susceptible. Preferential infection of the tissue of the respiratory tract occurred even when live virus was introduced intravenously or intracardially (Basarab and Smith, 1969). Preferential infection of respiratory tissue was also confirmed by Barber and Small (1974) by the introduction of a surgically formed, subcutaneous tracheal pouch. Virus infected both natural and implanted tracheal tissue regardless of route of inoculation. Passively administered ferret antibody did not prevent dissemination by the hematologic route.

Infection of the ferret with influenza is followed by an increase in nasal washing protein, transient appearance of neutralizing antibody in nasal washings, and a rapid rise in humoral antibody. After recovery from infection, ferrets are immune to reinfection with the homologous virus (Smith *et al.*, 1933; Francis and Stuart-Harris, 1938; Haff *et al.*, 1966; Marois *et al.*, 1971). Because this response so closely resembles that seen in man, interest has been renewed in the ferret as a convenient model for studying immunity and immunization methods. Potter *et al.* in a series of reports (1972a,b) and Potter (1973) described the absence of a protective effect of intramuscular administration of aqueous inactivated vaccine. Immunization employing adjuvant provided some protection associated with serum HI antibody titers, but immunity was not as complete as that resulting from natural infection. This, in general, parallels the human experience and suggests that failure to provide complete immunity may relate, in part, to the inability of the inactivated vaccine to consistently stimulate nasal antibody. Nasal antibody is regularly found after natural disease (Haff, 1973).

B. Rodents

The white Swiss mouse has been the most commonly used laboratory model for human influenza for over 40 years (Andrewes *et al.*, 1934; Francis, 1934). The advantages of the mouse are obvious; its small size and cost make laboratory studies possible which would be impractical with larger, more expensive animals, such as the ferret.

Unlike the ferret, the mouse is not highly susceptible to influenza viruses. Intranasal installation of infectious materials from man produces no overt disease in the mouse, although the virus may multiply in the lungs, bronchioles, trachea, and, less readily, in nasal tissue (Hirst, 1947a; Iida and Bang, 1963; Mulder and Hers, 1972). Because evidence of virus multiplication must be obtained by *in ovo* or *in vitro* titrations, the mouse offers no advantage for virus isolation. However, after a period of adaptation, usually requiring six or more serial passages of lung extracts, influenza A viruses cause gross pathological lung changes and/or death as early as 48 hours after intranasal inoculation. Influenza B viruses adapt less readily to the mouse lung. These overt pathogenic changes with influenza A represent selected genetic characteristics which are independent of the ability of the virus to grow in the mouse lung. High titers in the lungs may also be obtained with unadapted strains, but growth occurs without the accompanying pathology or lethal consequences (Hirst, 1947a).

A somewhat different pattern of infection is seen upon adaptation of egg-grown virus to mice. The first intranasal inoculation usually causes lung lesions and death, whereas the next several passages produce no pathological effect. This phenomenon is attributable to the toxicity of initial massive virus content of infected egg fluids. Very little infectious virus is produced in the mouse under these circumstances (Sugg, 1950). Specific lung lesions and deaths begin to occur after an additional four to ten serial passages of infected lung tissues.

The pulmonary pathology caused by influenza viruses in the mouse represents a true virus pneumonia and in many respects is similar to viral pneumonia in man (Loosli, 1949; Mulder and Hers, 1972). Earlier findings by light microscopy suggesting specific virus destruction of the alveolar cell lining were confirmed by Albrecht et al. (1963) by fluorescent antibody and by Plummer and Stone (1964) by electron microscopy. Although all cells in the respiratory tract are susceptible to virus infection, some evidence suggests that, as in man (see Chapter 13), the alveolar cells are the primary sites of virus multiplication (Albrecht et al., 1963). This peculiar ascendant course of respiratory infection may be more apparent than real. When an anesthetized animal is inoculated intranasally, the virus is introduced throughout the respiratory tract. Virus multiplication may occur more rapidly in the lungs than in the ciliated epithelial cells of the upper respiratory passages.

In sublethal infections the virus begins to clear from the lungs after about 7 days, which coincides with the appearance of humoral antibody. On healing, alveolar epithelium is replaced by ciliated bronchiolar columnar and cuboidal cells. Squamous metaplastic changes also occur (Baskerville et al., 1974).

Because airborne transmission from infected to noninfected animals readily occurs within a few days after exposure, the mouse has provided an excellent model for virus transmission studies (Schulman, 1969). The mouse has also been used extensively for studies of vaccines (Eddy, 1947; Kaye et al., 1969), mechanisms of immunity (Schulman et al., 1968), and antiviral drug studies (Davies et al., 1966; Suganuma and Ishida, 1973).

Influenza A strains will multiply readily in hamster lungs with minimal signs of disease (Friedewald and Hook, 1948). The few influenza B strains which have been examined were only slightly pathogenic, but lung lesions can be produced after adaptation (Friedewald and Hook, 1948; Davenport, 1951; Kilbourne et al., 1951). Because of the low pathogenicity of influenza viruses for hamsters, the use of these animals for experimental influenza studies was not vigorously pursued. Recently, however, the hamster has been found to be particularly suitable for evaluation of candidate temperature-sensitive vaccine strains (Mills and Chanock, 1971). It is one of the few laboratory animals with a body temperature of 37°C. Like the ferret, the hamster does not readily produce antibody in response to aqueous vaccines unless primed by prior infection with an influenza A virus (Potter *et al.*, 1973).

A few other rodent species have also been employed. Stuart-Harris (1937) reported that influenza virus could multiply in the turbinates of rats and guinea pigs, but did not destroy epithelium.

C. Nonhuman Primates

The use of nonhuman primates as experimental models for the study of influenza has met with variable success. As early as 1937, McIntosh and Selbie attempted to produce illness in rhesus and cercopithecus monkeys with the H0N1 virus, but without success. Experience with rhesus and cyno-molgus monkeys inoculated with A/FM/1/47 (H1N1) strain was similar. No clinical illness was observed, but typical necrosis and desquamation of the respiratory epithelium could be demonstrated (Verlinde and Mak-stenoieks, 1954).

Saslaw and Carlisle (1965) reported that more consistent clinical results could be achieved by using aerosol challenge, which they felt was more natural than the intranasal or intratracheal route. By this technique they were able to infect rhesus and cynomolgus monkeys with A/PR/8/34 (H0N1). Attempts to infect monkeys with an H2N2 strain and a type B strain were unsuccessful. Berendt (1974) also used small particle aerosols and reported virus shedding and seroconversions with all six rhesus monkeys challenged with the A/Hong Kong/68 (H3N2) virus. There was no overt clinical illness. All animals were refractory to rechallenge.

Kenya baboons (*Papio* sp.) were found to be susceptible to infection with an H3N2 strain similar to A/Hong Kong/68 (Kalter *et al.*, 1969). The virus was recovered from throat specimens, and seroconversions were demonstrated for inoculated animals as well as uninoculated animals in neighboring cages. Clinical disease was not apparent.

The gibbon appears potentially to be one of the better primate models for human influenza (Johnsen *et al.*, 1971). A small group of animals inoculated with the A/Hong Kong/68 strain failed to show evidence of disease, but 2 to 3 weeks later respiratory tract infections spread throughout the entire gibbon colony. Signs consisted of rhinitis, coughing, anorexia, depression, loss of weight, and gastrointestinal disturbances. Illnesses lasted an average of 3 to 6 days and convalescence was frequently prolonged. Four deaths occurred. The spectrum of clinical disease was remarkably similar to that seen in man. A second group of animals inoculated with A/Japan/305/57 (H2N2) failed to become infected.

Most influenza virus strains used to challenge nonhuman primates have been laboratory-adapted strains, either having undergone multiple passages in eggs, mice, or ferrets, or combinations thereof. Nonhuman primates may be no more susceptible to these probably attenuated strains than is man himself. Whether primates can be more readily infected with virus passaged directly from man remains to be seen. Serologic studies undertaken in African green (cercopithecus) and rhesus monkeys shortly after captivity showed a high incidence of H3 antibody beginning in 1968 (O'Brien and Tauraso, 1973). The report of Murphy *et al.* (1972) was also interesting; they described an outbreak of A/Hong Kong/68-like virus in progress among marmosets upon their arrival at the laboratory from Colombia. These findings indicate that primate infections with human influenza type A can occur, under certain conditions, but the high frequency of transmission may be unique for the Hong Kong virus.

D. Disease Patterns Altered by Immunosuppression

Manipulations which effect the immune systems of animals infected with influenza may be of interest in increasing sensitivity to infection in experimental animals and possibly making normally insusceptible hosts susceptible to infection. However, there have been relatively few reports of such studies, and the published data give rise to conflicting views. Singer *et al.* (1972) reported that in mice immunosuppressed by cyclophosphamide the severity of infection by A/PR8 virus was reduced. In contrast, Virelizier *et al.* (1974) found that cyclophosphamide-treated mice were considerably more susceptible than normal mice to the lethal effects of A/PR8 virus infection, the LD_{50} titer of a virus preparation being at least 100-fold higher in the treated than in normal mice. Mayer *et al.* (1973) also found that immunosuppression with cyclophosphamide much enhanced the neuravirulence of A/NWS. The results of these two studies suggest that humoral antibody is an important factor in recovery from infection in mice. Thymus-deprived mice were slightly more susceptible than normal mice to PR8 infection in the experiments reported by Virelizier *et al.* (1974). The studies of Portnoy *et al.* (1973) in bursectomized chickens showed that this procedure enhanced susceptibility to infection by fowl plague virus, and this finding was also taken as indicating the importance of humoral antibody in recovery from infection.

IV. Virus Isolation from Clinical Material

Specimens for virus isolation should be collected within the first 3 days after onset of disease. Chances for isolation diminish quickly after that, but in some cases virus may be recovered for 7 to 10 days. The best specimens for virus isolation are nasal washings. However, throat and nasal swabs are generally more convenient for the physician and less objectionable to the patient. Specimens for virus isolation should be kept cold at all times. They should be inoculated as soon as possible. If they cannot be inoculated within 48 hours after collection, they should be sealed and stored in dry ice or under low-temperature mechanical refrigeration ($-70°C$). In fatal cases of suspected influenza pneumonia, virus isolation may be attempted from lung tissue, tracheal mucosa, and blood. Isolation of the virus under these conditions has met with variable success (Dowdle and Coleman, 1974).

Types A and B influenza viruses may be grown in embryonated chicken eggs and in cell cultures from a variety of animals. The embryonated egg and rhesus or green monkey kidney tissue cultures are conceded to be the most sensitive hosts for isolation. Influenza C has been isolated only from the embryonated egg.

For maximum isolation in eggs, 10- to 11-day-old embryos are inoculated simultaneously intraamniotically and intraallantoically. Eggs are incubated at 33°C for 3 to 4 days, and samples of both amniotic and allantoic fluids are tested for the presence of virus by the addition of guinea pig or chicken erythrocytes. Guinea pig (for human Type O) erythrocytes were reported to be more sensitive than chicken erythrocytes for detecting H0N1 and H1N1 viruses in early egg passage. This observation does not apply to the current viruses which agglutinate avian and mammalian erythrocytes equally well. Chicken erythrocytes are preferred, however, since they settle much faster than mammalian erythrocytes, agglutination titers are easier to read, and they are less susceptible to nonspecific agglutination by mammalian sera. Two or three blind amniotic passages may be necessary in some instances to increase the titer of the virus to the level at which hemagglutination is detectable. If the virus grows or has been successfully adapted to growth in the allantoic cavity, amniotic inoculation is no longer necessary.

For isolation of influenza type C, 7-day-old embryonated eggs are inoculated intraamniotically and incubated at 33°C for 5 days. This virus does not readily replicate in the allantoic cavity even after extensive egg passages.

Rhesus or green monkey kidney cells in monolayer tube cultures are the most sensitive cell culture systems for isolation of influenza A or B. Nonspecific inhibition of influenza viruses by substances in culture media-containing serum can be a serious problem and must be avoided by washing the monolayers several times with serum-free medium and by using serum-free medium for virus isolation. Influenza A viruses grow less vigorously in cell culture than influenza B viruses. The cytopathogenic effects (CPE) consist of slowly vacuolating or lacy cells which degenerate or become detached from the glass. CPE is difficult to detect, not pathognomonic, and may not become apparent until after multiple passages. The presence of the virus may usually be detected by hemadsorption of guinea pig erythrocytes (Vogel and Shelokov, 1957) within 3 to 4 days after inoculation, which is well in advance of an obvious CPE.

Most influenza B isolates may be detected by hemadsorption or hemagglutination within 3 to 4 days after inoculation. CPE usually is also evident. Cells become progressively granular, swollen, and round; later they become pyknotic and fragmented, and the cell sheet is eventually destroyed. The appearance of CPE and the production of hemagglutination for both influenza A and B may be hastened by placing the tubes on a roller drum, although this does not increase the isolation rate.

Multiple uninoculated cell culture tubes should be maintained to rule out the presence of adventitious virus contaminants. Parainfluenza type 2 (SV5) is a hemadsorbing virus which is a frequent contaminant of rhesus monkey kidney cell cultures. Nonspecific adsorption of old erythrocytes is a characteristic feature of most kidney cell cultures and may erroneously suggest the presence of virus (Dowdle and Robinson, 1966). Therefore, only fresh erythrocytes should be used for hemadsorption. Most rhesus monkey kidney cell cultures also contain SV40 or SV13 ("foamy") viruses. Whereas the presence of these agents is undesirable and may interfere with interpretation of CPE, they do not appear to influence the sensitivity of the cell for isolation of influenza viruses.

It is difficult to assign values for efficiency of isolating influenza type A or type B by either tissue culture or eggs. Isolation rates for both types of viruses have varied throughout the years. In general, monkey kidney has been superior to eggs for isolating influenza B, but the degree of superiority has varied. Experience with influenza A suggests even wider variability, and for this type, eggs are more sensitive than cell cultures. For this reason, and because influenza viruses may vary biologically as well as antigenically, the most efficient method of isolation is not always predictable. Inoculation of primary rhesus or green monkey kidney cells as well as the amniotic and allantoic sac of the embryonated egg is recommended for isolation of the maximum number of type A and type B strains.

References

Albrecht, P., Blaškovič, D., Styk, B., and Koller, M. (1963). *Acta Virol. (Prague)* **7**, 405.

Andrewes, C. H., Laidlaw, P. P., and Smith, W. (1934). *Lancet* **2**, 859.

Barber, W. H., and Small, P. A. (1974). *Infec. Immunity* **9**, 530.
Basarab, O., and Smith, H. (1969). *Brit. J. Exp. Pathol.* **50**, 612.
Basarab, O., and Smith, H. (1970). *Brit. J. Exp. Pathol.* **51**, 1.
Baskerville, A., Thomas, G., Wood, M., and Harris, W. J. (1974). *Brit. J. Exp. Pathol.* **55**, 130.
Beare, A. S., and Keast, K. A. (1974). *J. Gen. Virol.* **22**, 347.
Becht, H. (1969). *J. Gen. Virol.* **4**, 215.
Berendt, R. F. (1974). *Infec. Immunity* **9**, 101.
Bernkoff, H. (1949). *Proc. Soc. Exp. Biol. Med.* **72**, 680.
Beveridge, W. I. B., and Burnet, F. M. (1946). *Med. Res. Counc. (Gt. Brit.), Spec. Rep. Ser.* **256**.
Blaškovič, P., Rhodes, A. J., and Labzoffsky, N. A. (1972a). *Arch. Gesamte Virusforsch.* **37**, 104.
Blaškovič, P., Rhodes, A. J., and Labzoffsky, N. A. (1972b). *Arch. Gesamte Virusforsch.* **39**, 299.
Burnet, F. M. (1940). *Aust. J. Exp. Biol. Med. Sci.* **18**, 353.
Burnet, F. M., and Bull, D. R. (1943). *Aust. J. Exp. Biol. Med. Sci.* **21**, 55.
Came, P. E., Pascale, A., and Shimonaski, G. (1968). *Arch. Gesamte Virusforsch.* **23**, 346.
Cherry, J. D., and Taylor-Robinson, D. (1970). *Appl. Microbiol.* **19**, 658.
Choppin, P. W. (1962). *Virology* **18**, 332.
Choppin, P. W. (1969). *Virology* **39**, 130.
Choppin, P. W., and Pons, M. W. (1970). *Virology* **42**, 603.
Davenport, F. M. (1951). *J. Immunol.* **67**, 83.
Davies, W. L., Grunert, R. R., and Hoffmann, C. E. (1966). *J. Immunol.* **95**, 1090.
Dimmock, N. J. (1969). *Virology* **39**, 224.
Dowdle, W. R., and Coleman, M. T. (1974). *In* "Manual of Clinical Microbiology" (E. H. Lennette, E. H. Spaulding, and J. P. Truant, eds.), 2nd ed., pp. 678–685. Amer. Soc. Microbiol., Washington, D.C.
Dowdle, W. R., and Robinson, R. Q. (1966). *Proc. Soc. Exp. Biol. Med.* **121**, 193.
Dowdle, W. R., Yarbrough, W. B., and Robinson, R. Q. (1963). *Pub. Health Rep.* **79**, 398.
Eddy, B. E. (1947). *J. Immunol.* **57**, 195.
Fazekas de St. Groth, S., and White, D. O. (1958). *J. Hyg.* **56**, 151.
Francis, T., Jr. (1934). *Science* **80**, 457.
Francis, T., Jr., and Stuart-Harris, C. H. (1938). *J. Exp. Med.* **68**, 813.
Franklin, R. M., and Breitenfeld, P. M. (1959). *Virology* **8**, 293.
Fraser, K. B. (1967). *J. Gen. Virol.* **1**, 1.
Friedewald, W. F., and Hook, E. W. (1948). *J. Exp. Med.* **88**, 343.
Fulton, F., and Armitage, P. (1951). *J. Hyg.* **49**, 247.
Gavrilov, V. I., Asher, D. M., Ratushkina, L. S., Zmieva, R. G., and Tumyam, B. G. (1972). *Proc. Soc. Exp. Biol. Med.* **140**, 109.
Gould, E. A., Ratcliffe, N. A., Basarab, O., and Smith, H. (1972). *Brit. J. Exp. Pathol.* **53**, 31.
Granoff, A. (1955). *Virology* **1**, 252.
Green, I. J. (1962). *Science* **138**, 42.
Green, I. J., Lieberman, M., and Mogabgab, W. J. (1957). *J. Immunol.* **78**, 233.
Grossberg, S. E. (1964). *Science* **144**, 1246.
Haas, R., and Wulff, H. (1957). *Z. Hyg. Infektionskr.* **143**, 568.

Haff, R. F. (1973). *Arch. Gesamte Virusforsch.* **40**, 168.

Haff, R. F., Schriver, P. W., Engle, C. G., and Stewart, R. C. (1966). *J. Immunol.* **96**, 659.

Hara, K., Beare, A. S., and Tyrrell, D. A. J. (1974). *Arch. Gesamte Virusforsch.* **44**, 227.

Heath, R. B., and Tyrrell, D. A. J. (1959). *Arch. Gesamte Virusforsch.* **8**, 577.

Henle, G., Girardi, A., and Henle, W. (1955). *J. Exp. Med.* **101**, 25.

Henry, C., and Younger, J. S. (1957). *J. Immunol.* **78**, 273.

Herbst-Laier, R. (1970). *Arch. Gesamte Virusforsch.* **30**, 379.

Hers, J. F. P. (1963). *Amer. Rev. Resp. Dis.* **88**, 316.

Hinz, R. W., and Syverton, J. T. (1959). *Proc. Soc. Exp. Biol. Med.* **101**, 22.

Hirst, G. K. (1941). *Science* **94**, 22.

Hirst, G. K. (1947a). *J. Exp. Med.* **86**, 357.

Hirst, G. K. (1947b). *J. Exp. Med.* **86**, 367.

Hoorn, B., and Tyrrell, D. A. J. (1969). *Progr. Med. Virol.* **11**, 408.

Hotchin, J. E. (1955). *Nature (London)* **175**, 352.

Hotz, G., and Bang, F. B. (1957). *Bull. Johns Hopkins Hosp.* **101**, 175.

Hoyle, L. (1968). "The Influenza Viruses." Springer-Verlag, Berlin and New York.

Iida, T., and Bang, F. B. (1963). *Amer. J. Hyg.* **77**, 169.

Johnsen, D. O., Woodling, W. L., Tanticharoenyos, P., and Karnjanaprakorn, C. (1971). *J. Infec. Dis.* **123**, 365.

Joss, A., Gandhi, S. S., Hay, A. J., and Burke, D. C. (1969). *J. Virol.* **4**, 816.

Kalter, S. S., Heberling, R. L., Vice, T. E., Lief, F. S., and Rodriguez, A. R. (1969). *Proc. Soc. Exp. Biol. Med.* **132**, 357.

Kaye, H. S., Dowdle, W. R., and McQueen, J. L. (1969). *Amer. J. Epidemiol.* **90**, 162.

Kilbourne, E. D., Anderson, H. C., and Horsfall, F. L. (1951). *J. Immunol.* **67**, 547.

Kilbourne, E. D., Sugiura, A., and Wong, S. C. (1964). *Proc. Soc. Exp. Biol. Med.* **116**, 225.

Ledinko, N. (1955). *Nature (London)* **175**, 999.

Lehmann-Grube, F. (1963). *Virology* **21**, 520.

Lehmann-Grube, F. (1964). *Arch. Gesamte Virusforsch.* **14**, 177.

Lehmann-Grube, F. (1965). *Arch. Gesamte Virusforsch.* **17**, 534.

Liu, O. C. (1955). *J. Exp. Med.* **101**, 677.

Liu, O. C. (1969). *In* "Diagnostic Procedures for Viral and Rickettsial Diseases" (E. H. Lennette, ed.), pp. 179–204. Amer. Pub. Health Ass., New York.

Loffler, H., Henle, G., and Henle, W. (1962). *J. Immunol.* **88**, 763.

Loosli, C. G. (1949). *J. Infec. Dis.* **84**, 153.

Low, I. E., Eaton, M. D., and Uretsky, S. B. (1962). *J. Immunol.* **89**, 414.

McIntosh, J., and Selbie, R. F. (1937). *Brit. J. Exp. Pathol.* **18**, 334.

Maeno, K., and Kilbourne, E. D. (1970). *J. Virol.* **5**, 153.

Marois, P., Boudreault, A., Difronco, E., and Pavilanis, V. (1971). *Can. J. Comp. Med.* **35**, 71.

Mayer, V., Schulman, J. L., and Kilbourne, E. D. (1973). *J. Virol.* **11**, 272.

Miller, G. L. (1944). *J. Exp. Med.* **79**, 173.

Mills, J. V., and Chanock, R. M. (1971). *J. Infec. Dis.* **123**, 145.

Mogabgab, W. J., Green, I. J., and Dierkhising, O. C. (1954). *Science* **120**, 320.

Mogabgab, W. J., Holmes, J. B., and Pelon, W. (1961). *J. Infec. Dis.* **108**, 312.

Morgan, C., Hsu, K. C., Rifkind, R. A., Knox, A. W., and Rose, H. M. (1961). *J. Exp. Med.* **114**.

Mostow, S. R., and Tyrrell, D. A. J. (1973). *Arch. Gesamte Virusforsch.* **43**, 385.

Mulder, J., and Hers, J. F. P. (1972). "Influenza," pp. 214–238. Walters-Noordhoff, Gröningen, The Netherlands.

Murphy, B. L., Maynard, J. E., Krushek, D. H., and Berquist, K. R. (1972). *Lab. Anim. Sci.* **22**, 339.

Nikitin, T., Cohen, D., Todd, J. D., and Lief, F. S. (1972). *Bull. W.H.O.* **47**, 471.

O'Brien, T. C., and Tauraso, N. M. (1973). *Arch. Gesamte Virusforsch.* **40**, 359.

Oxford, J. S., and Schild, G. C. (1968). *J. Gen. Virol.* **2**, 377.

Oxford, J. S., and Schild, G. C. (1974). *In* "Biology of Large RNA Viruses" (R. D. Barry and B. Mahy, eds.). Academic Press, New York.

Palese, P., and Schulman, J. L. (1974). *Virology* **57**, 227.

Palese, P., Bodo, A., and Tuppy, H. (1970). *J. Virol.* **6**, 556.

Pereira, H. G. (1961). *Advan. Virus Res.* **8**, 245.

Plummer, M. J., and Stone, B. S. (1964). *Amer. J. Pathol.* **45**, 95.

Porebska, A., Pereira, H. G., and Armstrong, J. A. (1968). *J. Med. Microbiol.* **1**, 145.

Portnoy, J., Bloom, K., and Merigan, T. C. (1973). *Cell. Immunol.* **9**, 251.

Potter, C. W. (1973). *Arch. Gesamte Virusforsch.* **42**, 285.

Potter, C. W., Oxford, J. S., Shore, S. L., McLaren, C., and Stuart-Harris, C. (1972a). *Brit. J. Exp. Pathol.* **53**, 153.

Potter, C. W., Shore, S. L., McLaren, C., and Stuart-Harris, C. (1972b). *Brit. J. Exp. Pathol.* **53**, 168.

Potter, C. W., Jennings, R., Rees, R. C., and McLaren, C. (1973). *Infec. Immunity* **8**, 137.

Reed, L. J., and Muench, H. (1938). *Amer. J. Hyg.* **27**, 493.

Roome, A. P. C. H., Dickinson, V., and Caul, E. O. (1971). *J. Clin. Pathol.* **24**, 487.

Rosztoczy, I., Toms, G. L., and Smith, H. (1973). *Lancet* **1**, 327.

Rutter, G., and Mannweiler, K. (1973). *Arch. Gesamte Virusforsch.* **43**, 169.

Rytel, M. W., and Sedmak, G. V. (1973). *Amer. J. Clin. Pathol.* **60**, 251.

Saslaw, S., and Carlisle, H. N. (1965). *Proc. Soc. Exp. Biol. Med.* **119**, 838.

Schäfer, W. (1955). *Z. Naturforsch. B* **10**, 81.

Schmidt, R. C., Maassab, H. F., and Davenport, F. M. (1974). *J. Infec. Dis.* **129**, 28.

Schulman, J. L. (1969). *Progr. Med. Virol.* **12**, 128.

Schulman, J. L., Khakpour, M., and Kilbourne, E. D. (1968). *J. Virol.* **2**, 778.

Shope, R. E. (1931). *J. Exp. Med.* **54**, 373.

Shope, R. E. (1934). *J. Exp. Med.* **60**, 49.

Simpson, R. W., and Hirst, G. K. (1961). *Virology* **15**, 436.

Singer, S. H., Noguchi, P., and Kirschstein, R. L. (1972). *Infect. Immunity* **5**, 957.

Skehel, J. J. (1972). *Virology* **49**, 23.

Skehel, J. J. (1973). *Virology* **56**, 394.

Smith, W., and Stuart-Harris, C. H. (1936). *Lancet* **2**, 121.

Smith, W., Andrewes, C. H., and Laidlaw, P. P. (1933). *Lancet* **2**, 66.

Soloviev, V. D., and Alekseeva, A. K. (1960). *Probl. Virol. (USSR)* **4**, 6.

Stuart-Harris, C. H. (1937). *Brit. J. Exp. Pathol.* **18**, 485.

Suganuma, T., and Ishida, N. (1973). *Tohoku J. Exp. Med.* **110**, 405.

Sugg, J. Y. (1950). *J. Bacteriol.* **60**, 489.

Sugg, J. Y., and Nagaki, D. (1955). *J. Immunol.* **74**, 46.

Sugiura, A., and Kilbourne, E. D. (1965). *Virology* **26**, 478.

Takemoto, K. K., and Fabisch, P. (1963). *Proc. Soc. Exp. Biol. Med.* **114**, 811.

Taylor, J. M., Hampson, A. W., and White, D. O. (1969). *Virology* **39**, 419.

Tobita, K., and Kilbourne, E. D. (1974). *J. Virol.* **13**, 347.

Toms, G. L., Rosztoczy, I., and Smith, H. (1974). *Brit. J. Exp. Pathol.* **55**, 116.

Tuppy, H., and Palese, P. (1969). *FEBS (Fed. Eur. Biochem. Soc.) Lett.* **3**, 72.

Tyrrell, D. A. J. (1959). *Nature (London)* **184**, 452.

Tyrrell, D. A. J., Bynoe, M. L., and Hoorn, B. (1965). *Brit. J. Exp. Pathol.* **46**, 370.

Verlinde, J. D., and Makstenieks, O. (1954). *Arch. Gesmate Virusforsch.* 5, 345.

Virelizier, J. L., Allison, A. C., and Schild, G. C. (1974). *J. Exp. Med.* **140**, 1559.

Vogel, L., and Shelokov, A. (1957). *Science* **126**, 358.

von Magnus, P. (1952). *Acta Pathol. Microbiol. Scand.* **30**, 311.

Votava, M., and Tyrrell, D. A. J. (1970). *Arch. Gesamte Virusforsch.* **29**, 253.

Watson, B. K., and Coons, A. H. (1954). *J. Exp. Med.* **99**, 419.

Webster, R. G. (1970). *Virology* **42**, 633.

Weller, T. H., and Coons, A. H. (1954). *Proc. Soc. Exp. Biol. Med.* **86**, 789.

Wilkinson, P. J., and Borland, R. (1972). *Nature (London)* **238**, 153.

Wong, S. C., and Kilbourne, E. D. (1961). *J. Exp. Med.* **113**, 95.

Wright, B. S., and Sagik, B. P. (1958). *Virology* **5**, 573.

10

Antigenic Variation of Influenza Viruses

Robert G. Webster and W. Graeme Laver

I. Introduction

Influenza type A virus is unique among agents infecting man in its capacity to change its antigenic identity so remarkably that the specific immunity established in response to infection by a particular strain may give little or no protection against viruses which subsequently arise. Because of this variation, influenza continues to be a major epidemic disease of man.

Two distinct kinds of antigenic variation have been demonstrated in influenza viruses, antigenic drift (Burnet, 1955) and major antigenic shift. The first consists of relatively minor changes that occur gradually within a family of strains, all of which are clearly related to each other with respect to both internal and surface antigens. Among influenza A strains infecting man, each successive variant replaces preexisting ones. This may be due to a selective advantage possessed by antigenic variants in overcoming immunological host resistance. Antigenic drift occurs in type B influenza viruses as well as in type A.

The second kind of antigenic variation, which has been described only for influenza type A, involves much more sudden and dramatic antigenic changes. These are referred to as major antigenic shifts. These major shifts, which occur at intervals of 10–15 years, (see Chapter 15) are marked by the appearance of antigenically "new" viruses to which the population has no immunity, and it is these viruses which cause the major pandemics of influenza.

These "new" viruses possess hemagglutinin and neuraminidase subunits which are completely different antigenically from those of viruses circulating in the human population just before the appearance of the new virus. The major shifts may involve one or both of the two surface antigens, and two influenza pandemics have been described which were caused by viruses within each of these two categories (see Chapter 15).

Influenza is also a natural infection of certain animals and birds. Viruses, which so far have been exclusively of type A, have been isolated from pigs, horses, and a wide variety of birds including chickens, ducks, turkeys, quail, pheasant, and terns (McQueen *et al.*, 1968; Pereira, 1969; World Health Organization, 1972).

It was once believed that the surface of the influenza virus particle consisted of a mosaic of antigens shared by all strains of a given type and that antigenic variation resulted from the displacement of given antigens from a prominent to a hidden position and vice versa. More recent evidence suggests an alternative mechanism for antigenic drift. It is now thought that gradual changes occur in the amino acids comprising the antigenic determinants on the hemagglutinin and neuraminidase subunits. These changes are the result of selection of mutants which show changes in the amino acid sequence of the polypeptides of the subunits which, in turn, are caused by mutation in the viral RNA.

The major antigenic shifts, where a "new" virus suddenly arises, probably involve a different mechanism. These "new" viruses have hemagglutinin and neuraminidase subunits which are completely unrelated, antigenically, to those of viruses circulating in the human population just before the appearance of the new strain. We think that a "new" virus does not arise by mutation from a preexisting human influenza virus, but that it is formed by genetic recombination between a human virus and one of the many type A influenza strains whose natural hosts are animals or birds. Following its appearance, the "new" virus replaces the "old" virus, which disappears completely from the human population.

Major antigenic shifts have not so far been detected in influenza B viruses. Pereira (1969) has suggested that the lack of major antigenic shift in type B influenza viruses may be a consequence of the absence of such influenza viruses in lower animals and birds.

Antigenic variation involves only the hemagglutinin and neuraminidase subunits; the internal proteins of the virus (the nucleoprotein antigen and the matrix or membrane M protein) are remarkably constant. Of the two variable surface antigens, the hemagglutinin is the more important, since antibody to this antigen neutralizes virus infectivity.

II. Historical Aspects of Influenza (see also Chapter 15)

A. Evidence of Antigenic Variation

Influenza-like illness has been frequently recorded in past centuries (Hirsch, 1883); the disease occurred either in a pandemic form affecting a very large proportion of the population and spreading over the entire world or it occurred as localized outbreaks. Until the virus was first isolated in 1933, it was impossible to tell with certainty whether these pandemics were caused by influenza viruses. However, characteristics of the epidemics described in historical writings suggest that they may well have been caused by influenza viruses. Although other infections produce many of the symptoms of influenza, only influenza viruses cause sudden epidemics that persist for a few weeks and equally suddenly disappear (Burnet and White, 1972). Serological evidence of influenza virus infections in elderly persons also provides evidence of previous influenza epidemics in the not so distant past (Mulder and Masurel, 1958).

German records place the earliest recognizable epidemic of influenza in 1170 (Hirsch, 1883), and from other historical records it has been possible to compile a fairly complete list of epidemics in Europe since 1500. Only the severe epidemics will be mentioned here. Further details are given by Hirsch (1883), Creighton (1891, 1894), Burnet and Clarke (1942), and Burnet and White (1972).

The epidemic of 1781–1782 first appeared in Asia in 1781 and spread through Russia to Europe by early 1782. Relatively few deaths occurred during this epidemic, but it was noteworthy in that it affected the middle-aged group rather than children and elderly people. Fairly severe epidemics also occurred in 1803, 1833, 1837, and 1847. The epidemic of 1847–1848 came from the east to Russia in March 1847 and reached Europe and England in the winter of 1847–1848. This epidemic caused a large excess of deaths, particularly among the elderly.

The pandemic of 1889 also spread across Europe from Russia reaching England and the United States in early 1890. The disease spread at a speed equivalent to human travel. Four waves of infection occurred after the appearance of this virus in 1889 in each of the ensuing years. The second and third waves caused high mortalities, particularly among infants and old people. Serological studies (Mulder and Masurel, 1958) and others (see review by Pereira, 1969) suggest that influenza viruses related to Asian, Hong Kong, and equine 2 were present at this time.

The most severe pandemic of influenza on record occurred in 1918–1919. The point of origin of this pandemic is less certain, but Burnet and Clarke (1942) suggest that the virus may have developed independently in Asia and in Europe or may have been brought to Europe by Chinese laborers. The pandemic occurred in waves and was responsible for the deaths of between 20 and 50 million people, principally young adults. It is probable that the 1918–1919 pandemic was due to a strain of influenza A virus related to the swine influenza virus. This was first suggested by Laidlaw (1935) and Shope (1936), but it is likely that the virus was transmitted from man to pigs rather than in the other direction. The extensive studies on the age incidence of antibody to the swine influenza virus in human sera by Davenport et al. (1953, 1964) and Hennessy et al. (1965) give evidence for a virus serologically related to swine influenza being the cause of the 1918–1919 epidemic.

The large number of deaths caused Burnet and Clarke (1942) to suggest that the virus may have had unusual virulence. Others (Zhdanov et al., 1958; Kilbourne, 1960) suggest that the conditions of war and absence of antibiotics may have been responsible for many deaths from secondary bacterial infection. It seems probable, however, that some mutants of the virus possessed high virulence, for the virus of the 1781 pandemic which also affected young adults, did not cause high mortality.

B. Antigenic Variation since 1933

Since the identification of the first influenza virus in 1933, which has been designated H0N1 (World Health Organization, 1971) antigenic shifts occurred in 1947 when the H1N1 viruses (e.g., A/FM/1/47) appeared, in 1957 when the H2N2 viruses (e.g., A/Singapore/1/57) appeared, and in 1968 with the appearance of the Hong Kong strain (A/Hong Kong/1/68). The antigenic shift in 1947 involved a change in the hemagglutinin antigen (H0N1 to H1N1); in 1957 both the hemagglutinin and the neuraminidase were completely different antigenically from the viruses in the preceding years (H1N1 to H2N2), and in 1968 the Hong Kong variant showed a major change in the hemagglutinin antigen (H2N2 to H3N2).

The Asian strain of influenza virus (H2N2) which appeared first in Kweichow province of China in 1957 possessed hemagglutinin and neuraminidase subunits which were completely unrelated antigenically to those of the H0N1 and H1N1 influenza viruses previously circulating in man. This virus strain caused the most widespread pandemic in history (Burnet and White, 1972) but did not cause a high excess mortality. The next and most recent influenza pandemic was caused by a virus (A/Hong Kong/68) which possessed neuraminidase subunits that were similar to those of the "old" A2/Asian viruses, and hemagglutinin subunits were completely different antigenically from those of the "old" Asian strains (Coleman *et al.*, 1968; Schulman and Kilbourne, 1969; Webster and Laver, 1972).

C. Common Features of Previous Pandemics

The pandemic nature of influenza in man indicates that at irregular intervals the population of the world has been exposed to viruses possessing new antigenic determinants. The information given above indicates that these pandemics frequently originate in southeast Asia and spread at the speed at which man travels. The majority of pandemics cause excess mortality in the very young and very old, but at least two pandemics (1781 and 1918) caused excess mortality in young adults.

III. Properties of the Influenza Virus Genome

Influenza virus has a segmented genome consisting of at least seven pieces of single-stranded RNA. This segmentation allows reassortment of the genome ("recombination") to occur during mixed infections (Chapter 7) with different strains and may be of key importance in antigenic variation of influenza virus. After mixed infection of cells with two different type A influenza viruses, recombinant viruses are formed with a high frequency. This high frequency of recombination between influenza A viruses was first demonstrated by Burnet (Burnet and Lind, 1949, 1951) and has been confirmed many times by other workers in the field (Hirst and Gotlieb, 1953, 1955; Simpson and Hirst, 1961; Simpson, 1964; Sugiura and Kilbourne, 1966). Recombination frequencies of up to 97% have been obtained.

This high frequency of recombination between influenza viruses allows antigenically hybrid viruses to be formed very readily during mixed infections in both *in vitro* and *in vivo* experiments. This was first shown biochemically by Laver and Kilbourne (1966), who found that a genetically stable recombinant virus X-7 isolated from cells mixedly infected with the NWS (H0N1) and RI/5+ (H2N2) strains of influenza possessed the hemagglutinin subunits of the H0N1 virus and the neuraminidase subunits of the H2N2 virus. Many other such recombinants of type A influenza viruses have subsequently been isolated and can, in fact, be made "to order" (Webster, 1970b) (see also Fig. 10.13). The creation of new strains of influenza by recombination between animal (or avian) and human influenza viruses is discussed in Section VII. Evidence has been obtained which suggests that the strains of virus which are the cause of influenza pandemics in man might arise naturally in this way. Recombination between influenza B viruses also occurs (Perry and Burnet, 1953; Perry *et al.*, 1954; Ledinko, 1955; Tobita and Kilbourne, 1974) but recombination with types A and B has never been demonstrated.

IV. The Hemagglutinin and Neuraminidase Subunits as Highly Variable Antigens

The hemagglutinin and neuraminidase activities of influenza viruses reside on separate subunits (Laver and Valentine, 1969; Laver, 1973) and form the layer of "spikes" on the surfaces of the virus particles (Fig. 10.1).

The hemagglutinin is the major surface antigen. It is responsible for the attachment of virus to cell receptors and for the induction of neutralizing antibodies. Variation in the hemagglutinin antigen allows epidemics of influenza to reoccur continually.

The enzyme neuraminidase constitutes the second virus-specific antigen on the surface of the influenza virus particle. It is completely unrelated antigenically to the hemagglutinin (Seto and Rott, 1966; Webster and Laver, 1967). Antibody to the neuraminidase does not neutralize virus infectivity (except at high cencentration), but it does slow down the release of virus from infected cells (Seto and Rott, 1966; Webster and Laver, 1967; Kilbourne *et al.*, 1968; Becht *et al.*, 1971; Dowdle *et al.*, 1974), and this antibody may play an important role in reducing viral replication *in vivo* and in preventing the spread of infection (Schulman *et al.*, 1968). Widespread variation in the neuraminidase also occurs, but variation in this antigen is possibly of lesser importance in the epidemiology of influenza.

The hemagglutinin subunits are rod-shaped glycoprotein structures, triangular in cross section, and of about 215,000 molecular weight (Fig. 10.2). They are "monovalent" and attach to cell receptors by one end only (Laver and Valentine, 1969). The isolated subunits are highly immunogenic when inoculated with adjuvant into animals. Each virus particle contains approximately 400 hemagglutinin subunits (Tiffany and Blough, 1970; Schulze, 1973; Laver, 1973).

The hemagglutinin subunits contain two species of polypeptides with molecular weights of approximately 25,000 and 55,000 (Compans *et al.*, 1970; Schulze, 1970; Laver, 1971; Skehel and Schild, 1971; Stanley and Haslam, 1971; Skehel, 1971, 1972; Klenk *et al.*, 1972). These are referred to as the heavy and light polypeptides—HA_1 and HA_2. The two chains are synthesized as a single large precursor polypeptide of about 80,000 molecular weight, which in certain host cells is cleaved to the light and heavy poly-

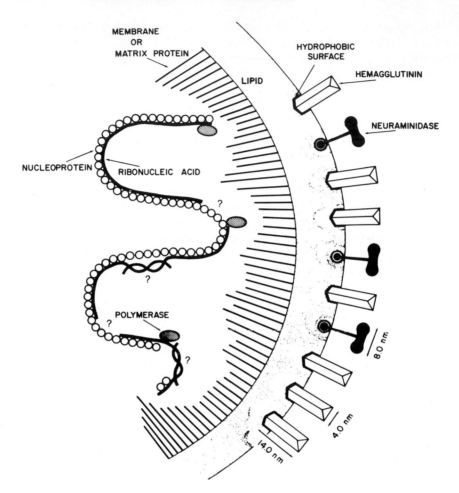

Fig. 10.1. Diagrammatic representation of a segment of an influenza virus particle. The hemagglutinin and neuraminidase subunits, which protrude as "spikes" from the surface of the virus are attached by their hydrophobic regions to the lipid envelope. The ratio of hemagglutinin to neuraminidase spikes varies from strain to strain (Webster *et al.*, 1968), but the relative distribution of these on the surface of the virus particle is not known. The orientation of the nucleo-protein RNA complex in the virion has not been fully elucidated; these complexes occur in segments when extracted from the virion but may be linked within the virion by labile bonds. Polymerase activity has been demonstrated within the core of the virion but the location is unknown.

peptides (Lazarowitz *et al.*, 1971, 1973; Skehel, 1972; Klenk *et al.*, 1972). In the intact subunits the heavy chain is joined to the light chain by disulfide bond(s) to form a dimer, and each hemagglutinin subunit is composed of two or three of these dimers (Laver, 1971).

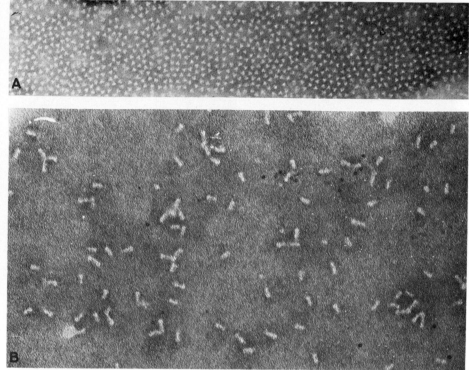

Fig. 10.2. Electron micrographs of the hemagglutinin subunits of influenza virus isolated from the SDS-disrupted virus particles by electrophoresis on cellulose acetate strips. (B) shows subunits in the presence of SDS, where they exist mostly as "monomers." (A) shows a collection of subunits viewed end-on and their triangular cross section is evident. ×240,000. (Electron micrographs were taken by Dr. Nick Wrigley.)

The hemagglutinin subunits possess hydrophilic and hydrophobic ends (Fig. 10.3). The hydrophilic end carries the biological activity of the subunit while the hydrophobic end is associated with the lipid of the virus envelope. The hydrophobic properties of the subunit seem to be associated with the C-terminal end of the light polypeptide chain (HA$_2$) (Skehel and Waterfield, 1975) (see Chapter 3).

The neuraminidase subunits are glycoprotein structures of about 240,000 molecular weight. They consist of a square, box-shaped head measuring $8 \times 8 \times 4$ nm and having a centrally attached fiber with a diffuse tail or small knob at its end (Fig. 10.4) (Laver and Valentine, 1969; Wrigley *et al.*, 1973). The isolated subunits have full enzymatic activity and are highly immunogenic when inoculated with adjuvant into animals. Each virus particle contains approximately 80 neuraminidase subunits (Schulze, 1973;

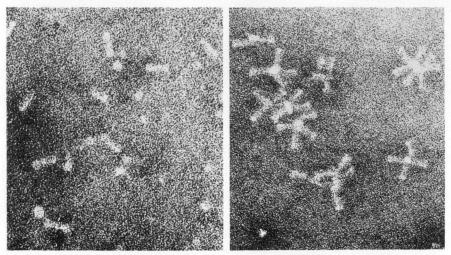

HEMAGGLUTININ SUBUNITS

IN SDS SOLUTION   SDS REMOVED

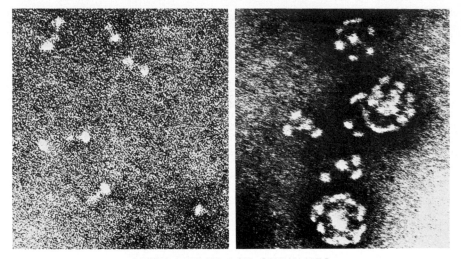

NEURAMINIDASE SUBUNITS

IN SDS SOLUTION   SDS REMOVED

Fig. 10.3. Electron micrographs of the isolated hemagglutinin (top) and neuraminidase (bottom) subunits in the presence of SDS (left) and after removal of the detergent (right). The hemagglutinin subunits were isolated from the HON1/Bel/42 strain of influenza, and the neuraminidase subunits from the HON2 recombinant virus X-7F1 (Webster *et al.*, 1968). The subunits were isolated from the SDS-disrupted virus particles by electrophoresis on cellulose acetate strips (Laver and Valentine, 1969) and eluted from the strips with water. For removal of SDS, the subunits were precipitated with cold ethanol and redissolved in saline. Electron micrographs were by Robin Valentine. From Laver (1973).

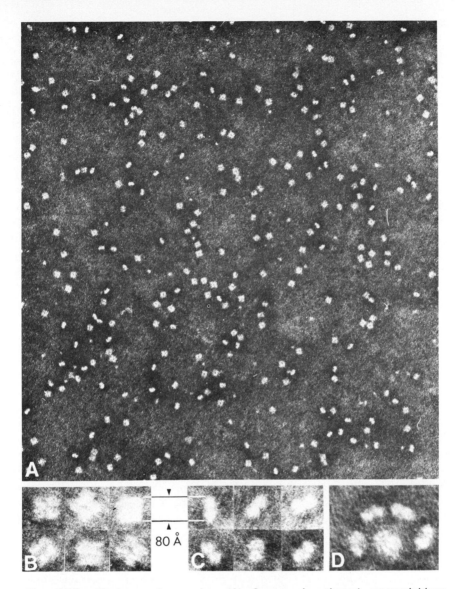

Fig. 10.4. Electron micrographs: (A) Square, box-shaped neuraminidase "heads" isolated by trypsin treatment from particles of B/LEE influenza virus showing both top and side views. (B) Six selected heads showing their square, box-shaped structure. Each head is clearly divided into four equal subunits. (C) Six heads shown side-on, each clearly having a division in the middle. (D) Complete neuraminidase subunits (consisting of heads and tails) isolated by electrophoresis from SDS-disrupted particles of B/LEE influenza virus. The subunits have aggregated by the hydrophobic tips of their tails in the way described in Fig. 10.3. The head of the subunits are oriented in such a way that their side views are shown, again with a clear subdivision in the middle. From Wrigley et al. (1973).

Laver, 1973). However, the amount of neuraminidase incorporated into particles of influenza virus is variable, depending on the strain of virus (Webster *et al.*, 1968; Webster and Laver, 1972; Palese and Schulman, 1974) and possibly also on the host cell in which the virus is grown (Laver, 1963).

The neuraminidase subunits consist of four glycosylated polypeptides of 60,000 molecular weight held together by disulfide bonds located in the fiber or tail (see also Chapter 4). With most strains the four polypeptides seem to be identical. However, in some strains the neuraminidase appears to consist of two species of polypeptide differing slightly in size (Webster, 1970a; Skehel and Schild, 1971; Bucher and Kilbourne, 1972; Laver and Baker, 1972; Lazdins *et al.*, 1972; Downie and Laver, 1973; Wrigley *et al.*, 1973).

The enzyme-active center and the antigenic determinants are located in different regions on the head of the neuraminidase subunits (Ada *et al.*, 1963; Fazekas de St. Groth, 1963) which possesses hydrophilic properties. The tail of the neuraminidase is hydrophobic and serves to attach the subunits to the lipid envelope of the virus (Laver and Valentine, 1969) (Fig. 10.3).

A. Segregation and Isolation of the Hemagglutinin and Neuraminidase Subunits of Influenza Viruses

Pure, intact hemagglutinin and neuraminidase subunits may be isolated from certain strains of influenza by electrophoresis on cellulose acetate strips after disruption of the virus particles with sodium dodecyl sulfate (SDS) (Laver, 1964, 1971; Laver and Valentine, 1969; Schild, 1970; Skehel and Schild, 1971; Webster and Laver, 1972; Downie and Laver, 1973). Successful isolation of either of these subunits by this technique depends on their ability to resist denaturation by SDS at room temperature. By this criterion influenza viruses can be divided into four groups:

1. Those with hemagglutinin subunits which resist denaturation by SDS. When these viruses are disrupted with SDS and electrophoresed on cellulose acetate strips all of the virus proteins except the hemagglutinin subunits migrate as anions. These hemagglutinins migrate as cations and can therefore be isolated in pure form and with full retention of biological activity under conditions which do not cleave covalent bonds [e.g., A/BEL/42 (H0N1)].
2. Those with neuraminidase subunits which resist denaturation by SDS. Pure, active neuraminidase subunits can be isolated from these viruses in the way described above (e.g., B/LEE/40).
3. Those in which neither the hemagglutinin nor the neuraminidase subunits resist denaturation by SDS. With these viruses all of the virus proteins

migrate as anions and neither of the surface subunits can be isolated in the way described above [e.g., A/NWS/33 (H0N1)].

4. Those in which both the hemagglutinin and neuraminidase subunits resist denaturation by SDS. With these viruses both subunits migrate as cations during electrophoresis and the two cannot be separated in this way [e.g., A/Singapore/1/57 (H2N2)].

The hemagglutinin and neuraminidase subunits of this last group of viruses can be isolated in the following way, illustrated in Fig. 10.5. An avian influenza virus was isolated (A/Shearwater/E. Aust./1/72, Hav6Nav5) which had SDS-stable hemagglutinin and neuraminidase subunits (Downie and Laver, 1973). These migrated together as cations during cellulose acetate electrophoresis (Fig. 10.5, top) and could not be separated in this way. Accordingly, the two kinds of subunits were segregated genetically into recombinant viruses (Webster, 1970b). For making the recombinants, parental viruses with hemagglutinin or neuraminidase subunits susceptible to denaturation by SDS were chosen. The SDS-stable avian virus hemagglutinin and neuraminidase subunits were then isolated from the SDS-disrupted recombinant virus particles by electrophoresis on cellulose acetate strips (Fig. 10.5, middle and bottom). Thus pure subunits could be obtained for chemical studies and for the preparation of "monospecific" antisera.

Hemagglutinin and neuraminidase subunits may also be isolated from certain strains of influenza by digesting the virus particles with proteolytic enzymes (Noll *et al.*, 1962; Seto *et al.*, 1966; Compans *et al.*, 1970; Brand and Skehel, 1972; Wrigley *et al.*, 1973). Liberation of the subunits from the virus particles in this way seems to result from the digestion of the hydrophobic ends of the polypeptide chains which are responsible for attaching the subunits to the lipid layer of the virus envelope. However, partial digestion of other regions of the hemagglutinin subunit must also occur, since hemagglutinin activity is destroyed and some antigenic determinants are lost.

B. Separation of the Hemagglutinin Polypeptides (HA$_1$ and HA$_2$)

The light and heavy chains of the hemagglutinin subunits can be separated by SDS–polyacrylamide gel electrophoresis. On a preparative scale, however, these are best separated by centrifugation on guanidine hydrochloride–dithiothreitol density gradients (Laver, 1971) done under conditions in which disulfide bonds are destroyed, or by gel filtration in guanidine hydrochloride–dithiothreitol solution (Webster, 1970a). The basis for the separation seems to be the strong hydrophobic property of the light poly-

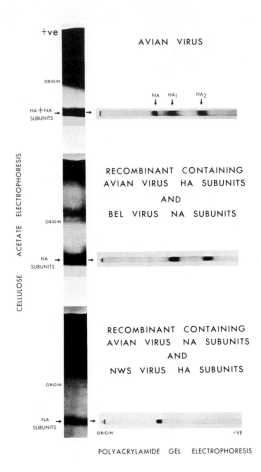

Fig. 10.5. Genetic segregation and isolation of the neuraminidase (NA) and hemagglutinin (HA) subunits of an avian influenza virus (A/Shearwater/E. Aust./1/72). The stained cellulose acetate strip at the top left shows the electrophoretic separation of the proteins of the avian virus after disruption of the virus particles with cold (20°C) SDS. The hemagglutinin and neuraminidase subunits of the avian virus were both stable in SDS solution, retained full biological activity, and migrated together as a single band during cellulose acetate electrophoresis. Polyacrylamide gel electrophoresis of the material in this band showed that it contained the polypeptides of the neuraminidase subunits and the heavy and light polypeptides (HA_1 and HA_2) of the hemagglutinin. The hemagglutinin and neuraminidase subunits of the avian virus were therefore segregated into recombinant viruses, the hemagglutinin into a virus containing AO/BEL/42 neuraminidase subunits, and the neuraminidase into a virus containing AO/NWS hemagglutinin subunits. When these hybrid viruses were disrupted with SDS, the only proteins which resisted denaturation by SDS were the HA and NA subunits of the avian virus, and these could then be isolated in pure form by electro-

peptide chain. During centrifugation in concentrated guanidine hydro-chloride–dithiothreitol solution, the light polypeptide sediments faster than the heavy chain, and during gel filtration the light chain emerges first, suggesting that even in this strongly dissociating medium the light chain does not exist as a monomer.

These remarks apply only to hemagglutinin subunits isolated from virus grown in cells in which proteolytic cleavage of the precursor hemagglutinin polypeptide, HA, to HA_1 and HA_2 is complete. Furthermore, the heavy and light polypeptides (HA_1 and HA_2) of hemagglutinin subunits isolated by proteolytic digestion cannot be separated in this way, probably because the hydrophobic regions of the light polypeptide are destroyed by the digestion (J. J. Skehel and W. G. Laver, unpublished).

C. Properties of HA_1 and HA_2

The light and heavy polypeptide chains of the (H0N1) BEL strain of influenza A virus were similar in amino acid composition, except that the heavy polypeptide contained considerably more proline than the light chain (Laver and Baker, 1972). However, maps of the tryptic peptides from the two chains were quite different, indicating that they had different amino acid sequences (Laver, 1971). Both polypeptide chains contained carbohydrate, but glucosamine analyses suggested that the heavy polypeptide contained much more carbohydrate than the light chain. The heavy chain was found to contain 9.4% N-acetylglucosamine as well as neutral sugars; thus, it probably contained about 20% carbohydrate.

D. Number of Different Virus-Specified Antigenic Determinants on the Hemagglutinin Subunits

The number of different virus-specified antigenic determinants on the hemagglutinin subunits of influenza virus is not known. (Host-specific determinants also exist on the hemagglutinin subunits.) Recent experiments,

---

phoresis on cellulose acetate (stained strips shown at middle and bottom left-hand side). The bands containing the avian virus hemagglutinin and neuraminidase subunits were eluted from the cellulose acetate strips with water, concentrated by ethanol precipitation, redissolved in hot (100°C) SDS and dithiothreitol, and electrophoresed on polyacrylamide gels. The stained gels confirmed that pure hemagglutinin and neuraminidase subunits had been isolated (from Downie and Laver, 1973).

however, have shown that the hemagglutinin subunits from the Hong Kong strain (H3N2) of human influenza possess at least two and possibly more different virus-specified antigenic determinants (Laver *et al.*, 1974). This was demonstrated in the following way: Hemagglutinin subunits were isolated from Hong Kong influenza virus (A/Hong Kong/68, H3 N2) and from its antigenic variant, A/Memphis/102/72, which arose as the result of antigenic drift. Immunodiffusion tests showed that the HK/68 subunits possessed at least two different kinds of antigenic determinants while the 1972 variant appeared to posses at least three different determinants (Fig. 10.6).

One of the antigenic determinants was common to the hemagglutinin subunits of A/Hong Kong/68 and A/Memphis/102/72 viruses. Antibody to this determinant cross-reacted in immunodiffusion, hemagglutination-inhibition, and neutralization tests with both viruses. Antibodies to another determinant showed no detectable serological cross-reactions between HK/68 and Mem/72 viruses. Thus it appeared that during antigenic drift, Hong Kong influenza virus had undergone a major antigenic change in this "specific" determinant. Evidence (Laver *et al.*, 1974) suggested that the different antigenic determinants were located on the same hemagglutinin subunit and that the virus particles did not possess a mixture of antigenically different subunits.

E. Location of the Host Antigen

Although early descriptions of a host antigen in influenza viruses (Knight, 1944, 1946) were received with a certain amount of scepticism, its existence is now firmly established. The presence of such antigen(s) has been revealed by a number of serological tests, including precipitation (Knight, 1944), immunodiffusion (Howe *et al.*, 1967), complement fixation (Smith *et al.*, 1955), hemagglutination inhibition (Knight, 1944; Harboe *et al.*, 1961; Harboe, 1963a) and by blocking of hemagglutination inhibition (Harboe, 1963b; Laver and Webster, 1966). The host antigen is composed largely of carbohydrate and is bound by covalent linkage to the polypeptides of the hemagglutinin and neuraminidase subunits. No host antigen (and no carbohydrate) is found attached to the internal proteins of the virus particle.

One of the puzzling features about the host antigen of influenza viruses is that it can be demonstrated in viruses grown in the allantoic sac of chicken and turkey embryos (Harboe, 1963a) but not, for example, in viruses grown in the allantoic sac of duck embryos, in mouse lungs, or in a variety of cultured cells. Viruses grown in these hosts were not inhibited at all in

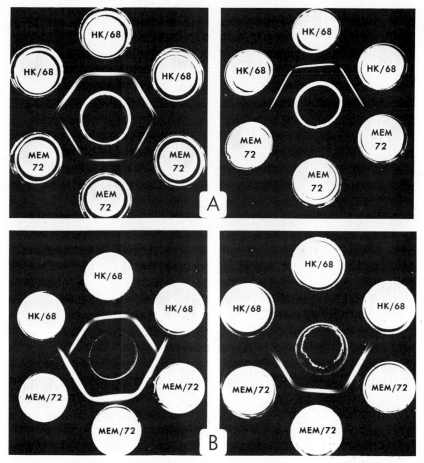

Fig. 10.6. Double immunodiffusion tests illustrating the preparation of antibody to the "specific" antigenic determinants on the hemagglutinin subunits of HK/68 and Mem/72 viruses. (A) On the left, center well, antiserum prepared against the isolated hemagglutinin subunits of HK/68 virus tested against particles of HK/68 and Mem/72 viruses disrupted with SDS, and on the right, center well, the same antiserum after absorption with intact particles of Mem/72 virus. (B) On the left, center well, antiserum prepared against the isolated hemagglutinin subunits of Mem/72 virus tested against particles of HK/68 and Mem/72 viruses disrupted with SDS, and, on the right, center well, the same antiserum after absorption with intact particles of HK/68 virus. In each case absorption of the sera with the heterologous virus removed the antibody reacting with the "common" determinant, leaving behind the antibody to the "specific" determinant(s).

hemagglutination-inhibition tests with antisera prepared against extracts of the uninfected host cells. It is probable that virus grown in these other cells contains host carbohydrate, but for some reason either this is not antigenic or antibody directed against it does not inhibit hemagglutination.

F. Role of the Host Antigen

The carbohydrate component may play a very important role in the assembly of the viral envelope. The way in which the isolated neuraminidase and hemagglutinin subunits aggregate in the absence of SDS suggests that these subunits possess both a hydrophobic and a hydrophilic end (Laver and Valentine, 1969), and it is possible that the host cell carbohydrate component gives the hemagglutinin and neuraminidase subunits their hydrophilic character at one end.

G. Antigenic Variation in the Hemagglutinin and Neuraminidase Subunits Detected by Using "Monospecific" Antisera

Until recently it was thought that the V antigen or envelope on the influenza virus particle was a single antigenic entity. This is clearly not the case. It is now known that the V antigen contains the hemagglutinin, neuraminidase, and host antigen of the virus. None of the earlier studies on antigenic relationships among the influenza viruses took this into account, so that, depending on the kind of test employed, a greater or lesser degree of cross-reaction between viruses was detected. Thus, the widely used strain-specific complement-fixation test detected cross-reactions between neuraminidase as well as hemagglutinin antigens, while hemagglutination-inhibition tests, in some cases, also detected cross-reactions between neuraminidase antigens. This is because "steric neutralization" of neuraminidase activity by antibody to the hemagglutinin (or vice versa) can occur with intact viruses (Laver and Kilbourne, 1966; Schulman and Kilbourne, 1969; Easterday *et al.*, 1969; Webster and Darlington, 1969).

Antigenic drift in the separate antigens of influenza can be studied after the antigens are separated from the virus particle (Webster and Darlington, 1969) or by genetic segregation of the antigens (Kilbourne *et al.*, 1967). Thus by using "monospecific" antisera to the two antigens, it is now possible to conduct detailed serological studies on antigenic drift in the individual antigens of influenza viruses.

V. Mechanism of Antigenic Drift (Minor Antigenic Variation)

A. Introduction

The two different patterns of antigenic variation observed among influenza A viruses, namely, the sudden appearance of new antigenic subtypes and the gradual drift within subtypes, are likely to be unrelated phenomena.

It is generally accepted that drift, the sequential replacement of human influenza A viruses by antigenically novel strains, results from the interplay of viral mutability and immunological selection (Table 10.1). The importance of this mechanism of selection is supported by the experimental production of antigenic variants by propagation of influenza viruses in the presence of subliming amounts of antiserum (Archetti and Horsfall, 1950; Isaacs and Edney, 1950; Burnet and Lind, 1949; Edney, 1957; Laver and Webster, 1968) or in partially immune animals (Gerber et al., 1955, 1956; Magill, 1955; Hamré et al., 1958). Epidemiological observations are also consistent with this mechanism, which offers a reasonable explanation for the disappearance of outmoded strains in human populations.

Several hypotheses have been proposed to explain the mechanism of antigenic drift. One proposal (Francis, 1952, 1955, 1960; Jensen et al., 1956; Jensen, 1957) suggests that the surface of the influenza virus consists of a mosaic of antigens shared by all strains of a given type but occurring in varying proportions or different situations in antigenically distinct strains. Antigenic variation would be a consequence of displacement of given antigens from a prominent to a hidden position on the viral envelope. An alternative hypothesis (Hilleman, 1952; Magill and Jotz, 1952; Andrewes, 1956, 1957; Takatsy and Furesz, 1957) is that antigens are gradually replaced in the course of variation. Both these hypotheses require the existence of a relatively large number of antigenically distinct protein molecules on the viral envelope. Jensen et al. (1956) estimated at 18 the number of anti-

Table 10.1 Antigenic Drift in the Hemagglutinin Subunits of Hong Kong Influenza Virus from 1968 to 1973

Virus strain	HI titers with antiserum to hemagglutinin subunits isolated from A/Hong Kong/1968 virus
A/Hong Kong/68	24,000
A/England/42/72	12,000
A/Memphis/102/72	4,800
A/Port Chalmers/73	2,400

gens arranged in different quantities and/or locations in each of a number of strains in a comprehensive collection of influenza A viruses available for study in 1953. Extension of these findings to the numerous new variants discovered since then would probably lead to the postulation of an even greater number of antigens in each virus, especially if it is accepted, as seems logical, that strains of human porcine, equine, and avian sources are part of the same complex. The existence of such a large number of distinct protein molecules in influenza viruses cannot be reconciled with the coding potential of the viral RNA (Laver, 1964). Furthermore, electron microscopic (Lafferty and Oertelis, 1963), immunochemical (Fazekas de St. Groth, 1961, 1962; Fazekas de St. Groth and Webster, 1963, 1964), and biochemical (Laver, 1964) evidence is more consistent with the existence of a very limited number of antigenically distinct protein molecules on the virus surface.

Recent experiments suggest that antigenic drift is the result of the selection by an immune population of mutant virus particles with altered antigenic determinants and, therefore, a growth advantage in the presence of antibody (Table 10.2). Furthermore, it has been shown that antigenic mutants isolated *in vitro* by selection with antibody have changes in the amino acid sequence of the polypeptides of the hemagglutinin subunits (Laver and Webster, 1968) (Fig. 10.7). Peptide maps have shown that changes in the amino acid sequence of both the heavy and light polypeptide chains also occur during natural antigenic drift (Fig. 10.8).

These results suggest that antigenic variation among influenza viruses is related to changes in the amino acid sequence of their antigenic proteins. Although some of the changes in sequence may have been random, having little or no effect on the antigenic determinants, it is likely that some of the alterations in amino acid sequence affected the antigenic determinants on the hemagglutinin subunits, making them less able to "fit" properly with the corresponding antibody molecules. The experiment did not show, how-

Table 10.2 Antigenic Drift *in Vitro*

Virus[a]	Number of passages in the presence of antiserum	HI titers of antisera to virus passaged		
		0 times	7 times	19 times
A/BEL/42 (H0N1)	0	12,600	4,500	390
	7	2,000	70,000	800
	19	560	4,400	30,000

[a] The A/BEL/42 (H0N1) strain of influenza virus was serially passaged in embryonated eggs in the presence of low avidity antiserum.

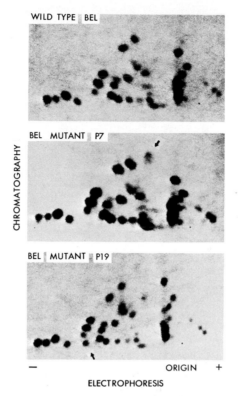

Fig. 10.7. Two-dimensional separation of the diffusible tryptic peptides from the hemagglutinin subunits of wild-type BEL virus and of the BEL antigenic mutants, P7 and P19. The peptides were mapped under the same conditions as in Fig. 10.8, and obvious differences between the 2 maps are indicated with arrows.

ever, whether the changes actually occurred in the antigenic determinants of the virus proteins, or in some other region of the molecule.

Influenza viruses show asymmetrical cross-reactions in hemagglutination inhibition tests. Fazekas de St. Groth (1970) has named viruses that behave in this way "senior" and "junior" strains. Furthermore, he has proposed (Fazekas de St. Groth, 1970) that during natural antigenic variation "senior" influenza viruses replace the "junior" strains. Little confirmatory evidence for the latter proposition has been presented.

B. Can Drift Be Anticipated?

The ability of influenza virus to undergo antigenic changes remains a major problem. Each new variant must be isolated and identified before

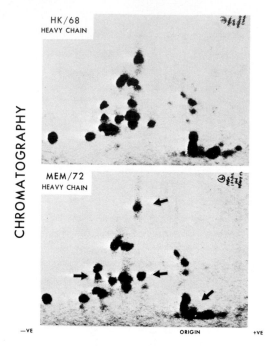

Fig. 10.8. Maps of the tryptic peptides (soluble at pH 6.5) from the heavy polypeptides (HA₁) of the hemagglutinin subunits of Hong Kong/68 influenza virus and its antigenic variant, A/Memphis/72 virus, which formed as the result of antigenic drift. Some differences between the two maps have been marked with arrows. These indicate that the two polypeptides differ slightly in amino acid sequence, but where these differences occur and how they affect the antigenic determinants on the hemagglutinin subunits is not known. Electrophoresis at pH 6.5 was followed by two rounds of ascending chromatography in a mixture of pyridine–isoamyl alcohol–water (35 : 35 : 30). Peptides were stained with ninhydrin.

any start can be made toward vaccine production, so that each new variant is able to infect a large number of people before vaccines are available to control it.

Attempts have therefore been made to anticipate antigenic drift in the laboratory before it occurs in nature, but this approach has so far met with only limited success. Claude Hannoun and Stephen Fazekas de St. Groth at the Pasteur Institute in Paris passaged the A/Hong Kong/68 (H3N2) strain in the presence of sublimiting concentrations of antiserum. After several such cycles of growth, they isolated a variant that no longer mutated antigenically under the experimental conditions. This variant, they postulated, represented the end point of evolution within the H3 subtype, and was thus a virus that would be expected to appear in the late 1970's. Support for this postulate was provided by the discovery that the London influenza variant first isolated in 1972 (A/ENG/42/72) was antigenically quite like the first mutant Hannoun and Fazekas de St. Groth had produced in their laboratory a year earlier (Fazekas de St. Groth and Hannoun, 1973).

It was hoped that vaccines produced from the final "senior" variant would provide protection against all H3 variants that might appear in man. However, type A viruses isolated subsequently in 1973 and 1974 (e.g., A/Port Chalmers/1/73) which were antigenically different from the A/England/42/72 strain were also significantly different from the artificially produced variant, suggesting that drift under natural conditions was not going in the direction anticipated.

In any case, the variant produced in the laboratory by passage in antiserum had undergone drift in the hemagglutinin only, whereas the naturally occurring variants drifted in both hemagglutinin and neuraminidase. Thus, this attempt to produce a "prospective" vaccine seems to have failed.

C. Possibility of Major Changes Occurring in Certain Antigenic Determinants during Antigenic Drift

It was shown in Section IV that the hemagglutinin subunits of Hong Kong influenza virus possess at least two distinct kinds of antigenic determinants and that during the evolution (by antigenic drift) of Hong Kong influenza, a virus was formed (A/Memphis/102/72) in which one of these antigenic determinants had undergone a major antigenic change (similar in magnitude to antigenic shift), while the other had drifted (Fig. 10.6). We have called the former the "specific" and the latter the "common" determinant for the two viruses (Laver *et al.*, 1974).

Antibody to the "specific" determinant did not show any cross-reactions between the two viruses in immunodiffusion, hemagglutination-inhibition, or in neutralization of infectivity tests. The other determinant(s) was common to the two viruses (although some antigenic drift had occurred in this determinant) and the cross-reactions found between HK/68 and Mem/72 viruses are due entirely to antibody to this "common" determinant(s).

Different animals responded to a different extent to the various determinants when immunized with the same preparation of isolated hemagglutinin subunits. This variation in response may explain the variable cross-reactions sometimes seen between two viruses when tested against different sera.

Despite the major antigenic change in one determinant, peptide maps of the heavy and light polypeptides (HA_1 and HA_2) of the hemagglutinin subunits of HK/68 and Mem/72 viruses were remarkably similar (Fig. 10.8), suggesting that relatively few changes had occurred in the amino acid sequence of these polypeptides during the evolution of Hong Kong virus and the formation of the Mem/72 variant. Changes occurred in the peptide maps of both the heavy (HA₁) and light (HA₂) polypeptide chains; some of these may have been random changes and others selected under antibody pressure.

D. Antigenic Variation in the Neuraminidase

Antigenic drift has been observed in the neuraminidase antigen of both influenza A and B viruses (Paniker, 1968; Schulman and Kilbourne, 1969; Schild et al., 1973; Curry et al., 1974). This probably occurs by the selection of mutants under antibody pressure which have altered amino acid sequences in the polypeptides of the neuraminidase subunits (Kendal and Kiley, 1973). So far, antigenic drift in the neuraminidase has not been achieved in the laboratory. Antibody to the neuraminidase does not neutralize virus infectivity; therefore, it is likely that the variation in this antigen is of lesser importance to the survival of the virus than variation in the hemagglutinin (Seto and Rott, 1966; Dowdle et al., 1974).

E. Antigenic Variation in Influenza B Viruses

Antigenic drift occurs among influenza B viruses to a similar extent as in type A influenza viruses, but the major antigenic shifts seen in these latter viruses have not been found among influenza B strains. Antigenic drift involves changes in both the hemagglutinin and neuraminidase antigens (Chakraverty, 1972a,b; Curry et al., 1974). The mechanism of antigenic variation in the B strains is presumably similar to that in influenza A viruses but biochemical studies have not been done.

F. Antigenic Variation in Avian and Animal Influenza Viruses

Antigenic variation among influenza viruses infecting lower animals and birds has not been studied in sufficient detail, and little information is available. Some results, however, do suggest that antigenic drift in animal or avian strains of influenza does occur but at a slower rate than in influenza viruses infecting man.

Antigenic drift has been observed with swine and equine 2 influenza viruses (Meier-Ewert *et al.*, 1970; Pereira *et al.*, 1972), but to date there is no evidence of antigenic drift among the avian influenza viruses. A possible reason for this is that avian species, especially domestic birds, usually have a shorter life span than man or horses. In man each successive variant of type A rapidly replaces the preexisting one completely, but in animals and birds, viruses differing from each other often circulate concurrently.

VI. Mechanism of Antigenic Shifts (Major Antigenic Variation)

During the other kind of antigenic variation, the surface subunits of the virus undergo major antigenic shifts. In these major shifts, sudden and complete changes occur in one or both of the surface antigens, so that "new" viruses arise to which the population has no immunity, and it is these viruses which cause pandemic influenza.

The human H2N2 influenza viruses offer a natural system for studying the molecular aspects of the major antigenic shifts. These viruses, which appeared in man in 1957, posessed hemagglutinin and neuraminidase subunits which were completely different antigenically from the hemagglutinin and neuraminidase subunits of the H1N1 strains. The H2N2 viruses underwent antigenic drift until 1968 when the "new" pandemic Hong Kong strain appeared. The A2 (H2N2) viruses and the Hong Kong (H3N2) strain both arose in China. Hong Kong virus possessed the same neuraminidase as the preceding A2 viruses, but the hemagglutinin differed antigenically (Coleman *et al.*, 1968; Schulman and Kilbourne, 1969). This was shown unequivocally by using specific antisera to the isolated hemagglutinin subunits of representative A2 influenza viruses grown in chick embryos. These "monospecific" sera were used in hemagglutinin-inhibition tests with the viruses grown in duck embryos (Webster and Laver, 1972), thus avoiding the problems of steric inhibition of hemagglutination by antibodies to the neuraminidase and host antigens which may occur when sera to whole viruses are used.

The results of these tests (Table 10.3) showed that there was no serological relationship between the hemagglutinin antigens of the "old" A2/Asian strains isolated between 1957 and 1968 and the Hong Kong (1968) virus. Little or no variation was found in three Hong Kong strains isolated during the first three years of the Hong Kong pandemic (Webster and Laver, 1972). Where then did the "new" hemagglutinin subunits of Hong Kong influenza come from? There seemed to be two possible origins for the "new" hemagglutinin subunits: either they were derived by mutation from those of a preexisting human influenza virus, or they came from some other source, such as an animal or avian influenza virus.

Table 10.3 Comparison of Hemagglutinins from Three Asian (H2N2) Strains and Three Hong Kong (H3N2) Strains Showing a Major Antigenic Shift

Antisera to hemagglutinin subunits isolated from viruses grown in chicken embryos	HI titer against intact viruses grown in duck embryos					
	Asian strains			Hong Kong strains		
	A2/Korea/68	A2/Ned/68	A2/Berk/68	A2/Aichi/68	A2/Qld/70	A2/Mem/71
A2/Korea/68	35,000	1,400	17,000	<20	<20	<20
A2/Ned/68	2,900	89,000	8,900	<20	<20	<20
A2/Berk/68	2,200	2,400	8,300	<20	<20	<20
A2/Aichi/68	<20	<20	<20	38,000	35,000	18,000
A2/Qld/70	<20	<20	<20	48,000	31,000	11,000
A2/Memphis/71	<20	<20	<20	9,400	9,400	9,200

A single mutation in an "old" A2/Asian influenza virus might have caused the polypeptide chains of the hemagglutinin subunits to refold in such a way as to expose completely new antigenic determinants. If the hemagglutinin subunits of Hong Kong influenza were derived by mutation in this fashion from the earlier A2 viruses, then the amino acid sequence of the polypeptides of the "old" and the "new" subunits would be similar. A complete shift in one antigenic determinant on the hemagglutinin subunits which occurred during antigenic drift was described earlier, and this "shift" in one determinant did not appear to be associated with any great overall change in the amino acid sequence of the hemagglutinin polypeptides. However, if the "new" hemagglutinin subunits did not arise by mutation and selection, but came instead from an animal or avian influenza virus, then their polypeptide chains might differ greatly in amino acid sequence from those of the "old" A2/Asian viruses.

Hemagglutinin subunits were isolated from three strains of A2/Asian influenza obtained in 1968 before the occurrence of the Hong Kong influenza pandemic and from three strains of Hong Kong influenza virus isolated in different parts of the world in 1968, 1970, and 1971. Because of antigenic drift, the three viruses isolated at the end of the A2/Asian era showed considerable antigenic variation. On the other hand, the three Hong Kong strains which were isolated during the first three years following the new pandemic showed almost no antigenic variation.

The hemagglutinin subunits isolated from each of these six virus strains were dissociated by treatment with guanidine hydrochloride and dithiothreitol, and their light and heavy polypeptide chains were separated by centrifugation (Laver, 1971). Each of the isolated polypeptide chains was digested with trypsin, and the tryptic peptides were mapped. The maps showed that the polypeptide chains from the hemagglutinin subunits of the "old" A2 viruses isolated in 1968 differed greatly in amino acid sequence from the polypeptide chains of the "new" Hong Kong strains (Figs. 10.9 and 10.10), suggesting that the "new" polypeptides were not derived by mutation from the "old" (Laver and Webster, 1972).

One explanation for this result is that a frame-shift mutation occurred, giving rise to polypeptides with a completely different sequence of amino acids. It seems unlikely, though, that even if such an event had occurred it would give rise to polypeptides able to form a functional hemagglutinin subunit. A second possibility is that mutations affecting mainly the basic amino acids might have occurred so that the tryptic peptide maps would be greatly different without any large change in the overall amino acid sequence of the polypeptides.

Evidence has now been obtained directly implicating certain animal (or avian) influenza viruses as possible progenitors of the Hong Kong strain

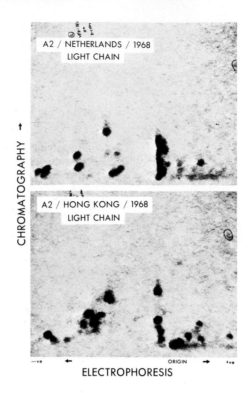

Fig. 10.9. Maps of the tryptic peptides (soluble at pH 6.5) from the light polypeptide chains (HA₂) of the hemagglutinin subunits of A2/Netherlands/68 influenza isolated before the occurrence of the Hong Kong influenza pandemic and of the light chains of A2/Hong Kong/68 influenza virus. The maps show that the light polypeptide chains from the hemagglutinin subunits of a virus isolated immediately before the Hong Kong influenza virus differ greatly in amino acid sequence from the light polypeptide chain of the Hong Kong influenza virus. Electrophoresis at pH 6.5 was followed by ascending chromatography in pyridine—isoamyl alcohol—water (35 : 35 : 30). The circle drawn in the top right-hand corner of each map shows the position of the phenol red marker added to the tryptic peptides before mapping.

of human influenza. Two strains of influenza virus, A/equine/Miami/1/63 (Heq2 Neq2) and A/duck/Ukraine/1/63 (Hav7 Neq2), isolated from horses and ducks in 1963, five years before Hong Kong influenza appeared in man, were found to be antigenically related to the Hong Kong strain (Coleman *et al.*, 1968; Masurel, 1968; Kaplan, 1969; Zakstelskaja *et al.*, 1969; Tumova and Easterday, 1969; Kasel *et al.*, 1969). The hemagglutinin subunits of the equine and duck viruses cross-reacted in hemagglutinin-inhibition and immunodiffusion tests with those of the Hong Kong strain of

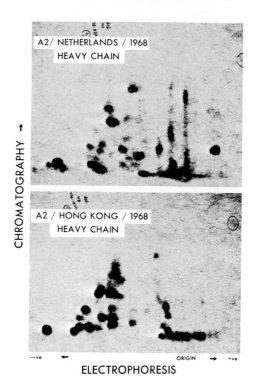

Fig. 10.10. Maps of the tryptic peptides from the heavy polypeptide chains (HA₁) of the hemagglutinin subunits of A2/Netherlands/68 and A2 Hong Kong/68 influenza viruses. The maps show many differences in amino acid sequence of the polypeptide chains.

human influenza A/Hong Kong/1/68 (H3N2). Furthermore, peptide maps of the light polypeptide chains from the hemagglutinin subunits of the equine, duck, and human viruses were almost identical, suggesting that the light chains from these three strains had practically the same amino acid sequence (Laver and Webster, 1973). These findings are highlighted in Fig. 10.11, which shows that the peptide maps of the light polypeptide chains from the hemagglutinin subunits of Hong Kong influenza and the equine 2 and duck/Ukraine influenza strains are almost identical and vastly different from the map of the light polypeptide chains from an "old" Asian/68 virus.

These results suggest that the equine and duck and the human Hong Kong viruses may have arisen, by genetic recombination, from a common ancestor and provide an alternative mechanism to mutation to explain the origin of Hong Kong influenza.

CHROMATOGRAPHY

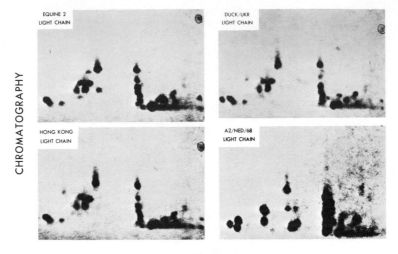

ELECTROPHORESIS

Fig. 10.11. Maps of the tryptic peptides (soluble at pH 6.5) from the light polypeptide chains (HA₂) of the hemagglutinin subunits of Hong Kong influenza virus compared with maps of the hemagglutinin light chains from equine 2 virus, duck/Ukraine virus, and an "old" A2/Asian (H2N2) strain (A2/Ned/68). These maps suggest that the hemagglutinin subunits of Hong Kong influenza came by genetic recombination from an animal or avian virus related to equine 2 and duck Ukraine viruses and that they did not come by mutation from an "old" A2/Asian strain.

The first suggestion that equine influenza viruses might be involved in human influenza pandemics came from observations made during the epidemic of 1693 (Molineux, 1695). Since then many authors have suggested animal or avian reservoirs as a source of human influenza viruses. In addition, the emergence of the Asian/57 influenza viruses and the Hong Kong variant and probably previous viruses from Asia (Chu, 1958; Andrewes, 1959; Kaplan and Payne, 1959; Francis and Maassab, 1965; Hoyle, 1968) have led many people to postulate the existence of an animal reservoir in China. Andrewes (1959) wonders if ". . . it is possible that influenza A is a virus imperfectly adapted to be forever a parasite of man, tending to die out, as it apparently did in the decades preceding 1889, yet starting afresh from time to time from a source in some unknown Central Asian host with which it stands in a stable relationship."

Recent studies have shown that sera from wild birds contain antibodies directed against antigens present on influenza viruses infecting man (World

Health Organization, 1972). Furthermore influenza viruses have recently been isolated from wild birds remote from human populations, suggesting that influenza is a natural avian infection and may have been so for many thousands of years (Downie and Laver, 1973).

An early suggestion that human pandemic influenza viruses arose from such animal or avian viruses by a process of recombination was made by Rasmussen (1964). Subsequently Tumova and Pereira (1965), Kilbourne (1968), and Easterday *et al.* (1969) obtained antigenic hybrid viruses by genetic recombination *in vitro* between human influenza viruses and avian or animal influenza strains. More recently Webster *et al.* (1971, 1973) have mimicked the emergence of a new pandemic strain of influenza in experiments *in vivo,* and these will be described later.

VII. Further Evidence to Support a Recombinational Event in the Origin of New Pandemic Influenza Viruses

The biochemical evidence given above does *not* support the theory that the hemagglutinin antigen of Hong Kong virus was derived by single step mutation from the previous Asian strains. We can therefore ask if there is any evidence from *in vitro* laboratory studies or from *in vivo* studies, or particularly from nature, that would support the theory that the new viruses arise by recombination.

A. *In Vitro* Evidence

Antigenic hybrids (recombinants) of many mammalian and avian influenza A viruses have been isolated after mixed infection of chick embryos or tissue cultures with different influenza A viruses (Tumova and Pereira, 1965; Kilbourne and Schulman, 1965; Kilbourne *et al.*, 1967; Kilbourne, 1968; Easterday *et al.*, 1969). These studies have been reviewed by Kilbourne *et al.* (1967) and by Webster and Laver (1971). It is now evident that recombinant influenza A viruses with the desired surface antigens (Webster, 1970b) or growth potential (Kilbourne and Murphy, 1960; Kilbourne *et al.*, 1971) or other biological characteristics (McCahon and Schild, 1971) can be made "to order."

Thus, "new" influenza viruses can be produced in the laboratory, but evidence that recombination and selection of "new" viruses can occur *in vivo* under simulated natural conditions has only recently been obtained (Webster *et al.*, 1971).

B. *In Vivo* Evidence

1. DEMONSTRATION OF RECOMBINATION *in Vivo*

Kilbourne (1970) pointed out that recombination between two different strains of influenza A viruses had not "yet been demonstrated in the intact animal—even under experimental conditions." In order to find out if recombination could occur *in vivo,* two systems were used. In the first only one of the parental viruses multiplied in the host animal, and in the second both parental viruses multiplied. Animals were inoculated with large doses of parental viruses, and on the third day, when at least one of the viruses had multiplied, the animals were killed. Lung suspensions were examined directly in the allantois on shell system for the presence of recombinant (antigenic hybrid) viruses, parental viruses being inhibited by specific antisera (Webser, 1970b).

In the first system pigs were inoculated with a mixture of swine influenza virus (A/swine/Wisconsin/1/67 [Hsw1N1]) and fowl plague virus (A/fowl plague virus/Dutch/27 [Hav1Neq1]) (FPV) (Fig. 10.12). The latter does not yield infectious virus after inoculation of pigs. Lung suspensions collected 3 days later contained parental viruses and the recombinant viruses possessing swine influenza virus hemagglutinin and FPV neuraminidase, swine(H)-FPV(N) (A/Hsw1-Neq1), and viruses possessing FPV hemagglutinin and swine influenza virus neuraminidase, FPV(H)-SW(N) (Hav1-N1) (Webster *et al.*, 1971).

In the second system where both viruses replicated, turkeys were infected with FPV and turkey influenza virus (A/turkey/ Massachusetts/3740/65 [Hav6N2]). Antigenic hybrids possessing turkey(H)-FPV(N) (Hav6-Neq1) and FPV(H)-turkey(N) (Hav1-N2) were isolated in the allantois on shell system as mentioned above.

There are two possible objections to the interpretation that the recombination described above occurred *in vivo*. The first is that the recombination might have occurred in the tissue culture system used for selection of viruses, and the second is whether the antigenic hybrids were genetically stable and not merely phenotypically mixed particles.

The first objection can be ruled out because the selection of antigenic hybrid viruses was done directly in very high concentrations of antibodies that would have neutralized the parental viruses. To provide more rigorous evidence that the antigenic hybrid viruses did not arise in the isolation procedures outside the infected hosts, it was necessary to plate the mixed yield from the lung suspension for plaque isolation and to characterize the virus stocks grown from plaque isolates. Twenty-five percent of the plaques isolated from the lung suspension of turkeys mixedly infected with FPV plus

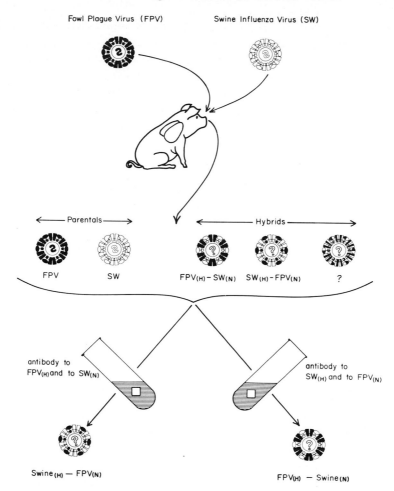

Fig. 10.12. Diagrammatic representation of genetic interaction of influenza "A" viruses *in vivo*. Pigs inoculated with fowl plague virus (FRV) and swine influenza virus (SW) were exsanguinated 3 days later. Lung suspensions contained high levels of SW and detectable levels of residual fowl plague virus, as well as antigenic hybrid viruses possessing FPV(H)-SW(N), SW(H)-FPV(N), and possibly other hybrids that were not detected. When this mixture of viruses was grown in the allantois on shell system in the presence of specific antibodies to FPV(H) and to SW(N) the antigenic hybrid possessing SW(H)-FPV(N) was isolated. The antigenic hybrids were genetically stable on cloning and caused infection in host animals. ▌, Hemagglutinin (H); ⋎, neuraminidase (N); ⌇, RNA. From Webster (1972).

turkey influenza virus neuraminidase were recombinant viruses. Hybrid viruses were not isolated from control cultures inoculated with artificial mixtures of both parental viruses.

The genetic stability of recombinant viruses was established by inoculation of host animals with the cloned antigenic hybrid viruses (Webster *et al.*, 1971). Thus, chickens inoculated with the antigenic hybrid virus possessing FPV(H)-turkey(N) (Hav1-N2) died of a fulminating infection, and the virus reisolated from the lungs of the birds 3 days later was a pure culture of virus possessing FPV(H)-turkey(N) (Hav1-N2). The other antigenic hybrid viruses were also reisolated from animals and were genetically stable.

2. NATURAL TRANSMISSION AND SELECTION

The above studies showed that two different strains of influenza A virus could recombine *in vivo* when they were simultaneously inoculated into the same animal. The simultaneous inoculation of animals with large doses of two different influenza A viruses, however, constitues an artificial system that probably would not occur in nature. To find out whether recombination could occur under more natural conditions, two different influenza A viruses were simultaneously allowed to spread in a flock of susceptible birds in the following way: Two turkeys infected with turkey influenza virus (A/turkey/Wisconsin/66 [Hav6N2][T/Wisc]) were placed in a flock of 30 susceptible sentinel turkeys. Two days later two turkeys infected with FPV were introduced into the same flock. Two of the sentinel turkeys were killed each day, and lung samples were assayed for the presence of each type of parental virus and for antigenic hybrid viruses in the allantois on shell system and by plaque isolation and virus identification (Webster *et al.*, 1971).

FPV rapidly spread through the sentinel birds and was detected three days after exposure; the turkey influenza virus was not detected until the ninth day after infected birds were put into the flock (Webster *et al.*, 1973). Antigenic hybrid viruses possessing FPV(H)-turkey(N) were detected on the tenth day after initial exposure and constituted the major virus population in the lung suspension of one of the birds tested. This type of experiment was repeated three times and in each experiments antigenic hybrids were isolated on the ninth to tenth day; the hybrids possessed FPV(H)-turkey(N), but the reciprocal hybrids were not isolated. The recombinant virus isolated probably had a growth advantage over the parental viruses, for in each experiment this virus was isolated as the predominant virus in one or more birds. For a "new" strain of influenza virus to arise in nature by recombination in this way and become an epidemic strain, it would be necessary for the "new" virus to have some selective advantage. This selective advantage could lie in possession of antigens to which the population at large was not immune, but the virus would also have to possess the capacity to transmit to susceptible hosts. Both possibilities were tested in the above experiments. Thus, normal birds were introduced at a time when recombinant viruses were present, but the recombinants failed to become the dominant strain, and all of the normal contact birds died of infection caused by parental FPV.

Recombination between different influenza A viruses of animal origin have also been demonstrated *in vivo* under conditions of natural transmission (Webster *et al.*, 1973). The Hong Kong strain of influenza virus (HK) isolated from pigs (Kundin, 1970) and swine influenza virus (A/swine/Wisconsin/67 [Hsw1 N1]) recombined in pigs after transmission from individually infected animals (Fig. 10.13). Recombinant influenza viruses possessing HK(H)-SW(N) and SW(H)-HK(N) were isolated from contact pigs. Both types of recombinants were genetically stable, caused mild respiratory infection in pigs, and the recombinant possessing HK(H)-SW(N) was naturally transmitted from pig to pig.

3. SELECTION AND TRANSMISSION OF A "NEW" INFLUENZA VIRUS *in Vivo*

If we postulate that new strains of influenza A viruses can arise by recombination in nature, it is essential to demonstrate how these viruses could be selected and become the dominant or new epidemic strain. A possible mechanism for selection would be for recombination and selection to occur in immune animals or birds. Recent experiments (Webster and Campbell, 1974) have shown that recombination and selection of a "new" strain of influenza virus can occur in turkeys that have low levels of antibodies to the hemagglutinin of one parental virus and to the neuraminidase of the other parental virus (Fig. 10.14).

Turkeys possessing low levels of antibodies to the hemagglutinin of turkey influenza virus (A/turkey/Wisconsin/66 [Hav6 N2]) and to the neuraminidase of FPV were mixedly infected with FPV and turkey influenza viruses. As well as both parental viruses, a recombinant influenza virus possessing FPV(H)-turkey(N) was present in the turkey tracheas 1 and 2 days after mixed infection. By the sixth day after mixed infection only the recombinant influenza virus [FPV(H)-turkey(N)] was present. The birds died on the seventh day after mixed infection and only recombinant influenza viruses possessing FPV(H)-turkey(N) were isolated. All viruses were isolated by limit dilution in the allantois on shell system or in embryonated eggs, and no antibody selection was used to select for recombinant viruses. Nonimmune birds introduced into the flock on the fifth day all died of a fulminating infection, and only recombinant influenza viruses were isolated from the contact birds.

Selection of recombinant influenza virus was not obtained following the

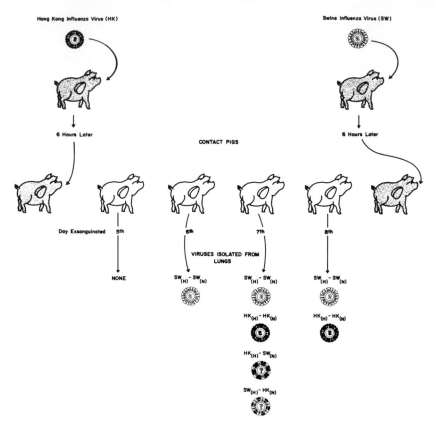

Fig. 10.13. Recombination between Hong Kong and SW influenza viruses under conditions of natural transmission. One pig was infected with HK influenza virus and a second pig was infected with SW influenza virus. Six hours later the infected animals were put into a room with four contact pigs. Beginning on the fifth day after introduction of the infected animals, one pig was exsanguinated each day and lung suspensions were examined for recombinant viruses as described in Materials and Methods. No viruses were detected in lung suspensions on the fifth day; on the sixth day parental SW virus was present, and on the seventh day both parental viruses and recombinant viruses possessing SW(H)-HK(N) and HK(H)-SW(N) were isolated. On the eighth day both parental viruses were present but no recombinant viruses were detected. From Webster *et al.* (1973).

mixed infection of either nonimmune or hyperimmune turkeys. Thus, mixed infection of birds that have low levels of antibodies to the hemagglutinin of one virus and to the neuraminidase of another provide ideal conditions for selection of recombinants. Following infection, both parental viruses replicated to a limited extent stimulating the immune system with elimination of the parental viruses. In this way recombinants can be selected and,

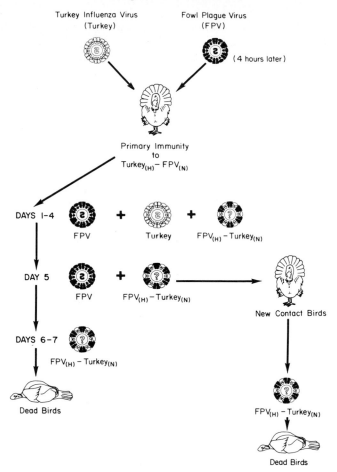

Fig. 10.14. Recombination, selection, and transmission of a new influenza virus *in vivo*. Turkeys with low levels of primary immunity to turkey/Wisconsin influenza virus hemagglutinin and to FPV neuraminidase were mixedly infected with parental FPV and turkey virus. On days 1–4, FPV, turkey/Wisconsin influenza virus, and a recombinant influenza virus possessing FPV(H)-turkey(N) were detected in tracheal swabs. On day 5 FPV(H)-turkey(N) was present in the tracheas with low levels of FPV; subsequently the recombinant influenza virus [FPV(H)-turkey(N)] became the dominant virus and killed the turkeys. Contact turkeys introduced on the fifth day all died with signs of CNS impairment, and only recombinant influenza virus [FPV(H)-turkey(N)] was isolated from the contact birds.

provided they possess the necessary properties of virulence and transmissability, can cause an epidemic of disease.

The above experiments were repeated twice; in each case recombinant influenza [FPV(H)-turkey(N)] viruses were selected but in one case the recombinants failed to transmit and cause disease in contact birds. A possible criticism of these experiments is that selective immunization against the hemagglutinin of one virus and against the neuraminidase of another virus would not occur in nature. On the contrary, inspection of the range of antigens in the avian influenza viruses will show that there are several influenza viruses that possess the same neuraminidase as FPV (e.g., A/chick/Germany "N"/49) and others that possess the same hemagglutinin as turkey/Wisconsin/66 (e.g., A/Shearwater/Australia/72). Thus, natural conditions might favor the emergence of new pandemic strains by the mechanisms proposed above.

These experiments demonstrate that recombination between different influenza A viruses can occur under relatively natural conditions and that the new viruses can have a selective advantage over both parents. The experiments do not establish that all new influenza viruses of lower mammals, birds, and humans arise by this mechanism but do establish that this is one method by which new viruses can occur.

C. Evidence for Recombination of Influenza Viruses in Nature

The above experiments leave no doubt that new strains of influenza virus can be produced *in vitro* and *in vivo* and suggest that a similar process might occur in nature. Is there any evidence, however, that recombination occurs in nature? The evidence is indirect and includes (1) antigenic relationships between influenza viruses from humans and from lower mammals and birds, and (2) the lack of a strict host range of influenza viruses.

1. ANTIGENIC RELATIONSHIPS BETWEEN INFLUENZA VIRUSES FROM HUMANS AND FROM LOWER MAMMALS AND BIRDS

Evidence suggesting that recombination between animal and human influenza viruses might occur naturally comes from the finding that some influenza viruses of man and of lower mammals and birds share similar if not identical surface antigens.

a. Antigenic Relationships Mediated through the Neuraminidase. The neuraminidase of some avian influenza viruses is antigenically closely related to the neuraminidase on earlier human influenza viruses. Thus, a virus from ducks (A/duck/Germany/1868/68 [Hav6N1]) possesses a neuraminidase that was very similar to the neuraminidase of the human H0N1 and H1N1 viruses (Schild and Newman, 1969). The influenza viruses from swine also possess a neuraminidase antigen that is closely related to the neuraminidase antigen from human H0N1 viruses (Meier-Ewert *et al.*, 1970). Similarly, a turkey influenza virus (A/turkey/Massachusetts/65 [Hav6N2]) possesses a neuraminidase that is similar to if not identical with the neuraminidase of the human H2N2 influenza viruses (Pereira *et al.*, 1967; Webster and Pereira, 1968; Schild and Newman, 1969). Other avian influenza viruses possess neuraminidase antigens closely related to the neuraminidase on equine-1 and equine-2 influenza viruses (Webster and Pereira, 1968; World Health Organization, 1971). Thus, the neuraminidase of fowl plague influenza virus (A/FPV/Dutch/27 [Hav1Neq1]) is similar to the neuraminidase on equine-1 influenza virus (A/equine/Prague/1/57 [Heq1Neq1]). These interrelationships have been utilized in a revised nomenclature for influenza viruses (World Health Organization, 1971). There are eight different subtypes of avian influenza viruses and four of these subtypes possess neuraminidase antigens closely related to neuraminidase antigens on human or equine influenza subtypes.

b. Antigenic Relationships Mediated through the Hemagglutinin Antigen. Fewer examples have been found of influenza virus from lower mammals and birds which have HA antigens related to that of human viruses. The interrelationships of the hemagglutinins of Hong Kong, duck/Ukraine/63, and equine-2 have been discussed above. Recently a virus isolated from ducks in Germany (A/duck/Germany/1225/74 [H2 Nav2]) was found to possess a hemagglutinin very closely related to the Asian influenza viruses. Thus, as more viruses are isolated, the number of interrelationships found are bound to increase.

2. HOST RANGE

Influenza A viruses do not always have strict host range specificity (see Easterday and Tumova, 1971; Webster, 1972). Thus, Hong Kong influenza virus has been isolated from pigs, dogs, cats, baboons, and gibbons. A/Hong Kong (H3N2) influenza viruses have also recently been isolated from chickens and a calf (Zhezmer, 1973). These viruses have been transmitted experimentally to calves and chickens; in each case the virus replicated in the host from which it was isolated. Thus the calf influenza virus caused respiratory infection in calves, and the chicken influenza virus replicated but did not show signs of disease in chickens (G. C. Schild, C. H. Campbell, and R. G. Webster, unpublished observation). Human strains of Hong Kong influenza viruses failed to replicate in chickens. In the case of Hong Kong influenza virus it is evident that this virus has been adapted to naturally infect other hosts and thus create conditions where double infection could occur and permit genetic interactions.

D. Summary of Available Evidence Supporting the View That New Strains of Influenza Virus Could Arise by Recombination

1. Pandemics of influenza in man are caused only by influenza A viruses, and only the influenza A viruses have been isolated from lower mammals and birds. Influenza B viruses will recombine *in vitro* but there may not be a pool of genetic information in nature that would permit a pandemic influenza B strain to emerge. Recombination between A and B influenza viruses has not been demonstrated.

2. Biochemical evidence presented above suggests that it is unlikely that "new" pandemic strains of influenza virus arise by direct mutation from preceding human influenza viruses.

3. New influenza viruses capable of causing a pandemic can occur by recombination and selection under experimental conditions *in vivo*.

4. Antigenic and biochemical relationships between the hemagglutinin and neuraminidase antigens of influenza viruses of man, lower animals, and birds suggest that genetic exchanges occur in nature.

The above evidence is circumstantial; more direct evidence would come if future human pandemic strains are found to have antigens identical to already isolated and characterized influenza viruses from domestic or wild animals and avian sources.

VIII. Future Antigenic Variation in Influenza Viruses and Possibilities of Anticipating Variation and Controlling the Disease (see also Chapter 15)

A. Possible Explanations for Cyclic Nature of Pandemics

Examination of antibodies in the sera of elderly people suggests that an influenza virus similar to the Hong Kong influenza virus occurred in man in earlier times and may have been the cause of the influenza pandemic at the end of the nineteenth century (see Section II). Low levels of antibodies to the hemagglutinins of equine-2 and Asian influenza viruses were also detected in the sera of elderly people. Antibodies to the neuraminidase of Hong Kong or Asian influenza viruses were not detected in the same antisera; while low levels of antibodies to equine-2 influenza virus neuraminidase were detected. This suggests that a virus having similar HA subunits and different NA subunits was responsible for the early and recent epidemics.

The epidemiological evidence has been interpreted to mean that the pandemic influenza viruses of man occur in cycles. The lack of evidence for the homologous neuraminidase makes it unlikely that the same Hong Kong influenza virus occurred at the end of the nineteenth century and again in 1968. It seems more likely that the influenza virus present at the end of the nineteenth century possessed a hemagglutinin subunit that bore some antigenic similarity to Hong Kong influenza virus but possessed a different neuraminidase antigen. From the serological evidence the neuraminidase could have been related antigenically to equine-2 neuraminidase. The recycling of influenza viruses may result from the emergence of viruses from an animal reservoir, either with or without a recombinational event, when herd immunity no longer precludes it from the human population.

Another phenomenon linked with the emergence of new strains of influenza is the apparent disappearance of the preceding strains. This may be due simply to the lack of interest in sampling for influenza viruses that are no longer a great public health hazard (Fenner, 1968), but this is an unlikely explanation, for experience has shown that human influenza viruses do not coexist in nature for any length of time. It is possible to explain the disappearance of strains that have arisen by antigenic drift in terms of self-annihilation; serological recapitulation would enhance earlier antibodies and prevent their spread. The disappearance of the senior strains (Fazekas de St. Groth, 1970) of each subtype after a major antigenic shift is more difficult to account for and no satisfactory explanation is available.

B. Possibilities of Control of Future Antigenic Variation in Influenza A Viruses

The biological, biochemical, and immunological evidence presented above only provides *circumstantial evidence* that major antigenic shifts in human influenza viruses occur by recombination. More definitive evidence would be obtained if recombination between different influenza viruses could be detected in nature leading to the appearance of a new pandemic strain. The rarity of this event virtually eliminates this possibility. An alternative approach to this problem is to isolate influenza viruses from animal and bird populations in advance of the occurrence of the next human pandemic strain; that is, to establish a bank of influenza viruses. After the appearance of the next human pandemic strain the virus could be compared with the viruses in the bank and evidence for its origin might be obtained. The wild animal and bird populations have largely been ignored as a source of new influenza viruses. The bird populations of the world have lived in high densities in their breeding colonies for much longer periods than animals or man.

It is of interest that eight different subtypes of avian influenza viruses have already been isolated; six of these are from domestic birds. This indicates that the logical place to start looking for influenza viruses in nature is in large bird colonies, particularly at the end of the nesting season. Such ecological studies might establish the number of different influenza virus subtypes that exist in nature and may eventually show how new strains originate. If there are a finite number of influenza A viruses, then in the future it may be possible to think in terms of control of the last remaining great plague of man.

Acknowledgments

This work was supported in part by U.S. Public Health Service Research Grant AI-08831 from the National Institute of Allergy and Infectious Diseases, General Research Grant RR-05584 from the National Institutes of Health, Childhood Cancer Research Center Grant CA-08480 from the National Cancer Institute, and The World Health Organization, and by ALSAC.

References

Ada, G. L., and Lind, P. E., and Laver, W. G. (1963). *J. Gen. Microbiol.* **32**, 225.
Andrewes, C. H. (1956). *Calif. Med.* **84**, 375.
Andrewes, C. H. (1957). *N. Engl. J. Med.* **242**, 197.
Andrewes, C. H. (1959). *In* "Perspectives in Virology" (M. Pollard, ed.), pp. 184–196. Wiley, New York.
Archetti, I., and Horsfall, F. L. (1950). *J. Exp. Med.* **92**, 441.
Becht, H., Hammerling, U., and Rott, R. (1971). *Virology* **46**, 337.
Brand, C. M., and Skehel, J. J. (1972). *Nature (London), New Biol.* **238**, 145.
Bucher, D. J., and Kilbourne, E. D. (1972). *J. Virol.* **10**, 60.
Burnet, F. M. (1955). "Principles of Animal Virology," 1st ed., p. 380. Academic Press, New York.
Burnet, F. M., and Clarke, E. (1942). "Influenza," Monogr. No. 4. Walter and Eliza Hall Inst., Melbourne.
Burnet, F. M., and Lind, P. E. (1949). *Aust. J. Sci.* **22**, 109.
Burnet, F. M., and Lind, P. E. (1951). *J. Gen. Microbiol.* **5**, 67.
Burnet, F. M., and White, D. O. (1972). "Natural History of Infectious Disease," 4th ed., pp. 202–212. Cambridge Univ. Press, London and New York.
Chakraverty, P. (1972a). *Bull. W.H.O.* **45**, 755.
Chakraverty, P. (1972b). *Bull. W.H.O.* **46**, 473.
Chu, C.-M. (1958). *J. Hyg., Epidemiol., Microbiol., Immunol.* **2**, 1.
Coleman, M. T., Dowdle, W. R., Pereira, H. G., Schild, G. C., and Chang, W. K. (1968). *Lancet* **2**, 1384.
Compans, R. W., Klenk, H. D., Caliguiri, L. A., and Choppin, P. W. (1970). *Virology* **42**, 880.

Creighton, C. (1891). "A History of Epidemics in Britain," Vol. 1. Cambridge Univ. Press, London and New York.

Creighton, C. (1894). "A History of Epidemics in Britain," Vol. 2. Cambridge Univ. Press, London and New York.

Curry, R. L., Brown, J. D., Baker, F. A., and Hobson, D. (1974). *J. Hyg.* **72,** 197.

Davenport, F. M., Hennessy, A. V., and Francis, T., Jr. (1953). *J. Exp. Med.* **98,** 641.

Davenport, F. M., Hennessy, A. V., Drescher, J., and Webster, R. G. (1964). *Cell. Biol. Myxovirus Infect., Ciba Found. Symp., 1964* pp. 272–287.

Dowdle, W. R., Downie, J. C., and Laver, W. G. (1974). *J. Virol.* **13,** 269.

Downie, J. C., and Laver, W. G. (1973). *Virology* **51,** 259.

Easterday, B. C., and Tumova, B. (1972). *Advan. Vet. Sci. Comp. Med.* **16,** 201.

Easterday, B. C., Laver, W. G., Pereira, H. G., and Schild, G. C. (1969). *J. Gen. Virol.* **5,** 83.

Edney, M. (1957). *J. Gen. Microbiol.* **17,** 25.

Fazekas de St. Groth, S. (1961). *Aust. J. Exp. Biol. Med. Sci.* **39,** 563.

Fazekas de St. Groth, S. (1962). *Advan. Virus Res.* **9,** 1.

Fazekas de St. Groth, S. (1963). *Ann. N.Y. Acad. Sci.* **103,** 674.

Fazekas de St. Groth, S. (1970). *Arch. Environ. Health* **21,** 293.

Fazekas de St. Groth, S., and Hannoun, C. (1973). *C.R. Acad. Sci., Ser. D* **276,** 1917.

Fazekas de St. Groth, S., and Webster, R. G. (1963). *J. Immunol.* **90,** 151.

Fazekas de St. Groth, S., and Webster, R. G. (1964). *Cell. Biol. Myxovirus Infect., Ciba Found. Symp., 1964* pp.246–271.

Fenner, F. (1968). *In* "Biology of Animal Viruses," Vol. 2, pp. 769–776. Academic Press, New York.

Francis, T., Jr. (1952). *Fed. Proc., Fed. Amer. Soc. Exp. Biol.* **11,** 808.

Francis, T., Jr. (1955). *Ann. Intern. Med.* **43,** 534.

Francis, T., Jr. (1960). *Proc. Amer. Phil. Soc.* **104,** 572.

Francis, T., Jr., and Maassab, H. F. (1965). *In* "Viral and Rickettsial Infections of Man" (F. L. Horsfall and I. Tamm, eds.), 4th ed., pp. 689–740. Lippincott, Philadelphia, Pennsylvania.

Gerber, P., Loosli, C. G., and Hamré, D. (1955). *J. Exp. Med.* **101,** 627.

Gerber, P., Hamré, D., and Loosli, C. G. (1956). *J. Exp. Med.* **103,** 413.

Hamré, D., Loosli, C. G., and Gerber, P. (1958). *J. Exp. Med.* **107,** 829.

Harboe, A. (1963a). *Acta Pathol. Microbiol. Scand.* **57,** 317.

Harboe, A. (1963b). *Acta Pathol. Microbiol. Scand.* **57,** 488.

Harboe, A., Borthne, B., and Berg, K. (1961). *Acta Pathol. Microbiol. Scand.* **53,** 95.

Hennessy, A. V., Minuse, E., and Davenport, F. M. (1965). *J. Immunol.* **94,** 301.

Hilleman, M. R. (1952). *Fed. Proc., Fed. Amer. Soc. Exp. Biol.* **11,** 879.

Hirsch, A. (1883). *In* "Handbook of Geographical and Historical Pathology," Vol. 1, p. 7. New Sydenham Society, London.

Hirst, G. K., and Gotlieb, T. (1953). *J. Exp. Med.* **98,** 53.

Hirst, G. K., and Gotlieb, T. (1955). *Virology* **1,** 221.

Howe, C., Lee, L. T., Harboe, A., and Haukenes, G. (1967). *J. Immunol.* **98,** 543.

Hoyle, L. (1968). *Virol. Monogr.* **4,** 1.

Isaacs, A., and Edney, M. (1950). *Brit. J. Exp. Pathol.* **31,** 209.

Jensen, K. E. (1957). *Advan. Virus Res.* **4,** 279.

Jensen, K. E., Davenport, F. M., Hennessy, A. V., and Francis, T., Jr. (1956). *J. Exp. Med.* **104,** 199.

Kaplan, M. M. (1969). *Bull. W.H.O.* **41,** 485.

Kaplan, M. M., and Payne, A. M. M. (1959). *Bull. W.H.O.* **20,** 465.

Kasel, J. A., Fulk, R. V., and Couch, R. B. (1969). *J. Immunol.* **102,** 530.

Kendal, A. P., and Kiley, M. P. (1973). *J. Virol.* **12,** 1482.

Kilbourne, E. D. (1960). *Ciba Found. Symp. Study Group* **4,** 1.

Kilbourne, E. D. (1968). *Science* **160,** 74.

Kilbourne, E. D. (1970). *Arch. Environ. Health* **21,** 286.

Kilbourne, E. D., and Murphy, J. S. (1960). *J. Exp. Med.* **111,** 387.

Kilbourne, E. D., and Schulman, J. L. (1965). *Trans. Ass. Amer. Physicians* **78,** 323.

Kilbourne, E. D., Lief, F. S., Schulman, J. L., Jahiel, R. I., and Laver, W. G. (1967). *Perspect. Virol.* **5,** 87.

Kilbourne, E. D., Laver, W. G., Schulman, J. L., and Webster, R. G. (1968). *J. Virol.* **2,** 281.

Kilbourne, E. D., Schulman, J. L., Schild, G. C., Schloer, G., Swanson, J., and Bucher, D. (1971). *J. Infec. Dis.* **124,** 449.

Klenk, H. D., Rott, R., and Becht, H. (1972). *Virology* **47,** 579.

Knight, C. A. (1944). *J. Exp. Med.* **80,** 83.

Knight, C. A. (1946). *J. Exp. Med.* **83,** 281.

Kundin, W. D. (1970). *Nature (London)* **228,** 857.

Lafferty, K. J., and Oertelis, S. (1963). *Virology* **21,** 91.

Laidlaw, P. P. (1935). *Lancet* **1,** 1118.

Laver, W. G. (1963). *Virology* **20,** 251.

Laver, W. G. (1964). *J. Mol. Biol.* **9,** 109.

Laver, W. G. (1971). *Virology* **45,** 275.

Laver, W. G. (1973). *Advan. Virus Res.* **18,** 57.

Laver, W. G., and Baker, N. (1972). *J. Gen. Virol.* **17,** 61.

Laver, W. G., and Kilbourne, E. D. (1966). *Virology* **30,** 493.

Laver, W. G., and Valentine, R. C. (1969). *Virology* **38,** 105.

Laver, W. G., and Webster, R. G. (1966). *Virology* **30,** 104.

Laver, W. G., and Webster, R. G. (1968). *Virology* **34,** 193.

Laver, W. G., and Webster, R. G. (1972). *Virology* **48,** 445.

Laver, W. G., and Webster, R. G. (1973). *Virology* **51,** 383.

Laver, W. G., Downie, J. C., and Webster, R. G. (1974). *Virology* **59,** 230.

Lazarowitz, S. G., Compans, R. W., and Choppin, P. W. (1971). *Virology* **46,** 830.

Lazarowitz, S. G., Compans, R. W., and Choppin, P. W. (1973). *Virology* **52,** 199.

Lazdins, I., Haslam, E. A., and White, D. O. (1972). *Virology* **49,** 758.

Ledinko, N. (1955). *J. Immunol.* **74,** 380.

McCahon, D., and Schild, G. C. (1971). *J. Gen. Virol.* **12,** 207.

McQueen, J. L., Steele, J. H., and Robinson, R. Q. (1968). *Advan. Vet. Sci.* **12,** 285.

Magill, T. (1955). *J. Exp. Med.* **102,** 279.

Magill, T. R., and Jotz, A. C. (1952). *J. Bacteriol.* **64,** 619.

Masurel, N. (1968). *Nature (London)* **218,** 100.

Meier-Ewert, H., Gibbs, A. J., and Dimmock, N. J. (1970). *J. Gen. Virol.* **6,** 409.

Molineux, I. (1695). *Phil. Trans.* **8**, 105ff.

Mulder, J., and Masurel, N. (1958). *Lancet* **1**, 810.

Noll, H., Aoyagi, T., and Orlando, J. (1962). *Virology* **18**, 154.

Palese, P., and Schulman, J. (1974). *Virology* **57**, 227.

Paniker, C. K. J. (1968). *J. Gen. Virol.* **2**, 385.

Pereira, H. G. (1969). *Progr. Med. Virol.* **11**, 46.

Pereira, H. G., Tumova, B., and Webster, R. G. (1967). *Nature (London)* **215**, 982.

Pereira, H. G., Takimoto, S., Piegas, N. S., and Ribeiro do Valle, L. A. (1972). *Bull. W.H.O.* **47**, 465.

Perry, B. T., and Burnet, F. M. (1953). *Aust. J. Exp. Biol. Med.* **31**, 519.

Perry, B. T., van den Ende, M., and Burnet, F. M. (1954). *Aust. J. Exp. Biol. Med.* **32**, 469.

Rasmussen, A. F. (1964). *In* "Newcastle Disease Virus" (R. P. Hanson, ed.), pp. 313–325. Univ. of Wisconsin Press, Madison.

Schild, G. C. (1970). *J. Gen. Virol.* **9**, 191.

Schild, G. C., and Newman, R. W. (1969). *Bull. W.H.O.* **41**, 437.

Schild, G. C., Henry-Aymard, M., Pereira, M. S., Chakraverty, P., Dowdle, W., Coleman, M., and Chang, W. K. (1973). *Bull. W.H.O.* **48**, 269.

Schulman, J. L., and Kilbourne, E. D. (1969). *Proc. Nat. Acad. Sci. U.S.* **63**, 326.

Schulman, J. L., Khakpour, M., and Kilbourne, E. D. (1968). *J. Virol.* **2**, 778.

Schulze, I. T. (1970). *Virology* **42**, 890.

Schulze, I. T. (1973). *Advan. Virus Res.* **18**, 1.

Seto, J. T., and Rott, R. (1966). *Virology* **30**, 731.

Seto, J. T., Drzeniek, R., and Rott, R. (1966). *Biochim. Biophys. Acta* **113**, 402.

Shope, R. E. (1936). *J. Exp. Med.* **63**, 669.

Simpson, R. W. (1964). *Cell. Biol. Myxovirus Infec., Ciba Found. Symp., 1964* pp. 187–206.

Simpson, R. W., and Hirst, G. K. (1961). *Virology* **15**, 436.

Skehel, J. J. (1971). *Virology* **44**, 409.

Skehel, J. J. (1972). *Virology* **49**, 23.

Skehel, J. J., and Schild, G. C. (1971). *Virology* **44**, 396.

Skehel, J. J., and Waterfield, M. D. (1975). *Proc. Nat. Acad. Sci. U.S.* **72**, 93.

Smith, W., Belyavin, G., and Sheffield, F. W. (1955). *Proc. Roy. Soc., Ser. B* **143**, 504.

Stanley, P., and Haslam, E. A. (1971). *Virology* **46**, 764.

Sugiura, A., and Kilbourne, E. D. (1966). *Virology* **29**, 84.

Takatsy, G., and Furesz, J. (1957). *Arch. Gesamte Virusforsch.* **4**, 344.

Tiffany, J. M., and Blough, H. A. (1970). *Virology* **41**, 392.

Tobita, K., and Kilbourne, E. D. (1974). *J. Virol.* **13**, 347.

Tumova, B., and Easterday, B. C. (1969). *Bull. W.H.O.* **41**, 429.

Tumova, B., and Pereira, H. G. (1965). *Virology* **27**, 253.

Webster, R. G. (1970a). *Virology* **40**, 643.

Webster, R. G. (1970b). *Virology* **42**, 633.

Webster, R. G. (1972). *Curr. Top. Microbiol. Immunol.* **59**, 75.

Webster, R. G., and Campbell, C. H. (1974). *Virology* **62**, 404.

Webster, R. G., and Darlington, R. W. (1969). *J. Virol.* **4**, 182.

Webster, R. G., and Laver, W. G. (1967). *J. Immunol.* **99**, 49.

Webster, R. G., and Laver, W. G. (1971). *Progr. Med. Virol.* **13**, 271.

Webster, R. G., and Laver, W. G. (1972). *Virology* **48**, 433.

Webster, R. G., and Pereira, H. G. (1968). *J. Gen. Virol.* **3**, 201.

Webster, R. G., Laver, W. G., and Kilbourne, E. D. (1968). *J. Gen. Virol.* **3**, 315.

Webster, R. G., Campbell, C. H., and Granoff, A. (1971). *Virology* **44**, 317.

Webster, R. G., Campbell, C. H., and Granoff, A. (1973). *Virology* **51**, 149.

World Health Organization. (1971). *Bull. W.H.O.* **45**, 119.

World Health Organization. (1972). *Bull. W.H.O.* **47**, 439.

Wrigley, N. G., Skehel, J. J., Charlwood, P. A., and Brand, C. M. (1973). *Virology* **51**, 525.

Zakstelskaja, L. J., Evstigneeva, N. A., Isachenko, V. A., Shenderovitch, S. P., and Efimova, V. A. (1969). *Amer. J. Epidemiol.* **90**, 400.

Zhdanov, V. M., Solovyev, V. D., and Epshtein, F. G. (1958). *Moscow Med.*

Zhezmer, V. Yu. (1973). *Vopr. Virusol.* **1**, 91.

11

Influenza Virus Characterization and Diagnostic Serology

G. C. Schild and W. R. Dowdle

I. Introduction

A. Unique Characteristics of Influenza as an Epidemiologic Problem and the Need for Influenza Surveillance

Antigenic variation is one of the most striking features of the influenza virus. It is thus hardly surprising that the study of this phenomenon has received considerable attention from the standpoint of its epidemiological implications and of the genetic and chemical properties of the virus. The different degrees to which influenza viruses of types A, B, and C undergo antigenic variation and the characteristic epidemiological behavior associated with these viruses have been described fully elsewhere (see Chapter 10). Only brief mention of the epidemiological behavior of human influenza viruses is required here to emphasise its major aspects. Pandemics of human influenza virus type A occur at irregular and infrequent intervals and are associated with major antigenic changes in the surface antigens of the virus, "antigenic shift." Between pandemics, outbreaks of lesser severity occur, and during this interpandemic period frequent minor, but progressive, changes termed "antigenic drift" in the surface antigens occur. In contrast, influenza virus type B is associated with restricted outbreaks of disease and undergoes only antigenic drift. It is characteristic that the appearance of a new variant of influenza virus type A or B in the population is followed by the rapid disappearance from the population of the formerly prevalent virus. The influenza virus thus presents epidemiological problems which are unique in terms of the pandemic nature of the disease, its unpredictability, and the constantly changing antigenic character of the infectious agent. In addition, it is becoming apparent that close epidemiological relationships exist between certain human influenza virus type A strains and human influenza, and it is well established that lower animals and birds form a reservoir of several different antigenic subtypes of influenza A viruses. Given these features it is clear that an understanding of the epidemiological behavior of influenza can only be achieved by intensive and continued international surveillance. Included in such surveillance is the identification of the antigenic characteristics of influenza viruses currently prevalent in human and nonhuman hosts; serological surveillance to reveal the degree of exposure to past and current influenza variants in human (and animal) populations; the probable level of immunity in the population, particularly in relationship to newly emerged variants; and the use of diagnostic serology. Besides its importance to epidemiological considerations, influenza surveillance is also of practical importance in attempts to control influenza. Immunoprophylaxis against influenza is practiced in several countries. To be effective influenza vaccines must contain virus strains that are antigenically identical, or closely related to currently prevalent strains. Surveillance is thus of practical importance in this respect, providing early evidence of the emergence of new variants of influenza type A or B virus and the identification of potentially susceptible populations. The laboratory methodology applicable to these problems is reviewed in this chapter.

B. WHO Influenza Surveillance Activities

In recognition of the worldwide epidemiological impact of influenza, the World Health Organization as long ago as 1947 initiated an international network of laboratories to effect influenza surveillance and established an Influenza Program. The surveillance activities were initially based on the establishment of an international influenza center in London together with a small number of centers in other countries. This program has now grown considerably in its range of activities and effectiveness and now includes 93 national influenza centers and over 70 additional collaborating laboratories in 61 different countries with two WHO international collaborating and reference centers situated in Atlanta and London.

The aims of the WHO program are severalfold. (1) To provide a system for the early detection and isolation of new antigenic variants of influenza virue and when appropriate provide warnings of probable future epidemic or pandemic activity based on the emergence of new antigenic varieties of virus. Recommendations on the composition of influenza vaccines also arise from these studies, and appropriate vaccine strains are distributed to influenza vaccine manufacturing agencies in several countries. (2) To document on a global basis the epidemic behavior and antigenic nature of prevalent virus strains. These studies involve both characterization of strains and sero-epidemiological surveys. Such investigations are essential to an improved knowledge of the ecology and natural history of influenza and of the origin of pandemic disease. (3) To provide reference reagents which are annually distributed to collaborating laboratories to facilitate the identification of virus isolates and provide reference standards between laboratories. (4) To encourage and coordinate studies on the ecology of influenza viruses in lower animals and birds as well as studies on the antigenic, biological, and genetic comparisons of human and animal influenza viruses. These investigations may be relevant to the origins of new human pandemic strains of influenza.

II. Summary of the Antigenic Components of Influenza Viruses

The antigenic composition of the influenza virus is among the best understood of the animal viruses so far investigated. Nevertheless our knowledge remains far from complete. The virus particle contains at least four virus-coded antigens. The two envelope proteins HA and NA take the form of spikes covering the virus surface attached by one end at the lipid membrane. Both the HA and NA are antigenically variable, and it is on the basis of the characterization of these two antigens that influenza viruses are divided into subtypes and variants (World Health Organization, 1971). Internally the particle contains several other components of which the two major ones are the NP which is closely associated with the RNA genome and the matrix (M) protein which underlies the lipid membrane and may form a matrix surrounding the NP–RNA complex. The antigenic nature of the HA, NA, NP (reviewed by Pereira, 1969; see also Chapter 10), and M (Schild, 1972) components of the virus is well established. The NP and M antigens are antigenically stable and type specific, providing the basis for the antigenic characterization of influenza viruses into types A, B (and C). The polypeptide composition of the influenza virus particle has been established by polyacrylamide gel electrophoresis and is described elsewhere (see Chapter 2). Seven polypeptides of molecular weights ranging from 25,000 to 94,000 daltons have been identified in the virus particle. Table 11.1 summarizes the estab-

Table 11.1 Polypeptide Composition and Antigens of the Influenza Virus[a]

Designation of polypeptide	Molecular weight of polypeptide	Approximate number of molecules per virus particle	Assignment to structural and antigenic properties of virus
P_1	94,000	<50	Minor internal proteins of the virus
P_2	81,000	<50	unknown antigenicity and function
NA	60,000	approx. 200	Envelope glycoprotein, neuraminidase antigen, antigenically variable
NP	53,000	approx. 1000	Internal protein, ribonucleoprotein antigen, antigenically stable, associated with RNA
HA_1	58,000	approx. 1000	Envelope glycoproteins, components of hemagglutinin antigen, heavy (HA_1) and light (HA_2) chains linked by disulfide bonds, antigenically variable
HA_2	28,000	approx. 1000	
M	25,000	approx. 3000	Internal protein, matrix protein antigen; antigenically stable; situated beneath lipid membrane of virus

[a] The values stated were determined for A/Hong Kong/1/68(H3N2) virus, X31 strain (Skehel and Schild, 1971). HA1 and HA2 are synthesized as a single polypeptide which is later cleaved to HA1 and HA2 in egg grown virus (see also Tables 2.1 and 2.2, Chapter 2).

lished relationships between these four antigenic components of the virus and the various species of structural polypeptides present in the virus particle.

Although, in general, little is known of the number, position, and chemical configuration of specific antigenic determinants of the various structural antigens of the influenza virus, recent studies (Laver *et al.,* 1974; Virelizier *et al.,* 1974) of the HA have clearly demonstrated that this antigen contains at least two groups of determinants, one of which changes antigenically during antigenic drift while other determinants are common for members of a given HA subtype.

The internal components P_1 and P_2 are present in small amounts in the virion and at present their antigenic characteristics are unknown.

In addition to the structural components of the virus, it is known (Skehel, 1973) that at least two other virus-coded products are synthesized in influenza-infected cells. The antigenic characteristics of these components have not been established, but it is possible that the nucleolar antigen identified by Dimmock (1969) in influenza-infected cells may relate to one of these polypeptides.

The properties of the antibodies directed against the major antigenic components of the influenza virus are discussed below, as are the methods employed in the antigenic characterization of influenza virus isolates. It is self-evident that a comprehensive view of the immune response to influenza must include assays of antibody to each of HA, NA, NP and M.

III. Methods of Antibody Assay

A. General Considerations

The methods available for the detection and assay of antibody to influenza virus antigens may be considered under two headings, namely, those which are multicomponent systems and those which are based on two component systems. Amongst the multicomponent methods are several which have been used routinely for many years, including virus neutralization tests, hemagglutination inhibition (HI), complement fixation (CF), and the more recently adopted neuraminidase inhibition (NI) test. Essentially multicomponent systems depend on testing serial dilutions of test sera with known doses of virus or viral antigen and employing an appropriate indicator system to measure the degree of reaction of antigen with specific antibody, i.e., susceptible host cells for virus neutralization, erythrocytes for HI, fetuin substrate for NI, and hemolysin-sensitized erythrocytes for CF tests. In some cases the system is made even more complex by the use of antibody to immunoglobulin either to enhance or to inhibit the primary antigen–antibody reaction. The advantage of these tests is that they may often be performed with rather low concentrations of crude virus antigen (e.g., infected allantoic fluids or crude antigen extracts). Their disadvantage is that in general they are tedious and time consuming to perform, and some of them are subject to nonspecific factors present in sera or lack specificity for antibody to particular antigens. These features will be discussed in detail below. More recently several two component systems have been adopted for routine use. These are immuno double diffusion (IDD) and single radial diffusion (SRD) techniques. These methods have the slight disadvantage of requiring the high concentrations of pure or semipurified antigens, but their advantage is that they are simple and rapid to perform, they are not subject to nonspecific factors in serum and can be made specific for particular virus antigens.

B. Antibody to the Hemagglutinin

1. NEUTRALIZATION

There are two basic immune mechanisms for inhibition of influenza virus replication. In the first, "true" or preincubation neutralization, the presence of antibody before virus inoculation prevents virus penetration of susceptible cells and thereby prevents replication. Only antibody to hemagglutinin is effective under these conditions. In the second mechanism, "apparent" or postincubation neutralization, the presence of antibody after virus penetration prevents release and spread of the newly emerging virus and thereby prevents *further* replication. Antibody to both hemagglutinin and neuraminidase are effective under these conditions. Apparent neutralization may result when virus–serum mixtures are added to susceptible cells and excess antiserum is not removed. Since hemagglutinin antibody causes preinoculation neutralization, any excess antibody remaining in the medium is probably of little consequence. However, the presence of excess neuraminidase antibody may cause apparent neutralization and lead to incorrect interpretations of hemagglutinin antigenic relationships.

The basic principles of the neutralization test for assay of hemagglutinin antibodies have been extensively reviewed (Lafferty, 1963; Fazekas de St. Groth and Webster, 1964). The neutralization tests most frequently used are those which require constant virus dosage and varying serum dilutions. Tests are usually conducted in mice, embryonated eggs, allantois on shell, or cell cultural monolayers. None of these systems are without disadvantages.

The mouse test requires the use of virus strains adapted through multiple passages to grow in mouse lungs and cause death (Eddy, 1947) or visible lesions (Schulman *et al.*, 1968). Protection of the immunized mouse is not an exclusive property of hemagglutinin antibodies. Antibodies to neuraminidase may protect equally as well. Thus, neutralization tests in mice must be performed under conditions where neuraminidase antibody is excluded (Schulman *et al.*, 1968). The inoculation of mice with serum–virus mixtures is probably more specific for hemagglutinin antibody (Kaye *et al.*, 1969), but even here the influence of residual neuraminidase antibody cannot be completely excluded. Neutralization tests in mice may also be performed with non-mouse-adapted strains by sacrificing the animals several days after inoculation and titrating the lungs in a susceptible system, such as eggs or tissue culture, for the presence of virus (Kilbourne and Horsfall, 1951).

In spite of its apparent simplicity, the neutralization test performed by inoculation of virus–serum mixtures into the allantoic cavity of the embryonated egg is fraught with problems. Test results may vary widely, depending upon the susceptibility of the egg to the virus strain and the susceptibility of the strain to nonspecific inhibitors. Because of the problems of the reproducibility, multiple replicates are required. The cost of materials and labor for a single neutralization test makes large cross-neutralization studies impractical.

In an effort to avoid the problems inherent in using the intact egg in the neutralization test, Fazekas de St. Groth and White (1958) devised a method for performing neutralization tests with bits of allantois on shell from embryonated eggs. The test is performed by adding small egg bits to wells in plastic trays containing a synthetic medium. Eighty or more bits may be obtained from a single egg. The test is simple, economic, and rapid; it is usually complete in 48 hours. With the large number of bits from a single egg, host variation within tests is reduced to a minimum. However, variation between tests is substantially affected by virus susceptibility of bits prepared from different eggs. This test is particularly sensitive for antibody to neuraminidase (Webster, 1970). Excess serum must be removed by washing the bits after virus adsorption. Influenza B strains grow poorly or not at all in this system.

The conventional neutralization test in monkey kidney cell culture offers a high degree of sensitivity and reproducibility. Host variation presents little problem, and most influenza A and B strains will multiply in this tissue without adaptation. The use of hemadsorption for assay of replicating virus makes this a sensitive test procedure (Shelokov *et al.*, 1958; Pereira, 1958; Johnson and Grayson, 1961). Because of the low virus dosage (32 to 300 $TCID_{50}$), it is highly sensitive to serum inhibitors. Pretreating sera to destroy nonspecific inhibitors of hemagglutination is recommended (Weinberger *et al.*, 1965). Likewise, the test is affected by the presence of antibody to neuraminidase (Dowdle *et al.*, 1974). Excess serum must be removed by washing cell monolayers after a suitable adsorption period (Kasel *et al.*, 1973).

2. HEMAGGLUTINATION INHIBITION (HI)

With the discovery by Hirst (1941) and McClelland and Hare (1941) that allantoic fluid from infected hen's eggs would agglutinate red blood cells, the HI test became the most widely used method for influenza antibody assay. There were several reasons for its popularity. First, the test was simple, requiring only erythrocytes and infected allantoic fluid. Second, the results of the test were shown to parallel those of the theoretically more desirable, but far more complex, neutralization test (Hirst, 1942).

Inhibition of hemagglutination(HA) is caused by attachment of antibody to the virus hemagglutinin. The antibody acts either to block hemagglutinin sites which are essential for adsorption to erythrocytes or to remove the virus from suspension through formation of virus–antibody aggregates. The antigenic site on the hemagglutinin molecule has not been located but may not be identical with the locus of attachment to the erythrocyte surface. Under the conditions of the standard HI test, which uses relatively dilute suspensions of virus (10^7–10^8 particles per 4 HA units), the contribution of the virus–antibody aggregates is probably negligible. Only those antibodies directed against the tips of the spikes are thought to be involved in inhibition, since the narrow spacing (7–8 nm) between the virion surface spikes very likely restricts penetration of the larger antibody molecule. The actual number of antigenic sites is not known.

The HI test in current use is basically that described by Hirst (1942) and later modified by Salk (1944). In its simplest form the antigen consists of supernatant fluids from infected tissue culture or extraembryonic fluids from infected eggs. The hemagglutinin content is determined first by testing serial twofold dilutions of infected fluid with a standard suspension of chicken, human, or guinea pig erythrocytes. The highest dilution of virus causing agglutination of erythrocytes is defined as 1 HA unit. Virus suspensions are adjusted to contain 4 HA units. This suspension is added to equal volumes of twofold serial dilutions of sera which have been treated to destroy nonspecific inhibitors. Equal volumes of the standardized suspension of erythrocytes are added. The test is read for inhibition of hemagglutination. The HI titer is defined as the highest dilution of serum which completely inhibits hemagglutination. Detailed procedures for the HI test are described elsewhere (Dowdle and Coleman, 1974; World Health Organization, 1959). The HA and HI test for influenza types A and B may be performed at room temperature. Tests with type C must be performed in the cold.

The HI test, like the HA test, can be performed with a variety of erythrocyte species over a wide range of pH values. The temperature is not critical for either test, except with influenza type C. Within limits, the HI titer of serum is inversely proportional to the amount of virus used in the test; that is, any variation in virus dosage results in approximately the same degree of change of serum titer (Hirst, 1942).

The test is highly reproducible. Hierholzer et al. (1969), using spectrophotometrically standardized cell suspensions, four units of virus, and treated antisera, determined day to day and within-run reproducibility with coded serum pairs. For all myxoviruses they found the reproducibility to be 80 to 90% for the exact titer and 100% for titers differing no more than one dilution. On an even larger scale, the microtiter HI test was evaluated in the WHO International Influenza Center, Atlanta, with 341 coded serum pairs and 6 diffterent antigens in 9 daily tests. Reproducibility for titers differing by no more than one dilution was 95% (World Health Organization, unpublished results). For most purposes this is a reasonably high degree of reproducibility.

Hahon et al. (1972) reported that by incorporating species-specific anti-immunoglobulin G (IgG) serum into the HI test influenza titers could be markedly increased, often as much as 32-fold. This phenomenon has also been observed for the assay of neuraminidase antibody by the hemagglutination inhibition test (Kendal et al., 1972; Holston and Dowdle, 1973; Dowdle et al., 1973). Because of this the specificity of the enhancement reported by Hahon et al. must remain in question. All tests were undertaken with wild-type viruses containing contemporary hemagglutinin and neuraminidase antigens. The possible role of neuraminidase antibody in the observed enhancement was not taken into consideration.

In spite of the many admirable characteristics of the HI test it has not been entirely satisfactory. Instances of disagreement between neutralization and HI test results and in HI results between laboratories and in the same laboratory are legion. The most common sources for disparity in results are (a) inadequate destruction of nonspecific inhibitors, (b) interference by anti-neuraminidase, (c) interference by anti-host antibodies, (d) variability among reference strains, (e) variability among erythrocytes, and, finally, (f) the simple mechanics of reading the test.

a. Nonspecific Inhibitors. Hemagglutination by influenza viruses may be inhibited by normal components of sera and body fluids from a wide variety of animals. Early attempts to classify these substances divided them into two groups: The Francis or α inhibitor (Francis, 1947), and the Chu or β inhibitor (Chu, 1951). A third group, the γ inhibitors, was described by Shimojo et al. (1958). The γ inhibitors were found largely in horse and guinea pig sera and were effective almost exclusively against the then newly emerged Asian (H2N2) viruses.

Attempts to further classify these three inhibitors according to their effects on type A and type B viruses led to conflicting results and confusion. In retrospect, the reasons for the confusion can be understood. Some sera may contain all three types of inhibitors (Shortridge and Lansdell, 1972), and the test viruses may consist of a population of inhibitor-sensitive particles and inhibitor-insensitive particles in varying proportions (Choppin and Tamm, 1960).

The major distinguishing characteristics generally accepted for the three groups of inhibitors and the virus types and subtypes affected are shown in Table 11.2.

Despite the different inhibitory effects on different virus strains, the nonspecific inhibitors in sera all appear to be glycoproteins and all seem to occur in the $\alpha2$-macroglobulin fraction as 18 S and 12 S components (Pepper, 1968; Shortridge and Lansdell, 1972). These findings suggest that the inhibitor-active prosthetic groups are probably carried on physically similar molecules. Additional evidence for this comes from findings that antisera prepared against active horse or human $\alpha2$-macroglobulin inhibitors cross-react with each other and with the $\alpha2$-macroglobulin in calf sera (Biddle and Shortridge, 1967).

The major differences between the α and γ inhibitors are that the γ inhibitor affects only the H2N2 and H3N2 virus strains and are generally insensitive to neuraminidase. The α inhibitor has a very broad spectrum of activity, but is highly sensitive to neuraminidase. Since both contain neuraminic acid, the difference between the two inhibitors may stem from differences in mo-

Table 11.2 Characteristics of Nonspecific Inhibitors of Influenza Virus Hemagglutination

Inhibitor type	Subtypes inhibited	Inactivation			Neutrali- zation
		Periodate	Neuramini- dase	Trypsin	
α	B, H0N1, H1N1, H2N2, H3N2,	+	+	$\pm$	−
β	H0N1, H1N1, H3N2 (late H2N2)	−	+	+	+
γ	H2N2, H3N2	+	−	+	+

lecular configuration which determines the accessibility of the virus enzyme to the substrate. A second possibility is that the differences between the two inhibitors are determined by the nature of the linkage of neuraminic acid to the adjacent sugar or the sugar itself (Cohen *et al.,* 1963).

Although much has been learned of inhibitor characteristics, the significance of the spectrum of inhibitor sensitivity exhibited by various influenza virus strains is little understood. Choppin and Tamm (1960) found that the inhibitor-sensitive and inhibitor-insensitive clones from the 1957 H2N2 strain were antigenically and morphologically identical. The only detectable difference between the two was that the inhibitor-insensitive particles failed to combine with the γ inhibitors in horse serum, whereas the inhibitor-sensitive particles combined with horse serum inhibitors with extraordinary firmness. The apparent change in sensitivity to nonspecific inhibitors with the H2N2 as well as with other strains seems to be primarily an alteration in binding efficiency with different neuraminic acid configurations.

In the diagnostic laboratory, variation in sensitivity to nonspecific inhibitors presents a practical problem in the identification of new isolates by the HI test. Patterns of nonspecific inhibition frequently vary with strains of a given subtype, presumably because most isolates are uncloned and represent varying mixtures of inhibitor-sensitive and inhibitor-insensitive particles. The two most commonly used procedures for removing the inhibitors from sera are potassium periodate (World Health Organization, 1959) and the receptor-destroying enzyme (RDE) described by Burnet and Stone (1947). Most RDE preparations consist of crude filtrates which may contain proteolytic enzymes in addition to neuraminidase. These contaminating enzymes in many instances may account for the broader effect of this preparation in comparison with purified neuraminidase. With some sera, particularly guinea pig sera, the only wholly effective treatment for removal of inhibitors is kaolin (Coleman and Dowdle, 1969). Since kaolin also removes immunoglobulins which may contain specific antibodies, it should not be used when other methods of removing inhibitors are effective. The effects of various treatment for removal of inhibitors for A/Hong Kong (H3N2) strains are shown in Table 11.3.

Other treatment procedures for destruction of nonspecific inhibitors have also been proposed, notably use of carbon dioxide and rivanol. The CO_2 procedure is not recommended because of variable results and frequent loss of specific antibody. Less is known of the mode of activity or effects of rivanol.

b. Anti-neuraminidase Antibody. Anti-neuraminidase antibody may inhibit hemagglutination, presumably through steric hindrance of the hemagglutinin (Schulman and Kilbourne, 1969). Inhibition by neuraminidase anti-

Table 11.3 A/Hong Kong/68 (H3N2) Hemagglutination Inhibitors in Normal Sera after Various Treatments[a]

Species	None	Heat	Trypsin	Periodate	Heat-Tryp.-Per.	RDE[c]	Kaolin
Monkey	—[b]	—	—	—	—	—	—
Goat	—	—	—	—	—	—	—
Chicken	—	+	—	—	—	—	—
Man	++	++	++	+	+	—	—
Ferret	++	++	+	—	—	+	—
Rabbit	++	++	+	++	+++	—	—
Guinea pig	+++	++++	++++	+++	+++	+++	—
Horse	++++	++++	++++	—	—	+++	++

[a] Adapted from Coleman and Dowdle (1969).
[b] HI titer range with chicken erythrocytes: —, <10; +, 11–20; ++, 21–80; +++, 81–320; ++++, ≥321.
[c] RDE, receptor-destroying enzyme.

body has been observed with the H2N2 and H3N2 strains, but it has not been demonstrated with the earlier A strains, H0N1 or H1N1 (W. R. Dowdle, unpublished results, 1973), or with influenza B strains (Tobita and Kilbourne, 1974). HI activity of anti-neuraminidase antisera may vary considerably with strains isolated since 1957 and may depend on the age and species of the erythrocyte, the animal, the method of serum treatment, and more importantly, the ratio of γ inhibitor-sensitive to γ inhibitor-insensitive particles (W. R. Dowdle, unpublished results). Only those strains which are sensitive to γ inhibitors are inhibited by anti-neuraminidase antibody.

Variation in hemagglutination inhibition by anti-neuraminidase antibody may be caused by variable synergistic effects of nondetectable levels of serum inhibitors. The addition of fetuin (W. R. Dowdle, unpublished results) or normal guinea pig sera (Kendal *et al.*, 1972) at concentrations too low to cause inhibition can enhance neuraminidase HI titers several hundredfold to several thousandfold. Under normal test conditions the levels of residual serum inhibitors may vary considerably. Where all nonspecific inhibitors have been destroyed neuraminidase HI occurs less frequently and at a much lower titer.

c. Anti-host Antibody. Hemagglutination of influenza viruses grown in the chick embryo may be inhibited by rabbit sera produced against antigens in normal chick allantoic fluid (Knight, 1944). This host antigen which is incorporated into the surface structures of both type A and type B strains was shown to be a carbohydrate (Haukenes *et al.*, 1965) with a molecular weight of the order of 15,000 (Laver and Webster, 1966). Host antigens have been demonstrated only with viruses grown in the allantoic sacs of chicken and turkey embryos (Harboe, 1963). They have not been demonstrated in viruses grown in duck embryos, mouse lungs, or a variety of cultured cells when they are used with antisera prepared against extracts of the normal host.

HI antibodies to host antigens have been shown to occur in sera from human recipients of egg-grown vaccine and in animals immunized with egg-grown virus. Host antibody is not normally found in chicken antisera, but it can be produced under certain conditions by prolonged immunization (Schoyen *et al.*, 1966). Viruses may vary both in their capacity to elicit egg host antibody upon immunization and in their sensitivity to host antibodies. Although antisera produced in ferrets immunized by infection with egg-grown viruses usually do not contain host antibodies, it is well to be aware that under certain conditions such antibodies may occur.

d. Reference Strains. The term "P-Q-R" coined by Van der Veen and Mulder (1950) has fallen into disuse during the past few years, probably because the term implies unnecessary compartmentalization, but it might be well to describe the phenomenon designated by the term here. Van der Veen and Mulder noted that in cross-hemagglutination inhibition tests, strains in an antigenic subgroup frequently show different patterns of inhibition with antibody. The P strains were inhibited to high titer with heterologous antisera. The Q strains gave low HI titers with both homologous and heterologous sera. The R strains were inhibited to high titers by both homologous and heterologous sera. The P-Q variation was said to be reversible, depending on the host (Isaacs *et al.*, 1952).

Choppin and Tamm (1960) suggested that variation in sensitivity to antibody might be due to the presence of two kinds of virus particles in varying proportions. They were able to isolate genetically stable substrains (+) which were highly sensitive to specific antibody and nonspecific inhibitors and substrains ("—") which had low sensitivity to specific antibody and nonspecific inhibitors. They suggested that the features of the surface structure of virus particles which determine antibody sensitivity may also determine sensitivity to specific inhibitors.

Recent experiences with influenza B/Hong Kong/5/72 has shown that at least one strain which had undergone 12 or more terminal dilution passages in chick embryos was threefold more sensitive than its parent to inhibition by antibody (unpublished results). The use of the most sensitive strains is essential for serologic surveys or vaccine studies.

e. Erythrocytes. Different HI test results have been reported with erythrocytes from different members of the same animal species. This is particularly true with chicken erythrocytes. Such variation may be avoided by preserving large batches of erythrocytes treated with glutaraldehyde (Bing *et al.*, 1967). However, the normal settling patterns of glutaraldehyde-treated cells are generally more difficult to read.

f. Reading.   Errors are very often made in interpreting erythrocyte settling patterns in low dilutions of serum. Frequently, high concentrations of protein will cause the cells to settle in a manner which suggests inhibition. This problem can be avoided if complete inhibition is judged by tilting the plates and observing whether the cells stream at the same rate as do the cell controls.

3. SINGLE RADIAL DIFFUSION (SRD)

The single radial immunodiffusion test provides a simple, two-component assay system for antibodies or antigens based on the principles first described by Mancini *et al.* (1965) of the direct visualization of the antibody–antigen reaction in a supporting matrix, usually an agar or agarose gel. One of the two reactants is incorporated uniformly throughout the matrix and the other reactant is introduced into discrete areas of the matrix from which it diffuses radially forming a visible disc of "precipitate" where the antigen and antibody have combined. Quantitation in this system is based on the existence of a direct relationship between the size of the disc of precipitate and the concentration of the diffusing reactant. In the application of the SRD test to the assay of antibody to viral antigens the appropriate antigen is distributed throughout the matrix and antisera for assay are added to wells in the matrix. This application of the test is thus the reverse of that described by Mancini *et al.* (1965) for the assay of immunoglobulin antigens.

The use of SRD tests to assay antibody to the surface antigens, HA and NA, of the influenza virus was described by Schild *et al.* (1972a). These workers found that SRD provided a simple, rapid, and accurate method for the assay of antibodies to influenza virus hemagglutinin and neuraminidase. The test is based on the incorporation of purified, intact influenza virus particles at a standard protein concentration (0.2 mg of viral protein per milliliter of gel) into an agarose gel. In practice a gel with a low setting temperature of 37°C (see Schild *et al.*, 1972a) is employed, since exposure of the viral antigen to temperatures much above 40°C may thus be avoided. With suitable antigen preparations addition of the influenza virus to the gel does not increase its opalescence once the gel has set although while a fluid, the suspensions are turbid. The gels are allowed to solidify in layers approximately 1.7 mm deep by adding 3 ml to microscope slides or more conveniently, to commercially available plastic chambers (e.g., Hyland immunoplates). Circular wells either 2.0 mm or 3.0 mm in diameter are cut in the gels to receive the test antiserum. Antisera for assay, 5 μl per 2.0 mm well or 10 μl per 3.0 mm well are transferred into the wells using calibrated micropipettes, and the SRD immunoplates are left in a moist chamber at room temperature for 16 hours to allow the antibody to diffuse from the wells and the immunological reaction to proceed. Zones normally reach maximum size within this time period. Under these conditions antibody to either of the two surface antigens, HA or NA, is capable of reacting with the intect virus particles giving zones which are opalescent when viewed with oblique illumination against a dark background. The zone diameter is measured with a micrometer eyepiece scale calibrated in 0.1 mm divisions and the zone annulus area is calculated. The zones are stable once formed and the plates may be soaked in phosphate-buffered saline for several days or weeks. Soaking the immunoplates intensifies the degree of opalescence of the zones and is thus recommended as a routine before reading the results. The influenza virus particles are unable to diffuse in agar or agarose gels (Schild and Pereira, 1969), and it appears that the reaction does not depend upon a precipitation phenomenon in the sense of the formation of immune aggregates, but rather on primary antigen–antibody binding. The zones of opalescence apparently result from an increase in the light scattering properties of the virus particles when coated with antibody molecules. However, physical basis of the mechanism involved has not been demonstrated. It is of interest that monovalent "half-molecules" of IgG prepared from anti-hemagglutinin serum react efficiently in SRD tests but fail to react in precipitin tests with hemagglutinin antigen (L. Haaheim and G. C. Schild, unpublished). This finding serves to confirm that the SRD reaction with intact influenza virus particles does not depend upon a precipitation. Figure 11.1 show the SRD reactions of anti-hemagglutinin and anti-neuraminidase sera in agarose gels and the dose–response curves for various dilutions of antiserum. A plot of zone annulus area (mm^2) against relative antibody concentration both on a linear scale is linear for both antiserum to hemagglutinin and neuraminidase. Thus, annulus area of the zone of opalescence may be taken as a direct measure of antibody concentration. A consistent finding is that the opalescent zones produced by antibody to HA are more intense (see Fig. 11.1) than those produced by anti-HA antibody. This probably reflects a higher density of HA subunits than of NA subunits on the virus surface; estimates from biochemical studies suggest that there are approximately 1000 hemagglutinin spikes and 200 neuraminidase spikes per virus particle (Skehel and Schild, 1971). In the antisera for assay antibody to both the hemagglutinin and neuraminidase of the test virus may be present and both antibodies will thus contribute to the SRD reaction. Where anti-hemagglutinin and anti-neuraminidase coexist, the zones produced by

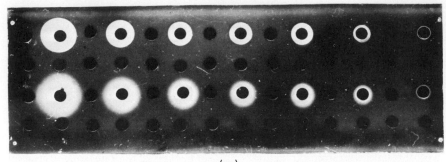

(a)

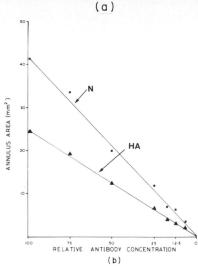

(b)

Fig. 11.1. (a) Shows the single radial diffusion reactions of anti-hemagglutinin and anti-neuraminidase sera in agarose gels containing A/Hong Kong/68 virus (0.2 mg virus protein per ml of agarose). Top: shows reactions of dilutions of anti-H3 rabbit serum. From left to right the wells contain sera diluted 1:1, 1:1.5, 1:2, 1:4, 1:8, and 1:16. Bottom: shows reactions of dilutions of anti-N2 rabbit serum. From left to right the wells contain sera diluted as for anti-H3 above. With serum dilution the intensity of the zones remains constant while their areas decrease. (b) shows typical single radial diffusion dose response plots antisera to hemagglutinin and neuraminidase HA, plot for anti-hemagglutinin serum. N, plot for anti-neuraminidase serum. Note that the dose response relationship differs from that of passive hemolysis tests (see Fig. 11.3).

each population of antibody overlap and are not additive. Thus the overall diameter of the zone reflects the concentration of the most abundant antibody, and the reaction cannot with certainty be attributed to either one of the antibodies. However, using appropriate recombinant (antigenic hydrid) influenza A viruses, antibody to hemagglutinin or neuraminidase may be assayed independently. Unfortunately this cannot be achieved for influenza B viruses because of the lack of distinct subtypes of hemagglutinin and neuraminidase antigens for B strains. Suitable test systems for the assay of antibody specific for the hemagglutinin and neuraminidase of the A/Hong Kong/1/68 (H3N2) virus are shown in Table 11.4 together with a summary of the applications of SRD to measure antibody to other influenza virus antigens. Using the recombination procedures described elsewhere in this book (see Chapter 10) recombinants appropriate for use in the assay of antibody to any influenza A hemagglutinin or neuraminidase subtype may be obtained.

Nonspecific inhibitors of the α and β type do not produce a reaction in the SRD test. Sera containing high levels of γ inhibitor, such as horse sera, may produce faint nonspecific zones due to this inhibitor. However, these are unstable and disappear after soaking the slides in saline for 24 hours. In contrast, zones produced by antibody are completely stable. It is thus not necessary to pretreat human or animal sera before testing. This has the advantage that sera may be tested undiluted thus increasing the sensitivity of the test.

Sera from a large range of species including man, ferret, rabbit, guinea pig, mouse, horse, and chicken containing antibodies to hemagglutinin have been found to perform satisfactorily in SRD tests. However, while postinfec-

Table 11.4 Single Radial Diffusion Systems for the Assay of Antibodies to Each of the Major Antigens of Influenza A/Hong Kong/1/68 (H3N2) Virus in Human Sera

Specificity of antibody to	Envelope antigens, intact virus[a]			Internal antigens disrupted virus Hav2Neq1[e]
	H3N2[b]	H3Neq1[c]	Heq1N2[d]	
Envelope proteins				
Anti-H3	+	+	−	−
Anti-N2	+	−	+	−
Internal proteins				
Anti-M	−	−	−	+[f]
Anti-NP	−	−	−	+[f]

[a] Treated with sodium sarcosyl sulfate.
[b] A/Hong Kong/1/68(H3N2) virus.
[c] Recombinant A/Hong Kong/1/68(H3)-equine/Prague/56(Neq1).
[d] Recombinant A/equine/Prague/56(Heq1)-Hong Kong/1/68(N2).
[e] A/chicken/Germany/N/49(Hav2Neq1).
[f] Antibody to internal NP (nucleoprotein) and M (matrix protein) can be clearly distinguished, since zones produced by the latter are of extremely high intensity.

tion sera present no problems of specificity, sera from animals hyperimmunized with chick embryo-grown influenza virus or with purified hemagglutinin may contain antibodies to chick "host" antigen, and such antibody may give opalescent zones in SRD tests which may give rise to misleading data. Antibody to "host" antigen may be completely removed by absorbing the sera with a heterotypic influenza virus, e.g., antisera to type A viruses are absorbed with a type B influenza virus suspension and vice versa, before testing (Schild et al., 1974b). This problem is also avoided by the use of anti-chicken antisera.

Although specific for antibody to distinct hemagglutinin (or neuraminidase) subtypes, the SRD test is broadly reactive within an HA (or NA) antigen subtype. It has been shown that antibody to each of the distinct groups of anigenic determinants of the hemagglutinin molecule is detectable by SRD (Virelizier et al., 1974) even though such antibodies may not always be readily detected by HI tests. The application of SRD to the independent assay of antibody to the distinct antigenic determinants of hemagglutinin was shown by Virelizier et al. to be of considerable value in studies of the immunological properties of hemagglutinin.

SRD tests for antibody assay employing purified virus may be rigidly standardized in terms of the antigen component by the use of highly purified virus of known protein concentration. For this purpose the degree of purity of the virus antigen may be established by polyacrylamide gel electrophoresis (Skehel and Schild, 1971). This approach may lead to a high degree of reproducibility in SRD tests performed in different laboratories and has led to the proposal of using SRD as a standard reference method for the assay of antibody to hemagglutinin and other viral antigens (Schild et al., 1974a). Statistical analyses of the performance of SRD tests for the assay of antibody to hemagglutinin and neuraminidase have been described elsewhere (Schild et al., 1973b) and indicate a high degree of accuracy and reproducibility. The test enables differences in antibody potency between samples as small as 35% to be detected with statistical significance on the basis of a single test for each sample. By performing two or more tests per sample differences of 20% or less may be resolved. In contrast, tests based on doubling dilution of test serum, for example HI tests, are able to discern difference of potency only if they are as great as two- to fourfold (i.e., 200–400%). Thus SRD is considerably more sensitive in detecting small changes in antibody levels.

In general the SRD test for the detection of antibody to hemagglutinin is marginally less sensitive than conventional HI tests, but sera with HI titers as low as 1 : 20 may give SRD reactions (Chakraverty et al., 1973; Mostow et al., 1975). However, SRD is more sensitive than H1 tests in detecting antibody rises (Mostow et al., 1975).

As described later in this chapter, SRD tests may be performed with disrupted influenza virus particles incorporated in gels. In such tests antibody to the internal, type-specific antigens of the virus, NP and M, produce opalescent zones. Since some preparations of influenza virus may undergo spontaneous degradation during their preparation or storage, it is necessary routinely to control immunoplates made with each batch of virus by testing on them antisera to NP and M. The presence of SRD reactions by these sera suggests the virus is degraded and that false positive reactions may thus be obtained. In practice this rarely occurs, and prepared immunoplates have been stored at 4°C for several months without harmful effects.

A further approach to the use of SRD for antibody assay is the incorporation in gels of purified hemagglutinin (or neuraminidase) antigens at standard concentration for the assay of their respective antibodies. It should be noted that with the use of soluble diffusible antigens the mechanism of the test is analogous to that described by Mancini *et al.* (1965) and dependent upon the formation of immune aggregates. Limited application of this approach in our laboratories has established its value as a research tool, but the method has been little exploited so far.

4. IMMUNO DOUBLE DIFFUSION (IDD)

A second example of a two-component serological technique for the detection of antibody to hemagglutinin, and other viral antigens, is the IDD test. The application of IDD techniques to the study of influenza antibodies was adopted only relatively recently. Styk and Hanna (1966) and Hanna and Hoyle (1966) found that precipitin lines corresponding to influenza NP antigen could be detected in conventional Ouchterlony double diffusion tests carried out in agar gels. Later these findings were extended to include the NA antigen (Schild and Pereira, 1969), the HA (Schild, 1970) and the M antigen (Schild, 1972). Figure 11.2 illustrates the production of precipitin lines corresponding to each of the four major antigenic components of the influenza virus. Since influenza virus particles are too large to diffuse in agar or agarose gels, precipitin tests must be performed using diffusible antigens isolated from virus particles of extracts of infected cells or by disrupting virus particles with appropriate detergents to release the diffusible antigen subunits. Among suitable detergents for this purpose are Nonidet P40, sodium dodecyl sulfate (Schild and Pereira, 1969), or sodium sarkosyl sulfate (Schild *et al.*, 1971). IDD techniques are of considerable value as qualitative tests for the identification of antibodies in test sera but are not readily adaptable to quantitative studies. In tests employing disrupted influ-

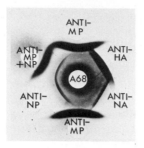

Fig. 11.2. Immuno double diffusion reactions of antisera to the four major antigenic components of the influenza virus. The center well (A68) contains purified A/Hong Kong/1/68(H3N2) (X31 strain) disrupted by the addition of sodium sarkosyl sulfate detergent to liberate diffusible antigenic components. Wells marked Anti-HA, Anti-NA, Anti-NP, and Anti-MP contain immune rabbit serum to the purified hemagglutinin and neuraminidase of A/Hong Kong/1/68 and to influenza A nucleoprotein and matrix protein antigens, respectively. When anti-NP and anti-MP are present together two precipitin lines form.

enza virus as antigen, test sera may give multiple precipitin lines. The identification of the specificity of the antibodies in such sera may be established by placing unknown antisera in peripheral wells in the agar gel with antisera to known antigenic components in adjacent wells. Continuity of the precipitin lines given by the unknown serum with reactions of known antisera enable the antibody to be identified. Thus, in a single test system, it is possible to obtain a rapid, qualitative estimate of the presence of antibody to each of the antigens of the influenza virus. Using other methods it would be necessary to apply several types of test to derive the same information.

IDD tests to detect antibody to purified hemagglutinin (or neuraminidase) antigens are subtype specific and specific for all members within a given subtype but not with different subtypes (Schild, 1970; Schild and Newman, 1969).

For the assay of antibody to hemagglutinin, IDD is considerably less sensitive than conventional HI tests or SRD tests. In general, precipitin reaction are given only with sera with HI titers of several hundred and SRD reactions of 5–7 mm^2 or greater (G. C. Schild, unpublished).

One disadvantage of IDD tests is that moderately high concentrations of antigens are required to obtain clearly defined precipitin lines. When disrupted virus particles are used as antigen, a concentration of virus of at least 1 mg per mg of viral protein is required and preferably higher concentrations. With purified antigens concentrations of at least 0.2 mg/ml are desirable.

IDD tests have been applied to a variety of purposes including seroepidemiological surveys and serodiagnosis of influenza and is studies of anti-genic variation. These applications will be described later in this chapter.

5. Complement Fixation (CF)

The CF test for the assay of antibodies to influenza surface antigens (Lief and Henle, 1959) has been preferred by many investigators because it is not affected by nonspecific inhibitors which beset the HI test. CF test results usually parallel those obtained by HI, but may exhibit a higher degree of strain specificity. Previous studies with this test have been performed without distinction between antibodies to the HA or NA antigens, since the antisera employed contained antibody to both these components and both antigens when reacting with appropriate antibodies. However, antibodies to the surface antigens may be assayed independently by the use of recombinants possessing genetically segregated antigens or by using purified antigen. The CF test is not suitable for assay for all animal sera because of high anti-complementary activity. Avian sera do not fix complement. The passive hemolysis (single radial hemolysis) technique described in Section III,B,6 is an adaptation of the complement fixation reaction to assay antibody to hemagglutinin.

6. Passive Hemolysis, Single Radial Hemolysis (SRH), for the Assay of Antibody to Hemagglutinin

More recently an assay system for antibody to hemagglutinin based on passive hemolysis of erythrocytes which have been "sensitized" by the addition of influenza virus particles or purified hemagglutinin has been described (Schild *et al.*, 1974c). The sensitized erythrocytes are lysed at 37°C in the presence of antibody to hemagglutinin and complement. For convenience the technique has been adapted for use as a single radial hemolysis (SRH) method in agarose gels using the following procedures. Ten percent suspensions of chicken erythrocytes in saline are treated with influenza virus using at least 300 HA units of virus per 1.0 ml of erythrocytes. This may be in the form of purified virus or crude allantoic fluids. In the latter case control erythrocytes are treated with uninfected allantoic fluid. After allowing time for virus to adsorb, the erythrocytes are thoroughly washed to remove unadsorbed antigen. The test may also be performed using purified HA preparations provided the purified antigen is capable of attaching to the erythrocyte surface. However, this approach has not been fully investigated.

SRH immunoplates are prepared by incorporating 0.3 ml of virus treated erythrocytes and 0.1 ml undiluted guinea pig complement in 2.6 ml of agarose at 42°C. The final concentration of erythrocytes in the gel is 2%

and that of complement 1:30. The suspension is then shaken to distribute evenly the erythrocytes and poured onto microscope slides or Hyland plastic immunoplates. Two mm diameter wells are cut in the gel for the acceptance of 5 μl volumes of test sera. Sera are heated at 56°C for 30 minutes before testing. Zones of complete or partial hemolysis are measured after incubating the plate at 37°C for 16 hours. The diameter of the zones are measured as for SRD tests. Sera are also tested on control plates containing normal cells or cells treated with uninfected allantoic fluids and the results given by sera producing lysis in control plates are discounted. In some cases such nonspecific hemolysis may be eliminated by adsorption of sera with chick erythrocytes or by further heating at 56°C.

Figure 11.3a shows the hemolysis reactions of a series of dilutions of antisera containing antibody to hemagglutinin in gel containing chicken erythrocytes sensitized with A/Port Chalmers/1/73 virus. The sizes of the zones of hemolysis decrease regularly with serum dilution. A plot of log zone diameter against log serum dilution approximates to linearity (Fig. 11.3b) and parallel plots are given by sera of different potencies. Undiluted sera with titers of 1:5120 in conventional HI tests give zones of hemolysis of 10–12 mm in diameter, those with HI titers of 1:256 give zones of approximately 6.0 mm, while sera with low HI titers of 1:10 to 1:15 give zones of 2.5–3.5 mm diameter. In detecting levels of anti-HA this test was found to be slightly more sensitive than conventional HI test and also more sensitive than HI tests in detecting changes in antibody levels. An advantage of this method is that for routine assessment of antibody levels sera need be tested only at one dilution, usually undiluted, and pretreatment of sera for testing is limited to heating at 56°C for 30 minutes. It is not necessary to remove nonspecific inhibitors of hemagglutination, as for HI tests, since these do not contribute to or interfere with hemolysis. A further advantage is that differences in the concentration of antigen on the erythrocytes up to two- to eightfold do not have a significant effect on zone area, and also the concentration of complement in the gel is not critical provided it is high enough to give lysis. Thus the method is readily standardized, and minor discrepancies in concentrations of reagents are not critical.

The passive hemolysis system was found in our studies to be specific for antibody to HA. Antibody to NA or the internal antigens of the virus, NP or M, do not produce hemolytic responses with erythrocyte coated with influenza virus particles. The method was effective in detecting antibody in human, ferret, rabbit, or goat sera, but thus far no hemolysis with mouse or chicken sera has been detected in tests using guinea pig complement even though these are potent in specific anti-HA antibodies. However, it is possible that the use of complement from other species would enable SRH tests to be used with antisera from a wider range of hosts. Hemolysis was found

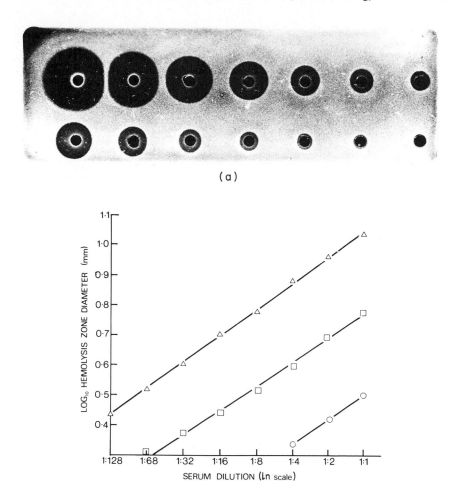

(a)

(b)

Fig. 11.3. Single radial hemolysis (passive hemolysis) reactions of human sera in agarose gel immunoplates containing guinea pig complement (final concentration 1 : 30) and chicken erythrocytes (1%) treated with A/Port Chalmers/1/73 virus. The clear areas represent zones of lysed erythrocytes produced by antibody to hemagglutinin. (a) Wells in the top row contain serial twofold dilutions (1 : 1 to 1 : 64) of a potent human serum having an HI titer of 1 : 2560 with A/PC/1/73 virus. The bottom row contains similar dilutions of a serum with an HI titer of 1:256. (b) Dose–response curves of serial dilutions of three samples of human sera of different HI antibody potencies. △, HI serum titer 1 : 2560; □, 1 : 256; ○, 1 : 20. A plot of $\log_{10}$ zone diameter against serum dilution (ln scale) gave parallel straight line relationships for each of these sera.

to be highly specific for the antigenic variety of hemagglutinin. No cross-reactions were detected between antibodies to different subtypes of hemagglutinin (H0, H1, H2 and H3). Furthermore, the test was found to be highly strain-specific (see Section) and may therefore be useful for the antigenic characterization of influenza virus variants. Preliminary investigations suggest that even in recently convalescent human sera it is essentially IgG antibodies which produce the hemolytic reaction.

The method of passive hemolysis may have wide applications for serological studies with virus antigens such as hemagglutinins which have a natural affinity for receptors on the erythrocyte surface. Antibody to rubella virus hemagglutinin is readily assayed by this method (G. C. Schild, unpublished) and this may be a useful diagnostic method for rubella infection. Additionally, antigens which do not normally attach spontaneously may be coupled to the erythrocyte surface by the use of appropriate reagents, making it potentially possible to use the method for detecting antibody to a wide range of antigens.

C. Antibody to Neuraminidase

1. Neuraminidase Inhibition (NI)

The NI test has been the most frequently used procedure for neuraminidase antibody assay and, in spite of its complexities, still remains the basic reference test for other assay systems. The test presently in use is based on methods for neuraminidase assay as described by Warren (1959) and Aminoff (1961) and on antibody assay by inhibition of enzyme activity as described by Ada et al. (1963) and Webster and Laver (1967). The sensitivity of the test for antibody has been increased by incubating virus, substrate, and antibody overnight as described by Downie (1970).

The current NI test procedure recommended by the World Health Organization (Aymard et al., 1973) consists of (1) assay of test virus for neuraminidase activity, (2) adjustment of virus dosage to a standard unit of neuraminidase activity, and (3) assay of antibody by testing serial dilutions of antiserum for inhibition of the standard unit of neuraminidase. There are five basic steps in the assay of neuraminidase. (a) Serial dilutions of virus are mixed with the substrate fetuin and incubated overnight at 37°C; (b) free N-acetylneuraminic acid (NANA) is released from fetuin by the action of neuraminidase; (c) NANA is converted to β-formylpyruvic acid by periodate oxidation; (d) chromophore of pyruvic acid is formed by the addition of thiobarbituric acid; and (e) this chromophore is extracted by organic solvents and its concentration determined by spectrophotometric analysis. From the potency of the neuraminidase activity thus determined, a standard virus dosage is calculated based on the optimal range of optical density for the NI test. The NI test is performed by incubating the standard viral neuraminidase dose with serial dilutions of normal and test sera. The inhibitory effect of serum on the neuraminidase activity is determined and the NI titer is calculated.

The concept of the NI test is relatively simple, but the manual labor required limits its application to only a few strains or a few antisera in any given test. Kendal and Madely (1969) proposed an automated technique which incorporated the thiobarbaturic acid method with a standard auto-analyzer. However, this technique has not been widely used.

Ziegler and Hutchinson (1972) described a coupled enzyme series for measuring neuraminidase activity spectrophotometrically in a single reaction system. Three enzymatic reactions proceed sequentially: viral neuraminidase acts on fetuin to release NANA, aldolase acts on the NANA to release pyruvate, and pyruvate is reduced to lactate by lactic acid dehydrogenase as nicotinamide adenine dinucleotide (NADH) is oxidized. The rate of reaction is determined by the change in adsorbance at 340 nm as the NADH is oxidized. Attempts to use this procedure for assay of neuraminidase antibodies have not been satisfactory (D. W. Ziegler and H. D. Hutchinson, personal communication).

The inhibition of neuraminidase activity by specific antisera was observed in very early studies to depend upon the size of the substrate (Fazekas de St. Groth, 1962). The substrate fetuin which is used in the NI test recommended by the WHO has a molecular weight of about 50,000. Enzymatic release of NANA from this relatively large molecule is strongly inhibited by specific antibody. On the other hand, sialolactose which has a similar neuraminic acid linkage (galactose), but a molecular weight of only 650, is not inhibited by the presence of antibody (Ada et al., 1963). This suggests that the action of antibody is directed not against the actual site of the enzyme activity but against an antigenic site probably some distance away (Fazekas de St. Groth, 1962). As with antigen–antibody interactions with the hemagglutinin of the intact influenza virus, presumably only those antibodies directed against the tips of the neuraminidase spikes are active. Therefore, the site of active enzymes must be either physically inaccessible to antibody or located elsewhere on the neuraminidase structure.

Since the actual site of neuraminidase activity appears to be inaccessible to antibody, it is quite possible that the enzymes for many influenza virus types are structurally similar. Support for this comes from the findings of Kendal and Madely (1969) which showed that viruses that appear to have antigenically different neuraminidases may have similar kinetic determinants. These findings applied not only to influenza A strains but extended to type B strains as well. Some influenza B strains could be placed in the same class as H0N1 strains on the basis of kinetic groupings.

Conditions for performance of the NI test should be carefully controlled. Changes in temperature over the range of 0° to 36°C have little or no effect on the interaction of influenza virus with antibody or virus with substrate, but virus enzymatic activity is wholly dependent on temperature (Fazekas de St. Groth, 1962). At 0°C, essentially all enzymatic activity ceases. NI tests are performed at 37°C.

The pH optima for neuraminidase activity may vary among strains, even among clones of the same strain, depending upon the substrate used. Because it is impractical to evaluate the optimum pH for every strain, a pH of 5.9 has been arbitrarily chosen for the NI test. As with the hemagglutinin, host carbohydrate is incorporated into the neuraminidase of viruses grown in the hen's egg (Ada et al., 1963). Therefore, antibodies to the host antigen may interfere with assays for specific antibodies. In addition, hemagglutinin antibody may cause low-level steric inhibition when intact viruses are used as a source of neuraminidase (Laver and Kilbourne, 1966; Easterday et al., 1969).

The reproducibility of the NI test for anti-influenza neuraminidase antibody is reasonably good. Hennesy and Davenport (1972) evaluated the reproducibility of the test by using 146 replications of two ferret antisera and two recombinant viruses. Differences ≥ 2.3-fold were considered significant. On the basis of similar studies in the WHO International Influenza Center, Atlanta, a threefold or greater change in antibody titer was found to be significant.

2. Neuraminidase Hemagglutination Inhibition (N-HI)

Hemagglutination by some influenza type A strains possessing the N2 antigens or recombinants thereof may be inhibited under certain conditions by potent anti-neuraminidase antibodies (Webster et al., 1968; Schulman and Kilbourne, 1969). Presumably, inhibition of hemagglutination by anti-neuraminidase antibodies occurs through interference with erythrocyte interaction by neighboring hemagglutinin spikes. The application of this phenomenon for assay of anti-neuraminidase antibody was first investigated by Kilbourne et al. (1968a) and later by Davenport et al. (1970) using the recombinant A/equine/Prague/1/56(Heq1)-RI/5/57(N2). Although the serologic study proved to be useful, the test was not particularly sensitive for detection of neuraminidase antibody. Sensitivity, however, could be greatly increased by adding specific anti-immunoglobulin antibody. Titers were enhanced 100-fold to 1000-fold. The mechanism of titer enhancement by anti-immunoglobulin has not been elucidated. Presumably, either anti-immunoglobulin increases the size of the neuraminidase–anti-neuraminidase antibody complex, thus enlarging the effective area of steric hindrance, or it causes aggregation of the virus–anti-neuraminidase antibody complexes. N-HI tests in which the recombinant A/equine/Prague/56(Heq1)-Hong Kong/16/68(N2) and anti-human IgG were used were found to be both sensitive and specific for assay of anti-human antibody (Kendal *et al.*, 1972; Holston and Dowdle, 1973).

However, the N-HI test may be highly variable. Alteration of erythrocyte composition or concentration virus dosage, the test serum, or the anti-immunoglobulin preparation may appreciably affect the test results. In the presence of some anti-immunoglobulins, a twofold change in virus dosage caused 100-fold variation in serum titer. The enhancement of N-HI titers by anti-immunoglobulin varied widely with different lots, in spite of similar potency values by other immunologic methods.

Recent studies suggest that the test is applicable only for influenza strains sensitive to γ (horse serum) inhibitors. Should the test strain consist of a mixture of inhibitor-sensitive and inhibitor-resistant particles, the N-HI titer may change from negative to a titer of several thousand by simply altering the virus dosage. As with other γ inhibitor strains, the titers are very likely influenced by nonspecific inhibitors present at levels too low to be detected. This may account for the variation in enhancing ability of various anti-IgG lots that appear to have similar immunological potency.

3. Indirect Hemagglutination (IHA)

The use of the IHA test as an alternative to the NI and the N-HI tests for assay of neuraminidase antibodies was reported by Holston and Dowdle (1973). Agglutination of sheep erythrocytes sensitized with purified neuraminidase (N2) subunits was shown to be specific and highly sensitive for N2 antibodies. The N-IHA test was at least equal to the N-HI tests for the detection of fourfold or greater antibody rises in paired sera from infected or vaccinated subjects. However, it was four times more sensitive than the other tests for detection of antibodies in sera before infection or vaccination.

The test is not restricted to the use of antigen subunits. It can be performed equally as well with chicken erythrocytes sensitized with purified intact viruses. Viruses for sensitization may be selected from recombinants containing the desired N antigens and irrelevant H antigens (I. S. Schwarzman, personal communication). Recent studies with such sensitized cells support the initial observation of Holston and Dowdle (1973) that the N-IHA test may not distinguish minor antigenic differences which may be detected by the NI test (W. R. Dowdle, unpublished data). The significance of the broader activity of antibodies in the N-IHA test is not clear, but certain fundamental differences between the two tests should be recognized. The NI test is an indirect method for assay of neuraminidase antibody. Inhibition of enzyme activity depends upon steric hindrance of the union between enzyme and substrate. The N-IHA test is a direct assay. Agglutination reflects direct binding of antigen by antibody. Differences in results between the two tests may indicate important fundamental differences between antibodies or between reactive antigenic sites.

4. Single Radial Diffusion (SRD)

The principles of the SRD test for the detection and assay of antibody to the surface antigens of the influenza virus have been described. Using SRD immunoplates containing intact influenza virus particles of the "wild-type" antibody to both hemagglutinin and neuraminidase is detected. However, by the use of gels containing intact recombinant influenza viruses (see Table 11.4) containing the appropriate neuraminidase antigens and irrelevant hemagglutinins the SRD test can be made specific to antibody to neuraminidase. This approach has been exploited by a number of studies involving antibody responses to vaccines and influenza infection (Molyneux et al., 1974; Mostow et al., 1974) and also in serological surveys (G. C. Schild, unpublished).

The SRD method may have an important theoretical advantage in anti-neuraminidase assays. It has been clearly shown by Dowdle et al. (1974) that antibody to neuraminidase does not depend on the neutralization of enzymatic activity for its biological properties, and furthermore it appears that the enzymatic site and the antigenic determinant of the neuraminidase are situated at different sites on the molecule. Thus tests of the ability of antibody to inhibit enzymatic activity are of doubtful significance and tests involving direct measure of antibody–antigen reactions, such as SRD, are preferable. In addition, the conventional NI test is extremely cumbersome, time consuming and subject to much variability.

For a given concentration of antibody reacting in the SRD test the size of the zone is influenced by the number of antibody molecules which react with each virus particle. Thus the zone intensity given by anti-neuraminidase antibodies is lower than for anti-hemagglutinin (Schild et al., 1972a) while the area of the anti-neuraminidase zones is generally greater than for anti-hemagglutinin. It follows therefore that for virus strains containing different numbers of neuraminidase molecules per particle such as the X7 and X7-F_1 strains (Webster et al., 1968) different SRD responses would be expected for given concentrations of antibody. This should be taken into account in the application of SRD tests and indeed SRD may be a useful tool for the examination of the relative abundance of the two surface antigens on the influenza virus surface.

5. IMMUNO DOUBLE DIFFUSION (IDD)

In spite of the fact that the neuraminidase is the minor antigenic component of the virus surface IDD tests employing detergent disrupted virions as antigen are effective in detecting precipitin reactions corresponding to the neuraminidase antigen (Schild and Pereira, 1969; Schild et al., 1971). However, the information obtained is qualitative rather than quantitative. The assignment of precipitin reactions detected in tests with unknown antisera as corresponding to neuraminidase antigen may be established by employing specific anti-neuraminidase sera in the test and seeking evidence of identity of the precipitin reactions. For detection of anti-neuraminidase antibody the conventional precipitin test is relatively insensitive and positive reactions are given only by sera with NI titers of several hundred or SRD zone areas of approximately 5 mm^2 or more. In general, IDD tests with neuraminidase antigens are broadly reactive as are those of hemagglutinin antigens and cross-reactions are detected between neuraminidase antigens of all members of a given subtype but not between subtypes (Schild and Newman, 1969).

6. NEUTRALIZATION

Neuraminidase antibody may cause apparent neutralization in the mouse (Schulman et al., 1968), in the chicken (Allan et al., 1971; Rott et al., 1974), and in cell cultures (Seto and Rott, 1966; Jaheil and Kilbourne, 1966; Webster and Laver, 1967; Kasel et al., 1973; Dowdle et al., 1974). Neuraminidase antibody does not prevent initiation of infection, but acts by inhibiting the release of virus from infected cells, thereby preventing virus spread.

In influenza virus plaquing systems, this means that neuraminidase antibody does not affect plaque number, but significantly reduces plaque size (Seto and Rott, 1966; Jahiel and Kilbourne, 1966). Limited studies have shown that the plaque size reduction tests can be useful for antigenic characterization of influenza A neuraminidase (Schulman and Kilbourne, 1969). The results generally paralleled those found with the NI test. Application of this test is restricted to those strains which may be adapted to form plaques. Many do not.

Neuraminidase antibody assay techniques based on postinfection neutralization tests with tissue culture (Dowdle et al., 1974) or with allantois on shell (Webster and Laver, 1967) deserve further study.

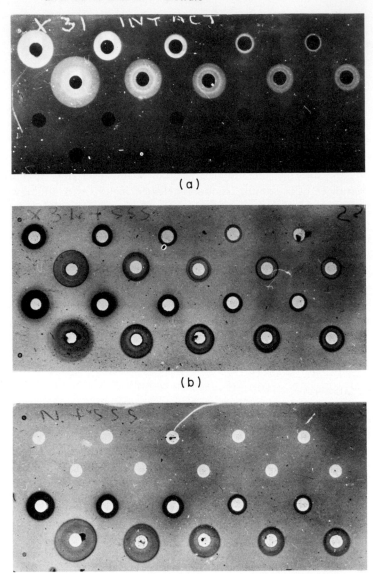

(a)

(b)

(c)

Fig. 11.4. Reactions of antisera to influenza A surface and internal antigens in immunoplates containing intact and disrupted virus as antigen. On each of the immunoplates (a), (b), and (c) the wells in the top row contain, left to right, serial twofold dilutions (1 : 1 to 1 : 16) of antiserum to A/HK/1/68 HA; the wells of in the second row contain similar dilution series of antiserum to A/HK/1/68 NA; the third row, dilutions of antiserum to influenza A M; and the fourth row, dilutions of antiserum to influenza A NP. Plate (a) contains intact A/HK/1/68 (X31) virus; plate (b) contains A/HK/1/68 virus disrupted by

7. Complement Fixation (CF)

The CF test (Lief and Henle, 1959) may be used for assay of antibody to the neuraminidase as well as to the hemagglutinin. Performance of the test would require the use of recombinants possessing gentically segregated surface antigens or the use of purified neuraminidase subunits. However, presumably because of the practical disadvantages of complement fixation tests in general this approach has not been exploited as a routine measure.

D. Antibody to the Internal Antigens of the Virus, NP and M

1. Single-Radial-Diffusion (SRD)

The influenza virus particle contains two internal type-specific antigens, the ribonucleoprotein (NP) or "soluble" antigen first described by Hoyle and Fairbrother (1937) and the matrix (M) protein (Schild, 1972). Of these, the M protein is the most abundant, there being approximately 3000 molecules of M and 1000 molecules of NP per virus particle (Skehel and Schild, 1971). The SRD test may be modified for the assay of antibody to these antigens (Oxford and Schild, 1974; Schild *et al.*, 1974c).

For such assays purified influenza virus preparations are disrupted by treatment with sodium sarkosyl sulfate detergent at a final concentration of 1.0% before addition to the gel at a concentration 0.2 mg virus protein per ml of gel. Figure 11.4 compares the SRD reactions of antisera to the four major antigens of the virus various test systems. With intact virus only antibody to surface antigens reacts, while with the disrupted homologous virus antibody to all four components react. However, if a disrupted influenza A virus with surface antigens of a different subtype is employed only antibody to the NP and M give reactions. For routine assays of NP and M antibodies in human sera an avian influenza A virus, such as A/chicken/Germany/'N'/49 (Hav2Neq1) may be employed (see Table 11.4), since antibody to the HA or NA antigens of this virus are not found in human sera. In this modification of the SRD test the antigens are rendered soluble and diffusible by the detergent, and opalescent zones are formed as a result of the formation of visible precipitates. The mechanism thus differs from that of SRD tests employing intact virus. The precipitates are not intense,

sodium sarkosyl sulfate detergent, and plate (c) contains a disrupted avian influenza A virus with surface antigens distinct from those of the A/HK/1/68 virus. The immunoplate (a) containing intact A/HK/68 virus detects only antibody to the surface antigens while plate (c), with disrupted avian influenza A virus, detects only antibody to the internal antigens, M and NP.

and the results of the tests are best read after staining the zones with a protein stain, e.g., Coomassie brilliant blue, after washing the immunoplates in saline for 24 hours to remove the unprecipitated antigen and serum proteins. As may be seen in Fig. 11.4 the zones produced by antibody to M are more intense than those produced by antibody to NP, and this feature is used to distinguish the two antibodies when both are present, using immune rabbit sera against M and NP for reference. When antibodies to NP and M are present in a single serum specimen, a composite reaction mune rabbit sera against M and NP for reference. When antibodies to M and a less intense outer zone produced by antibody to NP. It should be noted that the difference in intensities of zones due to M and NP reflect the higher concentration of M antigen in the virus and thus in the SRD gel. Because of this the sensitivity of the tests in detecting antibody to M is less than for NP. However, the test may be made sensitive for antibody to M by reducing the concentration of disrupted virus added to the gel fivefold (0.02 mg virus per ml). Under these conditions antibody to NP produces zones which are barely detectable due to the suboptimal concentrations of NP antigen, while anti-M antibody gives zones of strong intensity which can be readily measured. For each of these modifications of the SRD test, zone annulus area gives an approximately linear relationship with antibody concentration and the results are thus annulus areas. To establish reproducibility and specificity of the test it is necessary to test reference anti-NP and anti-M sera on each immunoplate.

The SRD technique has certain advantages over the more conventional CF technique for the assay of antibody to NP. First, it is more sensitive; this may be due in part to the fact that precipitin zones are given by all classes of immunoglobulin, while CF reactions are given only by antibodies belonging to certain immunoglobulin classes, namely, IgM and certain subclasses of IgG. Second, it is rapid and simple and may be performed with small volumes of untreated sera. Indeed "pin pricks" of whole blood may be placed directly in the wells for screening tests. Third, unlike CF tests, it is applicable to sera from a wide range of species. A disadvantage is that its application is at present limited to influenza A. Since all influenza B strains appear to belong to a single subtype reactions because the surface antigens cannot be eliminated by the use of strains with distinct surface antigens as for influenza A. However, it is possible to isolate the antigenically active NP and M of influenza virus either independently by electrophoretic separation (Schild, 1972) or in the form of virus cores (Skehel, 1971), and these procedures may be exploited to provide purified NP and M antigen preparations for use in antibody assays by SRD. Following the procedures employed by Pereira et al. (1972) for adenovirus hexon, the sensitivity of such tests could be enhanced considerably by the use of radioactively labeled antigens in combination with autoradiographic techniques. Such procedures would allow the test to be performed with very low concentrations of antigens.

2. Immuno Double Diffusion (IDD)

Antibody to both NP (Hanna and Hoyle, 1966; Schild and Pereira, 1969) and M (Schild, 1972) may be detected by immuno double diffusion tests using detergent-disrupted influenza virions as antigen. When multiple-precipitin lines are detected with an unknown antiserum, the identification of the precipitin reactions as corresponding to NP or M is established by the use of specific reference antisera to those antigens. As emphasized previously, the use of IDD test is of qualitative rather than quantitative value. Recently, Dowdle et al. (1974) described the preparation of M and NP antigen from infected allantoic fluids by precipitation of these proteins at a low pH. Such antigen preparations may be used for routine IDD tests to detect antibodies to NP and M.

3. Complement Fixation (CF)

For many years the complement fixation test was the only method available for the assay of antibody to the internal antigens of influenza virus. Initially CF tests were performed using the "soluble" or "S" antigen, essentially ribonucleoprotein, present in extracts of infected mouse lung tissue (Hoyle and Fairbrother, 1937; Lennette and Horsfall, 1940). Subsequently CF assays for antibody were routinely carried out using S antigen present in extracts of infected chick embryo chorioallantoic membranes (Lief and Henle, 1959). Standardized CF techniques for this purpose have been described elsewhere employing macrotests (Bradstreet and Taylor, 1962) or microtests (United States Public Health Service; 1965). It is now clear that there are two internal antigens of the virus particle, NP and M, and that both are present in preparations of S antigens. Nevertheless, the M is a minor component of the S antigen prepared from egg membranes by conventional methods, and although M antigen readily fixes complement on reaction with specific antibody (Schild, 1972), the low level of this component present in the CF antigen would suggest that anti-M antibody probably contribute little to the reactions obtained in conventional CF tests.

In assessing the results of CF tests note should be taken of the fact that only IgM and certain subclasses of IgG fix complement, and the absence of complement fixation reaction does not necessarily exclude the presence of antibody to the antigen used in the test. Indeed complement-fixing antibodies following influenza infection may be relatively short-lived and not detectable several months after infection. Antibody to the NP antigen detected by SRD does not decline as rapidly as CF antibody (G. C. Schild, unpublished).

4. Fluorescent Antibody

Using direct or indirect immunofluorescence techniques (see Liu, 1969), the fluorescent labeling of NP and M antigens in infected cells can be detected. Antibody to NP labels produces essentially nuclear fluorescence (Liu, 1955; Breitenfeld and Schafer, 1957), while antibody to M produces predominantly cytoplasmic fluorescence but also some nuclear fluorescence (Oxford and Schild, 1974). This method has been applied as a qualitative diagnostic test for the detection of influenza antibodies in postinfection human serum (de Silva and Tobin, 1973), but the procedure is technically exacting and difficult to control and has not been applied routinely.

E. Determination of Immunoglobulin Class of Influenza Antibodies

Current evidence suggests that after initial influenza infection or immunization of man, the immunoglobulin response parallels that seen with many other virus diseases (Dobrovalsky, 1971). That is, antibodies of the IgM class appear first and in the largest proportion and are replaced several weeks later by antibodies of the IgG class. This is also true of mice (Berlin, 1963), rabbits (Webster, 1968), and chickens (Heyward et al., 1972) immunized with influenza viruses.

Antibody responses to influenza in the adult human, however, are infinitely more complex because of the likelihood of reinfections with antigenically related influenza viruses and the phenomenon of "original antigenic sin" (Francis, 1953). Also, antibody responses to each of the four major virus antigens, HA, NA, M, and NP, are totally independent events.

Recent interest in serologic methods for the diagnosis of influenza at autopsy (de Silva and Tobin, 1973) or under conditions when only single serum specimens are available (Glick et al., 1970) has emphasized the need to document the normal patterns of immunoglobulin response to influenza and to develop reliable and practical techniques for determining immunoglobulin class.

The conventional procedures for serum fractionation, such as sucrose gradient centrifugation (Brakke, 1967) and molecular sieve chromatography (Heyward et al., 1972), are laborious and present formidable dilution problems, particularly if fractions are to be treated for destruction of nonspecific inhibitors before assay by HI or neutralization tests. As an alternative, direct identification of immunoglobulin class by specific anti-immunoglobulin anti-sera has been proposed. Fluorescein-labeled antisera against human IgA, IgG, and IgM have been used for staining influenza antigen–antibody complexes (Brown and O'Leary, 1971). This procedure, however, does not differentiate between antibodies that may be reactive with different virus antigens. The reliability of the indirect FA procedure for classification of the immunoglobulins requires further evaluation. A radioimmunoassay procedure similar to that described by Daugharty *et al.* (1972) seems to offer several theoretical advantages. The immunoglobulin class of antibody to each surface antigen could be assayed independently by using either selected antigenic recombinants or purified antigens. This has not yet been demonstrated. The sensitivity of this procedure for IgM assay may be seriously limited by preferential binding of IgG antibody over IgM (Daugharty, 1973).

IV. Recommended Procedures for the Assay and Characterization of Antigens

A. The Hemagglutinin

1. HEMAGGLUTININ ASSAY BY HI AND SRD TESTS

The most frequently applied systems for the hemagglutinin content of influenza virus preparations are based on their ability to agglutinate erythrocytes. These assays may be performed by a variety of methods such as the HA "pattern" assay in plastic plates (World Health Organization, 1959) or the CCA assay using a colorimeter to assess the degree of agglutination of erythrocytes (Miller and Stanley, 1944). These methods are simple to perform and provide information which is generally an adequate assessment of the viral content of a preparation. However, all such assays are subject to several disadvantages; the main disadvantage is that the results are dependent upon the physical state of the hemagglutinin in the test preparations in addition to its quantity, i.e., whether in the form of intact spherical or filamentous particles, as subviral particles, or pure HA which may be polyvalent or monovalent. Indeed the highly purified hemagglutinin obtained by Brand and Skehel (1972) by bromelain treatment of influenza particles fails to agglutinate erythrocytes although it is an excellent antigen. A further variable factor is the chicken erythrocytes which may vary considerably in their sensitivity to hemagglutinin. It is perhaps unfortunate that up until recently assays based on agglutination were the only ones available for research and routine purposes and also for the standardization of the potency of influenza vaccines. Now that techniques are available for the identification of the hemagglutinin polypeptides by polyacrylamide gel analysis (Skehel and Schild, 1971) or other physicochemical techniques, improved assay systems for the quantitative and qualitative assay of HA will no doubt be developed.

As an alternative to erythrocyte agglutination tests, SRD has been used to assay HA antigen. In the method described (Schild *et al.*, 1974a) antiserum to purified hemagglutinin is distributed throughout an agarose gel, and antigen preparations for HA assay are applied to wells after treatment by detergent to ensure that the HA antigen is present in a diffusible form. The area of the zone of opalescence produced by the reaction of HA antigen and antibody after diffusion gives a measure of the quantity of HA present. A considerable advantage of this assay system over those based on agglutination is that the physical state of the antigen plays no role in the reaction, since all the HA present is converted to diffusible subunits by treatment with detergent. Application of this method for the assessment and control of influenza vaccine potency has been proposed (Schild *et al.*, 1974a), and preliminary assessments of its value have given satisfactory results. Similar procedures could be used for any of the structural or nonstructural antigens of the influenza virus, provided that potent and specific antibody is available as is the case for NA, NP, and M (but not at present for the nonstructural components). As a further adaptation of SRD as a highly sensitive technique to detect minute quantities of hemagglutinin or other influenza antigens specific antiserum to the appropriate antigen may be radioactively labeled, e.g., with ^{125}I, and added to the gel in immunoplates. Samples of antigen for assay are added to wells and the resulting zones of antibody–antigen reaction are demonstrated by autoradiography after thoroughly washing the nonprecipitated radioactivity from the immunoplates. This method has been exploited for adenoviruses (Pereira *et al.*, 1972) to detect small concentrations of adenovirus hexon antigen. Its application to influenza might be of value in detecting small quantities of antigens in infected cultures or in body fluids of infected hosts. In the latter case it may be of value in studies of viremia or antigenemia accompanying influenza infections.

2. Hemagglutinin Characterization by HI and SRH Tests

Antigenic characterization of the hemagglutinins of influenza virus isolates in order to identify subtype and strain variations is routinely performed by HI tests. The performance of these tests had been described earlier in this chapter. Preliminary studies on new influenza virus isolates are conventionally performed by employing postinfection ferret sera or chicken sera using a chessboard pattern of tests. A typical pattern of cross-HI reactions with recently isolated influenza strains is shown in Table 11.5. Evidence of antigenic drift in the hemagglutinin (H3) antigens of the viruses of the Hong Kong subtype isolated between 1968 and 1974 can clearly be seen by the low, or negative, inhibition titers of the chronologically later isolates by antiserum to the 1968 strains. HI tests performed with post-infection ferret sera are highly sensitive in detecting evidence of minor antigenic differences between strains. However, these antisera may contain antibody to neuraminidase as well as to hemagglutinin, and such antibody may influence the results of the tests (Kilbourne, 1968). In order to eliminate the role of the neuraminidase antigen and to ascertain that the HI relates only to the HA antigen, antisera for use in HI tests may be prepared against recombinant influenza virus strains containing antigenically irrelevant neuraminidases (Schulman and Kilbourne, 1969).

A further aspect of the use of HI tests is to identify the hemagglutinin subtype of influenza strains. For this purpose potent hyperimmune antisera prepared against purified hemagglutinins or against recombinant influenza viruses containing irrelevant neuraminidases are preferable to postinfection sera. This is because the latter are narrowly specific and may not react with all the virus strains within a given hemagglutinin subtype (see Table 11.5). In contrast hyperimmune sera react broadly within a subtype but under appropriate test conditions are subtype specific. Such hyperimmune sera prepared against hemagglutinin from chick embryo-grown virus may contain antibody to chick "host" antigen which is cross-reactive between HA subtypes (Haukenes *et al.,* 1965) and may thus give false positive HI reactions. This may be eliminated by the use of virus in the HI tests which has been grown in duck eggs and does not contain the chick specific "host" antigen (Webster and Laver, 1972) or by removal of host antibody by adsorption of the sera by a heterotypic influenza virus (Schild *et al.,* 1974b).

The SRH test performed with postinfection ferret sera may be employed for the characterization of HA antigens of influenza isolates and is extremely sensitive in detecting antigenic differences between strains. The results of representative tests to compare A/Hong Kong/1/68 and its variants are shown in Table 11.6. When compared with the antigenic relationships detected between the same strains in HI tests (Table 11.5) it is clearly seen that the SRH is more narrowly specific. This method appears to be appropriate for routine use in characterization of HA antigens.

3. HEMAGGLUTININ CHARACTERIZATION BY IDD AND SRD TESTS

Applications of these tests to the characterization of the hemagglutinin antigens of influenza viruses may be illustrated by studies to compare

Table 11.5 Antigenic Cross-Reactions of Recent Influenza A Viruses as Indicated by Hemagglutination Inhibition Tests[a]

Virus strains	Reference strains				New variants		
	A/HK/ 1/68	A/HK/ 107/71	A/Eng/ 42/72	A/PC/ 1/73	A/Hann/ 61/73	A/P. Rico/ 1/74	A/Eng/ 635/74
A/Hong Kong/1/68	3840	480	3840	320	60	320	60
A/Hong Kong/107/71	160	7680	320	960	240	80	240
A/England/42/72	640	160	7680	1280	320	160	480
A/Port Chalmers/1/73	160	320	1280	2560	1280	480	640
A/Hannover/61/73	<40	240	1280	2560	2560	480	3840
A/Puerto Rico/1/74	120	120	160	640	120	1920	160
A/England/635/74	40	120	160	640	960	160	3840

[a] Using postinfection ferret serum.

Table 11.6 Antigenic Cross-Reactions of A/Hong Kong/1/68 and Its Variants Employing Postinfection Ferret Sera and Single Radial Hemolysis Tests[a]

Virus on chick erythrocytes	A/HK/ 1/68	A/Eng/ 42/72	A/PC/ 1/73	A/Eng/ 635/74
A/Hong Kong/1/68	41.9	4.3	<1	<1
A/England/42/72	3.5	35.3	8.5	2.1
A/Port Chalmers/1/73	<1	4.5	56.5	12.5
A/England/635/74	<1	<1	10.3	47.3

[a] Zone annulus areas of hemolysis (mm²).

A/Hong Kong/1/68(H3N2) virus with its variants A/England/42/72 and A/Port Chalmers/1/73. IDD tests were carried out with hyperimmune sera to the purified HA antigen (H3) of A/Hong Kong/1/68 virus, the antiserum was placed in the center well of the IDD pattern, and various test virus strains disrupted with detergent in the peripheral wells (see Fig. 11.5). All strains isolated from 1968 and 1973 gave precipitin reactions. However viruses containing hemagglutinins of other subtypes H0, H1, or H2, failed to react, illustrating the subtype specific nature of the IDD reactions. The reactions given by the successive variants A/Hong Kong/1/68, A/England/42/72, and A/Port Chalmers/1/73 did not show complete identity, however, and the antiserum to A/Hong Kong/1/68 hemagglutinin produced spurs between these strains tested in adjacent wells. The pattern of precipitin reactions thus confirmed that the HA of A/Port Chalmers/1/73 virus was of the same subtype (H3) as the prototype A/Hong Kong/1/68 virus and that the antigenic changes which have occurred in this antigen since 1968 were attributable to antigenic drift. To confirm that the hemagglutinins of A/Hong Kong/1/68 and A/Port Chalmers/1/73 viruses each contained antigenic determinants, i.e., strain-specific determinants (see Laver and Webster, 1974; Virelizier et al., 1974) which were not shared, cross-absorption experiments were performed. Antiserum to the HA of Hong Kong/68 virus was absorbed by the addition of purified A/Port Chalmers/1/73 virus to remove antibodies to antigenic determinants shared by both strains and the absorbed serum tested by IDD tests. No reaction was detected with the 1973 variant but distinct precipitin lines were found with 1968, 1971, and 1972 variants (see Figure 11.5). Similarly antiserum to the HA of Port Chalmers virus after absorption with Hong Kong/68 virus gave IDD reactions with the 1973 variant and with the 1972 variant but not with the 1968 and 1971 variants. The results of the absorption experiments indicated that the HA antigens of the 1968 and 1973 variants contained antigenic determinants

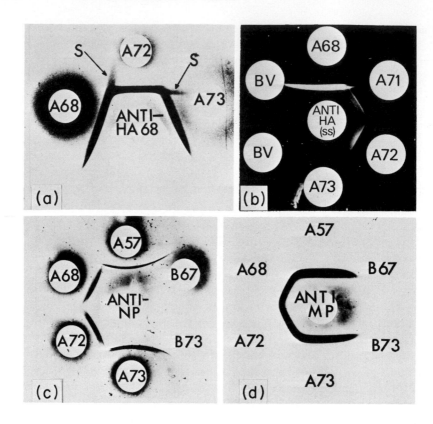

Fig. 11.5. Immuno double diffusion studies to show antigenic variation in the HA antigen of the Hong Kong virus from 1968 to 1973 and lack of variation in NP and MP antigens. Throughout the figures wells marked A68, A71, A72, and A73 contain purified influenza A/Singapore/1/57, A/Hong Kong/1/68, A/Hong Kong/107/71, A/England/42/72, and A/Port Chalmers/1/73 viruses, respectively, disrupted with sodium sarkosyl sulfate detergent. BV and B/73 represent wells containing influenza B/Hong Kong/8/73 virus, and B/67, containing B/Roma/1/67 virus. Wells marked Anti-HA 68 contain rabbit antiserum to the purified HA of A/Hong Kong/1/68 virus; Anti-HA 68 (SS), the same antiserum tested after adsorption with purified, concentrated A/PC/1/73 virus in order to obtain a strain-specific population of anti-HA antibody. ANTI-NP and ANTI-MP represent wells containing rabbit antiserum to purified NP and MP antigens. (a) shows evidence of progressive antigenic variation in the HA antigen in strains isolated from 1968 to 1973. Spurs (S) indicating antigenic determinants not shared by the HA antigens of the strains tested in adjacent wells are indicated. (b) After absorbing antiserum to A/HK/1/68 HA by the addition of purified, concentrated A/PC/1/73 virus a relatively strain-specific population of antibodies was remaining which reacted with A/HK/1/68 virus and intermediate strains isolated in 1971 and 1972 but failed to react with A/PC/1/73. This population of antibodies is directed against antigenically variable determinants

which were not shared and thus provided evidence that during antigenic drift certain antigenic determinants of the HA antigen underwent complete antigenic change while other determinants remained unaltered and provided the antigenic basis for the recognition of the antigen as H3.

The test strains were also compared by single radial diffusion. This technique enables a high degree of accuracy and reproducibility for antibody assays and was thus of value for the quantitation of antigenic differences between influenza variants (Schild *et al.*, 1973a). The comparative SRD reactions of anti-hemagglutinin, (or anti-neuraminidase) sera or postinfection ferret sera on immunoplates containing equivalent quantities of intact A/Hong Kong/1/68, A/England/42/72, and A/Port Chalmers/1/73 virus are shown in Table 11.7. Antisera to the purified hemagglutinin (and the purified neuraminidase) of A/Hong Kong/1/68 virus gave opalescent zones in tests with A/England/42/72 and A/Port Chalmers/1/73 viruses which were smaller than those given by the homologous virus. The zone areas in tests with A/Port Chalmers/1/73 were 34 and 13% of the homologous zones for the anti-hemagglutinin and anti-neuraminidase sera, respectively. This finding provides confirmatory evidence of a considerable degree of antigenic change in the HA (and NA) antigens from 1968 to 1973, and the method is of value as an additional analytical technique for antigenic variation in HA and NA. It is important in such studies that the hyperimmune sera employed should be exhaustively absorbed with a heterotypic influenza virus to remove antibody to "host" antigen which may otherwise produce nonspecific reactions in SRD tests.

The SRD method for the analysis of variant influenza virus hemagglutinins may also be combined with antibody absorption procedures (Schild *et al.*, 1973a) to remove antibody populations which are cross-reactive for the hemagglutinins of influenza variants within a subtype. Such a procedure enhances the sensitivity of the SRD test to distinguish between antigenic variants.

B. The Neuraminidase

Our present concepts of the antigenic relationships among the influenza A and B strains are based largely on findings with the NI test. Major reciprocal NI tests have been undertaken for influenza A strains of human

of HA which are not possessed by the 1973 variant. (c) and (d) represent precipitin reactions given by antisera to internal components of influenza A (NP and MP) and fail to show evidence of antigenic change in these antigens from 1957–1973. These antigens are distinct for influenza type A and type B viruses and form the basis of classification of influenza viruses into types.

Table 11.7 Serological Cross-Reactions of A/Hong Kong/1/68 (H3N2) with its Variants in Single Radial Immunodiffusion Tests[a]

Purified virus incorporated in immunoplate	Antisera to isolated A/Hong Kong/1/68 antigens				Postinfection ferret sera[b] to					
	Anti-pure H3 hemagglutinin (chick origin)		Anti-pure N2 neuraminidase (rabbit origin)		A/Hong Kong/1/68		A/England/42/72		A/Port Chalmers/1/73	
	Area	% homologous reaction	Area	% homologous reaction	Area	% homologous reaction	Area	% homologous reaction	Area	% homologous reaction
A/Hong Kong/1/68 (H3N2)	63.8	100	130	100	43.2	100	30.3	66	5.5	8.6
A/England/42/72 (H3N2)	34.8	55	56.5	43	13.4	31	45.7	100	37.1	58
A/Port Chalmers/1/73 (H3N2)	22.2	34	16.7	13	6.1	14	33.6	73	63.8	100

[a] Areas of opalescence (mm²) per 10 μl of serum.

[b] Zones given by postinfection sera reflect essentially antibody to hemagglutinin, since such sera are found to contain high levels of antibody to hemagglutinin and low amounts of antibody to neuraminidase.

(Paniker, 1968; Dowdle *et al.,* 1969) and animal origin (Schild and Newman, 1969; Tumova and Easterday, 1969; Madely *et al.,* 1971; Tumova and Schild, 1972). Major reciprocal NI tests have also been undertaken with influenza B strains (Chakraverty, 1972). It must be stressed, however, that many of these tests have been performed without regard to possible interference by hemagglutinin antibodies. Laver and Kilbourne (1966) and Easterday *et al.* (1969) have shown that hemagglutinin antibody may cause low-level steric inhibition of neuraminidase activity when intact viruses are used as a source of enzyme. The low-level antigenic relationships reported between strains in many instances must be considered provisional.

Some workers have attempted to avoid interference by antibodies to the hemagglutinin by pretreating the virus with pronase to destroy the hemagglutinin (Schild and Newman, 1969; Chakraverty, 1972) or by disrupting the virus with detergent (Laver, 1964). Because the efficiency of methods for destruction of hemagglutinin or disruption of the virus may vary widely with different strains, NI tests with whole viruses and monospecific neuraminidase antisera are recommended. Such sera may be prepared for influenza A strains through the use of virus recombinants possessing genetically segregated surface antigens (Schulman and Kilbourne, 1969; Webster, 1970) or with the isolated neuraminidase subunits (Webster and Laver, 1972). Monospecific antisera to the influenza B neuraminidase may be readily prepared from trypsin-released enzyme (Noll *et al.,* 1962; Curry *et al.,* 1974). Antigenic recombinants of influenza B strains are few (Tobita and Kilbourne, 1974) and not likely to be practical for production of monospecific antisera because of extensive cross-reactions among surface antigens.

The NI test is recommended by the WHO for antigenic characterization of neuraminidase (Aymard-Henry *et al.,* 1973). However, the acceptance of any procedure must be tempered by our lack of understanding of the role of neuraminidase antibody. In time the NI may not prove to be the most relevant test. Minor antigenic dissimilarities based on indirect evidence of enzyme inhibition may not be totally relevant to immunologic protection against disease.

For this reason, as well as for more practical considerations, the WHO has further recommended that neuraminidase subtypes be distinguished on the basis of NI and immunoprecipitin test results (World Health Organization, 1971). The immunoprecipitin (IDD) test is broadly reactive and may demonstrate antigenic relationships not apparent by other methods. For example, all neuraminidase within a subtype (N1 or N2) share a common precipitin line regardless of the antigenic dissimilarities seen by the NI test (Schild and Newman, 1969; Schild *et al.,* 1969). The neuraminidase of the classical swine virus shows little or no relationships to the human N1 strains by the NI test (Paniker, 1968) but is found to be identical by the immuno double diffusion (IDD) test (Schild *et al.,* 1972b). In instances where major antigenic differences within an NA antigen sybtype appear to exist by the NI test the IDD may show precipitin lines of partial identity (Schild *et al.,* 1973a; Curry *et al.,* 1974).

Other methods, such as single radial immunodiffusion (SRD) (Schild *et al.,* 1972a), the neuraminidase neutralization test (Dowdle *et al.,* 1974), and the N-IHA test (Holston and Dowdle, 1973), need to be investigated further to determine their applicability for characterization of the neuraminidase.

None of these procedures is satisfactory for assay of neuraminidase antigen potency. The SRD test seems to offer the greatest promise. In this test the neuraminidase antibody is incorporated into the agarose gel, and the antigenic content of the detergent-disrupted virus is assayed by the size of the zone opalescence surrounding the wells. Unlike the NI test, SRD does not depend upon enzyme activity for assay of antigen content. Also, disruption of the virus by detergent makes it unlikely that the test will be affected by virus aggregation or surface spatial relationships.

C. The Internal Components

Identification of influenza viruses is based on characterization of type-specific internal antigens and strain-specific surface antigens. In practice the internal antigen is rarely characterized. The usual laboratory procedure is to proceed immediately to identification of the isolates by the HI test using antisera prepared against current influenza type A and B (or C, if indicated strains. The antisera may fail to inhibit hemagglutination as a result of the presence of hemagglutinating bacteria, avian mycoplasma, some parainfluenza viruses, a mixture of virus types, or an antigenically novel influenza strain. Also, antisera may not be available for the various influenza subtypes which may be isolated from horses, pigs, and a variety of avian species.

In this event, suspected influenza viruses may be typed with specific antisera to the nucleoprotein (NP) or the matrix (M) protein. The type-specific CF test (Lief and Henle, 1959) for NP antigen has traditionally been used for this purpose. The test, however, is complex and time consuming and requires highly specific and expensive reagents which are often in short supply. For these reasons, it cannot be performed in many laboratories with limited resources. The immuno double diffusion test is recommended as a replacement for the CF test (Dowdle *et al.,* 1974). This test is rapid and simple and requires no special equipment or expensive reagents. The same test may be performed with anti-NP or anti-M antisera (see Fig. 11.5b and c). In limited studies the anti-M test appears to be slightly more sensitive than anti-NP, apparently because of the greater abundance of the M antigen in the virion. Also, less time is required for the precipitin line to develop because the small M molecule (20,000 MW) migrates rapidly in agar gels. The test requires only a single drop of test virus concentrate which may be obtained by simple precipitation with acid. Virus concentrates from the allantoic fluid contents of one egg are adequate for the test. Although it is recommended that allantoic harvests should have hemagglutinin titers of >40, some isolates have been typed by IDD from fluids with HA titers as low as 10.

The immuno double diffusion test, of course, does not permit quantitation of antigen. The CF test may be used for assay of NP antigens (Lief and Henle, 1959), but there are no reports of its applicability for assay of M antigen. In theory, the SRD test of Mancini et al. (1965) may be useful for assay of both antigens. This test is similar to that described previously for quantitation of the surface antigens (Schild et al., 1974a). Antibody is incorporated into the agarose gels and antigen added to the wells. The area of opalescent zones surrounding the wells should be proportional to the quantity of antigen. Further investigation of this procedure is required.

Tests which are most frequently used for identification and antigenic characterization of influenza viruses are summarized in Table 11.8.

V. Recommended Procedures for Immunologic Assay

A. Diagnosis

1. PAIRED SERA

By the time a child reaches school age, he has had at least one encounter with an influenza virus. For this reason, the presence of antibody in a single serum specimen may not be indicative of recent infection. Serologic diagnosis of influenza in most instances rests entirely on the demonstration of a significant increase in antibody titer between the acute serum collected at the onset of disease and the convalescent serum collected 2 or 3 weeks later. There are some exceptions, however, such as the presence of specific antibody after an outbreak of a totally new antigenic subtype or an antibody titer proven to be statistically higher than expected.

In theory, a significant rise in antibody titer by any serologic test with any antigenic component of the influenza virus is evidence of recent infection or immunization. In practice, it is somewhat more complex. Rises in antibody to all antigenic components do not occur with equal frequency, and various tests have different degrees of sensitivity.

Table 11.8 Summary of Tests for Antigenic Characterization of Influenza Viruses[a]

Test	Antisera	Test antigen	Antigen	Recommended use[b]		
				Type	Subtype	Strain
HI	Chicken (single injection)	Whole virus	HA[c]		++	+++
	Ferret (infection)	Whole virus	HA[c]		++	++++
	Rabbit (hyperimmune)	Whole virus	HA[c]		++++	+
SRH	Ferret (infection)	Whole virus	HA		+	++++
	Guinea pig (infection)	Whole virus	HA		+	++
NI	Chicken (single injection)	Whole virus	NA[c]		++	++
	Ferret (infection)	Whole virus	NA[c]		++++	++
	Rabbit (hyperimmune)	Whole virus	NA[c]		++++	+
SRD		Not recommended as routine procedure				
CF	Guinea pig (injection)	Whole virus "v"	HA/NA			+
	Anti-NP	CAM extract "s"	NP	+		
IDD	Anti-HA	Disrupted virus	HA		++++	++
	Anti-NA	Disrupted virus	NA		++++	++
	Anti-NP	Disrupted virus	NP	+		
	Anti-M	Disrupted virus	M	+		

[a] HI, hemagglutination inhibition; SRH, single radial hemolysis; NI, neuraminidase inhibition; CF, complement fixation; SRD, single radial immunodiffusion; IDD, immuno double diffusion; HA, hemagglutinin; NA, neuraminidase; NP, nucleoprotein; M, matrix protein; CAM, chorioallantoic membrane.

[b] The usefulness of the test for the indicated purpose is expressed on a scale of + (least useful) to ++++ (most useful).

[c] Serum containing high antibody titer to the second surface antigen (HA or NA) may in low dilutions and under certain conditions cause inhibition, presumably through steric hindrance. Test specificity achieved by selecting viruses or recombinant viruses with the required antigenic composition.

a. Antibody to Internal Components.   Since the influenza internal nucleo-proteins and matrix proteins do not undergo antigenic variation, serologic tests with these antigens are often considered useful when a virus emerges with a totally new complement of surface antigens. The need for tests to meet such an emergency is infrequent. Historically, the surface antigens of most new subtypes are characterized quickly, and reference strains are distributed rapidly and widely.

The major advantage of testing for antibody to the antigenically stable internal proteins is that fewer test antigens are required. Tests for NP antibody are particularly advantageous for those laboratories conducting routine CF tests for a variety of other respiratory diseases. One procedure can be used satisfactorily to detect antibody rises to multiple agents. The immuno double diffusion (IDD) test with NP antigen has proved useful for screening animal sera for evidence of infections which may have been associated with numerous known or unknown influenza viruses.

Serologic tests for nucleoprotein (NP) antibody have been used widely for diagnosis of human influenza ever since the original description of the influenza CF test by Fairbrother and Hoyle (1937). Early tests were generally performed with crude preparations of infected mouse lung, infected embryonated chick lung, or infected chorioallantoic membrane without regard to exact antigenic content. In more recent years the CF test has been performed with partially purified and concentrated NP antigen (Lief and Henle, 1959).

A precise value is difficult to assign for sensitivity of the NP CF test for serodiagnosis, but after years of experience by numerous laboratories several general conclusions can be drawn. Antibody response to NP at the time of initial infection in childhood is usually poor, occurs infrequently, and may disappear rapidly over a period of weeks or months. Later, in childhood and young adulthood, antibody response is rapid, occurs frequently, and tends to persist somewhat longer. After multiple infections in older adults, titers tend to persist at higher levels for longer periods of time and are less likely to show significant increases as a result of reinfection. These are only general impressions; actual titers and responses to infection can vary considerably with each individual.

In spite of early reports (Rosenbaum and Woolridge, 1956), the CF test for NP antibody has not proved to be a reliable index for distinguishing hemagglutinin antibody rises produced by infection from those produced by vaccination (Rapmund *et al.*, 1959). Some inactivated vaccines are quite efficient in stimulating NP antibody rises, especially vaccines prepared by disruption of the virus (Tauraso, 1972), and some infections fail to cause a rise.

There has been relatively little experience reported with single radial immunodiffusion for detecting diagnostic rises to the NP antigen, but recent studies with detergent-disrupted virus suggest that the test may be slightly more sensitive than CF (see below).

Diagnostic rises in NP antibody after infection can also be determined by immuno double diffusion tests (Styk *et al.,* 1968; Beard, 1970). The major disadvantage to this procedure is the inability to quantitate changes in antibody content precisely. However, in the studies of Schild *et al.* (1971), it was found to be as sensitive as conventional methods of serodiagnosis. The IDD is the test of choice for the examination of avian sera since they do not fix complement.

Tests for the M antigen have not been thoroughly investigated. SRD results with detergent-disrupted virus suggest that rises in matrix antibody in human sera occur only infrequently and may be associated with the severity of the disease (G. C. Schild, unpublished results).

b. Antibody to Surface Antigens.   Serodiagnosis by tests for antibody to surface antigens, unlike antibody to the internal antigens, may indicate, within broad limits, the probable infecting virus strain. However, rarely is more than one antigenic subtype or its closely related variant in circulation at any given time in a geographic location. This is particularly true for type A. Type B epidemics are frequently associated with strains exhibiting minor antigenic differences, but the magnitude of differences is such that differentiation of infecting strains by relative increases in antibody titer is usually not possible. In addition, rises in antibody to surface antigens are not always restricted to the infecting strain.

Anamnestic responses to earlier strains frequently occur, depending upon the previous immunologic experiences of the individual. In many instances antibody to a previous strain may increase at a faster rate and exceed the titer to the infecting strain. This was commonly observed after Hong Kong (H3N2) virus infection even with such remotely related antigen as those of the H2 hemagglutinin (Coleman and Dowdle, 1969; Satz *et al.,* 1970). Diagnostic efficiency can often be increased by including in the HI or strain-specific CF test strains recently prevalent as well as those currently prevalent.

Information as to the prevalence and titer of antibody against the surface antigens of contemporary strains is, of course, important for assessment of previous antigenic experience in the community and probable immunity to the current strain. This is discussed in Section V,B. The two possible advantages of serodiagnosis by assay for antibody to surface antigens are simplicity and sensitivity. At present, neither of these advantages applies to tests for antibody to the neuraminidase. The NI test is cumbersome and time consuming and is not suitable for testing the large number of sera usually encountered in diagnostic studies. The N-IHA, the N-HI, and the SRD offer the advantage of simplicity, but the sensitivity of these tests for diagnosis, as well as that of the NI test, has not been thoroughly evaluated.

Preliminary studies with the N-IHA, N-HI, and NI tests (Holston and Dowdle, 1973) indicate that the sensitivity of all three tests is somewhat less than for HI used for serodiagnosis. The N-IHA test was the most sensitive of the three, with 83% of the HI-positive paired sera demonstrating N-IHA antibody rises. The relative insensitivity of diagnostic tests for rises in neuraminidase antibody may be characteristic for that antigen. Kilbourne *et al.* (1968b) noted that whereas neuraminidase antibody frequently rose in response to infection, this was not a consistent event. Davenport *et al.* (1970) observed that antibody response after first exposure to the new neuraminidase N2 antigen was poor or nonexistent. Only after reinfection with a virus possessing a closely related neuraminidase was the antibody titer consistently elevated. The percentage of infected individuals showing diagnostic rises in antibody to the N2 (1957) antigen rose progressively from 3% after the Asian epidemic in 1957 to 96% in 1968. The low level of sensitivity from 1957 to 1966 may be related to the use of the N-HI test, but studies with the N-IHA and NI tests (W. R. Dowdle *et al.* unpublished results) tend to support Davenport's findings.

The HI test for antibody to the hemagglutinin has the advantages of both simplicity and sensitivity and, consequently, is one of the most commonly used procedures for serodiagnosis. The major disadvantage of the HI test is the required treatment of sera for removal of nonspecific inhibitors. To some extent this can be avoided by the selection of inhibitor-resistant test strains, but such strains may also have reduced sensitivity to antibody (Choppin and Tamm, 1960). The strain-specific CF test has been proposed as an alternate for assay of hemagglutinin antibody to avoid the problems of nonspecific inhibitors (Lief and Henle, 1959), but the advantage of simplicity offered by the HI test is then lost. Tests for hemagglutinin antibody that use SRD are also unaffected by the presence of nonspecific inhibitors. Present studies suggest that this test with selected recombinant antigens may under some conditions be a reasonable alternative to the HI (G. C. Schild, unpublished results).

The HI test for hemagglutinin antibodies may be more sensitive for serodiagnosis than the CF test for NP antibodies (Coleman and Dowdle, 1969), or it may be less so (Kalter *et al.*, 1959). In the first report 92% were detected by HI and 78% by CF. In the second, 67% were detected by HI and 89% by CF. Others also found that during the Hong Kong outbreak in 1968, the CF test for antibody to surface antigen was more sensitive for serodiagnosis than tests for antibody to the NP (Satz *et al.*, 1970). In the first two reports, approximately 10% of the positives would have been missed if only the more sensitive test had been used. The superiority of one of these tests over the other depends largely upon the age and previous antigenic experience of the individual, the strain used in the HI test, and the interval between drawing the acute and convalescent sera. Because all of these variables are interrelated, we recommend that both tests be used in parallel for maximum diagnostic efficiency.

Even when both serologic tests are used, diagnosis cannot always be assured. Figures vary widely, but a small percentage of subjects may be ill and shed virus but yet fail to respond with significant increases in antibody detectable by conventional serologic tests (Rapmund et al., 1959; Satz et al., 1970).

The results of direct comparisons of HI, CF and various applications of SRD tests (to detect antibody to HA, NA and NP) in seroepidemiological and serodiagnostic studies are further discussed in Section V,B.

2. UNPAIRED SERA

The diagnosis of influenza in an individual requires isolation of the virus and/or a rise in influenza antibody titer between the time the acute and convalescent sera are drawn. Isolation of the virus may require a week or longer. Serodiagnosis requires a minimum of 2 to 3 weeks for collection of paired sera. A diagnosis of an influenza outbreak, however, may be made in 24 hours by using groups of acute and convalescent sera collected from different individuals (Milstone et al., 1946; Grist et al., 1961). The principle of this test is based on the observation that by the time the presence of an outbreak is recognized, a number of persons in the community usually are already convalescent from the illness and a number of other persons are in the early acute stages. Ten or more acute specimens and ten or more convalescent specimens can usually be collected. Because influenza antibody titers may vary according to the age of the individual, persons in the acute and convalescent groups should be matched as closely as possible with respect to age and vaccination history.

Any acceptable serologic test may be performed. Geometric mean titers (GMT) are calculated for the acute and convalescent groups. If the GMT of antibody of the convalescent group is significantly greater (i.e., fourfold for HI or CF, 20% for SRID) than that of the acute group, then a diagnosis can be made. If the differences are less, then a statistical test for significance should be undertaken (Center for Disease Control, 1968). The cause of the outbreak should be confirmed when specimens for virus isolation or acute and convalescent serum pairs become available.

B. Seroepidemiological Surveys

The object of seroepidemiologic surveys is to test representative collections of sera for influenza antibodies in order to derive data on the epidemiological behavior of past and current influenza viruses and the immune status of the population. In such surveys HI tests and CF tests for antibody to NP antigen have been most widely applied. The former test is of value since it detects antibody which is subtype or strain specific and which is relevant as an index of the immune status of the population as well as of exposure. In contrast CF tests are type specific and are relevant to detecting evidence of exposure to infection rather than immunity. While antibody detected by HI tests is long lived, antibodies detected by CF are relatively short lived and usually indicate recent infection. Both HI and CF tests are of value but suffer to some extent from the practical disadvantages of being time consuming, requiring serial dilutions of test sera, and being subject to a number of nonspecific factors.

SRD techniques offer a simple and rapid procedure for assaying sera for antibody to the surface or internal antigens of influenza viruses. In addition immunoplates containing intact or disrupted influenza viruses in airtight chambers (e.g., Hyland immunoplates) are stable and can be transported readily between laboratories by ordinary mail. These methods are thus of considerable value in performing large-scale international surveys of influenza, and studies employing these procedures are in progress. One advantage is that standardized immunoplates prepared in a single center may be used for serological surveys in many countries, thus eliminating variations from laboratory to laboratory which are inevitably the case with HI and CF tests; also surveys may be carried out in areas where laboratory facilities are not available. An additional advantage is that very small volumes of serum or even whole blood obtained by finger puncture may be used in surveys.

SRD tests for antibody to the surface and internal antigens have been evaluated in a number of laboratories for sensitivity as seroepidemiological and serodiagnostic tools.

In surveys with human sera it was shown (Chakraverty et al., 1974) that SRDT with intact viruses in the gel was of comparable sensitivity to HI tests in detecting antibody. Sera with HI titers of 20 or greater in general produced opalescent zones of 2.5 mm diameter or more. However, in a small proportion of sera discrepancies in the results of HI and SRDT were observed. Seven percent of sera gave positive reactions on HI but not SRDT, and 4% gave responses in SRD but not HI tests.

Table 11.9 shows a summary of the results of testing acute and convalescent serum samples from persons with suspected A/Hong Kong/1/68 infections on immunoplates containing intact A/Hong Kong/68 virus (for the detection of anti-HA and anti-NA antibodies) and on plates containing disrupted avian influenza A virus (to detect antibodies to NP and M). Serological evidence of infection was clearly demonstrated by the acquisition or increase in areas of reaction zones in one or.both test systems. An increase

Table 11.9 Comparisons of Conventional Diagnostic Tests (HI and CF) and SRD Methods in the Serodiagnosis of Infection in Suspected Cases of (Clinical) Influenza due to A/Hong Kong/1/68 Virus

Number of serum pairs tested	Number and percent of individuals with diagnostic (at least 4-fold) antibody rises by conventional diagnostic tests		Number and percent of individuals with significant antibody (20% or greater increase in zone area) in SRD tests with stated antigens				
	CF tests[a]	HI tests[b]	NP[c]	HA, NA or both[d]	HA + NA	HA only[e]	NA only[f]
150	55 (37%)	80 (53%)	75 (50%)[a]	86 (57%)	75 (50%)	6 (7%)[h]	5 (5.8%)[h]

[a] Complement-fixation tests employing A/PR8/34 soluble NP antigen in extracts of infected egg membranes.
[b] Standard HI tests (World Health Organization, 1953) employing 8 HA units of influenza virus.
[c] SRDT with disrupted avian influenza A virus in immunoplates (see Table 11.2).
[d] SRDT with intact A/Hong Kong/1/68 (X31) virus in immunoplates.
[e] SRDT with recombinant containing A/Hong Kong/1/68 HA and an irrelevant NA (see Table 11.2).
[f] SRDT with recombinant containing A/Hong Kong/1/68 NA and an irrelevant NA (see Table 11.2).
[g] Only 22 of 75 individuals (30%) with antibody rises to NP had detectable anti-M in the convalescent serum.
[h] Percentages expressed as proportion of sera showing SRDT rises in tests with intact A/Hong Kong/1/68 virus (HA and/or NA).

in area of 35% was considered to be significant of an antibody rise. SRD with intact virus was slightly more sensitive than conventional HI tests in the diagnosis of infections and was the most sensitive of all the tests included in the study. It is of interest that when these tests were carried out with recombinant influenza A viruses with irrelevant HA or NA antigens to detect antibody to each of these antigens independently, a proportion of infected individuals developed only anti-HA or anti-NA antibody and not both. The detection by SRD of antibody rises to the NP and M antigens was more sensitive than conventional CF tests with influenza "soluble" NP. SRD indicated that of infected individuals who developed antibody to NP only approximately 30% also developed unequivocal evidence of antibody to M. Studies by Mostow et al. (1974) and Molyneux et al. (1974) have shown SRD to be effective in detecting antibody rises occurring in recipients of inactivated or live influenza vaccines.

Tests which are most frequently used for serodiagnosis or seroepidemiologic surveys of influenza are summarized in Table 11.10.

Table 11.10 Summary of Tests for Influenza Serology[a]

Test	Test antigens	Antibody detected	Recommended use[b]	
			Sero-diagnosis	Serosurvey
IDD	Disrupted virus	HA, NA[c]	++	+
	Disrupted virus	NP, M[b]	++	+
CF	CAM extract "s"	NP	++	
	Whole virus "v"	HA, NA	+++	
HI	Whole virus	HA[c,d]	++++	++++
NI	Whole virus	NA[c,d]		++++
N-IHA	NA	NA		++++
SRD	Whole virus	HA, NA[c]	++++	+++
	Disrupted virus	NP, M[c]	+++	

[a] IDD, immuno double diffusion; CF, complement fixation; HI, hemagglutination inhibition; NI, neuraminidase inhibition; N-IHA, neuraminidase-indirect hemagglutination; SRD, single radial immunodiffusion; CAM, chorioallantoic membrane; HA, hemagglutinin; NA, neuraminidase; NP, nucleoprotein; M, matrix protein.

[b] The usefulness of the test for the indicated purpose is expressed on a scale of + (least useful) to ++++ (most useful).

[c] Test specificity achieved by selecting viruses or recombinant viruses with the required antigenic composition.

[d] Serum containing high antibody titer to the second surface antigen (HA or NA) may in low dilutions and under certain conditions cause inhibition, presumably through steric hindrance.

C. Secretory Antibody

Assay of influenza secretory antibody has been limited exclusively to vaccine evaluations and to studies on the immune secretory system. Because of the complexity of the assay procedure, secretory antibody has no immediate application for influenza diagnosis. The protein content of nasal washings, unlike that of serum, may vary considerably depending upon the subject, the time of collection, and the technique used. In order for all specimens to be compared at the same immunoglobulin concentration, the washings should be concentrated and adjusted to the same IgA content as determined by radial immunodiffusion. The techniques for collection, treatment, and assay of secretory immunoglobulins have been extensively reviewed (Dayton *et al.*, 1969; Rossen *et al.*, 1971). Techniques for assay of influenza antibodies in nasal secretions are basically no different from those previously described for sera, except that IgA antibodies do not fix complement.

References

Ada, G. L., Lind, P. E., and Laver, W. G. (1963). *J. Gen. Microbiol.* **32**, 225.

Allan, W. H., Madeley, C. R., and Kendal, A. P. (1971). *J. Gen. Virol.* **12**, 79.

Aminoff, D. (1961). *Biochem. J.* **81**, 384.

Aymard-Henry, M., Coleman, M. T., Dowdle, W. R., Laver, W. G., Schild, G. C., and Webster, R. G. (1973). *Bull. W.H.O.* **48**, 199.

Beard, C. W. (1970). *Bull. W.H.O.* **42**, 779.

Berlin, B. S. (1963). *Proc. Soc. Exp. Biol. Med.* **113**, 1013.

Biddle, F., and Shortridge, K. F. (1967). *Brit. J. Exp. Pathol.* **48**, 285.

Bing, D. H., Weyand, J. G. M., and Stavitsky, A. B. (1967). *Proc. Soc. Exp. Biol. Med.* **124**, 1166.

Bradstreet, C. M. P., and Taylor, C. E. D. (1962). *Mon. Bull. Min. Health Pub. Health Lab. Serv.* **21**, 96.

Brakke, M. K. (1967). *In* "Methods in Virology" (K. Maramarosh and H. Kaprowski, eds.), Vol. 2, pp. 93–118. Academic Press, New York.

Brand, C. M., and Skehel, J. J. (1972). *Nature (London), New Biol.* **238**, 145.

Breitenfeld, P. M., and Schafer, W. (1957). *Virology* **4**, 328.

Brown, G. C., and O'Leary, T. P. (1971). *J. Immunol.* **107**, 1486.

Burnet, F. M., and Stone, J. D. (1947). *Aust. J. Exp. Biol. Med. Sci.* **25**, 227.

Center for Disease Control. (1968). "Influenza-Respiratory Disease Surveillance Report," No. 84, pp. 23–25. U.S. Public Health Service, Atlanta, Georgia.

Chakraverty, P. (1972). *Bull. W.H.O.* **46**, 473.

Chakraverty, P. M., Pereira, M. S., and Schild, G. C. (1973). *Bull. W.H.O.* **49**, 327.

Choppin, P. W., and Tamm, I. (1960). *J. Exp. Med.* **112**, 895.

Chu, C. M. (1951). *J. Gen. Microbiol.* **5,** 739.

Cohen, A., Newland, S. E., and Biddle, F. (1963). *Virology* **20,** 518.

Coleman, M. T., and Dowdle, W. R. (1969). *Bull. W.H.O.* **41,** 415.

Curry, R. L., Brown, J. D., Baker, F. A., and Hobson, D. (1974). *J. Hyg.* **72,** 197.

Daugharty, H. (1973). *J. Immunol.* **111,** 404.

Daugharty, H., Davis, M. L., and Kaye, H. S. (1972). *J. Immunol.* **109,** 849.

Davenport, F. M., Minuse, E., and Hennessy, A. V. (1970). *Arch. Environ. Health* **21,** 307.

Dayton, D. H., Small, P. A., Chanock, R. M., Kaufman, H. E., and Tomasi, T. B., eds. (1969). "The Secretory Immunologic System." U.S. Dept. of Health, Education and Welfare, and Public Health Service, NIH, Bethesda, Maryland.

de Silva, L. M., and Tobin, J. O'H. (1973). *J. Med. Microbiol.* **6,** 15.

Dimmock, N. J. (1969). *Virology* **39,** 224.

Dobrovolsky, M. G. (1971). *J. Hyg., Epidemiol., Microbiol., Immunol.* **15,** 148.

Dowdle, W. R., and Coleman, M. T. (1974). *In* "Manual of Clinical Microbiology" (E. H. Lennette, E. H. Spaulding, and J. P. Truant, eds.), p. 678. Amer. Soc. Microbiol., Washington, D.C.

Dowdle, W. R., Coleman, M. T., Hall, E. C., and Knez, V. (1969). *Bull. W.H.O.* **41,** 419.

Dowdle, W. R., Sarateanu, D., and Reimer, C. B., (1972). *J. Immunol.* **109,** 1321.

Dowdle, W. R., Downie, J. C., and Laver, W. G. (1974). *J. Virol.* **13,** 269.

Dowdle, W. R., Galphin, J. C., Coleman, M. T., and Schild, G. C. (1975). *Bull. W.H.O.* (in press).

Downie, J. C. (1970). *J. Immunol.* **105,** 620.

Easterday, B., Laver, W. G., Pereira, H. G., and Schild, G. C. (1969). *J. Gen. Virol.* **5,** 83.

Eddy, B. E. (1947). *J. Immunol.* **57,** 195.

Fairbrother, R. W., and Hoyle, L. (1937). *J. Pathol. Bacteriol.* **44,** 213.

Fazekas de St. Groth, S. (1962). *Advan. Virus Res.* **9,** 1.

Fazekas de St. Groth, S. (1967). *Cold Spring Harbor Symp. Quant. Biol.* **32,** 525.

Fazekas de St. Groth, S., and Webster, R. G. (1964). *Cell. Biol. Myxovirus Infec., Ciba Found. Symp., 1964* pp. 246–271.

Fazekas de St. Groth, S., and White, D. O. (1958). *J. Hyg.* **56,** 151.

Francis, T. (1947). *J. Exp. Med.* **85,** 1.

Francis, T., Jr. (1953). *Ann. Intern. Med.* **39,** 203.

Glick, T. H., Likosky, W. H., Levitt, L. P., Mellin, H., and Reynolds, D. W. (1970). *Pediatrics* **46,** 371.

Grist, N. R., Kerr, J., and Isaacs, B. (1961). *Brit. Med. J.* **2,** 431.

Hahon, N., Booth, J. A., and Eckert, H. L. (1972). *Appl. Microbiol.* **23,** 485.

Hanna, L., and Hoyle, L. (1966). *Acta Virol. (Prague)* **10,** 506.

Harboe, A. (1963). *Acta Pathol. Microbiol. Scand.* **57,** 317.

Haukenes, G., Harboe, A., and Mortensson-Egmund, K. (1965). *Acta Pathol. Microbiol. Scand.* **64,** 534.

Hennessy, A. V., and Davenport, F. M. (1972). *Appl. Microbiol.* **23,** 827.

Heyward, J. T., Coleman, M. T., and Dowdle, W. R. (1972). *Proc. Soc. Exp. Biol. Med.* **140,** 1289.

Hierholzer, J. C., Suggs, M. T., and Hall, E. C. (1969). *Appl. Microbiol.* **18,** 824.

Hirst, G. K. (1941). *Science* **94**, 22.

Hirst, G. K. (1942). *J. Exp. Med.* **75**, 47.

Holston, J. L., and Dowdle, W. R. (1973). *Appl. Microbiol.* **25**, 97.

Hoyle, L., and Fairbrother, C. (1937). *J. Hyg.* **37**, 512.

Isaacs, A., Gledhill, A. W., and Andrews, C. H. (1952). *Bull. W.H.O.* **6**, 287.

Jahiel, R. I., and Kilbourne, E. D. (1966). *J. Bacteriol.* **92**, 1521.

Johnson, P. B., and Grayson, J. T. (1961). *J. Infec. Dis.* **108**, 19.

Kalter, S. S., Casey, H. L., Jensen, K. E., Robinson, R. Q., and Gorrie, R. H. (1959). *Proc. Soc. Exp. Biol. Med.* **100**, 367.

Kasel, J. A., Couch, R. B., Gerin, J. L., and Schulman, J. L. (1973). *Infec. Immunity* **8**, 130.

Kaye, H. S., Dowdle, W. R., and McQueen, J. L. (1969). *Amer. J. Epidemiol.* **90**, 162.

Kendal, A. P., and Madeley, C. R. (1969). *Biochim. Biophys. Acta* **185**, 163.

Kendal, A. P., Minuse, E., and Davenport, F. M. (1972) *Z. Naturforsch.* **27**, 241.

Kilbourne, E. D. (1968). *Science* **160**, 74.

Kilbourne, E. D., and Horsfall, F. L. (1951). *J. Immunol.* **67**, 431.

Kilbourne, E. D., Laver, W. G., Schulman, J. L., and Webster, R. G. (1968a). *J. Virol.* **2**, 281.

Kilbourne, E. D., Christenson, W. N., and Sands, M. (1968b). *J. Virol.* **2**, 761.

Knight, C. A. (1944). *J. Exp. Med.* **80**, 83.

Lafferty, K. J. (1963). *Virology* **21**, 76.

Laver, W. G. (1964). *J. Mol. Biol.* **9**, 109.

Laver, W. G., and Kilbourne, E. D. (1966). *Virology* **30**, 493.

Laver, W. G., and Webster, R. G. (1966). *Virology* **30**, 104.

Laver, W. G., Downie, J., and Webster, R. G. (1974). *Virology* **59**, 230.

Lennette, E. H., and Horsfall, F. L. (1940). *J. Exp. Med.* **72**, 233.

Lief, F. S., and Henle, W. (1959). *Bull. W.H.O.* **20**, 411.

Liu, C. (1955). *J. Exp. Med.* **101**, 675.

Liu, C. (1969). *In* "Diagnostic Procedures for Viral and Rickettsial Infections" (E. H. Lenette, ed.), p. 179. Amer. Pub. Health Ass., New York.

McClelland, L., and Hare, R. (1941). *Can. Pub. Health J.* **32**, 530.

Madeley, C. R., Allan, W. H., and Kendal, A. P. (1971). *J. Gen. Virol.* **12**, 69.

Mancini, G., Carbonara, A. O., and Heremans, J. F. (1965). *Immunochemistry* **2**, 235.

Miller, G. L., and Stanley, W. M. (1944). *J. Exp. Med.* **79**, 185.

Milstone, J. H., Lindberg, R. B., Bayliss, B. M., DeCoursey, E., and Berk, M. E. (1946). *Mil. Surg.* **99**, 777.

Molyneux, M. E., Beare, A. S., Callow, K., and Schild, G. C. (1974). *J. Hyg.* (in press).

Mostow, S., Schild, G. C., Dowdle, W. R., and Wood, R. J. (1975). In preparation.

Noll, H., Aoyagi, T., and Orlando, J. (1962). *Virology* **18**, 154.

Oxford, J. S., and Schild, G. C. (1974). *In* "The Biology of Large RNA Viruses" (R. D. Barry and B. W. J. Mahy, eds.). Academic Press, New York (in press).

Paniker, C. K. J. (1968). *J. Gen. Virol.* **2**, 385.

Pepper, D. S. (1968). *Biochim. Biophys. Acta* **156**, 317.

Pereira, H. G. (1969). *Progr. Med. Virol.* **11**, 46.

Pereira, H. G., Machado, R., and Schild, G. C. (1972). *J. Immunol. Methods* **2**, 121.

Pereira, M. S. (1958). *Lancet* **2**, 668.

Rafelson, M. E., Schnier, M., and Wilson, V. W. (1963). *Arch. Biochem. Biophys.* **103**, 424.

Rapmund, G., Johnson, R. T., Bankhead, A. S., Herrman, Y. F., and Dandridge, O. W. (1959). *U.S. Armed Forces Med. J.* **10**, 637.

Rosenbaum, M. J., and Woolridge, R. L. (1956). *J. Infec. Dis.* **99**, 275.

Rossen, R. D., Kasel, J. A., and Couch, R. B. (1971). *Progr. Med. Virol.* **13**, 194.

Rott, R., Becht, H., and Orlich, M. (1974). *J. Gen. Virol.* **22**, 35.

Salk, J. E. (1944). *J. Immunol.* **49**, 87.

Satz, J., Prier, J. E., Riley, R., Schroek, W. D., Hrehorovich, V., and Deardorff, J. (1970). *Amer. J. Pub. Health* **60**, 2197.

Schild, G. C. (1970). *J. Gen. Virol.* **9**, 191.

Schild, G. C. (1972). *J. Gen. Virol.* **15**, 99.

Schild, G. C., and Newman, R. W. (1969). *Bull. W.H.O.* **41**, 437.

Schild, G. C., and Pereira, H. G. (1969). *J. Gen. Virol.* **4**, 355.

Schild, G. C., Winters, W. D., and Brand, C. M. (1971). *Bull. W.H.O.* **45**, 465.

Schild, G. C., Aymard-Henry, M., and Pereira, H. G. (1972a). *J. Gen. Virol.* **16**, 231.

Schild, G. C., Brand, C. M., Harkness, J. W., and Lamont, P. H. (1972b). *Bull. W.H.O.* **46**, 721.

Schild, G. C., Aymard-Henry, M., Chakraverty, P. M., Pereira, M. S., Dowdle, W. R., Coleman, M. T., and Change, W. K. (1973a). *Bull W.H.O.* **48**, 269.

Schild, G. C., Berryman, I. L., Pereira, H. G., and Aymard-Henry, M. (1973b). *Symp. Immunochem. Stand.* **20**, 39.

Schild, G. C., Pereira, H. G., Rothwell, D., and Berryman, I. L. (1974a). "Proceedings of the International Conference on Standardization of Diagnostic Materials," p. 243. Center for Disease Control, Atlanta, Georgia.

Schild, G. C., Virelizier, J. L., and Oxford, J. S. (1974b). *J. Gen. Virol.* (in press).

Schild, G. C., Virelizier, J. L., and Oxford, J. S. (1974c). *Proc. Miles Symp. Immunol., 8th,* 1974. In press

Schoyen, R., Harboe, A., and Wang, L. (1966). *Acta Pathol. Microbiol. Scand.* **68**, 103.

Schulman, J. L., and Kilbourne, E. D. (1969). *Proc. Nat. Acad. Sci. U.S.* **63**, 326.

Schulman, J. M., Khakpour, M., and Kilbourne, E. D. (1968). *J. Virol.* **2**, 778.

Seto, J. T., and Rott, R. (1966). *Virology* **30**, 731.

Shelokov, A., Vogel, J. E., and Chi, L. (1958). *Proc. Soc. Exp. Biol. Med.* **97**, 802.

Shimojo, H., Sugiura, A., Akao, T., and Enomoto, (1958). *Bull. Inst. Pub. Health, Tokyo* **7**, 219.

Shortridge, K. F., and Lansdell, A. (1972). *Microbios* **6**, 213.

Skehel, J. J. (1971). *Virology* **44**, 409.

Skehel, J. J. (1973). *Virology* **56**, 394.

Skehel, J. J., and Schild, G. C. (1971). *Virology* **44**, 396.

Styk, B., and Hanna, L. (1966). *Acta Virol. (Prague)* **10**, 281.

Styk, B., Hanna, L., and Sedilekova, M. (1968). *Acta Virol. (Prague)* **12**, 208.

Tauraso, N. (1972). *J. Infec. Dis.* **126**, 219.

Tobita, K., and Kilbourne, E. D. (1974). *J. Virol.* **13**, 347.

Tumova, B., and Easterday, B. C. (1969). *Bull. W.H.O.* **41**, 429.

Tumova, B., and Schild, G. C. (1972). *Bull. W.H.O.* **47,** 453.

United States Public Health Service. (1965). *U.S., Pub. Health Serv., Publ.* **1228.**

Van der Veen, J., and Mulder, J. (1950). *Onderz. Meded. Inst. Praev. Geneesk* No. 6.

Virelizier, J. L., Schild, G. C., and Allison, A. C. (1974). *J. Exp. Med.* **140,** 1559.

Warren, L. (1959). *J. Biol. Chem.* **234,** 1971.

Webster, R. G. (1968). *Immunology* **14,** 39.

Webster, R. G. (1970). *Virology* **42,** 633.

Webster, R. G., and Laver, W. G. (1967). *J. Immunol.* **99,** 49.

Webster, R. G., and Laver, W. G. (1972). *Virology* **48,** 433.

Webster, R. G., Laver, W. G., and Kilbourne, E. D. (1968). *J. Gen. Virol.* **3,** 315.

Weinberger, H. L., Buescher, E. L., and Edwards, V. M. (1965). *J. Immunol.* **94,** 47.

World Health Organization. (1953). *World Health Organ., Tech. Rep. Ser.* **64.**

World Health Organization. (1959). *World Health Organ., Tech. Rep. Ser.* **170,** 45.

World Health Organization. (1971). *Bull. W.H.O.* **45,** 119.

Ziegler, D. W., and Hutchinson, H. D. (1972). *Appl. Microbiol.* **23,** 1060.

12

Immunology of Influenza

J. L. Schulman

I. Introduction

Despite 40 years of extensive laboratory research and almost an equivalent period during which vaccines against influenza have been evaluated in human subjects, enormous gaps in our understanding of immune mechanisms in influenza persist. To a great extent, these deficiencies in our knowledge are a direct consequence of the unique and perplexing capacity of influenza virus for periodic major antigenic changes in its envelope glycoproteins (see Chapters 10 and 15). As new strains containing novel surface antigens appear, immunity that is dependent on antibodies directed to antigens contained in older strains is circumvented and pandemic disease results. Conversely, the presence of high titers of antibody to older strains in the sera and respiratory secretions of the majority of the population undoubtedly favors the emergence to predominance of novel strains once they appear.

A second area of uncertainty concerns whether immunity in influenza is mediated primarily by serum antibody or by secretory IgA antibody in the respiratory tract, and without precise knowledge of the relative importance of each it has been difficult to define the optimal method for immunization against influenza (see Kilbourne *et al.*, 1973, for review).

Finally, little is known about the role of immune mechanisms in *recovery* from influenza. Although there is an enormous body of evidence demonstrating that prior infection, active immunization with inactivated virus or passive administration of antibody prevents or modifies subsequent infection with antigenically related virus, the passive administration of antibody after infection has been established does not modify disease (Francis, 1941). However, there is insufficient evidence at present to permit an assessment of the contribution made by cell-mediated immune mechanisms in the process of recovery.

II. Expressions of Immunity

The definitive expression of antiviral immunity is the capacity of the immunized host to inhibit replication of the invading virus and consequently to prevent virus-induced disease. Operationally, immunity may function by preventing the initiation of infection under circumstances of exposure in which infection is likely, or alternatively, by sufficiently inhibiting or anatomically restricting virus replication after infection has occurred to prevent or modify illness. A third expression of immunity is observed in the protection afforded nonimmune individuals in a population by the presence of large numbers of immune people in the same population. Herd immunity requires that immune subjects are less likely to become part of the epidemic chain of infection and hence to serve as a source of infection for other (nonimmune) individuals. Such a requirement is met if the immune response reduces susceptibility to the acquisition of infection or modifies the infection in a manner that lessens the likelihood of subsequent transmission. In contrast, immune mechanisms that modify disease but do not prevent infection or its subsequent transmission have no effect on the epidemiology of disease in the nonimmune population. Immunity resulting from prior infection or immunization with inactivated influenza virus has been shown to produce all three effects: decreased susceptibility to the acquisition of infection, modified disease, and decreased risk of disease among nonimmune individuals in the same population.

A. Decreased Susceptibility to the Acquisition of Infection

Numerous epidemiologic studies have provided abundant evidence that individuals with hemagglutinating inhibiting (HI) antibody in their sera are not as likely as nonimmune individuals to become infected during influenza epidemics, as demonstrated by a lower proportion showing fourfold or greater antibody rise (Commission on Influenza, 1943; Davenport, 1961, review). For example, in an influenza outbreak among military recruits, Farník and Bruj (1966) found that 98% of men with initial HI antibody titers below 1:8 had a fourfold or greater rise in titer during the epidemic, whereas only 6.3% of men with initial titers of 1:64 or greater had serologic evidence of infection. In a similar study in a children's home, Moffet *et al.* (1964) found that fourfold or greater rises in antibody titers were observed in 70% of children with initial titers of less than 1:10, in 41% of those with titers of 1:10–1:40, and in 2.4% of children with initial titers of 1:80 or greater. Similar evidence has been obtained from carefully controlled experimental infection of volunteers (Francis *et al.,* 1944; Henle *et al.,* 1946; Alford *et al.,* 1966; Morris *et al.,* 1966). Moreover, the relationship of serum antibody titers and resistance to challenge infection does not depend on whether the antibody derives from prior infection or subcutaneous immunization with inactivated virus (McDonald *et al.,* 1962; Andrews *et al.,* 1966; Beare *et al.,* 1968). Figure 12.1 summarizes cumulative experience in England with influenza A and B virus challenge in volunteers, and in both cases demonstrates an inverse linear relationship (over a wide range) between prior levels of serum HI antibody and the likelihood of becoming infected following experimental challenge.

A similar relationship repeatedly has been demonstrated in experimental studies in mice where it also has been shown that the concentration of virus needed to initiate infection increases in direct proportion to the dose of inactivated virus used for immunization (Fig. 12.2, Schulman and Kilbourne, 1971).

B. Modified Infection

In addition to reducing the risk of acquiring infection, the prior possession of antibody to surface antigens of influenza virus has been shown by an impressive body of evidence to be associated with less severe disease if infection does occur (see Davenport, 1961, for review). In experimental animals,

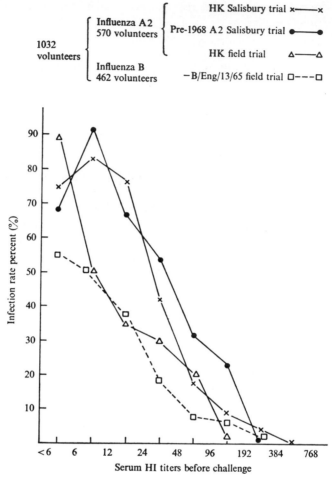

Fig. 12.1. Infection rate of volunteers challenged with various influenza viruses in relation to their prechallenge titers or homologous serum HI antibody. From Hobson *et al.* (1973). *J. Hyg., Camb.* Copyright 1973 Cambridge University Press. Reproduced by permission.

this increased resistance is expressed by lower pulmonary virus titers, decreased lung lesions, and lower mortality following challenge. Figure 12.3 illustrates the course of infection in unimmunized mice and animals injected 4 weeks previously with a small dose of inactivated virus, following challenge with a sufficient dose of aerosolized virus to infect all animals in both groups. It is evident that immunization was associated with lower peak virus titers, more rapid disappearance of virus from the lungs, less extensive pulmonary disease, and a heightened antibody response following infection.

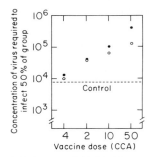

Fig. 12.2. Effect of graded doses of Aichi (○) and X-31 (●) vaccines on the quantity of virus required to infect 50% of mice by aerosol. Modified from Schulman and Kilbourne (1971).

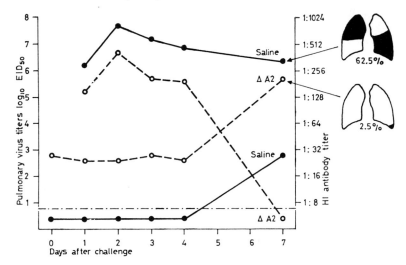

Fig. 12.3. Effect of intraperitoneal immunization of mice with formalin inactivated A/Japan/304/57 (H3N2) virus on pulmonary virus titers, lung lesions, and antibody response after homotypic challenge. From Schulman (1970).

Similar observations have been made in human subjects infected during epidemics or by experimental challenge. For example in the same study of military recruits referred to previously, not only was serological evidence of infection inversely related to prior serum antibody levels, but among those with proven infection, the incidence of febrile illness was likewise inversely related to antibody titers (Farník and Bruj, 1966). Similarly, in a study of the effects of vaccine in a group of volunteers experimentally challenged with Aichi(H3N2) virus, Couch *et al.* (1971) found that among subjects with documented infection, the incidence of illness was considerably reduced among those who had been immunized.

C. Effects of Immunity on Transmission

The effects of immunity on spread of infection to nonimmune members of a population (herd immunity) have not been studied nearly as extensively as have its effects on infection and disease. However, the limited data available from laboratory studies and epidemiologic observations suggest that at least under some circumstances, immune mechanisms may profoundly influence transmission.

Immunized volunteers have been shown to be less readily infected (Couch *et al.*, 1971), and if infected to shed lower quantities of virus in their nasal secretions than control subjects following experimental challenge (Couch *et al.*, 1971, 1974). Presumably if a large enough proportion of any population is immune, spread of influenza among nonimmune individuals is reduced both by a decrease in the total number of susceptibles in the population and by reduced transmission by immune people who are infected. Evidence that these effects actually may be operative during natural epidemics of influenza was provided by Monto *et al.* (1969) and is illustrated in Fig. 12.4. These investigators conducted a mass immunization program among school age children in Tecumseh, Michigan in advance of the outbreak of Hong Kong influenza in 1968–1969. The incidence of respiratory disease during the ensuing epidemic was lower in Tecumseh than in Adrian, a nearby community of comparable size and demographic composition in which no immunization program was carried out. Moreover, when respiratory illness was examined with respect to age-specific rates, it was noted

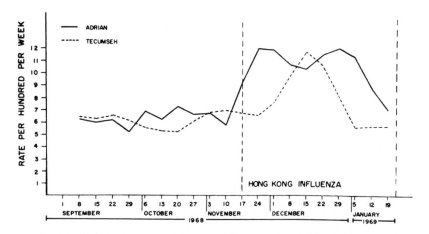

Fig. 12.4. Effect of mass immunization of school children with influenza vaccine on the incidence of the respiratory illness in a community. Tecumseh, immunization program; Adrian, control population. From Monto *et al.* (1969).

that the greatest differences were found in illness rates of persons aged 20–30 in the 2 communities, suggesting that immunization of children in Tecumseh appreciably lowered the incidence of influenza among the parents of that community. Data obtained from this experiment support the hypothesis advanced by Francis (1967) suggesting that mass immunization of children, in whom influenza epidemics generally begin, might diminish the intensity of epidemics in the general population.

III. Immune Responses Mediated by Antibody Specific for Hemagglutinin and Antibody Specific for Neuraminidase

For many years immunity to influenza had been considered to be the direct expression of effects mediated by antibody measured in hemagglutinin inhibition assays. With the recognition that influenza viruses contain 2 virus-coded glycoprotein antigens in their envelopes, attention was focused on attempts to segregate and independently study immune effects mediated by antibody to each of the 2 antigens. By employing antigenically hybrid recombinant strains (Chapters 7, 10, and 15) and isolated, purified proteins as antigens, the relative contributions to immunity made by the 2 kinds of antibody have been defined.

A. Antibody to Hemagglutinin

1. Resistance to Infection

It is clear in retrospect from an impressive body of evidence gathered over the past 40 years that antibody specifically directed toward the hemagglutinin of influenza viruses is capable of neutralizing the virus *in vitro* and of rendering an immune host less susceptible to acquisition of infection with virus containing the same hemagglutinin.

Experimental studies have demonstrated that mice immunized with a recombinant virus containing a hemagglutinin identical to that in the virus used for challenge, but a different neuraminidase, are as resistant to the acquisition of infection as mice immunized with virus containing both antigens (Schulman *et al.*, 1968).

2. Modified Disease

It is also evident that antibody specific for hemagglutinin can modify or prevent disease if infection does occur. Following challenge with large doses of virus, mice with antibody to hemagglutinin engendered by active or passive immunization have 100- to 1000-fold lower peak pulmonary virus titers than control animals and absent or markedly reduced lung lesions. Although comparable experiments have not yet been conducted in man, the close correlation of levels of serum HI antibody and reduced severity of disease in immune subjects infected with influenza virus, strongly suggest that antibody to hemagglutinin not only reduces the likelihood of infection but may prevent disease when infection does occur.

3. Transmission

The effects of antibody specific for hemagglutinin on transmission of influenza infection in man have not been clearly defined. It is obvious that individuals with HI antibody who are resistant to the acquisition of influenza virus infection cannot participate in the chain of infection; consequently, the risk of infection for other members of the population is reduced. However, it is not clear whether people with HI antibody; once infected, are less likely to transmit infection to others. On the one hand, it would seem likely that lower virus titers in such people would be accompanied by a lessened likelihood of spreading infection. However, the limited evidence bearing on this question derives from experiments in animals, and paradoxically indicates that mice immunized with inactivated virus or passively given antibody to hemagglutinin, if infected, are as effective in transmitting infection as unimmunized controls (Schulman, 1967).

4. Mechanism of Action of Antibody to Hemagglutinin

Antibody to hemagglutinin exerts its effects by preventing the attachment of virus to cells. As a result, viral infectivity *in ovo* or in cell culture is reduced. Presumably infection is prevented or modified in the intact host by a comparable neutralizing effect.

B. Antibody to Neuraminidase

1. Resistance to Infection

There is some controversy as to whether antibody specific for neuraminidase increases resistance to the acquisition of infection. In view of the fact that neuraminidase activity does not influence virus attachment or penetration (Chapter 4) it would seem unlikely that antibody to neuraminidase would be capable of preventing infection. This assumption is given support by the observation that extremely high concentrations of antibody to neuraminidase are required to neutralize virus *in ovo* or in cell culture (Kilbourne *et al.*, 1968). Furthermore, mice with passively or actively acquired antibody to the neuraminidase of a challenge virus are as readily infected as control animals (Schulman, 1970). Additional evidence to the same effect comes from studies with volunteers with varying levels of antibody to the neuraminidase of a challenge virus but none to its hemagglutinin. Following challenge, the frequency of laboratory confirmed infection was as high in subjects with antibody to neuraminidase as in volunteers with none (Murphy *et al.*, 1972; Couch *et al.*, 1974).

On the other hand, Monto and Kendal (1973) observed that during the 1968–1969 outbreak of Hong Kong influenza in a population lacking antibody to the hemagglutinin of the new virus, increasing titers of antibody to neuraminidase were associated with a lower incidence of serologically proven infection. It should be noted that although the differences in this study were statistically significant, the magnitude of the reduction of the infection rate in people with anti-neuraminidase antibody was considerably less than that which has been observed with antibody to hemagglutinin. In another study in which resistance to infection was assessed by discriminant analysis of infection rates and titers of hemagglutinin and neuraminidase antibody, resistance was most closely correlated with levels of antibody to neuraminidase (Slepushkin *et al.*, 1971). It is difficult to reconcile the differences in the results obtained in these various studies, but the preponderant evidence at present suggests that resistance to the initiation of infection is much more closely associated with antibody to hemagglutinin than with antibody to neuraminidase.

2. MODIFIED DISEASE

If the relationship of antibody to neuraminidase and resistance to initiation of infection remains controversial, its effects in modifying disease have been clearly demonstrated. In experimental animals, immunization with purified isolated neuraminidase is associated with reduction of pulmonary virus titer and less extensive lung lesions after challenge with virus containing the same neuraminidase (Schulman *et al.*, 1968). Moreover, passive immunization of mice with rabbit antiserum to neuraminidase produces identical effects, thus establishing that the increased resistance is mediated by specific antibody. Similar effects have been observed in human subjects with naturally acquired antibody to neuraminidase (Murphy *et al.*, 1972; Monto and Kendal, 1973), or in volunteers immunized with inactivated virus possessing the same neuraminidase antigen as that contained in the challenge virus, but a different hemagglutinin antigen (Couch *et al.*, 1974).

3. Transmission

As is the case with antibody to hemagglutinin, the effects of antibody to neuraminidase on transmission have not been extensively studied. Mice immunized passively with antibody to neuraminidase prior to experimental infection are less effective in transmitting infection to previously uninfected cagemates than unimmunized infectors. In contrast, as indicated above, animals immunized passively with antibody specific for hemagglutinin do not have a reduced capacity for transmission after experimental infection (Schulman, 1970).

As illustrated in Fig. 12.5, specific immunization of volunteers against the neuraminidase antigen of a challenge virus is associated with significantly lower titers of virus in nasal secretions following challenge (Couch *et al.*, 1974), but no comparable study has been made of the effects of antibody specific for hemagglutinin on virus excretion after infection.

4. Mechanism of Action of Antibody to Neuraminidase

There is still some uncertainty concerning the mechanism by which antibody to neuraminidase moderates influenza virus infection in the intact host. As the function of viral neuraminidase began to be elucidated (see Chapter 4) it was thought that specific antibody sterically blocked the access of neuraminidase to high molecular weight substrate at the cell surface, and hence

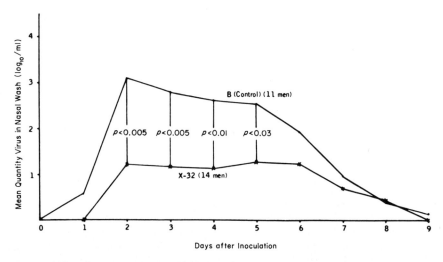

Fig. 12.5. Effect of neuraminidase-specific immunization with X-32 (Heq1N2) virus on quantity of virus shed in nasal wash specimens after infection of volunteers with H3N2 virus. From Couch *et al.* (1974).

interfered with the release of newly synthesized virus from the cell surface. Subsequently, experiments with univalent antibody cast doubt on this hypothesis, in that unlike bivalent antibody, concentrations of univalent antibody which inhibited neuraminidase *in vitro* had no demonstrable effect on virus release during single cycle replication (Becht *et al.*, 1971). As a consequence, it was suggested that antibody to neuraminidase does not influence virus replication by specific inhibition of viral neuraminidase activity, but binds virus to the cell surface by bridging antigenic sites on virus particles to similar sites on the cell membrane. However, in later experiments with univalent antibody, an effect on multicycle virus replication was observed (Kilbourne *et al.*, 1975), demonstrating that the effects of antibody to neuraminidase may be mediated at least in part by its effects on sialidase activity. Regardless of the relative importance of these 2 mechanisms, it is clear that antibody to neuraminidase does not block the attachment or penetration of virus into cells, but by either or both of the two mechanisms, discussed above, inhibits or delays the release of virus from infected cells and thereby prevents infection of adjacent cells.

C. Relative Importance of Antibody to Hemagglutinin and Antibody to Neuraminidase in Immunity

Table 12.1 summarizes currently prevalent assumptions regarding the specific effects of antibody to hemagglutinin and antibody to neuraminidase on influenza virus infection. It should be clear from the preceding discussion that the validity of some of these assumptions is far from definitively established, especially those concerning the effects of both kinds of antibody on transmission. However, from the mass of experimental and epidemiologic data available, several generalizations seem warranted.

In the first place, from a variety of different kinds of evidence, it seems abundantly clear that antibody to hemagglutinin provides a more powerful

Table 12.1 Effects of Antibody to Hemagglutinin and Antibody to Neuraminidase in Immunity to Influenza

	Specific antibody to	
Effect	Hemagglutinin	Neuraminidase
Prevention of infection	+	0
Modified illness	+	+
Herd immunity		
Fewer susceptibles	+	0
Decreased transmission	0	+

defense against influenza than antibody to neuraminidase. In experimental studies, animals possessing antibody only to the hemagglutinin of a challenge virus may resist infection, and if infected have far greater reductions in pulmonary virus titers than if the challenge virus contains only a neuraminidase antigen in common with the virus used for immunization. Convincing evidence also can be derived from naturally occurring outbreaks of epidemic influenza. With the appearance of Hong Kong influenza (H3N2) virus in 1968, man was confronted with a new variant containing a novel hemagglutinin antigen and a neuraminidase antigen similar to that present in viruses which had been prevalent for several years. Although the morbidity and the mortality of the ensuing pandemic were lower than in 1957–1958 when both surface antigens were new, widespread influenzal disease occurred in populations which had experienced repeated exposures to viruses with related neuraminidases. It is likely that individuals with higher titers of neuraminidase antibody escaped illness, but it is evident that illness was not prevented in a great number of people with prior immunological experience with a neuraminidase common to that in the new variant (see Chapter 15). In comparison, artificial immunization or prior infection with virus containing a hemagglutinin similar to that in the prevalent strain is protective in the majority of people, and the occurrence of pandemic influenza appears to require the appearance of virus with a novel hemagglutinin, regardless of whether or not the neuraminidase has changes as well. On the other hand, antibody to neuraminidase in sufficiently high titer does modify disease, even if it does not prevent infection,* and this "second line" of defense may play a particularly important role when antigenic changes in hemagglutinin have occurred. Moreover, although the evidence on this point is not conclusive, it is possible that antibody to neuraminidase may have a specific effect not shared by antibody to hemagglutinin in reducing virus shedding and subsequent transmission.

IV. Comparison of Effects of Immunity Produced by Infection and by Parenteral Immunization with Inactivated Virus

Francis (1941) suggested many years ago that resistance to influenza was more closely related to antibody in nasal secretions than to serum antibody.

* Recently, attempts have been made to take advantage of the fact that antibody to neuraminidase does not inhibit infection but does prevent subsequent disease to prepare neuraminidase-specific inactivated virus vaccines. According to this concept of "infection-permissive" immunization (Kilbourne et al., 1972, 1975) infection-induced immunity without the penalty of consequent disease would result from monospecific neuraminidase immunization and subsequent exposure to natural infection.

Later, Fazekas de St. Groth and Donnelley (1950) demonstrated that mice immunized by intranasal inoculation of inactivated virus were more resistant to influenza virus challenge than parenterally immunized mice. More recently, several studies in experimental animals have revealed a dissociation between serum antibody levels and resistance. Mice immunized by prior infection cannot be reinfected with up to 1000 MID_{50} of the same virus for at least 1 year, while mice immunized by injection of inactivated virus are uniformly infected with lower doses of challenge virus although they have comparable serum antibody titers (Schulman and Kilbourne, 1967). Similarly, Potter *et al.* (1973a) observed greater resistance in ferrets immunized by infection than in ferrets with equivalent serum antibody titers derived by injection of inactivated virus.

Observations in human subjects have provided conflicting data, in part depending on the nature of the study. Experiments in which the protective effects of live virus vaccines have been compared with those of parenteral vaccines have suggested, in general, a primary role for secretory antibody (Beare *et al.*, 1968), while analyses of antibody titers in respiratory secretions and sera and their correlations with infection rates and disease have produced variable results (see Kilbourne *et al.*, 1973, for summary).

Although definitive evidence is not at hand, the available evidence suggests that infection-induced immunity against influenza is more protective and more durable than immunity resulting from parenterally administered vaccines which have been in use up to now, and it is likely that this difference reflects the specific stimulation of local 11 S IgA antibody. Parallel observations with other virus infections of the respiratory tract suggest strongly that immunization procedures which are capable of producing a local secretory IgA antibody response provide more effective immunity (Smith *et al.*, 1966). However, parenterally administered influenza vaccine particularly in immunologically primed people may provide an efficient stimulus for the production of secretory antibody, and it may not be appropriate to assume that attenuated live virus vaccines or intranasal administration of inactivated vaccine will prove to be the most efficient method for influenza immunization. It is also necessary to emphasize that measurements of 11 S IgA antibody in nasal secretions may not provide the most sensitive or accurate reflection of local immunity. Precise knowledge is not available regarding the natural route of infection with influenza virus in man. If infection is initiated in the lower respiratory tract, antibody titers in bronchial secretions may be more important than nasal antibody. In one study where these considerations were taken into account, the ratio of IgG to IgA in human bronchioalveolar washings was found to be 2.5:1 in contrast to a ratio of 1:3 in nasal washings. Aerosol administration of inactivated virus vaccine produced a threefold increase of antibody titers in bronchial fluids, whereas parenteral administration of the same vaccine produced an increase only in serum antibody titers (Waldman *et al.*, 1973). While still indicating a specific local response to antigenic stimulation, these results imply that IgG, and not IgA, may be of greater importance in the lower respiratory tract.

V. Effect of Antigenic Drift on Immunity

The unique capacity of influenza viruses for periodic major and minor changes in its envelope antigens has been discussed in Chapter 10. There is no doubt that the major "shifts" in the antigenic structure of the hemagglutinin of influenza A viruses occurring approximately every decade circumvent the protective effects of immune mechanisms and are associated with pandemic influenza. The consequence of the minor "drift" in antigenic structure of hemagglutinin and neuraminidase which occur within the epoch of a particular influenza A subtype are less well understood. As new variants appear which are not identical to prototype strains, antibody made in response to the original strain is less reactive in serologic assay, and a greater proportion of the population is found to be lacking detectable antibody to the new variant. As a result, officials responsible for determining vaccine formulae are confronted with the difficult problem of deciding whether the magnitude of antigenic change warrants revision of vaccine composition, and uncertainty is created as to whether people previously infected with the prototype strain are adequately protected against the new variant.

Unfortunately, data bearing on these questions are limited and have led to conflicting conclusions, in part because the independent variation of hemagglutinin and neuraminidase antigens and the protective effects of antibody to neuraminidase have not been fully taken into account.

A. Antigenic Drift of Hemagglutinin

It is very likely that gradual changes in the antigenic structure of the hemagglutinin is essential for the survival of influenza viruses. Undoubtedly, as a consequence of these changes people who would be resistant to *infection* with the antecedent variant of the prototype strain are infected and transmit the infection to other susceptible members of the population. However, it is not at all certain whether resistance to *disease* is equally compromised by minor antigenic changes in hemagglutinin. Experimentally it has been shown that mice immunized with 1968 H3N2 virus are less resistant to infection with a recombinant virus containing a hemagglutinin derived from a later variant than they are to infection with a recombinant virus with the homotypic hemagglutinin. However, with the doses of challenge virus employed (100 MID_{50}), pulmonary virus titers were markedly reduced and lung lesions were prevented even after infection with virus containing a dissimilar hemagglutinin (Schulman, 1973). There have not been any comparable studies in man in which the protective effects of antibody to neuraminidase have been excluded, but observations made after immunization with vaccine containing prototype strains of virus have provided evidence of protection against disease caused by later variants, almost comparable in effectiveness to that seen when the vaccine strain and the epidemic strain contain identical hemagglutinins (Meiklejohn, 1958; Stiver *et al.,* 1973; Hoskins *et al.,* 1973). Influenza B virus does not undergo the marked antigenic changes in its hemagglutinin characteristics of influenza A viruses, but gradual antigenic "drift" of its hemagglutinin does occur. Presumably, the survival of the virus is favored by these antigenic alterations, but the observation that influenza B virus does not usually cause severe disease in adults in part may be related to the residual protective effects of antibody derived from exposure to previous strains. The point of these speculations is not to imply that resistance to disease is not compromised by minor antigenic changes in hemagglutinin, but to suggest that resistance to *infection* may be more profoundly affected.

HIERARCHY OF INFLUENZA A VIRUSES

Taking a somewhat different view of antigenic variation, Fazekas de St. Groth (1969) suggested that an asymmetric relationship exists among strains within a single subtype, such that more cross-reactivity in HI tests is observed when antibody to later ("senior") strains is tested against earlier ("junior") virus than is seen with the reciprocal titration. Speculating on these observations, Fazekas proposed that an ideal vaccine would be one containing the most senior strain which can be isolated after serial passage in the presence of antibody. A vaccine containing a variant of H3N2 virus has been prepared, but whether the laboratory variant will prove to be antigenically identical to variants which emerge in nature and whether the vaccine will prove to be more effective than conventional vaccines remain to be determined (see discussion in Chapter 10). It is significant that antigenic variation among different isolates has been found to be more pronounced at the end of a subtype era than at the beginning (Dowdle *et al.,* 1974), suggesting that it may be extremely difficult to predict in advance which variant is likely to be predominant 5–10 years after the introduction of a new subtype.

B. Antigenic Drift of Neuraminidase

Major changes in the antigenic structure of neuraminidase appear to occur less frequently in influenza A viruses than do major antigenic "shifts" of hemagglutinin, but gradual minor antigenic alterations of neuraminidase independent of those taking place in the hemagglutinin antigen have been identified. The immunological and epidemiological significance of antigenic drift in neuraminidase has not been defined, but it has been shown experimentally that mice immunized with isolated purified 1957 N2 neuraminidase have greater reductions in pulmonary virus titers following challenge with a virus containing the identical neuraminidase than after challenge with virus containing a nonidentical (1968) N2 neuraminidase (Schulman, 1970). If antibody to neuraminidase plays an important role in reducing transmission of influenza, then mutants with antigenically altered neuraminidase would be expected to have some selective advantage.

VI. Heterotypic Immunity

The classification of influenza A viruses into subtypes is based upon serological cross-reactivity in tests of hemagglutination inhibition (HI) and neuraminidase inhibition (NI) (World Health Organization Committee on Influenza Virus Nomenclature, 1971). With considerable justification, immunity mediated by antibody to hemagglutinin is regarded as subtype specific, i.e., limited to strains of virus reactive with the antibody in conventional HI tests. However, there is some evidence to suggest that subtle antigenic similarities may be present in the hemagglutinins of viruses which do not cross-react in HI or neutralization tests. For example, antibody to isolated H0 hemagglutinin has been shown to be reactive with disrupted H1N1 virus in immunodiffusion assay (Schild, 1970; Baker *et al.*, 1973) and in single radial diffusion tests (Chapter 11). Indeed, cross-reactions of H0 and H1 antigens can be detected in HI tests with certain virus strains (Sugiura and Kilbourne, 1966). The documented vaccine failures associated with the appearance of variants with markedly different hemagglutinin antigens make it evident that immune mechanisms based on these subtle antigenic relationships are not very potent. Nevertheless, it is possible that prior experience with viruses of one subtype may influence the immune response to virus of another subtype.

From the pioneer experiments in immunity to influenza carried out in England and the United States, it was clear that immunization of animals by infection of influenza A virus of one subtype increased resistance to challenge with virus of a different subtype in the absence of demonstratable neutralizing antibody to the heterotypic strain. In the light of present knowledge it is possible that this increased resistance was due in large part to antigenically related neuraminidases in the two viruses. Subsequently, Henle and Lief (1963) observed that after repeated infections of guinea pigs with H1N1 virus, neutralizing antibody reactive with Hsw1N1, H0N1, and H2N2 viruses was obtained. Experiments in mice indicated that even a single infection with H0N1 virus conferred partial resistance to H2N2 virus challenge, and that the antibody response to the H2 hemagglutinin was more pronounced in the animals previously infected with the heterotypic virus (Schulman and Kilbourne, 1965). Similar observations of an enhanced antibody response in animals "primed" by prior heterotypic infection have been made in ferrets (McLaren and Potter, 1974), and in hamsters. Potter *et al.*, (1973b) transferred the capacity for a primed response with spleen cells from previously infected animals. Taken together, these observations suggest that the hemagglutinins of influenza A viruses of different subtypes share common minor antigenic determinants. Although this antigenic relatedness is not evident in conventional serological tests or reflected by significant heterotypic resistance in man, it probably does play a role in the broadened antibody response seen after multiple infections and in potentiating the immune response to infection or immunization with heterotypic virus. It should be noted that it is not clear whether this effect requires prior infection with a heterotypic strain or whether similar results can be achieved by parenteral injection of vaccine given in multiple doses or with adjuvant (Hennessy, 1967).

VII. Original Antigenic Sin

A. Hemagglutinin Antigen

Another expression of antigenic relatedness among the hemagglutinin antigens of influenza A viruses of different subtypes is seen in the phenomenon of original antigenic sin (Francis *et al.*, 1953). Briefly, this term has been coined to summarize the characteristic antibody response following sequential experience with viruses of different subtypes: Upon exposure to virus containing a new hemagglutinin, antibody is produced which reacts in HI test not only with the new strain but also with the virus which provided the primary antigenic stimulation. Furthermore, antibody to the new strain can be removed by adsorption with the virus to which the subject was first exposed, but adsorption with the new strain only removes antibody reactive with that strain. The strain of original antigenic sin is age related, Hsw1N1 for those born between 1918–1930, H0N1 for people born between 1930–1947, etc. As a result, assays of sera of people of different ages produce characteristic "profiles" of HI antibody titers against viruses of different subtypes (Davenport *et al.*, 1953). Although it was originally believed that original antigenic sin is part of the antibody response to all influenza A viruses, more recent evidence indicates that exposure to H2N2 strains did not evoke an antibody response to earlier subtypes (Webster, 1966). The immunological basis for this phenomenon has recently been elucidated with influenza virus antigens (Virelizier *et al.*, 1974a). The results were in accord with previous studies of a comparable phenomenon with chemically defined antigens which indicated that the effect is probably due to cross-stimulation of an enlarged population of cross-reactive B memory cells remaining after the primary antigenic stimulation (Eisen *et al.*, 1969).

B. Neuraminidase Antigen

Recent data make clear that the phenomenon of original antigenic sin also is operative in the response to neuraminidase. Age-related profiles similar to those seen with antibody titers to hemagglutinin have been obtained with neuraminidase antibody (Kendal *et al.*, 1973). Moreover, unpublished experiments in the author's laboratory indicate that immunization with H3N2 virus evokes an antibody rise to N1 (PR/8) neuraminidase in persons born before but not in those born after 1957.

VIII. Cell-Mediated Immunity in Influenza

The possibility that cell-mediated immunity plays a role in the pathogenesis of influenza is only now beginning to be explored. The fact that resistance can be transferred by inoculation of sera from immune animals prior to challenge makes it clear that *prevention* of infection and disease can be accomplished with antibody alone. However, antibody given later in the course of infection does not modify disease, and it is possible that *recovery* from infection may be influenced by cell-mediated immune mechanisms.

Cellular immune responses to influenza virus antigens have been demonstrated in laboratory animals and in man following infection or injection of inactivated virus, but their effect on resistance to subsequent infection is difficult to evaluate because of the antibody response which is simultaneously elicited. Loosli *et al.* (1953) found that mice immunized passively by repeated intraperitoneal injections of rabbit antiserum were protected against a lethal challenge of homologous virus, but 3 weeks later these animals lacked demonstrable antibody in their sera and respiratory secretions. Nevertheless these animals were partially resistant to a second challenge with the same virus. Small *et al.* (1973) obtained similar results in passively immunized ferrets and speculated that the partial resistance to a second challenge in animals immunosuppressed by passive administration of antibody might be mediated by cellular immune mechanisms. Conflicting evidence has been obtained in other experiments with immunosuppressed animals. Hirsch and Murphy (1968) found that injection of rat anti-mouse lymphocyte serum did not influence survival of mice infected with influenza virus. On the other hand, Singer *et al.* (1972) observed increased survival of influenza-infected mice given cyclophosphamide, despite the suppression of an antibody response and the persistence of higher titers of virus in the lungs, and attributed the results to depression of cellular immune response. In a more recent experiment, Suzuki *et al.* (1974) demonstrated that injection of rabbit antiserum to mouse lymphocytes was associated with increased survival and decreased lung lesions in mice infected with low doses of H2N2 virus, and concluded that the cellular immune response to influenza virus was detrimental to the host despite the fact that virus persisted for longer periods and antibody titers were lower in immunosuppressed animals. The separation of the effects of antibody and cell-mediated immunity in recovery from influenza is further complicated by the recent demonstration that T lymphocytes are required for an antibody response to specific determinants on influenza virus hemagglutinin (Virelizier *et al.,* 1974b). In the absence of definitive data derived by reconstitution of T cell-deficient animals with normal and immune lymphocytes, it is virtually impossible to resolve these conflicting results, and the effects of cell-mediated immune response to influenza virus (particularly its effects in man) remain undefined.

IX. Summary

Specific antibody reactive with the surface antigens of influenza virus has the capacity to inhibit infection and to prevent disease if infection does occur. In particular, adequate titers of antibody directed to hemagglutinin provides an effective defense against influenza, but antibody to neuraminidase also may modify illness and may play a specific role in preventing transmission. Unfortunately, these immune mechanisms are circumvented by the unique capacity of influenza viruses for periodic major antigenic change, and to a lesser extent are compromised by less extensive alterations in antigenic structure. Although it is likely that immunity against influenza reflects events taking place at the surface of the respiratory epithelium, the relative importance of secretory and serum antibody has not been fully defined. Finally, the role of immune mechanisms in recovery from infection, in particular the effects of cell-mediated immunity in recovery and pathogenesis of disease remain obscure.

References

Alford, R. H., Kasel, J. A., Gerone, P. J., and Knight, V. (1966). *Proc. Soc. Exp. Biol. Med.* **122,** 800.

Andrews, B. E., Beare, A. S., McDonald, J. C., Zuckerman, A. J., and Tyrrell, D. A. J. (1966). *Brit. Med. J.* **1,** 637.

Baker, N., Stone, H. O. and Webster, R. G. (1973). *J. Virol.* **11,** 137.

Beare, A. S., Hobson, D., Reed, S. E., and Tyrrell, D. A. J. (1968). *Lancet* **2,** 418.

Becht, H., Hammerling, V., and Rott, R. (1971). *Virology* **46,** 337.

Commission of Influenza. (1943). Armed Forces Epidemiologic Board.

Couch, R. B., Douglas, R. G., Jr., Fedson, D. S., and Kasel, J. A. (1971). *J. Infec. Dis.* **124,** 473.

Couch, R. B., Kasel, J. A., Gerin, J. L., Schulman, J. L., and Kilbourne, E. D. (1974). *J. Infec. Dis.* **129,** 411.

Davenport, F. M. (1961). *Amer. Rev. Resp. Dis.* **83,** Part 2, 146.

Davenport, F. M., Hennessy, A. V., and Francis, T., Jr. (1953). *J. Exp. Med.* **98,** 641.

Dowdle, W. R., Coleman, M. T., and Gregg, M. B (1974). *Progr. Med. Virol.* **17,** 91.

Eisen, H. N., Little, J. R., Steiner, L. A., and Simms, E. E. (1969). *Isr. J. Med. Sci.* **5,** 338.

Farník, J., and Bruj, J. (1966). *J. Infec. Dis.* **116,** 425.

Fazekas de St. Groth, S. (1969). *Bull. W.H.O.* **41,** 651.

Fazekas de St. Groth, S., and Donnelley, M. (1950). *Aust. J. Exp. Biol. Med. Sci.* **28,** 61.

Francis, T., Jr. (1941). *Harvey Lect.* **37,** 69.

Francis, T., Jr. (1967). *Med. Clin. N. Amer.* **51,** 781.

Francis, T., Jr., Pearson, H. E. Salk, J. E., and Brown, P. N. (1944). *Amer. J. Pub. Health* **34,** 317.

Francis, T., Jr., Davenport, F. M., and Hennessy, A. V. (1953). *Trans Ass. Amer Physicians* **66,** 231.

Henle, W., and Lief, F. S. (1963). *Amer. Rev. Resp. Dis.* **88,** 379.

Henle, W., Henle, G. Stokes, J., Jr., and Maris, E. P. (1946). *J. Immunol.* **52,** 145.

Hennessy, A. V. (1967). *Sci. Publ., PAHO, (Pan-Amer. San. Bur.)* No. 147, P669.

Hirsch, M. S., and Murphy, F. A. (1968). *Lancet* **2,** 37.

Hobson, D., Curry, R. L., Beare, A. S., and Ward-Gardner, A. (1973). *J. Hyg.* **70,** 767.

Hoskins, T. W., Davies, J. R., Allchin, A., Miller, C. L., and Pollock, T. M. (1973). *Lancet* **2,** 116.

Kendal, A. P., Minuse, E., Maassab, H. F., Hennessy, A. V., and Davenport, F. M. (1973). *Amer. J. Epideminol.* **98,** 96.

Kilbourne, E. D., Laver, W. G., Schulman, J. L., and Webster, R. G. (1968). *J. Virol.* **2**, 281.

Kilbourne, E. D., Schulman, J. L., Couch, R. B., and Kasel, J. A. (1972). *Proc. Int. Congress Virol., 2nd, 1971* pp. 118–119.

Kilbourne, E. D., Butler, W. T., and Rossen, R. D. (1973). *J. Infec. Dis.* **127**, 220.

Kilbourne, E. D., Palese, P., and Schulman, J. L. (1975). *Perspect. Virol.* **9**, 99.

Loosli, C. G., Hamre, D., and Berlin, B. S. (1953). *Trans. Ass. Amer. Physicians* **66**, 222.

McDonald, J. C., Zuckerman, A. J., Beare, A. S., and Tyrrell, D. A. J. (1962). *Brit. Med. J.* **1**, 1036.

McLaren, C., and Potter, C. W. (1974). *J. Hyg.* **72**, 91.

Meiklejohn, G. (1958). *Amer. J. Hyg.* **67**, 237.

Moffet, H. L., Cramblett, H. G., and Dobbins, Jr. (1964). *J. Amer. Med. Ass.* **190**, 806.

Monto, A. S., and Kendal, A. P. (1973). *Lancet* **1**, 623.

Monto, A. S., Davenport, F. M., Napier, J. A., and Francis, T., Jr. (1969). *Bull. W.H.O.* **41**, 537.

Morris, J. A., Kasel, J. A., Saglam, M., Knight, V., and Loda, F. A. (1966). *N. Eng. J. Med.* **274**, 527.

Murphy, B. R., Kasel, J. A., and Chanock, R. M. (1972). *N. Engl. J. Med.* **286**, 1329.

Potter, C. W., Jennings, R., and McLaren, C. (1973a). *Arch. Gesamte Virusforsch.* **42**, 285.

Potter, C. W., Jennings, R., Rees, R. C., and McLaren, C. (1973b). *Infec. Immunity,* **8**, 137.

Schild, G. (1970). *J. Gen. Virol.* **9**, 191.

Schulman, J. L. (1967). *J. Exp. Med.* **125**, 467.

Schulman, J. L. (1970). *Prog. Med. Virol.* **12**, 128.

Schulman, J. L. (1973). *Symp. Ser. Immunobiol. Stand.* **20**, 106.

Schulman, J. L., and Kilbourne, E. D. (1965). *J. Bacteriol.* **89**, 170.

Schulman, J. L., and Kilbourne, E. D. (1971). *J. Infec. Dis.* **124**, 463.

Schulman, J. L., Khakpour, M., and Kilbourne, E. D. (1968). *J. Virol.* **2**, 778.

Singer, S. H., Noguchi, P., and Kirschstein, R. L. (1972). *Infec. Immunity* **5**, 957.

Slepushkin, A. N., Schild, G. C., Beare, A. S., Chinn, S., and Tyrrell, D. A. J. (1971). *J. Hyg.* **69**, 571.

Small, P. A., Jr., Waldman, R., Gifford, G., and Bruno, J. (1973). *Symp. Ser. Immunobiol. Stand.* **20**, 238.

Smith, C. B., Purcell, R. H., Bellanti, J. A., and Chanock, R. M. (1966). *N. Engl. J. Med.* **275**, 1145.

Stiver, H. G., Graves, P., Eickhoff, T. C., and Meiklejohn, G. (1973). *N. Engl. J. Med.* **289**, 1267.

Sugiura, A., and Kilbourne, E. D. (1966). *Virology* **29**, 84.

Suzuki, F., Ohya, J. and Ishida, N. (1974). *Proc. Soc. Exp. Biol. Med.* **146**, 78.

Waldman, R. H., Gaclol, N., Olsen, G. N., and Johnson, J. E., III. (1973). *Symp. Ser. Immunobiol. Stand.* **20**, 222.

Webster, R. G. (1966). *J. Immunol.* **97**, 177.

World Health Organization Committee on Influenza Virus Nomenclature. (1971). *Bull. W.H.O.* **45**, 119.

Virelizier, J. L., Allison, A. C., and Schild, G. C. (1974a). *J. Exp. Med.* **140**, 1571.

Virelizier, J. L., Postlethwaite, R., Schild, G. C., and Allison, A. C. (1974b). *J. Exp. Med.* **140**, 1559.

13

Influenza in Man

R. Gordon Douglas, Jr.

I. Introduction

The intent of this chapter is to describe influenza virus infections as they occur in man, for it is the resultant morbidity and mortality which makes influenza such an important medical and public health problem. Because

395

of the nature of this book, there is no discussion of treatment or differential diagnosis as may be found in textbooks of medicine. Furthermore, experimental infections in volunteers are emphasized because there is a great deal more quantitative information available concerning experimental than natural infections. Hopefully, this data is applicable to naturally occurring infections. Finally, much related material in regard to antibody response, diagnostic methods, and the role of host factors in the epidemiology of influenza has been discussed in detail elsewhere, and is mentioned only briefly here.

II. Naturally Occurring Influenza Virus Infection in Man

A. Uncomplicated Influenza

1. PATHOLOGY AND PATHOGENESIS

The mechanism of transmission is discussed elsewhere (Chapter 15). Influenza virus is deposited on the mucous blanket lining the respiratory tract or directly in the alveolus. In the former site, it is exposed to mucoprotein receptors similar to N-acetylneuraminic acid receptors on the erythrocyte and respiratory tract epithelial cell. Binding of virus to mucus leads to protection of epithelial cells against infection. However, through the action of the neuraminidase, the virus can presumably break this bond and in the process liquify mucus. Specific locally secreted IgA antibodies and nonspecific inhibitors of viral replication would exert their role before virus attachment occurs. If not prevented by one of these mechanisms, virus attaches to the surface of a respiratory epithelial cell and then intracellular replication cycle is initiated.

Most of the data concerning the pathology of influenza has been obtained from fatal cases. However, nasal exudate smears and tracheal biopsies have been studied in uncomplicated cases (Mulder and Hers, 1972). Presumably the major site of infection is the ciliated columnar epithelial cell. The first alteration is disappearance of the elongated form of these cells. These cells become rounded and swollen, and the nucleus shrinks, becomes pyknotic, and fragments. Vacuolization of the cytoplasm may occur. As the nucleus disintegrates, the cytoplasm shows inclusion bodies and the cilia are lost. Immunofluorescence with anti-influenza virus antibody reveals bright staining predominately in the cytoplasm of epithelial cells most of which were cylindrical ciliated cells (Tateno *et al.*, 1966).

Studies of the trachea and bronchi of fatal cases reveal similar cytopathology (Mulder and Hers, 1972). In addition, evidence of bronchitis and tracheitis are prominent: increased permeability of vascular capillary walls, hyperemia, edema, and polymorphonuclear cellular infiltration of the tunica propria and submucosa. Mononuclear cells are also found regularly in the tunica propria and submucosal region around mucous glands, but cellular infiltration is not massive. Phagocytosis of degenerate epithelial cells by these leukocytes is observed. The basement membrane is not affected.

2. INFLUENZA A VIRUS INFECTION

The incubation period is characteristically 2 days but may vary from 1 to 4 days. As shown in Table 13.1, in most cases, the onset is abrupt and

Table 13.1 Symptoms in Proven Adult Cases of Influenza A Virus Infection

Symptoms	H0N1 1937, 1939, 1941 (60 cases)[a]	H1N1 1947 (76 cases)[b]	H2N2 1957 (30 cases)[c]
Sudden onset	75[d]	67	46
Systemic symptoms			
Chilliness	80	85	64
Feverishness	—[e]	99	71
Headache	85	86	72
Myalgia	60	60	62
Malaise	87	—	67
Anorexia	71	—	37
Respiratory symptoms			
Sneezing	—	—	67
Nasal obstruction	80	—	52
Nasal discharge		70	82
Sore throat	48	49	62
Hoarseness	10	—	37
Cough	88	97	90
Sputum	31	32	41
Other			
Photophobia	20		—
Nausea	17	29	4
Vomiting		9	7
Diarrhea	—	4	0
Abdominal pain	—	15	0

[a] From Stuart-Harris (1961).
[b] From Kilbourne and Loge (1950).
[c] From Jordan et al. (1958).
[d] Percent with indicated symptom.
[e] No data.

many patients can pinpoint the hour of onset. At the onset, systemic symptoms predominate. Most frequently observed are feverishness, chilliness, headache, myalgias, malaise, and anorexia. Headache or myalgia is usually the most troublesome symptom, and the severity of these symptoms is related to the height of the fever. Myalgias may be most severe in the long muscles of the back but often involve the extremities as well. Arthralgias, not frequently commented on earlier, have been a common finding since the appearance of the H3N2 virus (Knight *et al.*, 1970). Respiratory symptoms, especially dry cough or nasal discharge, are almost always present at the onset but are overshadowed by the systemic symptoms. Nasal obstruction, hoarseness, and dry or sore throat may also be present, but these symptoms tend to become more prominent as the disease progresses. Ocular symptoms, when present, are helpful in arriving at a diagnosis of influenza and include photophobia, tearing, burning, and pain on moving the eyes.

Physical findings are presented in Table 13.2. The most important finding is fever, which usually rapidly rises to a peak of 100° to 106°F within 12 hours of onset, coincident with the development of systemic symptoms. Fever is usually continuous but may be intermittent especially if antipyretics are

Table 13.2 Physical Findings in Proven Adult Cases of Influenza A Virus Infection

Signs	H0N1 1937 (82 cases)[a]	H1N1 1947 (76 cases)[b]	H2N2 1957 (30 cases)[c]
Maximum temperature			
100°F			13[d]
100°–101.9°F	101.2°F (average)	101.3°F (average)	58
≥102°F			29
Flushed face	67	58	24
Conjunctival abnormalities	89	66	56
Nasal discharge	22	52	20
Nasal injection/edema	—[e]	—	64
Nasal obstruction	51	—	—
Pharyngeal infection	73	72	68
Pharyngeal exudate	1	0	0
Cervical adenopathy	—	22	8
Rhonchi and/or rales	20	4	0

[a] From Stuart-Harris (1961).
[b] From Kilbourne and Loge (1950).
[c] From Jordan *et al.* (1958).
[d] Percent with indicated symptoms.
[e] No data.

administered. It is usually lower on the second and third days than on the first day, and as the fever diminishes the systemic symptoms subside. Classically, the duration of fever is 3 days, but it may last from 1 to 5 or more days. In a small percentage of cases, a second fever spike occurs on the third or fourth day resulting in a diphasic fever curve.

On physical examination early in the course of illness the patient appears toxic, the face is flushed and the skin hot and moist. The eyes are watery, reddened, and the palpebral fissure narrowed as a result of edema of the lids contributing to the characteristic facies. Thin clear nasal discharge is commonly observed, but nasal obstruction is less common. The mucous membrane of the nose and throat are hyperemic, but pharyngeal and tonsillar exudate are not observed. Small tender cervical lymph nodes are palpated in some cases. If the chest is examined frequently, transient scattered rhonchi or localized areas of rales may be detected in many cases. However, as indicated in Table 13.2, persistent signs in the chest are found in less than 20% of cases.

During the second and third days of illness as the systemic signs and symptoms diminish, the respiratory complaints and findings become more obvious. By the fourth day, the illness is predominantly respiratory. Cough is the most frequent and troublesome symptom and may be accompanied by substernal pain or burning. Nasal obstruction and discharge and pharyngeal pain and injection are also common. Such symptoms and signs usually persist 3 to 4 days, but cough commonly persists longer. A long convalescence is common. Cough, lassitude, and malaise may last 1 or 2 weeks after disappearance of other manifestations.

Data presented in Tables 13.1 and 13.2 show the constancy of the clinical manifestations of influenza A infection in spite of significant changes in the surface antigens of the virion.

The above description of the classical influenza syndrome applies to the most easily recognized cases of influenza virus infection. However, during an influenza outbreak, other respiratory tract syndromes are frequently associated with influenza virus infection, such as common colds, pharyngitis, laryngitis, and tracheobronchitis, or systemic illness without any respiratory symptoms. Furthermore, subclinical cases occur. In a study of 46 proven infections, 33 patients developed the influenza syndrome, 3 developed "fever only," and 10 were subclinical infections (Kilbourne *et al.,* 1951).

3. Influenza B Virus Infection

Stansfield and Stuart-Harris (1943) studied clinical illness in an outbreak of influenza B infection and their findings are presented in Table 13.3. When the frequency of occurrence of these symptoms is compared to those pre-

Table 13.3   Frequency of Symptoms in Proven
Influenza B Virus Infections[a,b]

Sudden onset	78%
Systemic symptoms	
Chilliness	82%
Sweating	91%
Headache	83%
Myalgia	75%
Malaise	80%
Dizziness	58%
Respiratory symptoms	
Nasal obstruction and discharge	66%
Sore throat	42%
Hoarseness	12%
Cough	92%
Sputum	24%
Other	
Photophobia	14%
Nausea and vomiting	29%

[a] From Stansfield and Stuart-Harris (1943).
[b] 24 cases.

sented in Table 13.1, it is apparent that they closely resemble those described for influenza A infections and consist of a 3-day febrile illness with predominant systemic symptoms.

Although most authorities agree with the above conclusions, some others feel that influenza B infection may be somewhat milder. Nigg *et al.* (1942) found that cases of influenza B infection tended to have more coryza and less myalgia than influenza A, but these differences were small, and Taylor *et al.* (1942), who studied 23 cases of influenza B infection, felt that they were less severe than influenza A infections and that sweating, myalgias, sputum production and eye findings were more commonly encountered in patients infected with influenza A virus.

4. INFLUENZA C VIRUS INFECTION

In contrast to influenza A and B viruses, influenza C infection results in predominantly afebrile upper respiratory illnesses in man, and such illnesses occur infrequently. In a study by Hilleman *et al.* (1962) of acute respiratory disease in children, 0.6% were due to influenza C. None of 155 illnesses among adults with upper respiratory illnesses were due to influenza C virus infection. Mogabgab (1963) showed in a serologic study that influenza C infection was associated with 10 of 713 (1.4%) afebrile upper respiratory illnesses in university students, 6 of 412 (1.5%) in airmen, and 2 of 45 (4.44%) in industrial workers.

5. INFLUENZA IN CHILDREN

As discussed in Chapter 15, influenza infection is most common in children, although the resulting illness is milder and the incidence of pulmonary complications is considerably less than in adults. Jordan *et al.* (1958) studied the clinical findings of influenza A infection in children, and these findings are shown in Tables 13.4 and 13.5. The symptoms observed in children are quite similar to those in adults (Tables 13.1 and 13.2) except for a higher incidence of nausea and vomiting and a lower incidence of myalgias among children. Maximal temperatures tended to be higher among children, and cervical adenopathy was observed more frequently among children than adults.

Table 13.4 Symptoms of Proven Influenza A Infection in Children 0–14 Years of Age[a]

	H1N1 95 cases	H2N2 45 cases
Sudden onset	65[b]	66
Systemic symptoms		
Chilliness	55	37
Feverishness	91	93
Headache	60	81
Myalgia	18	33
Malaise	73	68
Anorexia	71	69
Respiratory symptoms		
Sneezing	40	38
Nasal obstruction	47	54
Nasal discharge	73	67
Sore throat	43	62
Hoarseness	29	22
Cough	76	86
Sputum	22	19
Other		
Nausea	—	23
Vomiting	24	26
Diarrhea	11	2
Abdominal pain	—	31

[a] From Jordan *et al.* (1958).
[b] Percent with indicated symptoms.

Table 13.5   Signs of Proven Influenza A Infection in Children
0–14 Years of Age[a]

Signs	H1N1 95 cases	H2N2 45 cases
Maximal temperature		
100°F	5	11
100°–101.9°F	17	39
≥102°F	79	60
Flushed face	38	28
Conjunctival abnormalities	40	61
Nasal discharge	48	38
Nasal injection/edema	46	50
Pharyngeal infection	50	60
Pharyngeal exudate	0	1
Cervical adenopathy	45	38
Rhonchi and/or rales	0	2

[a] From Jordan et al. (1958).

6. Clinical Laboratory Findings

Smorodintseff et al. (1937) reported, in the 1936 outbreak in Leningrad, leukocytosis in $\frac{1}{3}$ of cases on the first day of illness. Leukopenia was a constant finding appearing on the second or third day of illness with counts as low as 3000 per mm³. By the tenth to eleventh days, the leukocyte count had returned to normal. Changes in the differential count were also observed: lymphopenia on the first 2 days of illness, then lymphocytosis, neutropenia most pronounced on the fifth day of illness, eosinopenia, and monocytosis.

Other studies have reported either leukocytosis or leukopenia (Hughes, 1938; Stuart-Harris, 1965). The apparently conflicting results probably depend on the time in the course of illness when blood counts were performed.

7. Alterations in Bacterial Flora

Jordan et al. (1958) studied the bacterial flora of the pharynx in 308 persons, 47% of whom acquired influenza A infection in the 1957 (H2N2) outbreak. Comparison of preepidemic and postepidemic throat cultures revealed no significant changes in prevalence of streptococci, pneumococci, staphylococci or Hemophilus influenzae. Furthermore, bacterial flora present at the time of proven influenza illness did not differ from that present in persons negative for influenza infection, and this is shown in Table 13.6. When preepidemic illness cultures were compared to postepidemic cultures,

Table 13.6   Changes in Pharyngeal Flora of Persons with Influenza[a,b]

Organisms postepidemic culture	Organisms present or absent	Influenza positive[c] Preepidemic		Influenza negative[d] Preepidemic	
		+	0	+	0
Streptococcus	+	1 (0.7)	3 (2.1)	—	6 (3.7)
	—	1 (0.7)	136 (96.5)	1 (0.6)	155 (95.7)
Staphylococcus	+	3 (2.1)	15 (10.6)	2 (1.2)	9 (5.6)
	—	15 (10.6)	108 (76.6)	15 (9.3)	136 (84.0)
Pneumococcus	+	1 (0.7)	11 (7.8)	1 (0.6)	23 (14.2)
	—	3 (2.1)	126 (89.4)	5 (3.1)	133 (82.1)
Hemophilus influenzae	+	0 (—)	4 (3.6)	0 (—)	2 (1.6)
	—	1 (0.9)	106 (95.5)	3 (2.4)	120 (96.0)

[a] From Jordan *et al.* (1958).

[b] Data given as number of changes, percent of changes in parentheses.

[c] 141 individuals cultured for streptococci, staphylococci and pneumococci; 111 individuals cultured for *Hemophilus influenzae*.

[d] 162 individuals cultured for streptococci, staphylococci and pneumococci; 125 individuals cultured for *H. influenzae*.

insignificant changes were observed with respect to streptococci and *H. influenzae*. However, 10.6% persons acquired staphylococci, but this was balanced by 10.6% who lost this organism. For pneumococci, acquisition was actually higher for individuals who did not have influenza (14.2% versus 7.8%).

In contrast to the above findings, several investigators have noted positive relationships between influenza and change in bacterial flora. Kilbourne and Loge (1950) detected an increase in the proportion of patients carrying β-hemolytic streptococci coincident with the decline of an influenza A (H1N1) outbreak as shown in Fig. 13.1, which culminated in a frank epidemic of streptococcal pharyngitis.

In addition, a positive relationship between meningococcal infection and influenza virus infection has been established. During a study of a simultaneous outbreak of meningococcal meningitis and influenza A virus infection, Young *et al.* (1972) demonstrated a positive association between serological evidence of influenza infection and serologic evidence of infection or nasopharyngeal carriage of *Neisseria meningitidis*. Both this study and others previously reported (Lal *et al.*, 1963 Eickhoff, 1971), suggest that influenza is associated with spread of meningococci. These authors suggest that influenza may directly effect the host in a manner that enchances the likelihood of acquisition of meningococci after exposure to these bacteria.

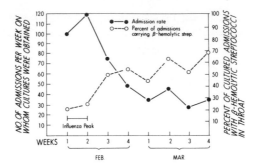

Fig. 13.1. Increase in proportion of patients carrying streptococci following an outbreak of influenza A (H1N1) infection. From Kilbourne and Loge (1950).

8. Pulmonary Function in Uncomplicated Influenza

Significant but reversible restrictive ventilative defects have been observed in uncomplicated influenza. Kennedy *et al.* (1965) performed a study of pulmonary function in 30 recruits with proven influenza, and demonstrated a transient but significant reduction in forced expiratory volume (in 0.75 seconds) and in derived voluntary ventilation. During the 1967–1969 A influenza (H3N2) epidemic, Johanson *et al.* (1969) performed serial pulmonary function studies on 10 previously normal healthy adults with uncomplicated nonpneumonic influenza. The ratio of residual volume to total lung capacity was slightly increased in 6 patients. The forced vital capacity of 4 patients was less than 85% of their predicted. In addition, arterial pO_2 was low in 7 patients and was associated with an increased alveolar–arterial oxygen tension difference. Administration of a bronchodilator aerosol produced no significant changes. Horner and Gray (1973) studied 20 patients 2 to 4 weeks after acute clinical influenza, which was unproven but occurred during the epidemic of 1968. The diffusing capacity for carbon monoxide was found to be reduced on initial measurement with a return to normal in all but 4 subjects within 2 to 3 months later.

Camner *et al.* (1973) studied tracheobronchial clearance in patients with influenza using a Teflon aerosol tagged with technetium-99. Clearance was significantly lower among 6 patients during illness than 9 healthy subjects, and this difference had disappeared at 1 month. Picken *et al.* (1972) tested three subjects with influenza B infection, proven serologically, and showed normal flow rates and airway resistance but development of frequency-dependent compliance believed to signify evidence of small airway involvement which persisted for 2 months.

Recently, Hall *et al.* (1974) reported alterations in peripheral airway resistance in subjects with proven influenza A/Port Chalmers/73 H3N2 infec-

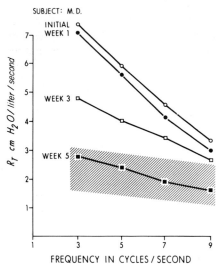

SUBJECT: M.D.

Fig. 13.2. A case report of frequency dependency characteristics of pulmonary resistance following uncomplicated influenza A (H3N2) infection. Hatched area represents usual normal levels. R_t, total pulmonary resistance, tested at varying frequencies. From W. J. Hall and R. G. Douglas, Jr. (unpublished data).

tion. Highly abnormal frequency dependency of total pulmonary resistance was noted in 9 of 13 normal adults with peak physiological abnormalities at 3 to 10 days after onset of illness. An example of such alterations is shown in Fig. 13.2. All subjects reverted to normal 3 to 5 weeks after acute illness.

These data indicate that apparently uncomplicated influenza is frequently accompanied by abnormalities in pulmonary function that are probably related to viral invasion of lower respiratory tract despite normal chest X-ray and physical examination.

9. VIRUS SHEDDING

a. Collection of Specimens.   In many instances the diagnosis of influenza can be determined on clinical grounds especially if it is known that an influenza epidemic exists in the community. However, for cases with unusual manifestations or of unusual severity, or to prove existence of influenza in a community, specific diagnosis is desirable. The preferred method for making a diagnosis in individual cases is virus isolation, because of the time lag required for serodiagnosis due to the requirement for convalescent sera. The likelihood of recovering influenza virus from most cases diminishes after 3 days; thus, specimens should be collected as soon as possible after onset of symptoms. Specimens may be collected from the nasopharynx, by swabbing or washing techniques. In addition, sputum or tracheal aspirates are excellent specimens, if available. Nasopharyngeal washings have been shown to be the optimal specimens in volunteers who are trained to perform the procedure. However, for single collections from patients we recommend a combined nose–throat swab. A dry cotton swab is inserted into the nasal cavity until resistence is met, and the nasal membranes are then swabbed vigorously with a twirling motion. With a second dry cotton swab, the tonsillar crypts and the posterior pharyngeal wall are swabbed vigorously. Both swabs are placed together in a vial of veal infusion broth containing 0.5% bovine albumin or other suitable transport media, such as cold tryptose broth with 0.5% gelatin. If the specimen needs to be shipped to a laboratory, it should be shipped on ice if the period of transportation will be less than 48 hours. Otherwise, it should be frozen at $-70°C$ and shipped on dry ice. Details of serological and virus isolation methods are presented in Chapters 9 and 11.

At the present time, there are sufficient laboratories based in hospitals and state health facilities in the United States so that viral isolation procedures are available to nearly every physician. In addition the Center for Disease Control in Atlanta, Georgia will accept specimens for virus isolation providing they are properly collected as outlined above. The possibility of more rapid diagnosis by immunofluorescence has been explored, but this method is not widely used. Tateno *et al.* (1965) have shown that immunofluorescence can lead to a diagnosis of influenza A and B virus infections within a few hours.

b. Virus Shedding Patterns.   Influenza virus is readily isolated from most cases of influenza providing the above techniques are used. Wingfield *et al.* (1969) isolated influenza virus from 93 of 95 serologically confirmed cases using pharyngeal swab specimens collected on 2 consecutive days. Togo *et al.* (1970) reported virus recovery from 48 normal adults undergoing naturally occurring influenza. Throat swabs and washings were obtained daily for 5 days, and tested for influenza virus in embryonated hens eggs. Between 63 and 100% of persons shed virus for each of the days tested, and, in contrast to most studies, they did not note a decrease in the number of patients shedding after the second day.

Knight *et al.* (1970) showed a high yield of positive cultures early in illness, and a decrease in frequency subsequently in a group of adult males undergoing naturally occurring influenza, and these results are shown in Fig. 13.3. This finding is more in keeping with the clinical experience that recovery of influenza virus is unusual after 3 or 4 days. In addition, and also shown in Fig. 13.3, quantities of virus shed in respiratory secretions rapidly fell from their initial mean peak, 3.0 $\log_{10}$ TCID$_{50}$* per milliliter.

---

* TCID$_{50}$, 50% tissue culture infectious dose.

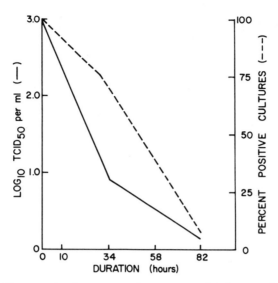

Fig. 13.3. Changes in frequency of recovery of influenza A (H3N2) virus (---) and quantities recovered (———) from throat swabs of patients according to duration of illness. From Knight *et al.* (1970).

c. Viremia. Since influenza virus was first demonstrated in extrapulmonary tissues of man, the occurrence of viremia has been suspected, and evidence to support this view was reviewed by Blattner (1959). In view of the predominance of systemic symptoms and the frequency of occurrence of chills, one might expect to find viremia in a large percentage of cases. Viremia, however, has only been reported in a few isolated cases. Naficy (1963) reported isolation of influenza virus from the throat wash specimen and clotted blood obtained on the second hospital day of a 40-year-old patient with a classical influenza syndrome with no complications. Isolations were made in rhesus monkey kidney cells, and embryonated hens eggs. Lehmann and Gust (1971) isolated Hong Kong influenza virus (H3N2) from the blood of two patients suffering from primary influenza viral pneumonia. One patient died and the virus was recovered from lung, liver, and spleen tissue as well as nasopharyngeal swab and tracheal swab at post mortem examination. It is of interest in this report that blood specimens were collected in heparin and sedimented in 1% dextran. Both plasma and the leukocyte fraction were tested and both yielded influenza virus. Khakpour *et al.* (1969) reported isolation of influenza virus. Khakpour *et al.* (1969) reported isolation of influenza A virus from a patient with uncomplicated influenza. Lozhkina *et al.* (1969) reported isolations from 3 patients on the third or fourth day after the onset of clinical symptoms. An additional case was reported of recovery of influenza A virus from postmortem serum obtained from the pulmonary vein (Wellings *et al.*, 1973). Several reports of unsuccessful attempts to isolate virus from blood have been published, notably that by Kilbourne (1959) and by Minuse *et al.* (1962). A study by Gresser and Dull reported by Naficy (1963) of 9 patients showed inability to isolate virus from washed leukocyte fractions. It is likely that the viremia in influenza is quite transient, and ability to detect it may be in part related to the presence or absence of serum inhibitors.

10. Interferon

Gresser and Dull (1964) looked for interferon in nasal washings of 13 patients in the acute phase of influenza. A virus inhibitor with characteristics of interferon was detected in 5 specimens from 4 patients. It was usually found in association with influenza virus, and was most easily demonstrated during the first 2 days of illness. Patients were retested during convalescence and viral inhibitor was not found. Ray *et al.* (1967) found an interferon-like inhibitor in the sera of 2 of 2 patients with influenza A infection, and 3 of 7 with influenza B infection. Interferon was detected on the first, second, and third day after the onset of illness and the titer was 4 or 8 I.U. All patients with circulating inhibitor were febrile at the time of collection of serum.

In contrast, Baron and Isaacs (1962) failed to detect interferon in human lung tissue obtained from 11 fatal cases of influenza viral pneumonia and speculated that the fatal outcome may have been related to its absence.

11. Antibody Response

Detailed information concerning the protective effect of antibody is presented in Chapter 12. Here, we are concerned primarily with the development of antibodies following naturally occurring influenza. Antibodies to influenza virus develop in the sera of most infected persons within a few weeks of onset of infection. Antibodies may be detected by complement fixation (CF), hemagglutination inhibition (HI), hemadsorption inhibition neutralization (N-HI), plaque reduction, or enzyme inhibition. For most clinical and epidemiologic purposes CF and HI tests are used.

Wingfield *et al.* (1969) showed that 35 of 46 (76%) patients developed N-HI antibodies 21 days after onset of illness in response to infection with influenza A (H3N2). The geometric mean titer rise was 27.8. In a study by Knight *et al.* (1970) of 16 patients with uncomplicated influenza A (H3N2) infection, all responded, and the geometric mean rise in neutralizing antibody titers was 64-fold. Neutralization tests are somewhat more sensitive indicators of infection than HI tests, and the latter are more sensitive than CF tests. In a study by Oker-Blom *et al.* (1970) of 59 proven infections with influenza A (H3N2), 42 were detected by CF and HI, 13 by HI only, and 4 by CF only.

The development of serum antibodies and antibodies in respiratory secretions to influenza A (H3N2) was studied by Togo *et al.* (1970) in 37 patients. At 21 days, 87% had developed fourfold or greater neutralizing antibody responses to serum; 49% in sputum and 27% in nasal washings. The time course of development of serum and sputum antibodies is shown in Fig. 13.4. The mean initial serum neutralizing antibody titer was 1:7 and at 21 days was 1:264, a mean titer increase of 40-fold. HI antibody responses were similar. Geometric mean titers of 1:275 were observed at 21 days, a mean titer increase of 12-fold.

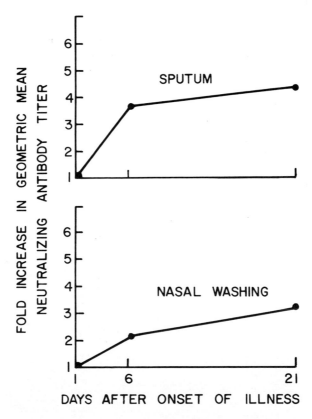

Fig. 13.4. Increase in geometric mean neutralizing antibody titers in sputum and nasal washings following influenza A (H3N2) virus infection. From Togo *et al.* (1970). *J. Amer. Med. Ass.* **211,** 1149–1156. Copyright 1970, American Medical Association.

With the recent advent of interest in antibodies to specific surface proteins, it will be of interest to observe if development of these antibodies parallels those previously described.

B. Pulmonary Complications

1. PNEUMONIA

Two kinds of pulmonary complications are well recognized: primary influenza viral pneumonia and secondary bacterial infection. Bacterial infection occurring after influenza was frequently observed in 1918, and this observation has been recorded may times subsequently. The syndrome of primary influenza virus pneumonia became well documented first in the 1957–1958 outbreak.

Louria *et al.* (1959) studied 33 hospitalized patients prospectively during the 1957 influenza A (H2N2) outbreak. Six patients who contracted influenza infection developed a relentless course of continued fever, leukocytosis, dyspnea, hypoxia, and cyanosis following the classical influenza syndrome, and a case report of one of these patients is shown in Fig. 13.5. Five of 6 died with a fulminating diffuse hemorrhagic pneumonia. Influenza virus was isolated directly from the lungs of 4 of these patients who died within 10 days of onset, and pre- and postmortem culture of blood and lungs failed to reveal bacteria. Six of these patients had underlying cardiovascular disease, 4 had rheumatic heart disease.

Autopsies performed on 4 patients revealed markedly congested, heavy, dark red lungs. The mucosa of the trachea and bronchi was strikingly hyperemic. On microscopic examination, tracheitis, bronchitis, and bronchiolitis

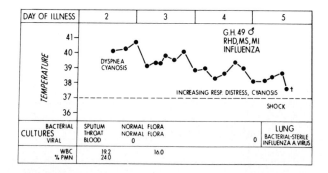

Fig. 13.5.   Case report of a volunteer with primary influenza viral pneumonia. From Louria *et al.* (1959).

with hyperemia, hemorrhage, slight cellular infiltrate, and loss of ciliated epithelium were constant findings. Alveolar exudate, consisting of both neutrophils and mononuclear cells, and hemorrhage were common. Pulmonary arteries and veins were normal, and there was no evidence of myocarditis.

A second group of 15 patients developed clear-cut bacterial pneumonia. Pneumonia occurred late in the course of influenza, usually after a period of improvement from the classic influenza syndrome resulting in a biphasic fever pattern. With the development of pneumonia, the signs and symptoms were typical of bacterial pneumonia. The pneumonitis was localized, and the etiology was pneumococcal in 8, staphylococcal in 3, *Hemophilus influenzae* in 1, and mixed bacterial in 3. Only one patient died. In contrast to the patients with primary influenza viral pneumonia, only 3 patients had underlying cardiovascular disease, all of which were rheumatic heart disease.

The third major group consisted of 9 patients who had concomitant pulmonary infection with influenza virus and bacteria. Three had pneumococcal, 3 staphylococcal, and 3 mixed bacterial infections. Five patients had underlying cardiovascular disease, 3 of which were rheumatic. Three patients died. The final 3 patients had only transient pulmonary signs and no radiographic evidence of pneumonia.

In the same epidemic, Martin *et al.* (1959) reported 20 cases of staphylococcal pneumonia complicating influenza, confirming the importance of this organism as a secondary bacterial invader in cases of influenza. Eleven of their patients had underlying diseases, which included bronchial asthma, chronic bronchitis, and obesity as well as rheumatic and other forms of cardiovascular disease. Nine of these patients died. Other reports have also stressed the importance of this organism as a cause of secondary bacterial pneumonia or mixed pneumonia following influenza virus infection, and have shown that it may occur in persons with no underlying disease.

More recent reports of pneumonia occurring in the 1968–1969 (H3N2) pandemic have confirmed and extended these observations. Schwarzmann *et al.* (1971) studied 108 cases admitted during a 3-week outbreak of influenza and compared them to all patients admitted with pneumonia in the previous year in the absence of influenza in the community. As shown in Table 13.7, there was a threefold increase in the proportion of cases of staphylococcal pneumonia during the influenza outbreak; however, *Pneumococcus* remained the organism most frequently isolated from patients with pneumonia in both periods, and the relative frequencies of *Hemophilus influenzae* and other gram-negative bacteria remained unchanged. Most patients (79 and 82%) had underlying disease, and the only difference observed was a higher proportion of patients with congestive heart failure in the influenza epidemic. Serological evidence for influenza infection was established in 74% of 42 patients tested who were admitted during the epidemic, but such tests

Table 13.7   Etiology of Bacterial Pneumonia during H3N2 Influenza A Outbreak as Compared to Preceding Year[a]

	Number of patients with indicated bacterial etiology	
	---	---
Bacterial etiology	During influenza outbreak[b] 1968–1969	Preceding year[c] (no influenza)
Pneumococcus	52 (48%)	103 (62%)
Staphylococcus	21 (19%)	10 (6%)
Staphylococcus and other	7 (7%)	7 (4%)
Hemophilus influenzae	12 (11%)	14 (8%)
Other gram negative	16 (15%)	33 (30%)
Totals	108	167

[a] From Schwarzmann *et al.* (1971). *Arch. Intern. Med.* **127,** 1037–1041. Copyright 1971, American Medical Association.
[b] 3 week period only.
[c] 12 month period.

were not carried out during the nonepidemic period. Overall mortality was similar, 21 and 24%, respectively. These findings suggest that epidemic influenza increases the pneumonia attack rate, but that the same patient is at risk.

Bisno *et al.* (1971) reported on 106 patients admitted to the hospital during the same epidemic and compared their results to those observed 1 year later, when only $\frac{1}{3}$ as many patients with pneumonia were admitted. During the epidemic, 84% of patients with pneumonia had serological evidence of influenza. Their findings were similar to those of Schwarzmann *et al.* (1971) in that *Pneumococcus* was the most frequent bacterial pathogen, that staphylococcal pneumonia was unusually common during the influenza outbreak, and that the underlying conditions were a much broader spectrum than those categorized by Louria *et al.* (1959) and included pulmonary disease, diabetes mellitus, renal disease, alcoholism, and pregnancy as well as cardiovascular disorders. No cases of primary influenza viral pneumonia were seen in Schwarzmann's series and only one probable case in Bisno's study. It is clear, however, that such cases occurred in the Hong Kong (H3N2) outbreak. Burk *et al.* (1971) reported four cases, one in a patient with mitral stenosis, two in patients with nephrotic syndrome on corticosteroid therapy, and one in a 34-year-old, healthy female. Newton-John *et al.* (1971) reported 10 cases occurring in 335 adult patients with pneumonia. Thus, it appears that the incidence of primary influenza viral pneumonia is low, probably just a few percent of the total cases of pneumonia, the vast majority of which are bacterial or mixed viral and bacterial in origin. Others have shown that the spectrum of primary influenza viral pneumonia is broader than the original description, and includes mild segmental pneumonia (Kaye *et al.*, 1962).

The question of the frequency of involvement of the respiratory tract has been answered in part by Fry (1951, 1958, 1959). As shown in Table 13.8, in five epidemics he observed chest complications to vary between 3 and 20% of cases. The incidence of such complications is age related, and this is shown in Table 13.9. As indicated 9.5% of patients were observed to have chest complications. From age 5 to 50 the rate was low, but increased progressively after the age of 60. Most of the complications were bronchitis or segmental pneumonia. Only 1% had lobar pneumonia, and all were over age 30.

2. ACUTE LOWER RESPIRATORY TRACT DISEASE OF CHILDREN

The contribution of influenza to lower respiratory tract disease in children appears to be much smaller than in adults. In a prospective study in a pediatric group practice by Glezen *et al.* (1971), it was shown that influenza A virus was a very infrequent cause of pneumonia or bronchiolitis in children. From 1963 through 1969 only 5 isolates of influenza virus were obtained from 1714 patients with pneumonia or bronchitis, 8 from 899 patients with tracheobronchitis and 11 from 502 patients with croup. In regard to influenza B, 14 isolates were obtained from patients with pneumonia and

Table 13.8 Comparative Rates of Chest Complications of Influenza Epidemics[a]

	Year and type of influenza				
	1950–1951 A	1953 A	1955 B	1957 A	1959 A + B
No. influenza cases	223	264	150	930	849
Total chest complications	43 (20%)	29 (11%)	15 (10%)	28 (3%)	80 (10%)
Pneumonia[b]	37 (17%)	17 (7%)	11 (7%)	18 (2%)	50 (6%)
Acute bronchitis	6 (3%)	12 (5%)	4 (3%)	10 (1%)	30 (4%)

[a] From Fry (1959). *Brit. Med. J.* **2,** 135–138. Reproduced by permission.
[b] Based on X-ray or physical findings.

Table 13.9 Distribution of Chest Complications in a General Practice[a]

Complication	0–4	5–9	10–19	20–29	30–39	40–49	50–59	60–69	70+	Total
Lobar pneumonia[b]	—	—	—	—	1	1	1	3	1	7
Segmental pneumonia[c]	3	9	5	3	2	3	5	6	6	43
Acute bronchitis	6	1	—	1	2	3	4	6	7	30
Total	9	10	6	4	5	7	10	15	14	80
% of all cases of influenza	12	8	4	4	4	7	10	36	73	9.5

Column group header: Age (years)

[a] From Fry (1959). *Brit. Med. J.* **2**, 135–138. Reproduced by permission.
[b] X-ray evidence of pneumonia.
[c] Persistent rales.

bronchiolitis, 21 from patients with tracheobronchitis, and 6 from patients with croup. It is of interest that influenza B was most commonly isolated between the ages of 3 and 8, whereas over 50% of the influenza A virus isolates were obtained from children under 2 years of age.

In another prospective study by Foy *et al.* (1973) in preschool children, influenza A and B were each isolated from 1% of 210 patients with croup. Influenza viruses were rarely isolated in spite of sharp epidemics of influenza A (H3N2) during the study period. Serological rises were shown to influenza A and B, respectively, among 3.2 and 1.2% of 249 patients with pneumonia, 9 and 3% of patients with tracheobronchitis, and 3.7 and 1.8% of patients with croup.

Others (Howard *et al.*, 1972) have pointed out that croup associated with influenza A virus infection is more severe than that associated with para-influenza virus or respiratory syncytial virus infections resulting in more frequent hospitalizations and tracheostomies.

3. Acute Exacerbation of Chronic Bronchitis

Influenza viruses are among the etiological agents associated with exacerbations of chronic bronchitis, an important association since such episodes may result in deterioration of pulmonary function. Carilli *et al.* (1964) described 46 illnesses in 24 patients, 4 of which were associated with influenza A virus infection. Stark *et al.* (1965) obtained serological evidence of influenza B virus infection in 9 of 185 (4.9%) of exacerbation of bronchitis. Eadie *et al.* (1966) showed serological evidence of influenza A in one case, and influenza C in 2 cases of exacerbations of bronchitis among 75 episodes. Stenhouse (1967) presented serological evidence of influenza A infection in 4 cases, and influenza B in 2 patients among 34 patients with 79 acute respiratory illnesses.

C. Reye's Syndrome

Reye *et al.* (1963) reported 21 pediatric cases of a disease with a high mortality rate characterized by acute encephalopathy with fatty degeneration of the viscera. Typically, the fulminating disease was preceded by a minor prodromal illness. Serum glutamic oxalacetic transaminase (SGOT) and glutamic pyruvic transaminase (SGPT) levels were markedly elevated, and hypoglycemia and hypoglycorrhachia were frequently present. Cerebral edema and fatty degeneration of the liver dominated the pathological picture.

Although diverse etiologies have been suggested, the most frequent epidemiological association has been with influenza B virus infection. In addition, Norman *et al.* (1968) isolated influenza B virus from a liver biopsy specimen obtained from a patient with Reye's syndrome. Although originally believed to be a rare disease, it has been recognized with considerable frequency in recent years. In a selective epidemiological study, Glick *et al.* (1970) detected 62 cases from parts of the United States and Puerto Rico over a 30-month period. Epidemic patterns appeared in February and March 1969, concurrent with outbreaks of influenza B infection. In January and February 1971, 36 children in New England and New York State were hospitalized with Reye's syndrome at the time of a documented outbreak of influenza B virus infection (Center for Disease Control, 1971). The age of the patients ranged from 3 to 16 years, 13 patients were male and 24 female, and 58% died. Evidence of influenza B virus infection was obtained in 7 of 12 patients tested.

In the winter of 1973–1974 in the United States, a total of 286 cases were reported from 28 states and the District of Columbia (Center for Disease Control, 1974a,b). The peak onset of disease occurred in February 1974, and was associated with an outbreak of influenza B virus infection in the middle section of the United States. The vast majority of patients had preceding upper respiratory illness 3 to 10 days prior to the onset of protracted nausea and vomiting. The mortality rate was 36%.

D. Myositis and Myoglobinuria

Myalgia is a characteristic feature of the classical influenza syndrome. Occasionally, myositis and myoglobinuria occur. Middleton *et al.* (1970) reported 26 children with severe leg pain associated with walking occurring 1 to 5 days after subsidence of upper respiratory symptoms. Effected leg muscles were tender on palpation, and serum creatinine phosphokinase (CPK) levels were elevated. No neurological changes were evident. Influenza B virus infection was proved in 20 cases and influenza A in one.

Simon *et al.* (1970) reported a case of serologically proved influenza A (H3N2) infection during the 1968–1969 outbreak in a 27-year-old man who, on the second day of a typical influenza-like illness with severe myalgias, developed dark brown urine containing myoglobin, an SGOT of 2660 units, and a CPK of 3920 units. A second case was reported (Minow *et al.*, 1974) during the influenza epidemic of 1972–1973 in a 28-year-old woman who on the third day of a typical influenza syndrome developed diffuse muscular pain, generalized weakness with swelling of the extremities, myoglobinuria, a SGOT of 1920 units, a SGPT of 560 units, and a CPK of 15,000 IU/ml. Muscle biopsy showed necrosis of individual muscle fibers with a mononuclear cell infiltrate. Influenza infection was established by a rise in complement fixing antibodies.

E. Central Nervous and Cardiac System Involvement

The occurrence of encephalopathy and fatty liver (Reye's syndrome) associated with influenza B virus infection has already been discussed. Sporadic case reports have appeared in the literature of other diseases of the central nervous system, such as Guillain-Barré syndrome, transverse myelitis, or encephalitis without liver involvement. Central nervous system involvement has occurred followed by a variable symptom-free interval an acute febrile illness characteristic of influenza, and the association has been supported by high or falling antibody titers to influenza A virus. Most reported cases have occurred during documented influenza A virus outbreaks. Wells (1971) reported serological evidence of infection with influenza A virus in 5 cases with transverse myelitis, one with Guillain-Barré, one with myeloradiculopathy, and one with subdural empyema during the winter of 1968–1969. The latter case was a presumed bacterial superinfection.

In regard to Guillain-Barré syndrome, Wells *et al.* (1959) reported 2 fatal cases with postmortem isolation of influenza A virus from lungs and cerebrospinal fluid which occurred during the 1957–1958 pandemic. Other reports indicate that even if some cases of Guillain-Barré may be associated with influenza A virus infection, the proportion resulting from influenza virus infection is small. Melnick and Flewitt (1964) in their study of 52 cases, showed serological evidence of influenza A infection in 4, influenza B in 2, and influenza C in 1 patient. These frequencies were not higher than those noted in 817 controls. Leneman (1966) reviewed reports of 1100 cases; 638 had antecedent infectious diseases, 83 were influenzal syndromes, and 259 were infections of the respiratory tract. In 8 cases there was serological evidence of influenza virus infection. Thus, while not proved, it seems likely that some cases of encephalitis, transverse myelitis, and Guillain-Barré syndrome may follow influenza virus infections. In this regard, Asbury *et al.* (1969) compared the pathological features of Guillain-Barré syndrome to those of experimental allergic neuritis and suggested that Guillain-Barré syndrome is a cell-mediated immunological disorder which may be triggered by a prior infection; thus, the absence of well-documented isolations of influenza virus from the central nervous system could be explained.

Recently, Edelen *et al.* (1974) reported the occurrence of encephalopathy, pericarditis, or both in 18 patients in Fairbanks, Alaska during an outbreak of influenza A/England/42/72 (H3N2). Eight of 12 patients who were tested showed evidence of influenza virus infection and no evidence of infection with other viruses.

Although myocarditis was observed clinically and pathologically during the 1918 outbreak, other observers more recently have been unable to document myocarditis despite careful study (Louria et al., 1959). Both influenza A and B rarely have been serologically associated with myopericarditis (Adams, 1959; Edelen et al., 1974), and influenza A virus has been recovered from pericardial fluid (Woodward et al., 1960; Hildebrandt et al., 1962).

F. Congenital Malformations

These are numerous reports in the literature concerned with the question of whether influenza virus infection of pregnant mothers leads to congenital malformations. Some reports suggest such a relationship, particularly in regard to anencephaly, and other CNS malformations (Coffey and Jessop, 1959, 1963; Doll et al., 1960). Transplacental passage of virus has been demonstrated in a fatal case of influenza during the last trimester of pregnancy (Yawn et al., 1971). Analysis of larger populations looking for prematurity, excess infant deaths, or malformation have failed to reveal any relationship to epidemic influenza (Hardy et al., 1961; Hewitt, 1962; Widelock et al., 1963; Leck et al., 1969). Thus, while it may be possible that there is a small risk of producing anencephaly in the fetus if the mother contracts influenza in the first trimester, the extent of the risk is very small, particularly when the frequency of infection of pregnant women during epidemics is considered.

G. Specific Therapy: Amantadine

The chemoprophylactic use of amantadine has been discussed elsewhere (Chapter 10). Several placebo-controlled double-blind studies have shown a mild but definite therapeutic benefit of amantadine in uncomplicated influenza, but no trials in influenza viral pneumonia have been performed. Togo et al. (1970) showed more rapid defervesence, and improvement in symptoms in amantadine-treated subjects as compared to controls in an outbreak of naturally occurring influenza. Similar findings were observed using amantadine and rimantadine by Wingfield et al. (1969). Knight et al. (1970) also showed more rapid improvement of patients receiving amantadine. In addition, they observed a more rapid decrease in titers of virus in throat swab specimens among amantadine-treated patients as compared to placebo-treated controls.

III. Experimental Influenza Virus Infections in Man

A. Effect of Dose and Route of Inoculation

In most of the early studies, influenza virus was administered by spraying aerosols of heterogenous particle diameters into the nasopharynx, probably resulting in inoculation of both the upper and lower respiratory tracts. In these studies, it was difficult to reproduce influenza in humans with instillation of virus into the nasopharynx alone (Henle *et al.*, 1946; Smorodintseff *et al.*, 1937; Francis *et al.*, 1944). However, more recent studies have shown conclusively that nasopharyngeal inoculations result in production of the classical influenza syndrome. This discrepancy may have several explanations: the use of subjects who possessed antibody, variation in clinical response due to virus strain, passage history of the inoculum, and dose as well as route of inoculation. Most experimental studies with influenza virus in recent years have employed methods of inoculation which deposit virus containing suspensions in the upper respiratory tract, either nose drops or coarse sprays into the nose, pharynx, or both (Couch *et al.*, 1974; Murphy *et al.*, 1973b). In general, the inoculum has contained fairly large doses of virus, usually between 10^4 and 10^6 TCID$_{50}$.

A limited amount of data is available on the infectivity of influenza viruses for humans deposited in the upper respiratory tract, and estimates of the 50% human infectious dose (HID$_{50}$) vary somewhat from strain to strain but in two instances have been shown to be 127 and 320 TCID$_{50}$ for influenza A/Aichi/68 (H3N2) (Couch *et al.*, 1971, 1974). In these studies, the inoculum consisted of second passage material in human embryonic kidney cells. The HID$_{50}$ also varies with the antibody status of the host so that the most meaningful data will be obtained from inoculation of volunteers with absent anti-neuraminidase and anti-hemagglutinin antibodies to the virus in question, and this has not usually been possible in the past because of the lack of availability of these specific antibody assays. Once infection occurs, there appears to be little effect of doses ranging from 10^3 to 10^9 TCID$_{50}$, except perhaps for a shortening of the incubation period with the larger doses. That is, the severity of the resulting illness is independent of dose if infection has occurred.

In regard to aerosol inoculations, early work by Smorodintseff *et al.* (1937), Burnet and Foley (1940), Francis *et al.* (1944), Henle *et al.* (1943, 1946), and others showed that the influenza syndrome could be reliably reproduced in volunteers inoculated by inhalation of atomized allantoic fluid harvests containing influenza virus. Large doses were atomized, 10^6 to 10^{10} egg or mouse infectious doses, but no information is available concerning the aerosol particle size, the site of deposition, or quantity inhaled and deposited. Despite these limitations, these studies showed conclusively that an illness could be produced experimentally in man with symptoms and signs that closely resembled naturally occurring influenza.

Limited data are available concerning influenza resulting from inoculations with aerosols which have been carefully characterized. Again, such inoculations resulted in infection and illness which closely resembled naturally occurring influenza, and some data is available concerning infectivity for man. Alford et al. (1966) administered varying doses of influenza virus contained in a homogenous aerosol with a mean particle diameter of 1.5 μm, an aerosol which was shown to be retained predominantly in the lower respiratory tract. The HID_{50} of influenza A/Bethesda/10/63 (H2N2) administered by this route was estimated to be 0.6 to 3 $TCID_{50}$ based on a titration experiment performed in 10 volunteers with low or absent serum neutralizing antibodies to influenza virus. Thus, it appears that the human lower respiratory tract is 40 to 500 times more sensitive than the upper respiratory tract to infection with influenza A viruses, although the same inoculum has not been titered by both routes of administration. This finding supports the contention that the majority of naturally occurring cases occur by the aerosol route.

Review of published data concerning the two methods of inoculation reveals other differences in clinical responses. In most studies with aerosol inoculations, the incubation period has been 12–48 hours, whereas with nasopharyngeal instillations the incubation period is somewhat longer, 2 to 3 days. Published descriptions of illness indicate that symptoms last briefer periods of time and are less severe following nasopharyngeal inoculation. There are two instances where the same inoculum was given by the differing routes. Henle et al. (1946) gave three different strains of influenza A and one of B to volunteers. Fifty-eight of 65 receiving inoculations by inhalation developed febrile responses, whereas only 2 of 16 receiving 10^8 and 10^9 chick embryo infectious doses of the same inocula by nasal instillation became febrile. In contrast, Alford et al. (1966) noted identical clinical responses to aerosol inoculation of 1 to 5 $TCID_{50}$ as compared to 80,000 to 180,000 $TCID_{50}$ nasopharyngeally, except for a shorter incubation period with the aerosol inoculation. It is most likely, in addition, that lower respiratory tract symptoms and cough are less following intranasal inoculations. In all other respects, the clinical responses are indistinguishable. At the present time most inoculations of human volunteers are performed by intranasal drops rather than by aerosols, primarily for reasons of safety. That is, the possibility of development of lower respiratory tract disease is considered to be less following nasal than following aerosol inoculations. Doses administered are between $10^{3.0}$ and $10^{5.0}$, a sufficient multiple of the HID_{50} to ensure adequate infectivity.

B. Effect of Tissue Culture and Egg Passage

Bull and Burnet (1943) originally suggested that since influenza viruses were inherently genetically unstable, tissue culture or egg passage would lead to less virulent strains, an advantage in terms of development of live attenuated vaccine but a hindrance to development of model infections in man which mimic naturally occurring disease. Several investigators have noted loss of infectivity for man following two to four passages in embryonated hens eggs. Zhdanov (1966) observed a reduction in virulence for humans after four to eight passages in chick embryos and later a loss of human infectivity after 12 to 16 passages. The number of passages needed for these changes can be detected only in volunteer trials, since there are no reliable laboratory markers by which they can be predicted. Other investigators have been unable to duplicate this work. Beare *et al.* (1968) tested an A/Leningrad/4/65 (H3N2) strain and two B strains, B/England/13/65 and B/England/101/62, each passaged 20 to 30 times in eggs, and rates of infection and illness were unchanged with passage. In the studies of Henle *et al.* (1943, 1946) and Burnet and Foley (1940) multiple egg-passaged material resulted in high frequency of illness responses. This discrepancy may reflect factors other than passage history, namely, strain variation, dose, or route of inoculation.

Animal-passaged influenza viruses generally have been shown to retain virulence for man. In particular, passage in ferrets (1–8 passages) and mice (≥ 15 passages) results in virulent inocula (Henle *et al.*, 1943, 1946; Francis *et al.*, 1944), although the final material was usually prepared in embryonated hens eggs.

Most investigators agree that tissue culture passage results in less attenuation of human virulence and infectivity than egg passage (Knight *et al.*, 1965). Thus, currently most investigators are working with low passage material grown in human embryonic or bovine kidney cell cultures (Couch *et al.*, 1974; Murphy *et al.*, 1973a). Rhesus monkey cell cultures are not suitable for preparation of inocula for human volunteers because of the large number of adventitious viruses known to contaminate such cultures.

C. Effect of Strain Variation

Some of the previously mentioned observed differences between inocula which cannot be explained by dose, route of inoculation, or tissue culture or animal passage may be due to differences between strains. Henle *et al.* (1946) demonstrated shorter incubation periods (12–24 hours) with the PR-8 strain of influenza A (H0N1) and two strains of influenza B than with the F-99 strain of influenza A (H0N1) virus (36–48 hours). In addition, with F-99 virus an inverse relation between level of preinoculation antibodies and febrile response was observed, but not with Lee (B) or PR-8. Other investigators have not noted differences between strains other than those subjected to genetic manipulation (mutation, cold adaptation, recombination). In any event, it should be apparent that these differences are minor, and the characteristic clinical syndrome does not vary from strain to strain or year to year.

D. Other Factors

Zhdanov and Ritova (1963) stated that their volunteers in Russia experienced more clinical reactions in winter than in summer, presumably, a climatic effort. In contrast, Beare *et al.* (1968) in England showed similar rates of illness among volunteers inoculated May through September as compared to those inoculated October through April.

E. Signs and Symptoms

A summary of recent experience with experimental influenza in normal volunteers is shown in Table 13.10. As indicated, doses of $10^{3.0}$ to $10^{5.0}$ $TCID_{50}$ resulted in infection of 50 to 90% of volunteers with low or absent antibody to the virus used for inoculation, and of those infected, 40 to 70% developed febrile influenza syndrome, 10% developed afebrile upper respiratory symptoms, and 27% were asymptomatic.

The incubation period to the onset of illness may vary from 1 to 3 days but, as noted previously, tends to be shorter with aerosol inoculation. Occasionally incubation periods of from 3 to 6 or 7 days have been observed, a result which may in part be explained by failure to infect with a low dose nasal challenge, and the occurrence of person to person transmission resulting in secondary infection. In part, however, such prolonged incubation periods may result from primary inoculation, since they have been observed in studies where volunteers were isolated from one another.

Illness is quite similar to that which has been described for naturally occurring influenza. A case report of a volunteer who developed the typical influenza syndrome following inoculation with influenza A/Udorn/307/72 (H3N2) virus is shown in Fig. 13.6. As indicated, the onset of illness was

Table 13.10 Illness Responses of Volunteers Inoculated with Influenza A H3N2 Strains

Method	Tissue culture[a]	Dose (TCID$_{50}$)	No. of volunteers	No. infected	Afebrile coryza and/or pharyngitis	Influenza syndrome	Reference
Coarse spray	BK$_4$	$10^{5.0}$	21	19	3	11	Murphy et al., 1972b
Coarse spray	HEK$_2$	$10^{4.5}$	7	7	1	6	Murphy et al., 1973b
Nose drops	HEK$_2$	$10^{3.0}$	14	11	2	4	Couch et al., 1971
Nose drops	HEK$_2$	$10^{3.0}$	13	11	0	10	Couch et al., 1974
Nose drops	HEK$_2$	$10^{3.2}$	10	5	1	3	R. G. Douglas, Jr. (unpublished observation)
Nose drops	HEK$_2$	$10^{4.0}$	15	8	0	3	R. G. Douglas, Jr. (unpublished observation)
Nose drops	HEK$_2$	$10^{4.5}$	8	5	3	2	R. G. Douglas, Jr. (unpublished observation)
Totals			88	66	9	39	

[a] BK, bovine kidney; HEK, human embryonic kidney. Subscript refers to number of passages.

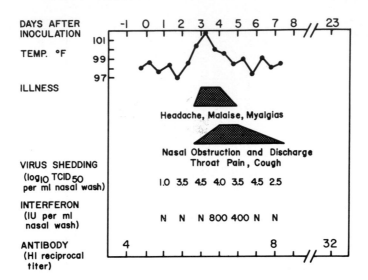

Fig. 13.6. Case report of a volunteer inoculated by nose drops with 1000 TCID$_{50}$ influenza A/Udorn/72 (H3N2) virus. N, negative.

abrupt on the night of the second day after inoculation. Symptoms at that time included feverishness, chills, headache, malaise, myalgia, and anorexia. In some cases, particularly following nasal inoculation, mild premonitory nasopharyngeal symptoms may be present for 1 or 2 days before systemic symptoms develop. The temperature reached its peak within 12 hours of onset, and the maximal temperature may vary from 100° to 104°F. During the early febrile stage of illness, systemic symptoms predominate. However, dry cough may be present, and mild, thin, clear nasal discharge or throat pain may occur. Fever is diminished on the second and third days of illness, and commonly disappears on the fourth day but may last from 1 to 5 days. Fever may be intermittent, but is usually continuous as shown, and in some cases the occurrence of a second peak on the third day or fourth day produces a diphasic temperature course. This was particularly seen in the early studies (Henle *et al.*, 1946; Francis *et al.*, 1944). As fever and systemic symptoms diminish, the respiratory symptoms usually increase in severity. Frequently, the cough becomes productive of small amounts of white sputum; nasal obstruction, nasal discharge, sore throat, and hoarseness are observed. Nausea and vomiting may occur in a small percentage of cases, but they are not predominant manifestations and are attributable to systemic reactions. Abdominal pain and diarrhea are not observed.

On physical examination early in the course of illness, the volunteers showed signs of toxicity. The face is flushed and is hot and moist. Injection of the conjunctiva, watering of the eyes, and narrowing palpebral fissures are commonly observed. Slight nasal obstruction and thin, clear nasal discharge are frequently observed. The mucous membranes of the nose and pharynx are commonly injected but exudate is seldom present. Small cervical nodes may be palpated especially if throat pain is a prominent symptom. Transient scattered rhonchi and expiratory fine rales may be detected, particularly in volunteers with moderate cough, but persistent signs in the chest are not found. The respiratory symptoms usually disappear by the fifth to seventh day of illness, although cough may persist longer.

In afebrile cases, the systemic symptoms, such as myalgias, headache, and malaise generally do not occur. Illness may predominantly involve the throat in which case throat pain, pharyngeal injection without exudate, and mild cervical adenopathy are observed; or the nose, in which case thin, watery nasal discharge, nasal obstruction, and boggy edematous membranes are observed; or a combination of any and all of the above symptoms and signs may occur.

In infected but asymptomatic volunteers, physical signs of illness are also absent.

F. Clinical Laboratory Findings

Smorodinsteff *et al.* (1937) described leukocytosis in $\frac{1}{3}$ of patients at the onset of illness for 1 day followed by a decrease in white blood cell counts to less than 6000 per mm³ persisting for 3–5 days in 25 of 72 volunteers challenged with influenza A virus. This observation has been confirmed and extended in subsequent studies. Henle *et al.* (1943) noted leukocytosis up to 15,000 per mm³ at the onset of illness, usually the second day after inoculation, due to an increase in circulating neutrophils. The total white count then rapidly dropped, and leukopenia, sometimes as low as 1500, was observed lasting 2 to 4 days. A relative lymphocytosis was observed on the fourth to the eighth days. They also detected leukopenia of 5000 or below among subjects who did not become ill, some of whom developed antibody responses.

Douglas *et al.* (1966) studied leukocyte responses among 38 volunteers inoculated intranasally with influenza virus A/Bethesda/10/63 (H2N2). Twenty-one of 38 of these volunteers became ill 2 to 4 days after inoculation. Infection occurred in 19 of 21 men who became ill, and in 14 of 17 who were not ill. An example of the circulating leukocyte response is shown in Fig. 13.7. As shown, among ill volunteers, neutrophilia occurred on the second day after inoculation followed by neutropenia on the sixth day. Lymphocytes fell on the first day of illness and, in some volunteers, rose on day 6 above the preinoculation levels. Total leukocyte counts exceeded

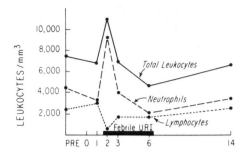

DAYS AFTER INOCULATION

Fig. 13.7. Serial changes in peripheral white cell counts in a representative volunteer inoculated with influenza A/Bethesda/10/63 (H2N2). From Douglas *et al.* (1966).

10,000 per mm³ (maximum 12,000) at the onset of illness in 8 of 21 men who were ill, and 2 of 17 who were not ill. Total leukocyte counts less than 5000 were noted later during illness in three volunteers. These changes were shown to be significant, but there were no significant changes in volunteers who were not ill. In addition, significant changes in eosinophil and monocyte counts did not occur, and serial study of hematocrit and hemoglobin values revealed no change. The erythrocyte sedimentation rate is elevated transiently in ½ of the subjects.

Further significant changes were observed in lymphocyte counts prior to the development of illness, which varied according to the severity of illness. Twelve volunteers developed maximal oral temperatures of $\geq 38°C$ and were considered more severely ill than 9 men whose maximal temperatures were less than 38°C. Among more severely ill volunteers, lymphocytes increased (+540 average change) from preinoculation to day 1, but in milder cases decreased, (−170). In more severely ill men, lymphocytes fell sharply (−1100) from day 1 to day 2 and in milder cases fell slightly (−110).

Evaluation of hepatic (SGOT, SGPT, alkaline phosphatase, bilirubin) and renal (urinalysis, serum creatinine, and urea nitrogen) function showed no alterations during or after infections as compared to those obtained prior to infection.

G. Quantitative Virus Shedding Patterns

Influenza A virus has been isolated from the nasal or oral cavities by a variety of means. Earlier studies tended to employ throat swabs, gargles, or nasal swabs. More recently, nasal washes (NW) have been predominantly used. In one study (R. B. Couch and R. G. Douglas, Jr., unpublished observation) comparison of NW, throat swab, sputum, throat gargle, anterior oral secretions, and nose swab specimens each collected daily from 6 volunteers inoculated intranasally with influenza A/Hong Kong/68 (H3N2) was performed. Figure 13.8 shows the data obtained. As indicated, NW specimens were the most consistently positive, and these specimens have been used for most of the quantitative studies. The superiority of the NW is likely to be due to the fact that the NW procedure obtains approximately 1 ml of secretions from the nasal passages and posterior pharynx, whereas swab specimens are limited to a single area and swabs become saturated with 0.15 ml secretions. However, the superiority of NW may reflect the early site of replication in the nasopharynx in experimental infection, since only during the first 2 days is it clearly superior to other specimens. Sputa are more difficult to collect from volunteers without cough, since they require inhalation of saline or expectorants to promote sputum production; and anterior oral secretions, in addition to containing less virus, are relatively toxic for tissue cultures.

As shown in Fig. 13.9, quantitation of virus in NW by titration in rhesus monkey kidney cultures reveals a characteristic pattern. Virus is detected in moderate quantities on the first day after inoculation, and quantities rise rapidly to peak titers of 3.0 to 7.0 $\log_{10}$ $TCID_{50}$/ml on the second day, then fall off somewhat more slowly. Virus is no longer detectable sometime around the fifth to tenth day after inoculation. As shown in Fig. 13.6 there

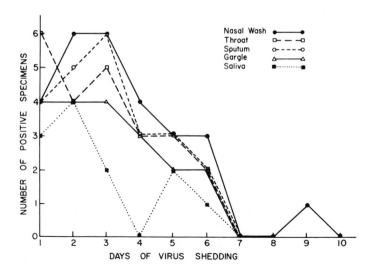

Fig. 13.8. Comparative frequency of isolation of influenza A (H3N2) virus from 5 different specimens each collected daily from six infected volunteers. From R. G. Douglas, Jr. and R. B. Couch (unpublished observations).

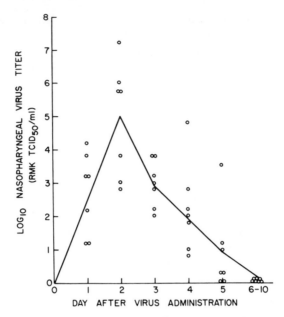

Fig. 13.9. Quantities of influenza A (H3N2) recovered from NW specimens obtained daily after inoculation from 7 infected volunteers. RMK, rhesus monkey kidney. From Murphy *et al.* (1973b). *J. Infec. Dis.* **128**, 479–487. Copyright 1973, University of Chicago Press. Reproduced by permission.

is a close correlation between illness and quantitative shedding. A definite relationship has been established between the degree of viral replication and severity of illness. Couch *et al.* (1971) was able to show a significant positive correlation between mean quantity of virus per positive specimen and severity of illness. In addition, Murphy *et al.* (1973a) demonstrated a correlation between the maximal titer of virus in NW and fever score, an objective evaluation of influenza illness that includes the degree and duration of temperature elevation.

Stanley and Jackson (1966) have reported viremia during induction of influenza in volunteers with influenza A/Bethesda/10/63 (H2N2) but confirmation of this work has not been published. Eleven of 23 specimens of laked blood collected during the incubation period yielded influenza virus when tested in embryonated eggs. The viremia occurred approximately 1 day before virus shedding from the nasopharynx, and 2 days before symptoms. Proof of the human origin of the viruses recovered was obtained by repeated reisolation from the original specimens, and infection in the volunteers was confirmed serologically. The virus isolates were confirmed as influenza A with properties similar to those of the challenge strain.

H. Interferon Response

Infection of volunteers with influenza viruses is accompanied by development of interferon in respiratory secretions and serum specimens. Results of studies by Jao *et al.* (1970) in regard to the occurrence of interferon in nasal washings after challenge of volunteers with influenza A/Bethesda/10/63 (H2N2) virus are shown in Fig. 13.10. Eight of 15 adult males who became infected after inoculation developed detectable interferon in NW specimens, and eight developed detectable interferon in serum. A total of 10 volunteers developed an interferon response, and six had detectable interferon in both sites. Nine of the 10 volunteers with interferon shed virus in nasal secretions, had clinical illness, and developed fourfold rises in serum neutralizing antibodies. As shown in Fig. 13.10, shedding of virus preceded by 1 to 2 days the appearance of interferon in both the nasal secretions and serum. Viral shedding correlated closely with illness as previously described. Duration of viral shedding after the rise of interferon to peak titers was variable, but in some volunteers it persisted beyond the rise and

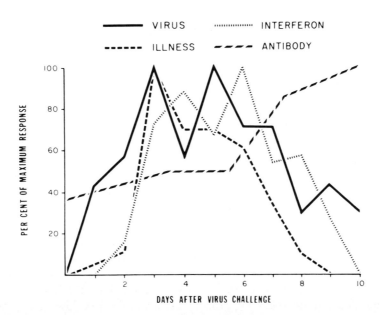

Fig. 13.10. Correlation of clinical, virological, and serological responses with detection of interferon in NW of volunteers infected with influenza A/Bethesda/10/63 (H2N2) virus. Peak frequency of virus shedding, peak titers of interferon and antibody, and peak severity of illness are considered as 100%. From Jao *et al.* (1970). *J. Infec. Dis.* **121,** 419–426. Copyright 1970, University of Chicago Press. Reproduced by permission.

disappearance of interferon. Of special interest in the study is the observation that clinical symptoms improved as interferon reached peak titers. It is possible, therefore, that interferon was active in the recovery process, especially the initial symptomatic improvement between the third and sixth day before any significant serum antibody response was demonstrable. There is a correlation between the rise of specific antibody in the serum and the rather abrupt secondary decline in symptoms and elimination of both shedding of virus and secretion of interferon which occurred after the first week.

Murphy *et al.* (1973b) has also demonstrated interferon in nasal secretions of 6 of 7 volunteers undergoing experimental infection with influenza A/Bethesda/68 (H3N2). He observed maximal individual titers of interferon nasal washes of 6000 units/ml and maximal geometric mean titer of 30 units on day 3. If one estimates a dilution factor of 1:10 in collection of nasal washes, the maximal titer of interferon induced is calculated to be 60,000 units. Interferon titers usually remained elevated for 6 days, after which interferon was detected on days 7 and 8 in only 2 of the 7 men. They noted a strong statistical association between maximal amount of virus shed and maximal titer of interferon in NW. Thus, although the temporal relation between appearance of interferon and recovery is apparent, it should be noted that the quantities of interferon are directly related to the degree of viral replication and severity of illness.

I. Antibody Responses

N-HI, HI, and CF antibodies develop in the sera of volunteers experimentally infected, and are usually first detected during the second week after inoculation. Detailed discussion of these antibodies and their detection is presented in Chapter 11 and 12, and the present discussion will be confined to the development and function of such antibodies in infected volunteers. As shown in Fig. 13.11, some volunteers developed detectable increases in antibody titer as soon as 7 days after inoculation. N-HI antibody usually reaches peak titers at the end of the second week after inoculation and rises only slightly higher in the ensuing interval. As discussed previously, the development of detectable serum antibodies correlates with cessation of the lingering symptoms of influenza. The development of HI, CF, and anti-neuraminidase antibodies (Fig. 13.12) parallels the development of N-HI antibodies.

The role of these antibodies in protection against infection is discussed in Chapter 12. More recently Murphy *et al.* (1972b) showed a relationship between anti-neuraminidase antibody and protection against illness experimentally induced by influenza A/Hong Kong/1968 (H3N2). As shown in

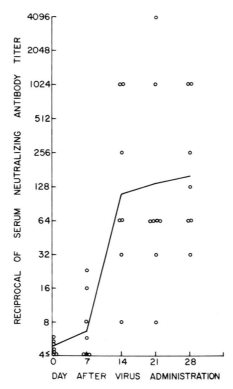

Fig. 13.11.   Serum neutralizing antibody response of 7 volunteers infected with influenza A (H3N2). Solid line indicates geometric mean. From Murphy *et al.* (1973a). *J. Infec. Dis.* **128**, 479–487. Copyright 1973, University of Chicago Press. Reproduced by permission.

Table 13.11, seven volunteers who did not become ill following challenge had significantly higher titers of anti-neuraminidase antibody than did those who developed febrile illness. In addition, the average number of days of shedding virus was significantly greater among those without anti-neuraminidase antibody. As shown in Table 13.12, a significant inverse relationship was shown between serum anti-neuraminidase antibody and clinical response.

The pattern of nasal secretory antibody response is shown in Fig. 13.13. It is apparent that development of nasal secretory N-HI antibodies parallels the serum response. Near peak titers are reached 14 days after inoculation, and some rise in mean titer is observed thereafter. Antibody also develops in sputum and saliva. Mann *et al.* (1968) reported that change in antibody titers over a period of 4 weeks tended to be similar in sputum and nasal wash specimens. Sucrose density gradient centrifugation of nasal

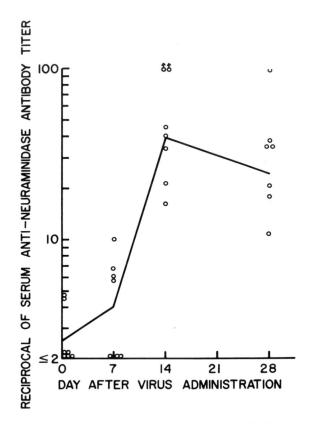

Fig. 13.12. Serum anti-neuraminidase antibody response of 7 volunteers (same as Fig. 13.8). Solid line indicates geometric mean. From Murphy *et al.* (1973a). *J. Infec. Dis.* **128,** 479–487. Copyright 1973, University of Chicago Press. Reproduced by permission.

wash specimens containing neutralizing activity indicate that the antibody which develops in secretions is primarily associated with 11 S immunoglobulin A (IgA) (Alford *et al.*, 1967b). Waldman *et al.* (1968, 1969) has shown, in comparative studies of antibody in sputum, saliva, and NW specimens collected from infected volunteers, that antibody in all of these secretions is primarily associated with IgA, and that similar concentrations of antibody are present in sputum and nasal wash specimens when they are equilibrated to the same IgA concentration. However, less antibody is detected in saliva.

In addition, and this is shown in Fig. 13.14, changes in secretory IgA occur (Rossen *et al.*, 1970). There is a rise in nasal secretion IgA content which occurs during illness which is not accompanied by a rise in NW N-HI

Table 13.11 Effect of Serum Anti-neuraminidase Antibody on Response of Volunteers to Intranasal Administration of Influenza A (H3N2) Virus[a]

Clinical response	No. of men	No. infected	Mean prechallenge serum ANAb[b] titer[c]	Prechallenge neutralizing antibody titer		No. of mean without antibody	Average day of virus shedding
				Serum	Nasal		
No illness	7	7	9.3	2.3	2.2	1	2.1
Afebrile illness	6	5	3.0	1.5	1.4	3	2.7
Febrile illness	8	8	1.3	1.6	1.6	7	6.1

$\left.\begin{array}{c} 9.3 \\ 3.0 \\ 1.3 \end{array}\right\} p < 0.01$[d]

$p < 0.01 \left\{ \begin{array}{c} 2.1 \\ 2.7 \\ 6.1 \end{array} \right\} p > 0.01$

[a] From Murphy *et al.* (1972b). *N. Engl. J. Med.* **286**, 1322–1332. Reprinted by permission.
[b] ANab, anti-neuraminidase antibody.
[c] Tested against HeqN2 (68) enzyme.
[d] Student *t*-test.

Table 13.12   Relation between Serum Anti-neuraminidase
Antibody Titer and Clinical Response to Influenza
A (H3N2) Virus[a]

Serum ANAb[b] titer	Men not ill	Men ill afebrile and febrile	Totals
<1:4	1	10	11
>1:4	6	4	10

$p < 0.05$, Fisher exact test (2-tailed)

[a] From Murphy *et al.* (1972b). *N. Engl. J. Med.* **286,** 1329–1332.
Reprinted by permission.
[b] ANAb, Anti-neuraminidase antibody.

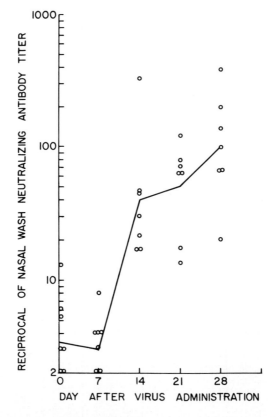

Fig. 13.13. Nasal wash neutralizing antibody response of 7 volunteers
(same as Figs. 13.8 and 13.9). Solid line indicates geometric mean. From
Murphy *et al.* (1973a). *J. Infec. Dis.* **128,** 479–487. Copyright 1973, University of
Chicago Press. Reproduced by permission.

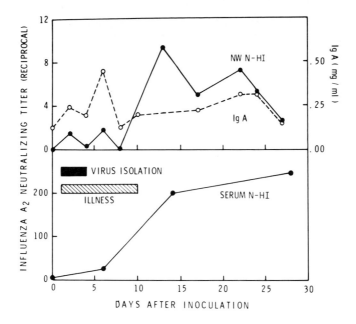

Fig. 13.14. Changes in NW IgA and neutralizing activity compared to virus isolation, illness, and serum neutralizing antibody response in 15 volunteers infected with influenza A (H2N2) virus. From Rossen *et al.* (1970). *J. Amer. Med. Ass.* **211**, 1157–1161. Copyright 1970, American Medical Association.

activity. NW N-HI antibody titers precede and then are accompanied by a second rise in nasal IgA concentration occurring 3 to 4 weeks after inoculation. As the NW antibody titer falls, IgA concentration returns to preillness values.

Rossen *et al.* (1970) compared the rate of occurrence of N-HI activity for four infected volunteers with high baseline nasal IgA concentrations, and four with low baseline concentrations. The men with high baseline levels exhibited a 7-day advantage in appearance of neutralizing activity. None of four with high baseline levels developed illness, whereas three of the four with low baseline did. Thus, the baseline level of respiratory secretion IgA may be another important determinant of the illness response.

The relative proportion of antibody found in respiratory secretions and in serum is determined in part by the route of inoculation. In extensive studies of antibody formation in respiratory secretions and serum, Kasel *et al.* (1969) showed that volunteers developed antibody in respiratory secretions more frequently and to a greater magnitude when given inactivated influenza virus vaccine intranasally than subcutaneously. Conversely, serum antibody developed more frequently and in higher titers when inactivated virus was given by the subcutaneous route than by the nasopharyngeal route.

Table 13.13 Neutralizing Antibody Responses in Nasal Wash and Serum to Inactivated Influenza Virus Vaccines[a]

Vaccine	Vaccination method	Mean maximum fold increase in antibody	
		Nasal wash	Serum
HK/68[b]	Nasopharyngeal (twice)	3.1	4.9
	Subcutaneous	1.0	6.3
A/64[c]	Nasopharyngeal	11.3	7.1
	Subcutaneous	3.2	35.9

[a] From Couch *et al.* (1969b).
[b] The majority lacked preexisting antibody.
[c] All had preexisting serum antibody.

However, differences in quantities of antibody in the two sites appear to be related to whether the individual is experiencing first or repeat exposure to the virus, and this is shown in Table 13.13. Volunteers experiencing first exposure to A/Hong Kong/68 (H3N2) virus developed more serum than nasal wash antibody regardless of how they received the vaccine. In contrast, in those individuals experiencing repeat exposure to influenza A/64 (H2N2), a striking disparity in antibody response in the two sites was observed that was related to route of administration. These latter findings are similar to those of Waldman *et al.* (1969) who also demonstrated protection against reinfection following administration of influenza vaccine by the aerosol route.

Much support has accumulated concerning the protective role of secretory antibodies in the respiratory tract. Data obtained in volunteer studies indicate an important role for both serum and secretory antibodies, and it has not been possible to dissociate their effects completely. Couch *et al.* (1969b) performed challenge studies of volunteers vaccinated either by the subcutaneous or by the nasal route. As shown in Table 13.14, equal proportions of volunteers in each group developed antibody in both sites. Following challenge with 3000 $TCID_{50}$ of influenza A/Hong Kong/68 (H3N2) 1 month after vaccination, virus shedding was similar in both vaccine groups as shown in Table 13.15. However, if only volunteers who developed an antibody response to vaccination are compared to controls, less infection occurred in the two vaccinated groups, particularly so in the nasal vaccination group. Illness occurred exclusively in volunteers with three or more isolates, only one of whom had developed antibody following vaccination. The relation of antibody titer to occurrence of infection is shown in Table 13.16. As

Table 13.14 Neutralizing Antibody Responses 4 Weeks following Vaccination with Influenza A_2/Hong Kong/68[a]

Vaccine group	Number of volunteers	Nasal wash antibody		Serum antibody	
		Number fourfold rise	ln titer	Number fourfold rise	ln titer
Nasal	12	4	2.75	9	3.25
Subcutaneous	9	2	2.5	8	4.22
Control	14	0	0	0	0

[a] From Couch *et al.* (1969b).

Table 13.15 Effects of Route of Vaccination on Virus Isolations from Volunteers after Nasal Inoculation with Influenza A_2 (H3N2)[a]

Group	Number of volunteers	Number of volunteers with indicated number of isolates[b]							
		0	1	2	3	4	5	6	7
Nasal vaccination	12	8	—	1	*1*	*1*	—	*1*	—
Subcutaneous vaccination	9	5	2	—	1	—	*1*	—	—
Control	14	6	1	—	1	1	1	3	1

[a] From Couch *et al.* (1969b).
[b] An italic number indicates man who did not develop serum antibody after vaccination. Yates mean score tests: Total group; nasal vs. control $p > 0.20$; subcutaneous vs. control $p > 0.15$. Those with antibody: nasal vs. control $p < 0.05$; subcutaneous vs. control $p = 0.07$.

shown, although frequency of infection was significantly higher among those without detectable serum antibody, infection occurred at all antibody levels. Similar comparisons of infection rates according to nasal secretion antibody titer revealed the same trend, although since so few volunteers possessed detectable nasal secretion antibodies that statistical proof was not obtained. The possible additive effects of nasal secretion to serum antibody are shown in Table 13.17. Only one individual possessed nasal secretion antibody and no serum antibody, and he became infected. The presence of serum antibody and no nasal secretory antibody was associated with a reduction in infection when compared with those who lacked antibody in both sites. When antibody was present in both sites, a still further reduction in the frequency of infection occurred, suggesting an additional protective effect occurred when both were present.

Table 13.16   Occurrence of Infection in Relation to Antibody Titer at Time of Nasal Inoculation with Influenza A_2 (Hong Kong Variant)[a,b]

Neutralizing antibody titer	Infection in relation to serum Ab titer		Infection in relation to NW Ab titer	
	Number of men	Number of infections[c]	Number of men	Number of infections
<4	17	11	28	14
4–8	8	3	6	2
16–32	5	1	1	0
≥64	5	1	—	—

[a] From Couch *et al.* (1969b).
[b] Frequency of infection in those with antibody vs. those with no antibody (exact tests): on basis of serum antibody, $p = 0.05$; on basis of NW antibody, $p = >0.30$.
[c] As determined by virus isolation.

Table 13.17   Relation of Location of Antibody to Occurrence of Infection with Influenza A_2 (Hong Kong Variant)[a]

Group		Number in group	Number infected[b]	Percent infected
Serum Ab	NW Ab			
Absent	Absent	16	10 (7)	62
Absent	Present	1	1 (1)	—
Present	Absent	12	4 (1)	33
Present	Present	6	1 (1)	17

[a] From Couch *et al.* (1969b).
[b] Numbers in parentheses are numbers ill.

Secretory antibodies probably do not persist as long as serum antibodies (see Fig. 13.10). Although published data on serial specimens is not available to document this contention, it is commonly observed that persons with histories of influenza in the remote past usually have undetectable levels of nasal secretory antibodies with detectable or even high levels of serum antibody.

J. Effect on Bacterial Flora

Alterations in bacterial flora of the upper respiratory tract have not been extensively studied in the volunteer model infection. Smorodintseff *et al.* (1937) reported serial bacteriological examination of 48 volunteers before inoculation and on various days after inoculation with influenza A (H0N1) virus. There were no quantitative or qualitative changes in bacterial flora in the upper respiratory tract in response to virus inoculation. Most investigators working with experimental influenza in man have reported absence of purulent complications following influenza, such as otitis media, acute purulent sinusitis, or pneumonia. Certainly the number of volunteers that have been inoculated in the combined studies far exceeds the expected frequency of bacterial complications (see Section II,B). However, the age group involved, that is, normal adults in good health between the ages of 18 and 30 have the lowest frequency of expected bacterial complications. In addition, other factors, such as route of inoculation, tissue culture passage, may serve to attenuate influenza illness and reduce the frequency of resulting bacterial complications.

K. Influenza B Virus Infection

A mild febrile systemic illness resembling that seen in milder cases of influenza A infection has been produced in volunteers using an inoculum of influenza B virus. Francis *et al.* (1944) inoculated volunteers intranasally with a spray containing varying doses of influenza B virus. Twenty-seven of 30 subjects developed febrile illnesses characterized by an incubation period of 10 to 24 hours, a sudden onset with chilly sensations, loss of appetite, nausea, and malaise. Only 2 complained of headache and 1 of myalgias. Respiratory symptoms, such as cough, coryza, and sore throat, were absent. Seven of the illnesses were considered moderately severe requiring bed rest, and 20 had temperatures of 101°F or higher. In the majority, signs and symptoms of illness disappeared within 24 to 48 hours. Of 30 uninoculated contact controls, 11 developed significant serological changes indicating person to person transmission of infection.

Henle *et al.* (1943) administered the Lee strain of influenza B to volunteers. All 22 who inhaled a spray containing 10^9 chick embryo infectious doses developed febrile illnesses. Only 1 of 6 given the same material intranasally became febrile. In 79%, the onset was in 13 to 24 hours, in 13% in 25 to 36 hours, and in 8% in 37 to 48 hours. White cell counts were depressed on the third day following inoculation, and 3 of 19 tested were below 6000 cells/mm³. Virus was isolated from only 2 volunteers, but fourfold antibody responses were detected in 18 of 25 tested. Symptoms lasted less than 48 hours. No person to person transmission was detected among 10 contact controls.

Beare *et al.* (1968) obtained similar results with influenza B/England/ 101/62 virus in that illness was mild and of short duration. They inoculated 46 volunteers intranasally who possessed varying antibody levels in influenza B virus. Virus was recovered from 25, antibody responses were detected in 30, and 19 became ill.

L. Influenza C Infection

In contrast to influenza A and B viruses, inoculation of volunteers with influenza C has resulted in afebrile common cold-like illnesses. Joosting *et al.* (1968) inoculated 12 volunteers with influenza C/Johannesburg/1/66. The inoculum was prepared in organ cultures of human embryo trachea, and contained $10^{5.7}$ egg infectious doses. Influenza C virus was recovered from nasal washings of eleven. Four developed fourfold rises in antibody titer by HI and 4 by CF tests. A febrile upper respiratory tract illness was observed in 6 volunteers. No systemic symptoms developed. Eleven additional volunteers were inoculated with pooled nasal secretions obtained from volunteers in the first experiment at the time they developed symptoms. A dose of $10^{4.25}$ EID_{50} was administered. Influenza C virus was recovered from 6 volunteers; 3 developed fourfold antibody responses by HI test and 4 by CF test. Two developed afebrile common colds, and one a febrile illness which may have been due to intercurrent cystitis. The mean incubation period, 4 days, was longer than that observed for experimental influenza A or B infections. Coryza, sore throat, headache, and malaise were very common symptoms, but cough and myalgias were absent. The average duration was 6 days. The infrequency of antibody responses is of interest. Only 8 of 17 volunteers shown to be infected by virus isolation developed HI or CF antibody responses.

M. Infection of Volunteers with Animal Influenza Virus

The influenza syndrome has been reproduced in man using viruses of swine and equine, but not avian origin. Beare *et al.* (1972) showed that influenza viruses of swine origin readily infected human volunteers. Seven volunteers were inoculated with $10^{5.5}$ egg infectious doses of influenza A/swine/Taiwan/7310/70, a virus antigenically related to human A/Hong Kong/68 (H3N2) virus, and probably derived from human H3N2 virus. Three shed virus from nasal secretions, and these three became ill. Symptoms were relatively mild and confined to nasal obstruction and discharge. Four developed fourfold HI antibody responses, and five showed significant anti-neuraminidase antibody responses. Antibodies to the hemagglutinin and neuraminidase of the human A/Hong Kong/68 virus were detected as well as to the antigens of the swine/Taiwan virus.

In contrast, evidence of infection by virus isolation or antibody rise was detected in only 2 of 13 volunteers challenged with swine/Wisconsin/66 virus and in 5 of 14 challenged with swine/Manitoba/67 virus, and symptoms were very mild or absent. It was of interest that these strains were not antigenically related to human strains, but were antigenically related to the prototype swine/Iowa/15/30 strain.

Alford *et al.* (1967a) administered influenza A/equine/2/Miami/1/63 virus to human volunteers. This strain had been recovered from a naturally infected horse, and been shown to infect 100% and to cause febrile illness in 63% of antibody-free ponies. It was tested in volunteers after 1, 2, or 3 human passages, after 10 human embryonic kidney cell culture passages, or after 6 passages in Chincoteague ponies. None of the inocula produced differing results. In summary, 4 of 33 volunteers became ill with brief systemic illnesses accompanied by fever. Virus was recovered from 21 of 33 volunteers, and neutralizing antibody responses to the infecting virus were detected in the sera of 21 volunteers. Forty-seven to 71% of those infected also developed antibody responses to influenza A (H2N2) viruses as well as to homologous virus. The human-passaged material retained its ability to produce infection and illness in ponies. Four of 4 ponies developed fever (maximum 103.2° to 105°F; normal equine temperature up to 102°F) for 1 to 7 days, shed virus for 5 to 7 days, and developed antibody responses.

More severe illness in humans using the same equine virus was reported by Couch *et al.* (1969a). The inoculum used had the following passage history: egg 5, human embryonic kidney 2, man 1, human embryonic kidney 4, man 1, human embryonic kidney 3. Thirteen of 15 volunteers became ill. Three developed afebrile upper respiratory illnesses, 10 febrile upper respiratory and systemic illnesses with maximum fever from 101° to 103°F, beginning on the second or third day after inoculation. Two of these had lower respiratory illness as well manifested by paroxysmal coughing, substernal discomfort, and tenderness of the trachea. When illnesses were compared to naturally occurring influenza A illnesses, it was noted that fever was of shorter duration (mean 1.3 days), nasal discharge and obstruction were slightly more frequent, and there was slightly less frequent occurrence of cough and sore throat among the volunteers infected with equine virus infection.

IV. Summary and Conclusions

In this chapter I have described the course and complications of naturally occurring and experimentally induced influenza in man. Emphasis has been

Table 13.18 Comparison of Natural and Experimental Influenza Infections in Man

	Natural infection with indicated influenza type			Experimental infection with indicated influenza type and method of inoculation					
				A		B	C	Equine	Swine
	A	B	C	Aerosol	Nasal	aerosol	nasal	coarse spray	nasal
Occurs in outbreaks	Yes	Yes	No	—	—	—	—	—	—
Incubation period	1–4 days	?	?	12–48 hrs	2–3 days	12–36 hrs	4 days	2–3 days	3–4 days
Sudden onset	Yes	Yes	No	Yes	Yes	Yes	No	Yes (nasal Sx may precede)	No
Cough	+++[a]	+++	+	+++	+	No	No	++	No
Other respiratory symptoms	+++	++	++	+++	++	No	+	+++	+
Fever (°F)	101–102	101–102	No	101–102	100–101	101–102	No	101–103	No
Systemic symptoms	+++	++	No	+++	++	++	No	++	No
Leukocytosis/leukopenia	+/+	?	?	+/+	+/+	?/+	?	?	?
Duration	3 days fever, 7 days resp. Sx[b]	3 days fever, 7 days resp. Sx	Several days	3 days fever, 7 days resp. Sx	1–2 days fever, 5 days resp. Sx	2 days fever, 2 days total	6 days	1 day fever, 4–5 days resp.	2–4 days
Complications	Pneumonia (viral and bacterial), croup, CNS	Reye's syndrome, croup	None	NR[c]	NR	NR	NR	NR	NR

[a] +, ++, +++, are increasing grades of severity.
[b] Sx, symptoms.
[c] NR, none reported.

placed on experimental infections because of availability of quantitative data which is often lacking in regard to naturally occurring infections. A summary of some of the major findings is shown in Table 13.18.

As indicated, naturally occurring influenza A virus infection is characteristically a 3-day febrile illness with an abrupt onset, moderately severe systemic symptoms and cough, followed by several days of respiratory symptoms. The illness remains constant despite major or minor changes in the surface glycoproteins of the virion. The major complications are pulmonary, and consist of primary viral pneumonia, secondary bacterial pneumonia, and pneumonia of mixed etiology. Influenza B virus infections result in similar illnesses, although systemic symptoms may be of lesser severity. The major complication of influenza B virus infection is the occurrence of Reye's syndrome. In contrast, influenza C virus infections occur only sporadically and infrequently, and result in afebrile common cold-like illnesses without systemic symptoms.

Typical influenza illness has been produced in normal volunteers by aerosol inoculation of influenza A virus, and a slightly milder illness by nasal inoculation. Less experience is available with influenza B virus, and a febrile systemic illness of short duration has been observed. Experimentally induced influenza C virus infections result in afebrile common cold syndromes similar to those described for naturally occurring influenza C virus infections.

In addition to experimentally induced infections with influenza viruses of human origin, infection and illness have been produced in human volunteers using viruses derived from animals. Infections with viruses of equine origin have resulted in febrile systemic illnesses closely resembling naturally occurring influenza A virus infection, whereas illnesses resulting from infection with viruses of swine origin have been milder and restricted to respiratory symptoms.

References

Adams, C. W. (1959). *Amer. J. Cardiol.* **4,** 45.

Alford, R. H., Kasel, J. A., Gerone, P. J., and Knight, V. (1966). *Proc Soc. Exp. Biol. Med.* **122,** 800.

Alford, R. H., Kasel, J. A., Lehrich, J. R., and Knight, V. (1967a). *Amer. J. Epidemiol.* **86,** 185.

Alford, R. H., Rossen, R. D., Butler, W. T., and Kasel, J. A. (1967b). *J. Immunol.* **89,** 724.

Asbury, A. K., Aranson, B. G., and Adams, R. D. (1969). *Medicine (Baltimore)* **48,** 173.

Baron, S., and Issacs, A. (1962). *Brit. Med. J.* **1,** 18.

Beare, A. S., Bynoe, M. L., and Tyrrell, D. A. J. (1968). *Brit. Med. J.* **2,** 482.

Beare, A. S., Schild, G. C., and Hall, T. S. (1972). *Bull. W.H.O.* **47,** 493.

Bisno, A. L., Griffin, J. P., Van Epps, K. S., Niell, H. B., and Rytel, M. W.(1971). *Amer. J. Med. Sci.* **261,** 251.

Blattner, R. J. (1959). *J. Pediat.* **55,** 113.

Bull, D. R., and Burnet, R. M. (1943). *Med. J. Aust.* **1,** 389.

Burk, R. F., Schaffner, W., and Koenig, M. G. (1971). *Ann. Intern. Med.* **127,** 1122.

Burnet, F. M., and Foley, M. (1940). *Med. J. Aust.* **2,** 655

Camner, P., Jarstrand, C., and Philipson, K. (1973). *Amer. Rev. Resp. Dis.* **108,** 131.

Carilli, A. D., Gohd, R. S., and Gordon, W. (1964). *N. Engl. J. Med.* **270,** 123.

Center for Disease Control. (1971). "Morbidity and Mortality Weekly Report," Vol. 20, No. 12, pp. 101–102. U.S. Dept. of Health, Education and Welfare, Atlanta, Georgia.

Center for Disease Control. (1974a). "Morbidity and Mortality Weekly Report," Vol. 23, No. 9, p. 87. U.S. Dept. of Health, Education and Welfare, Atlanta, Georgia.

Center for Disease Control. (1974b). "Morbidity and Mortality Weekly Report," Vol. 23, No. 12, p. 115. U. S. Dept. of Health, Education and Welfare, Atlanta, Georgia.

Coffey, V. P., and Jessop, W. J. E. (1959). *Lancet* **2,** 935.

Coffey, V. P., and Jessop, W. J. E. (1963). *Lancet* **1,** 748.

Couch, R. B., Douglas, R. G., Jr., Riggs, S., and Knight, V. (1969a). *Nature (London)* **224,** 512.

Couch, R. B., Douglas, R. G., Jr., Rossen, R., and Kasel, J. A. (1969b). *In* "The Secretory Immunologic System" (P. A. Small, Jr. *et al.,* eds.), pp. 93–112. U.S. Govt. Printing Office, Washington, D.C.

Couch, R. B., Douglas, R. G., Jr., Fedson, D. S., and Kasel, J. A. (1971). *J. Infec. Dis.* **124,** 473.

Couch, R. B., Kasel, J. A., Gerin, J. L., Schulman, J. L., and Kilbourne, E. D. (1974). *J. Infec. Dis.* **129,** 411.

Doll, R., Hill, A. B., and Sakula, J. (1960). *Brit. J. Prev. Soc. Med.* **14,** 167.

Douglas, R. G., Jr., Alford, R. H., Cate, T. R., and Couch, R. B. (1966). *Ann. Intern. Med.* **64,** 521.

Eadie, M. B., Stott, E. J., and Grist, N. R. (1966). *Brit. Med. J.* **2,** 671.

Edelen, J. S., Bender, T. R., and Chin, T. Y. (1974). *Amer. J. Epidemiol.* **100,** 79.

Eickhoff, T. C. (1971). *J. Infec. Dis.* **123,** 519.

Foy, M., Cooney, M. K., Maletzky, A. J., and Grayston, J. T. (1973). *Amer. J. Epidemiol.* **97,** 80.

Francis, T., Jr., Pearson, H. E., Salk, J. E., and Brown, P. M. (1944). *Amer. J. Pub. Health Nat. Health* **34,** 317.

Fry, J. (1951). *Brit. Med. J.* **2,** 1374.

Fry, J. (1958). *Brit. Med. J.* **1,** 259.

Fry, J. (1959). *Brit. Med. J.* **2,** 135.

Glezen, W. P., Loda, F. A., Clyde, W. A., Jr., Senior, R. J., Sheaffer, C. I., Conley, W. G., and Denny, F. W. (1971). *J. Pediat.* **48,** 394.

Glick, T. H., Likosky, W. H., Levitt, L. P., Mellin, H., and Reynolds, D. W. (1970). *Pediatrics* **46,** 371.

Gresser, I., and Dull, H. B. (1964). *Proc. Soc. Exp. Biol. Med.* **115,** 192.

Hall, W. J., Douglas, R. G., Jr., Roth, F. K., and Cross, A. S. (1974). *Program Abstr., 14th Intersci. Conf. Antimicrob. Ag. Chemother.* p. 309.

Hardy, J. M. B., Azarowicz, E. N., Mannini, A., Medearis, D. M., and Cooke, R. E. (1961). *Amer. J. Pub. Health Nat. Health* **51,** 1182.

Henle, W., Henle, G., and Stokes, J., Jr. (1943). *J. Immunol.* **46,** 163.

Henle, W., Henle, G., Stokes, J., Jr., and Maris, E. P. (1946). *J. Immunol.* **52,** 145.

Hewitt, D. (1962). *Amer. J. Pub. Health Nat. Health* **52,** 1676.

Hildebrandt, H. M., Maassab, H. F., and Willis, P. W., III. (1962). *Amer. J. Dis. Child.* **104,** 179.

Hilleman, M. R., Hamparian, V. V., Ketler, A., Reilly, C. M., McClelland, L., Cornfeld, D., and Stokes, J., Jr. (1962). *J. Amer. Med. Ass.* **180,** 445.

Horner, G. J., and Gray, F. D., Jr. (1973). *Amer. Rev. Resp. Dis.* **108,** 866.

Howard, J. B., McCracken, G. H., Jr., and Luby, J. P. (1972). *J. Pediat.* **81,** 1148.

Hughes, D. L. (1938). *Med. Res. Counc. (Gt. Brit.), Spec. Rep. Ser.* **228,** 87.

Jao, R. L., Wheelock, E. F., and Jackson, G. G. (1970). *J. Infec. Dis.* **121,** 419.

Johanson, W. G., Pierce, A. K., and Sanford, J. P. (1969). *Amer. Rev. Resp. Dis.* **100,** 141.

Joosting, A. C. C., Head, B., Bynoe, M. L., and Tyrell, D. A. J. (1968). *Brit. Med. J.* **2,** 153.

Jordan, W. S., Denny, F. W., Badger, G. F., Curtiss, C., Dingle, J. H., Oseasohn, R., and Stevens, D. A. (1958). *Amer. J. Hyg.* **68,** 190.

Kasel, J. A., Horne, E. B., Fulk., R. B., Togo, Y., Huber, M., and Hornick, R. B. (1969). *J. Immunol.* **102,** 555.

Kaye, D., Rosenbluth, M., Kook, E. W., and Kilbourne, E. D. (1962). *Amer. Rev. Resp. Dis.* **85,** 9.

Kennedy, M. C. S., Miller, D. L., and Peason, A. J. (1965). *Brit. J. Dis. Chest* **59,** 10.

Khakpour, M., Saidi, A., and Naficy, K. (1969). *Brit. Med. J.* **2,** 208.

Kilbourne, E. D. (1959). *J. Clin. Invest.* **38,** 255.

Kilbourne, E. D., and Loge, J. P. (1950). *Ann. Intern. Med.* **33,** 371.

Kilbourne, E. D., Anderson, H. C., and Horsfall, F. L., Jr. (1951). *J. Immunol.* **67,** 547.

Knight, V., Kasel, J. A., Alford, R. H., Loda, F., Morris, J. A., Davenport, F. M., Robinson, R. Q., and Buescher, E. L. (1965). *Ann. Intern. Med.* **62,** 1307.

Knight, V,. Fedson, D., Baldini, J., Douglas, R. G., Jr., and Couch, R. B. (1970). *Infec. Immunity* **1,** 200.

Lal., H. B., Narayan, T. K., Kalra, S. L., and Lal, R. (1963). *J. Indian Med. Asst.* **40,** 113.

Leck, I., Hay, S., Witte, J. J., and Greene, J. C. (1969). *Pub. Health Rep.* **84,** 971.

Lehmann, N. I., and Gust, I. D. (1971). *Med. J. Aust.* **2,** 1166.

Leneman, F. (1966). *Arch. Intern. Med.* **118,** 139.

Louria, D. B., Blumenfeld, H. L., Ellis, J. T., Kilbourne, E. D., and Rogers, D. E. (1959). *J. Clin. Invest.* **38,** 213.

Lozhkina, A. N., Dreizia, R. S., and Ketiladze, E. A. (1968). *Rev. Roum. Inframicrobiol.* **541,** 269.

Mann, J. J., Waldeman, R. H., Togo, Y., Heiner, G. G., Dawkins, A. T., and Kasel, J. A. (1968). *J. Immunol.* **100,** 725.

Martin, L. M., Kunin, C. M., Gottlieb, L. S., and Finland, M. (1959). *AMA Arch. Intern. Med.* **103,** 532.

Melnick, S. C., and Flewett, T. H. (1964). *J. Neurol., Neurosurg. Psychiat.* [N.S.] **27**, 395.

Middleton, P. J., Alexander, R. M., and Szymanski, M. T. (1970). *Lancet* **2**, 533.

Minow, R. A., Gorbach, S., Johnson, B. L., and Dornfeld, L. (1974). *Ann. Intern. Med.* **80**, 359.

Minuse, E., Willis, P. W., III, Davenport, F. M., and Francis, T., Jr. (1962). *J. Lab. Clin. Med.* **59**, 1016.

Mogabgab, W. J. (1963). *Ann. Intern. Med.* **59**, 306.

Mulder, J., and Hers, J. F. (1972). "Influenza." Walters-Noordhoff, Gröningen, The Netherlands.

Murphy, B. R., Chalhub, E. G., Nusinoff, S. R., and Chanock, R. M. (1972a). *J. Infec. Dis.* **126**, 170.

Murphy, B. R., Kasel, J. A., and Chanock, R. M. (1972b). *N. Engl. J. Med.* **286**, 1329.

Murphy, B. R., Chalhub, E. G., Nusinoff, S. R., Kasel, J., and Chanock, R. M. (1973a). *J. Infec. Dis.* **128**, 479.

Murphy, B. R., Baron, S., Chalhub, E. G., Uhlendorf, C. P., and Chanock, R. M. (1973b). *J. Infec. Dis.* **128**, 488.

Naficy, K. (1963). *N. Engl. J. Med.* **269**, 964.

Newton-John, H. F., Bennett, N., and Forbes, J. A. (1971). *Med. J. Aust.* **2**, 1160.

Nigg, C., Ecklund, C. M., Wilson, D. E., and Crowley, J. H. (1942). *Amer. J. Hyg.* **35**, 265.

Norman, M. G., Lowden, J. A., Hill, D. E., and Bannatyne, R. M. (1968). *Can. Med. Ass. J.* **99**, 549.

Oker-Blom, N., Hovi, T., Leinikki, P., Palosuo, T., Pettersson, R., and Suni, J. (1970). *Brit. Med. J.* **3**, 676.

Picken, J. J., Niewoehner, D. E., and Chester, E. H. (1972). *Amer. J. Med.* **52**, 738.

Ray, C. G., Gravelle, C. R., and Chin, T. D. H. (1967). *J. Pediat.* **71**, 27.

Reye, R. D. K., Morgan, G., and Baral, J. (1963). *Lancet* **2**, 749.

Rossen, R. D., Butler, W. T., Waldman, R. H., Alford, R. H., Hornick, R. B., Togo, Y., and Kasel, J. A. (1970). *J. Amer. Med. Ass.* **211**, 1157.

Schwarzmann, S. W., Adler, J. L., Sullivan, R. J., and Marine, W. M. (1971). *Arch. Intern. Med.* **127**, 1037.

Simon, N. M., Rouner, R. M., and Berlin, B. S. (1970). *J. Amer. Med. Ass.* **212**, 1704.

Smorodintseff, A. A., Tushinsky, M. D., Drobyshevskaya, A. I., Korovin, A. A., and Osetroff, A. I. (1937). *Amer. J. Med. Sci.* **194**, 159.

Stanley, E. D., and Jackson, G. G. (1966). *Trans. Ass. Amer. Physicians* **79**, 376.

Stansfield, J. M., and Stuart-Harris, C. H. (1943). *Lancet* **2**, 789.

Stark, J. E., Heath, R. B., and Curwen, M. P. (1965). *Thorax* **20**, 124.

Stenhouse, A. C. (1967). *Brit. Med. J.* **3**, 461.

Stuart-Harris, C. H. (1961). *Amer. Rev. Resp. Dis.* **83**, 54.

Stuart-Harris, C. H. (1965). "Influenza and other Virus Infections of the Respiratory Tract," 2nd ed., pp. 1–248. Williams & Wilkins, Baltimore, Maryland.

Tateno, I., Suzuki, S., Nakamura, S., and Kawamura, A., Jr. (1965). *Jap. J. Exp. Med.* **35**, 383.

Tateno, I., Kitamoto, O., and Kawamura, A., Jr. (1966). *N. Engl. J. Med.* **274**, 237.

Taylor, R. M., Parodi, A. S., Fernandez, R. B., and Chialovo, R. J. (1942). *Rev. Inst. Bacteriol. Dep. Nac. Hig. (Argent.)* **11**, 44.

Togo, Y., Hornick, R. B., Felitti, V. J., Kaufman, M. I., Dawkins, A. T., Jr., Kilpe, V. E., and Claghorn, J. L. (1970). *J. Amer. Med. Asso.* **211**, 1149.

Waldman, R. H., Mann, J. J., and Kasel, J. A. (1968). *J. Immunol.* **100**, 80.

Waldman, R. H., Mann, J. J., and Small, P. A. (1969). *J. Amer. Med. Asso.* **207**, 520.

Wellings, F. M., Skinner, J. J., Lewis, A. L., and Seabury, C. J. (1973). *CDC Influenza-Resp. Dis. Surv.* **88**, 10.

Wells, C. E. C. (1971). *Brit. Med. J.* **1**, 369.

Wells, C E. C., James, W. R. L., and Evans, A. D. (1959). *AMA Arch. Neurol. Psychiat.* **81**, 699.

Widelock, D., Csizmas, L., and Klein, S. (1963). *Pub. Health Rep.* **78**, No. 1, 1–11.

Wingfield, W. L., Pollack, D., and Gninert, R. R. (1969). *N. Engl. J. Med.* **281**, 579.

Woodward, T. E., McCrumb, F. R., Jr., Carey, T. N., and Togo, Y. (1960). *Ann. Intern. Med.* **53**, 1130.

Yawn, D. H., Pyeatte, J. C., Joseph, M., Eichler, S. L., and Garcia-Bunuel, R. (1971). *J. Amer. Med. Ass.* **26**, 1022.

Young, L. S., LaForce, F. M., Head, J. J., Feeley, J. C., and Bennett, J. V. (1972). *N. Engl. J. Med.* **287**, 5–8.

Zhdanov, V. M. (1966). *Proc. Int. Conf. Vaccines Against Viral & Rickettsial Dis. Man, 1st, 1966,* pp. 9–15.

Zhdanov, V. M., and Ritova, V. V. (1963). *Fed. Proc., Fed. Amer. Soc. Exp. Biol.* **22**, 1800.

14

Animal Influenza

B. C. Easterday

I. History

A. Influenza-like Diseases in Animals

The term *influenza* has been used to describe various kinds of acute respiratory and generalized diseases of several animal species, especially horses, for many years. The extent to which such conditions may have been caused by influenza viruses is not known. While it is quite apparent that some of the influenza described in horses was not caused by influenza virus, descriptions of epizootics among horses as far back as the fourth and fifth centuries

449

attracted considerable attention because of the marked morbidity rate, rapid spread, and wide distribution (Van Es, 1932). Epizootics of great magnitude occurred in Europe in 1881–1883 and in the United States in 1872–1873 and 1900–1901.

Several authors (Youatt, 1843; Gardenier, 1900; Hodgins and Haskett, 1901) have described influenza of horses in considerable detail. Synonyms for influenza included catarrhal fever, epidemic catarrh, distemper, pink-eye, and epizooty. Many of the descriptions were appropriate to the equine influenza of today caused by type A influenza viruses. Knowledge about the disease included: the cause was "germs floating in the air"; it was more common in spring and fall; young horses were more disposed to infection; it was common where horses were congregated; one attack was "self-protective"; cough, fever (105°F), and debility were common; and it spread over large districts and sometimes whole countries.

It is evident, however, from descriptions of several authors (Hayes, 1904; Kelser, 1927; Van Es, 1932) that not all of the influenza was due to type A influenza virus. They indicated that the disease could be transmitted by intravenous or subcutaneous inoculation of blood from diseased horses, that blood was virulent for at least $3\frac{1}{2}$ months, that semen was virulent 4 years after the stallion recovered, and that infectious virus remained after several months when blood was stored at refrigerator temperature. None of these observations are consistent with the properties of influenza viruses and their host–virus relationships.

The cause of equine influenza was established "as an ultramicroscopic, filterable virus" (Kelser, 1927) and an "equine influenza virus" that was isolated from cases of equine influenza in 1941 has been shown to be the equine rhinopneumonitis virus (a herpesvirus). It is also likely that the viral arteritis virus (an unclassified RNA virus) was responsible for some of the conditions called influenza. Both of these infections are readily transmitted by the parenteral inoculation of blood from infected horses.

Reference to influenza of other species appears infrequently in some of the old literature. Hayes (1904) included a short description of diseases of cattle "resembling influenza" and indicated that "many have observed among cattle, peculiar, epizootic, morbid conditions which resemble equine influenza." Gardenier (1900) described influenza of sheep as a disease "due to causes which seem to exist at times over extended portions of the country, and is liable to affect a large number of animals at a time." It seemed to be an ill-defined upper respiratory disease associated with cold damp weather. Occasional reference to canine influenza is most likely canine distemper, a specific viral disease of dogs, other Canidae, and Mustelidae.

There are many respiratory disease conditions among animals that are similar to influenza, as is the case in man. Several bacteria and viruses have been associated with these conditions. For example, so-called "shipping fever" of cattle is a respiratory disease complex associated with the shipping of cattle. Several infectious agents have been incriminated in this disease complex including, e.g., *Pasteurella multocida* and *P. hemolytica, Chlamydia,* parainfluenza-3 virus, bovine viral diarrhea virus, infectious bovine rhinotracheitis virus.

Respiratory disease is as common in swine as it is in other species, and many respiratory conditions of swine that are reported as influenza are due to other causes (Nakamura *et al.,* 1972). The term "hog flu" or swine influenza was applied to a new disease among swine in Iowa and Illinois in 1918 in which the signs and epizootic characteristics were similar to influenza that was epidemic in man at the time (Dorset *et al.,* 1922). No infectious agent was identified until 1930 when Shope (1931b) isolated the swine influenza virus.

While the term influenza has been used freely to describe respiratory disease of undetermined cause among mammals, it has not been used commonly for describing respiratory disease among avian species. A condition among young geese in Hungary called gosling influenza was found to be caused by a reovirus and *Hemophilus anserisepticus* (Csontos and Miklovich-Kis Csatári, 1967a,b). It was not until type A influenza viruses were isolated from ducks in England and Czechoslovakia in 1956 that the term influenza found its way into the avian disease literature.

It remains that the term influenza should not be used to describe respiratory disease of animals unless the causative agent is identified and known to be an influenza virus. It is interesting to read about and speculate on the circulation of influenza viruses among animals in the past, however, such speculation must be flavored with caution.

B. Chronology of the Appearance and Identification of Influenza Viruses in Animals

The fowl plague virus (Hav1Neq1), identified as a type A influenza virus in 1955 (Schafer, 1955) based on the nature of the ribonucleoprotein (RNP), had caused serious disease problems among poultry for many years. The disease was reported in Italy in 1878 and known to be caused by a "filterable virus" since 1900 (Stubbs, 1965).

The viral cause of swine influenza was demonstrated by Shope (1931b) in 1930 in his experiments to determine the cause and means of transmission. Three years later, the viral nature of influenza in man was demonstrated by Smith *et al.* (1933) when they infected ferrets with nasopharyngeal washings from human beings with influenza.

While the swine influenza virus continued to circulate among pigs particularly in north central United States, there were no other influenza viruses recovered from animals for nearly 20 years. A virus called N virus (Hav2N1) was recovered from chickens in Germany in 1949 and was considered to be an avirulent form of the fowl plague virus (Dinter and Bakos, 1950). Ten years later, it was found that the N virus has the type A influenza RNP (Rott and Schafer, 1960). In 1952, a virus isolated from ducklings with central nervous system disease in Manitoba was designated only as a "filterable" hemagglutinating agent distinct from Newcastle disease virus (Walker and Bannister, 1953). Subsequently, this virus was also shown to be a type A influenza virus (Mitchell *et al.*, 1967).

Thus, during the first 20 years after the viral etiology of influenza was established, only three influenza viruses were recovered from animals, i.e., swine, chickens, and ducks. Those three viruses plus the fowl plague virus constituted a prelude to an animal influenza era that began in 1956.

Three distinct type A viruses were recovered from animals in 1956; from ducks in England and from horses and ducks in Czechoslovakia. The two duck viruses, A/duck/Eng/56 (Hav3Nav1) and A/duck/Czech/56 (Hav4Nav1), were antigenically distinct from each other and from any previously known viruses (Koppel *et al.*, 1956; G. B. Simmins and F. D. Asplin, personal communication, 1956, as cited by Roberts, 1964). These viruses caused respiratory disease and sinusitis with considerable morbidity. The virus, A/equine/Prague/56 (Heq1Neq1), was recovered from horses during an epizootic of respiratory disease, and it was also antigenically distinct from all other type A viruses (Sovinova *et al.*, 1958). Heller *et al.* (1956) reported that horses convalescent from respiratory disease in Sweden had antibodies against the type A RNP (known as "soluble" antigen at the time). The extent, if any, that type A influenza virus infections were present among horse populations prior to 1955 remains a matter of speculation.

No other new influenza virus infections of animals were reported until 1959. During the period of 1959–1963 several new viruses were recovered from various avian species and horses. The first of these viruses, A/chicken/Scotland/59 (Hav5N1), was from chickens in Scotland suffering from a fowl plague-like disease. In 1960, 1961, and 1963 at least five viruses were recovered from ducks in the Soviet Union (Easterday and Tumová, 1972a). The A/duck/England/62 (Hav4Nav1) virus was recovered from ducks in England on the same farm from which the A/duck/England/56 (Hav3Nav1) virus was recovered, however, the A/duck/England/62 virus was similar to the A/duck/Czech/56 virus (Hav4Nav1). During this same period of 1959–1963 a virus, A/tern/S. Africa/61 (Hav5Nav2), was isolated from common terns (*Sterna hirundo*) in South Africa (Becker, 1966). The virus was responsible for a fowl plague-like disease with a high mortality rate among the terns. Subsequently, it was shown that the A/tern/S. Africa/61 virus and the A/chicken/Scot/59 viruses were similar (Pereira *et al.,* 1965). The Hav5 hemagglutinin is common to both viruses. There was much speculation about the epizootiology of these two viruses because of the migration patterns of the tern. While free-flying birds were reported to have been infected with the fowl plague virus (Stubbs, 1965), the A/tern/S. Africa/61 was the first evidence that free-flying birds were infected with other influenza viruses.

Two new viruses, one from turkeys and one from horses, were identified in North America in 1963 (Lang *et al.,* 1965; Land and Wills, 1966; Waddell *et al.,* 1963). Other than fowl plague and the A/duck/Canada/52 virus, no other influenza viruses had been identified among avian species in North America. The virus from turkeys, A/turkey/Ontario/3724/63 (Hav6Neq2), originally called Wilmot virus, was responsible for respiratory disease and decreased egg production among turkeys in Ontario. The virus, A/equine/Miami/1/63 (Heq2Neq2), was recovered from horses with respiratory disease in Miami, Florida in January of 1963 and spread throughout the United States during the succeeding 5 months. It was also during that period that the A/equine/Prague/1/56 (Heq1Neq1) virus was isolated in the United States. There was serological evidence that the virus, Heq1Neq1, or a closely related virus had infected horses in North America as early as 1957.

Subsequent to the recovery of the A/turkey/Ontario/3724/63 virus, many viruses have been isolated, mainly from turkeys, throughout North America, e.g., in 1964 from turkeys in California and Ontario; 1965 from turkeys in Massachusetts and Ontario; 1966 from turkeys in Wisconsin, California, and Ontario; 1967 from turkeys in Minnesota, Washington, and Ontario; 1968 from turkeys in Washington and Wisconsin; 1969 from ducks in Pennsylvania; 1970 from turkeys in Minnesota. During the same time period, many viruses were recovered from several species in other parts of the world. A chronology of the recovery and identification of avian influenza viruses from 1927–1970 has been provided by Easterday and Tumová (1972a).

There was additional evidence for the infection of wild birds with influenza viruses in 1968 when antibody was demonstrated among geese in North America (Easterday *et al.,* 1968). Subsequently antibodies have been found and viruses have been recovered from several wild avian species, e.g., shearwaters on the Great Barrier Reef (Downie and Laver, 1973), wild ducks in California (Slemons *et al.,* 1974), sea birds off the Norwegian coast (G. C. Schild, personal communication, 1973), and wild birds in the Soviet Union (Zakstel'skaja *et al.,* 1972; Slepuskin *et al.,* 1972; D. K. Lvov, personal communication, 1974). Furthermore, several influenza viruses have been recovered from a variety of exotic avian species imported into the United States (Slemons *et al.*, 1973; B. C. Easterday, unpublished data, 1973).

Another era of influenza began in 1970 when Hong Kong (H3N2) influenza virus was recovered from swine in Taiwan (Kundin, 1970). Antibody against the Hong Kong virus had been demonstrated in swine serum in Hungary in 1969; and it has been demonstrated in swine serum throughout the world since that time. The Hong Kong influenza virus has been recovered from several nonhuman species (see Section IV,D).

It is probable that with the present interest and technology influenza viruses will continue to be isolated from a variety of nonhuman mammalian and avian species. New hemagglutinins and neuraminidases, different from the existing 15 hemagglutinins and 9 neuraminidases, are also likely to be identified.

II. Influenza Viruses from Animals

A. Antigenic Spectrum

A revised system of nomenclature of influenza viruses that provides for designating the three major antigens of the virus, the RNP, hemagglutinin and neuraminidase, was presented in 1971 (World Health Organization, 1971). Prior to that time, the system of classification and nomenclature was based on the nature of the RNP and hemagglutinin. The second surface antigen, the neuraminidase, is readily characterized antigenically, and it is known that the hemagglutinin and the neuraminidase undergo antigenic changes independently. The present system, a revision of the prior system, provides for designating the three major antigens and the host, place, and year of origin.

So far viruses containing the type B RNP have not been recovered from animals, other than one report of isolation from horses (Compagnucci *et al.*, 1969). Of the 15 known hemagglutinins found in the type A viruses, 12 have been identified in various nonhuman animal species, and all of the 9 neuraminidases have been identified in viruses recovered from animals. The type A influenza virus hemagglutinins and neuraminidases and their host of origin are indicated in Table 14.1. Examples of the antigenic spectrum and mix of hemagglutinin and neuraminidase antigens among the animal influenza viruses are listed in Table 14.2.

Table 14.1 The Hemagglutinins and Neuraminidases of the
Type A Influenza Viruses[a]

Species of origin	Hemagglutinin	Neuraminidase
Human	H0, H1, H2, H3	N1, N2
Swine	Hsw1	(N1)[b]
Equine	Heq1, Heq2	Neq1, Neq2
Avian	Hav1, Hav2, Hav3, Hav4, Hav5, Hav6, Hav7, Hav8	Nav1, Nav2, Nav3, Nav4, Nav5

[a] There is no species designation if the antigen is of human origin, e.g., H0 is the first hemagglutinin obtained from human beings, and Heq1 is the first hemagglutinin identified from horses. The host designation refers to the source of the virus in which the antigen was first characterized. H, hemagglutinin; N, neuraminidase.

[b] The neuraminidase contained in the swine influenza virus is similar if not identical to the N1 neuraminidase of human origin. So far, no neuraminidase unique to swine has been identified.

B. Host Range

At best it can be said that the natural host range is extremely broad for influenza viruses in general. For any one virus, however, the range may be limited with regard to infection and/or disease. Natural and experimental host ranges have been given by Hoyle (1968) and Easterday and Tumová, (1972a,b).

Viruses have been recovered from more than 25 avian species and there is serological evidence for infection of several others. The host range is extremely variable, and it is unwise to speculate on the host range based on the species of origin and/or antigenic composition. The ability of the Hong Kong influenza virus (H3N2) to infect a variety of species (e.g., swine, chickens, dogs, cattle) under natural conditions appears to be unique among the influenza viruses isolated from human beings.

There has been a tendency to assume that a virus isolated from one avian species will be infectious and/or pathogenic for very wide range, if not all, avian species. There has also been a tendency to assume that viruses that are similar antigenically are similar biologically. Slemons and Easterday (1972) showed that a virus, A/turkey/Ont/7732/66 (Hav5N?) that is highly pathogenic for turkeys (all experimentally infected birds die) has low infectivity and/or no pathogenicity for four other species (quail, ducks, pheasants, and pigeons). They also showed that another virus of turkey origin, with the same hemagglutinin, A/turkey/Wis/1/68 (Hav5N?), produced no disease in experimentally infected turkeys and the other four species. Similarly, Beard and Easterday (1973) reported that the A/tur-

Table 14.2   Examples of the Antigenic Spectrum, Chronological Distribution, and Mix of Animal Influenza Viruses

Species of origin	Virus	Antigenic composition
Swine	A/swine/Iowa/15/30	Hsw1N1
	A/swine/Merotin/57	Hsw1N1
	A/swine/Wis/1/67	Hsw1N1
	A/swine/Wis/1/72	Hsw1N1
Equine	A/equine/Prague/1/56	Heq1Neq1
	A/equine/Wis/1/69	Heq1Neq1
	A/equine/Miami/1/63	Heq2Neq2
	A/equine/Switzerland/65	Heq2Neq2
	A/equine/Wis/2/69	Heq2Neq2
Avian	A/fowl plague/Dutch/27	Hav1Neq1
	A/chicken/Brescia/02	Hav1N1
	A/turkey/Oregon/71	Hav1Nav2
	A/turkey/England/63	Hav1Nav3
	A/chicken/Germany "N"/49	Hav2Neq1
	A/duck/England/56	Hav3Nav1
	A/duck/Czech/56	Hav4Nav1
	A/chicken/Scotland/59	Hav5N1
	A/tern/S. Africa/61	Hav5Nav2
	A/turkey/Ontario/63	Hav6Neq2
	A/turkey/Mass./65	Hav6N2
	A/shearwater/Australia/70	Hav6Nav5
	A/duck/Ukraine/1/63	Hav7Neq2
	A/turkey/Ontario/6118/68	Hav8Nav4

[a] Many more swine and equine influenza strains have been isolated than indicated, but there are no other antigen combinations than those listed. The list of avian influenza viruses provides only examples and is not intended as an inclusive list of all of the viruses isolated from avian species (World Health Organization, 1971).

key/Ore/71 (Hav1Nav2) virus, containing the hemagglutinin of fowl plague and the neuraminidase of the A/tern/S. Africa/61 virus, was avirulent for chickens. Both the fowl plague and tern virus are highly pathogenic for chickens.

III. The Disease

A. Swine

1. The Natural Disease

Typical swine influenza is a herd disease and is commonly observed in north central United States in the autumn, winter, and early spring. The descriptions of the disease, as provided by early writers (Dorset *et al.,* 1922; McBryde, 1927; Shope, 1931a), are excellent and appropriate to the disease as it appears in north central United States today. Dorset *et al.* (1922) described the disease as follows: "The onset is sudden, and all or a large part of the herd will quickly develop the gravest symptoms . . . The herd was so sick that they could be walked among and even kicked without forcing them to move. Recovery is about as rapid and as surprising as the attack . . . The state of severe illness remained practically unchanged until the sixth day when there was a remarkable change in the condition. Practically the entire herd was up and eating, and a large number were in the yard moving briskly about and apparently recovered." McBryde (1927) commented on the sudden onset of the disease with "an entire herd coming down, as a rule, within a day or two." The signs described by those writers and the signs observed now are almost exclusively referable to the respiratory tract. Sick animals have labored, jerky, or thumpy breathing. Many individual animals rest on the sternum with the forelegs extended in an effort to facilitate breathing. There is a paroxysmal and hard cough particularly when animals are disturbed and forced to move. Such coughing spells are occasionally so severe and prolonged as to induce vomiting. Conjunctivitis and nasal discharge are common, and body temperatures of 105°F or higher are not uncommon. Characteristically the animals suffer a considerable loss of weight. The acute phase of the disease usually has passed within 5 to 7 days, and improvement in condition is as marked and rapid as the onset of the disease.

Nakamura *et al.* (1972) observed these typical signs on many farms in Wisconsin, isolated the virus, and demonstrated antibodies in the pigs following the disease. They also observed respiratory disease of pigs in which the herd disease was not typical of the disease described above from which they isolated the swine influenza virus and demonstrated antibodies following the disease. On such farms an occasional pig may have the typical signs. There were other cases where the disease was considered to be typical, clinical swine influenza; however, the virus could not be isolated, and there was no serological evidence for infection with the swine influenza virus. In other cases the signs were extremely mild, and it was only by chance that such conditions were shown to be related to infection with the swine influenza virus. Nakamura *et al.* (1969) reported evidence of infection with this virus among swine on farms in New York and Massachusetts, where there were no typical signs of the disease reported by the owners, indicating that inapparent infections may be common. Nakamura (1972) has also described swine influenza antibody among pigs in Hawaii without signs of disease.

Menšik (1962) reported the frequent occurrence of dead and mummified fetuses and dead piglets soon after birth when the sow was infected during pregnancy. The swine influenza virus could be isolated from the organs of the stillborn pigs and from the placental tissue of the sow. Young and Underdahl (1949a,b, 1950a,b) reported that pigs farrowed by dams inoculated with influenza virus before conception had a lower mortality rate than pigs farrowed by control dams. Conversely, pigs farrowed by dams inoculated during the first month of pregnancy had higher mortality rates than those from control dams. Veterinarians and herd owners in southern Wisconsin have expressed the opinion that litters are often small from sows that had influenza during pregnancy and that the pigs are small and have poor viability. Other aspects of swine influenza are described in more detail by Easterday (1970).

Since the mortality rate with swine influenza is so low (1–5% depending on age) there are very few descriptions of the lesions based on necropsy observations in naturally infected pigs. There are no remarkable lesions in any organ other than the lung. When pneumonia occurs it is usually confined to the apical and cardiac lobes, with the affected purple-red pneumonic areas being sharply demarcated from the nonpneumonic areas. The bronchial and mediastinal lymph nodes may be enlarged and congested. When the pneumonia is more severe and more extensive, fibrin is obvious in the bronchial exudate and there is accumulation of fibrin on the pleural surfaces of the lung and thoracic wall. The histological changes in naturally infected pigs do not seem to be different from the lesions that have been described under experimental conditions. A description of the histological changes as they occur sequentially is given in Section II,A,2.

2. The Experimental Disease

The course and signs of disease under experimental conditions vary greatly. Shope (1931b) reported that a mild disease which he called "filtrate disease" developed when pigs were exposed only to the swine influenza virus. Generally there was no febrile response, but occasionally a few pigs had fever for 1 day. There was moderate and transient lassitude and some loss in appetite for a period of up to 3 days, and occasionally a slight cough and a moderate to marked leukopenia. When the pigs were infected with a mixture of the swine influenza virus and *Hemophilus influenzae suis,* the signs and course of the disease and infection were similar to those described under natural conditions (Section III,A,1). Nayak *et al.* (1965) reported that when pathogen-free miniature pigs, 1 week old, were exposed to the swine influenza virus there was an increase of rectal temperature of 2°F or more within 24 hours after exposure. The body temperature was usually normal again by the fourth or fifth day after exposure. Nakamura (1967) reported a very wide range in response in experimental infections from no signs of disease to febrile response with loss of appetite, some coughing, and some prostration.

The sequential development of the lesions has been described in experimental infections by Nayak *et al.* (1965). They found the gross changes limited to the lungs and the mediastinal lymph nodes. There was consolidation within 24 hours most frequently involving the tips of the right apical and intermediate lobes. By the fourth day the diaphragmatic lobes were obviously involved, and regression of the consolidated areas was evident on the sixth and seventh days with subsequent total recovery except for a few small lobular areas that remained consolidated and discolored. The mediastinal lymph nodes were usually hyperemic and enlarged.

Shope (1931a), Urman *et al.* (1958), and Nayak *et al.* (1965) have reported the microscopic lesions in considerable detail. Obvious microscopic changes were observed within a few hours after exposure. By 8 hours there was general congestion of lung parenchyma and thickened alveolar septa due to vasodilation and infiltration of neutrophils. Some degenerative changes were evident in the epithelium of small bronchi at this time. By 16 hours there was focal atelectasis and focal necrosis of the bronchial epithelium. There was a widespread lobular atelectasis with compensatory emphysema 24 hours after infection. Small bronchi were completely or partially filled with exudate containing mostly neutrophils by the third day. At this time there was also focal coagulative necrosis in some alveoli and some early hyperplasia of bronchial epithelium. By the fourth day there were signs of repair apparent, and the cellular character of exudate had changed from mostly neutrophilic to mononuclear cells. By day 5 there was thickening of alveolar septa, interstitial pneumonia, and hyperplasia of bronchial epithelium. By the ninth day there was maximal cellular reaction in the bronchial epithelium, alveolar septa, and the peribronchial and perivascular areas.

Using immunofluorescent techniques there was evidence of viral antigen in bronchial epithelial cells within 2 hours after infection. By the sixteenth hour there were large fluorescent areas of bronchial epithelium. Some bronchi were completely fluorescent and contained fluorescent exudate by the twenty-fourth hour. Staining was intense through 72 hours after infection and then diminished and disappeared from the bronchial mucosa by the ninth day. Antigen was also detected in the alveolar septa within 4 hours after infection, and at 24 hours there were numerous fluorescent cells in the alveoli and alveolar ducts. The fluorescent staining in the alveoli also disappeared by the ninth day. Antigen was also detected in the lower portion of the trachea near the bifurcation and was most evident 48 hours after infection. The antigen could not be detected in the trachea after the fourth day. Occasional fluorescence was observed in the epithelium of the turbinates and mediastinal lymph nodes. Fluorescent cells were not detected in the tonsil, larynx, liver, and kidney.

Nayak *et al.* (1964) found that pigs with lungworms, either prepatent or patent, reacted more severely to influenza virus than did pigs without lungworms. Lung consolidation was more extensive in the pigs with lungworms plus virus than with either alone.

B. Equine

1. The Natural Disease

Bryans (1964), Gerber (1970), and Bryans and Gerber (1972) have provided excellent descriptions of equine influenza. The signs of disease in horses infected with either of the two subtypes of equine influenza virus are approximately identical, except that the equine 1 virus (Heq1Neq1) usually causes a milder disease than the equine 2 (Heq2Neq2) virus. The equine 2 virus is more likely to be pneumotropic and generally more virulent than the equine 1 virus. Bryans (1964) described the signs of disease in horses as follows: "They consist of pyrexia, dry cough, and serous nasal efflux. Almost all become depressed. Inappetance and obvious generalized muscular soreness and dependent edema occur in a few cases. A temperature peak varies from slightly above normal to as high as 105°F. Fever lasts 1 to 5 days. There may be a cough for only 2 or 3 days or it may persist for as long as three weeks. The virus may be isolated from the upper respiratory tract during the early stage of disease." The incubation period is usually considered to be 2–3 days. A cough that is dry, harsh, and usually nonproductive is a very common sign. A moderate amount of nasal discharge which is serous, eventually mucous and later occasionally mucopurulent is observed although there is little rhinitis. Gerber (1970) emphasized that equine influenza is not an upper respiratory disease. Fever is common, and Gerber (1970) indicated that the equine 2 virus is associated with a higher level of fever in a greater percentage of cases than the equine 1 virus.

Horses that are allowed to rest recover from the disease without serious complications; however, those that are worked within a few days following the acute phase of the disease are more likely to have recurrence of fever and prolonged signs of disease. Complications and sequelae of equine influenza include purulent pharyngitis, purulent conjunctivitis, sinusitis, chronic laryngitis, laryngeal paralysis, chronic bronchiolitis with alveolar emphysema, and chronic bronchopneumonia. The most common complicating factor is infection with hemolytic streptococci, usually *S. zooepidemicus.*

The lesions with equine influenza have not been well defined because the mortality rate has been low. Gerber (1970) provides a tabular summation of the histological lesions due to the equine 2 virus. These include vacuolation and erosions in the nasal mucosae of young foals and subacute laryngitis and tracheitis in adults. Epithelial proliferation in alveoli, erosive bronchitis, and hyaline membranes have been observed in the lungs of young foals. In adults there is diffuse subacute interstitial pneumonia, peribronchitis, periarteritis, bronchitis, and bronchopneumonia. Involvement of other organs has included myocarditis and encephalopathy.

2. Experimental Infections

The course, signs, and lesions of experimental infections with the equine 2 virus have been similar to the natural infections. Experimental infections with the equine 1 virus seem to be more difficult to accomplish and are less frequently reported. Blaškovič *et al.* (1966) reported on the pathogenesis of experimental infections of horses with the equine 1 virus. They were able to infect horses with and without mild signs of disease, e.g., fever, cough, and nasal discharge. The most prominent signs of disease and good recovery of virus were in those horses that had been subjected to about 12 hours of windy conditions at $-15°$ to $-18°C$. While the precise pathogenesis was not determined they found that virus could be recovered from tissues of the respiratory tract up to the eighth day after exposure. When horses were exposed in another experiment after a 20 minute gallop at an ambient temperature of $15°$ to $18°C$, there were no signs of disease or recovery of virus.

Blaškovič *et al.* (1969) have also reported on experimental infections of horses with the equine 2 virus. Following intranasal infection they observed fever, nasal discharge, laryngitis and heavy cough, and secondary bacterial infection with purulent rhinitis, and pulmonary complications in some. Contact infection was also observed.

Chincoteague ponies were infected with the equine 2 virus given by atomizer and intratracheal inoculation (Cameron *et al.*, 1967). Virus was recovered from 22 of 24 exposed ponies and 15 of the 24 were febrile. There were other signs of disease including inactivity, anorexia, rapid breathing rates, and dry cough only in those animals with high fever. The signs of disease subsided as the body temperature returned to normal. Antibody response was definite but low, as had been observed in natural cases and in the experiments done by Blaškovič *et al.* (1969) There was, however, no equine 1 antibody response, which was in contrast to the reports of Blaškovič *et al.* (1969) and Dowdle *et al.* (1964). Cameron *et al.* (1967) took their findings as evidence that the ponies had had no previous encounter with the equine 2 virus.

C. Avian

1. The Natural Disease

The signs, course, and lesions of influenza virus infections among avian species are extremely variable depending, e.g., on the species affected, the infecting virus, environmental factors, age, sex, concurrent infections. The infections may be inapparent or result in highly fatal disease with mortality approaching 100%. The various signs among the various species have included coughing, sneezing, rales, sinusitis, excessive lacrimation, edema of the head and face, diarrhea, central nervous system involvement with paralysis, decreased egg production, decreased feed consumption, inactivity, huddling, and ruffled feathers. Any of these signs may be observed alone or in various combinations. Examples of the extreme variation in the nature of disease due to infection with avian influenza viruses are described for several species: ducks (Roberts, 1964; Rinaldi et al., 1965; Hwang et al., 1970), chickens (Stubbs, 1965; Rinaldi et al., 1968), terns (Rowan, 1962; Becker, 1966), turkeys (Wells, 1963; Bankowski and Conrad, 1966; Lang and Wills, 1966; Olesiuk et al., 1967; Lang et al., 1968a,b; Smithies et al., 1969a,b), pheasant (Rinaldi et al., 1967a), quail (Coturnix) (Rinaldi et al., 1967b), and in several species by Easterday and Tumová (1972a,b).

A major problem among turkeys in North America is the severe effect of influenza viruses on reproductive efficiency. Infection in turkey breeding flocks is commonly characterized by a precipitous drop in egg production, with or without signs of respiratory tract involvement. In some cases the loss in egg production is permanent. The same virus that causes the reproductive failure in the adult birds may cause severe respiratory disease among young birds on the same farm with mortality of up to 25%.

While there have been several influenza viruses isolated from wild avian species, there have been no signs of disease or lesions observed except for the disease and high mortality rate among terns in South Africa in 1961 (Rowan, 1962; Becker, 1966). Other than the birds being obviously ill the only other sign reported was profuse diarrhea. The significant lesions were inflammation of the lower intestine and marked cloudiness of the air sacs.

The lesions observed in many avian species are as varied with regard to location and severity as are the signs, nature, and course of the disease. Lesions observed in both natural and experimental infections are considered together here. On one end of the scale, influenza viruses have been isolated from birds in which there were no obvious gross signs or lesions. On the other end of the scale a variety of congestive, hemorrhagic, transudative, and necrobiotic changes have been described in infections with high mortality rates caused by viruses such as fowl plague, chicken/Scotland/59, tern/South Africa/61, turkey/England/63, and turkey/Ontario/7732/66. Sinusitis of varying degrees of severity and character has been described in ducks, turkeys, chickens, quail, partridge, and pheasants (Easterday and Tumová, 1972a,b).

The descriptions of the microscopic changes associated with avian influenza virus infection have been limited primarily to those conditions in which there have been severe overt disease and obvious gross changes. Fowl plague virus causes lesions throughout the body. These include edema, hyperemia, hemorrhage, and perivascular lymphoid cuffing particularly in the myocardium, spleen, lungs, and brain and to a lesser extent in liver and kidney. Jungherr *et al.* (1946) described the lesions of fowl plague in considerable detail. Foci of necrosis were observed in the spleen, liver, lung, kidney, and pancreas in decreasing order of frequency. Small necrotic foci have been found in the brain within 24 hours after exposure and then advanced, being accompanied by signs of encephalitis, e.g., perivascular lymphoid cuffing, vascular-glial reactions, and neuronal degeneration. Lesions in chickens infected with the tern/South Africa/61 and chicken/Scotland/69 viruses, included focal necrosis and lymphoid infiltration in the spleen, brain, eyes, ocular muscles, comb, skeletal muscles, and myocardium (Uys and Becker, 1967). After 5 or 6 days diffuse encephalitis in both the cerebrum and cerebellum was observed with the "tern" virus. Generally, the disease and lesions were more severe with the "tern" virus than with the chicken/Scotland/59 virus.

Extensive and severe lesions have been reported in turkeys infected experimentally with the turkey/Ontario/7732/66 virus. Electrocardiographic changes with this infection were subtle but definite and appeared to be related to the severe myocarditis that was observed (McKenzie *et al.,* 1972). Pancreatitis with extensive necrosis of acinar cells has been a striking lesion observed with experimental infections of turkeys with turkey/Ontario/6213/66 and turkey/Ontario/7732/66 virus (Rouse *et al.,* 1968; Narayan *et al.,* 1969a). Degenerative and necrotic changes with these two viruses have also been observed in other organs including liver, brain and meninges, myocardium, and cutaneous tissues. Microscopic lesions seen in the sinus of ducks and turkeys include cell degeneration, epithelial hyperplasia, infiltration of heterophils, and acute inflammation of the lamina propria (Rinaldi *et al.,* 1966a,b). Hwang *et al.* (1970) found catarrhal tracheitis and air sacculitis in ducks. The precise effect of influenza virus on the reproductive tract of turkeys has not been determined.

2. EXPERIMENTAL INFECTION

Experimentally, the same range in signs, nature, and course has been observed as under natural conditions. There is no pattern or generalization to be made about the nature of the avian influenza virus–host combination.

Viruses having the same or similar antigenic character are often quite different biologically, particularly with regard to virulence. It must be kept in mind that virus that is particularly virulent for one avian species will not necessarily be virulent for another avian species (Slemons and Easterday, 1972).

IV. Epizootiology

A. Swine

It is assumed that swine influenza virus has been present in midwestern United States since the disease was first observed in 1918. Typically, outbreaks of swine influenza begin in late September and increase in number rapidly through October and then begin to diminish in number through November, December, and the remainder of the winter. The appearance of these local epizootics is often coincidental with the onset of autumn rains and marked diurnal fluctuations of temperature. The changing meteorological factors and management procedures that take place in that time of year are believed to be stressful situations which contribute to the precipitation of the disease. These outbreaks are not associated with the movement of animals, and instead of rapid spread from herd to herd the observations suggest the virus is widely seeded among herds and that the disease appears almost simultaneously on many farms.

It is common that all of the pigs on a farm appear to become ill at the same time; however, observant owners have reported that one or a few pigs were ill 2–5 days before the herd disease appeared. For many years it was assumed that after the disease ran its course on individual farms and the area by midwinter it disappeared until the next autumn and the cycle was repeated. This disappearance and reappearance of a highly contagious disease on a seasonal basis intrigued many investigators. The major question was concerned with how and where the virus survived during the interepizootic period.

In studies, by the author and colleagues on swine influenza in southern Wisconsin over the past 14 years, it is clear that swine influenza occurs throughout the year. While the typical swine influenza is most common during the fall and early winter, respiratory disease associated with influenza virus infection occurs throughout the year. In midwestern United States the swine influenza virus has been recovered from pigs in every month of the year except June. Others (Scott, 1941; Woods and Simpson, 1964) have also indicated that infection and disease may occur throughout the year.

Respiratory disease of swine that does not have all the characteristics of classical influenza may be caused by swine influenza virus. Nakamura *et al.* (1972) have reported on the recovery of swine influenza viruses from such cases.

Nakamura (1967) and Nakamura *et al.* (1972) have offered the hypothesis that pigs upon convalescence from the acute infection may become carriers of the virus and serve as a means for perpetuation of the virus in nature. Their hypothesis was based on epizootiological and serological observations and not on the isolation of the virus from asymptomatic pigs. Experiments done by Blaškovič *et al.* (1970) support the hypothesis of a persistent or carrier state with animals being occasional or intermittent shedders of the virus. They found that susceptible animals placed in contact with pigs that had been infected 3 months before became infected and the virus was isolated from them. Susceptible animals introduced 42 days, 6, 9, and 12 months after the initial exposure did not become infected.

Shope (1941a,b, 1943a,b, 1955) had previously proposed a complicated mechanism for the interepizootic survival of the swine influenza virus. He offered the hypothesis that the swine lungworm was capable of harboring the swine influenza virus, that it served as an intermediate host and transmitted the virus from pig to pig, and that the virus remained latent or occult in the lungworm in the pig until there was a stressful or provocative stimulus that led to the release of the virus. Shope was intrigued by the disappearance of the disease during the interepizootic period and the sudden and widespread reappearance of the classical disease every autumn. In an attempt to determine where and how the virus survived he considered that swine might have been carriers of swine influenza. He discarded that possibility, however, because "at that time no way of introducing swine influenza virus into swine was known that did not cause either infection or the acquisition of immunity" (Shope, 1941a). He concluded that infected swine became immune and eliminated the possibility that the virus could remain in the immune animal. Since that time there are numerous reports describing the persistence of various kinds of viruses in the immune host and the presence of circulating antibody.

There was skepticism about this very complicated means for the interepizootic maintenance of the virus almost as soon as the hypothesis was published. Blakemore *et al.* (1941) indicated that "the indefinite nature of the symptoms sometimes shown and the possibility of animals already carrying the infection, unknown to the investigators, the lungworm theory cannot be accepted as a complete explanation." Others have expressed doubts over the years. In 1950 Andrewes stated: "One thing worries me about Shope's experiment: such a complex association between creatures of four species has the hallmark of an ecologic happy family, the result of eons of evolution.

Yet neither the pig nor the earthworm concerned is native to the United States and swine influenza is asserted never to have been known to the middle west before 1918. It would be odd if swine influenza, which is not known to survive so long anywhere else (except in the virologist's dry ice container), should just happen to find the interior of a lungworm an ideal resting place. I feel that either there is something wrong with the facts as presented or we ought to be looking more earnestly for some similar mechanism to explain the survival of human influenza viruses."

The Shope hypothesis is as follows: Lungworms (*Metastrongylus*) present in the lung at the time of infection with influenza become infected with the virus and the virus is passed in the ova of the lungworm. The embryonated lungworm ova are deposited in the bronchioles of the pig, coughed up, swallowed and passed in the feces. The ova are then ingested by the earthworm, a necessary intermediate host for the lungworm, hatch and the larvae develop to the third or infective larval stage in the earth worm. These third stage or infective larvae contain the influenza virus. Eventually the earthworm is eaten by a pig, the lungworm larvae are released, there are two more developmental stages, and the larvae migrate from the intestines of the pig via the vascular system and lymphatics to the lungs where they become adults. Under the most optimal conditions this cycle may be completed in a little more than a month but the cycle may take as long as 3 years for completion. Generally the swine infested with the lungworms carrying the "masked virus" or "occult" or latent virus do not develop swine influenza immediately upon the lungworms reaching the lungs. The animals remain normal until such time as there is some provocative stimulus, such as the onset of cold inclement weather or a change in the management and practice, at which time the virus is released and produces disease.

One of the puzzling aspects of Shope's hypothesis is that the virus has never been demonstrated directly in the lungworm, lungworm larvae, lungworm ova, or the earthworm. While Shope provided an imaginative approach to explain the interepizootic survival of the swine influenza virus, investigators have not found it necessary to propose such a complex biological system to explain the survival of influenza viruses among human, equine, and avian populations. Many aspects of the epizootiology and epidemiology of influenza of the various species remain obscure, and certainly the Shope lungworm hypothesis and the recovered carrier hypothesis are not mutually exclusive.

The precise methods and mechanisms of transmission of the swine influenza virus have not been determined. The virus is found readily in the nasal and pharyngeal secretions during the febrile period. It is assumed that this is the main if not the only source of virus for transmission to susceptible hosts. The main method of transmission is probably by the airborne route

but not over great distances. Experimentally, pigs can be infected by introduction of virus into the nasal passages or by exposure to aerosols of influenza virus generated as described by Beard and Easterday (1965). Viremia
may be detected irregularly and with increasing difficulty with increasing
age (Walker, 1971). Menšik (1962) has reported intrauterine transmission
of the disease when pregnant sows have been infected, but Renshaw (1970)
and Walker (1971) failed to demonstrate intrauterine transmission by exposure of sows intranasally and by aerosol at various stages of pregnancy. When
they introduced virus directly into the uterus, the fetuses became infected
and there was some abnormal development, fetal wastage, abortion, and the
delivery of weak and stunted pigs.

The precise role that environment plays in swine influenza is unknown.
As indicated above, there is considerable circumstantial evidence that environmental and climatic factors may precipitate the disease in the autumn
and early winter. Numerous outbreaks are often coincidental with sudden
changes in climate, such as the onset of cold, rainy nights in the fall along
with the lack of preparedness on the owner's part in having housing available for the pigs to escape the elements. Menšik (1960) described the influence of what he termed microclimate on the course of experimental swine
influenza. He observed that pigs kept in a cold damp concrete facility with
a temperature of $1°$ to $10°C$ and a relative humidity of 95 to 100% were
more susceptible and developed more severe disease than pigs provided with
insulated shelter but allowed to run outside when the temperature varied
from $-13°$ to $+2°C$ and the relative humidity was 75 to 85%. Experiments,
not previously reported, done at the University of Wisconsin have attempted
to determine the effect of climatic conditions on the course of swine influenza. In one experiment pigs were exposed to the virus and after 2 and
3 days they were exposed overnight to temperatures of $-15°$ to $-20°C$
and sprayed intermittently with water. There was no exacerbation of disease
and the signs were no different than those in their counterparts kept at
$+18°C$ during the course of the experiment. In another experiment, pigs
were exposed to temperatures in the range of $+1°$ to $+4°C$ in environmental chambers and sprayed with water in an attempt to simulate cool,
rainy autumn days There were no differences in the course of the disease
among these pigs and their counterparts held at constant $+18°C$. While
Nakamura (1972) observed the presence of swine influenza antibody among
pigs in Hawaii, there is no evidence that the typical disease occurs there
among pigs. Furthermore, swine influenza antibody has been found in swine
serum collected in southern United States (B. C. Easterday, unpublished
data, 1973), but the literature does not record evidence of the clinical disease
in pigs in that area.

Swine influenza may be suspected with any acute respiratory disease involving pigs particularly in the fall or early winter. A clinical diagnosis of influenza can be only presumptive as is the case in any species. Nakamura *et al.* (1972) have described conditions identical to typical swine influenza in which there was no evidence that the disease was caused by the swine influenza virus. They also described respiratory disease not typical of swine influenza but which proved to be due to infection of that virus.

Serological surveillance for swine influenza is relatively easy. It is necessary only to go to slaughter houses and collect blood at the time of slaughter and test the serum for the presence of swine influenza antibody. In the large progressive slaughter houses in north central United States, pigs are identified as to their area of origin and in many cases by their farm of origin. Nakamura *et al.* (1972) collected serum from pigs at slaughter at various times of the year and found that approximately 60% of all sows and "heavys" (1 or more years old) going to slaughter had antibody to swine influenza virus. On the other hand, market pigs or butchers (5–7 months old) were only 23–30% positive for swine influenza virus antibody. They also noted that the levels of antibody were significantly higher in the older pigs. Pirtle (1973) reported that 34% of 73 herds of swine tested had swine influenza antibody. In those 73 herds, 53% of 15 breeder herds and 30% of 58 butcher herds had antibody. He also noted that in herds in which there were no signs of influenza-like disease, 14% of the serum samples collected had antibody. In herds where there were signs of influenze-like disease reported, 29% of the serum samples had antibody. Another method of surveillance in the United States has been to test serum that has been collected in such disease control programs as those for brucellosis and hog cholera. Large numbers of serum samples may be available at state diagnostic laboratories for testing.

The economic importance of this disease has not been determined on a nationwide or a worldwide basis. In areas where the disease occurs annually swine producers absorb considerable loss in the form of delayed weight gains, increased time to market, cost of medication, and increased mortality rates of suckling pigs. Death losses are usually very low except in suckling pigs. It is reasonable to estimate that the cost of influenza per pig is approximately $5.00 based on increased time to market, medication, veterinary care, and more feed consumption.

B. Equine

The epizootiological features of equine influenza are not unlike those observed in human influenza. The pattern, incidence, and nature of the disease among horses as in other populations is influenced by the level of herd immunity and by the antigenic and biological characteristic of the virus. While there may be some areas of the world where equine influenza has not been a problem, the disease has been of epizootic proportion in every major subdivision of the world.

Bryans and Gerber (1972) emphasize that "the pattern of disease produced by equine influenza viruses is governed mainly by the immunity that has developed as a result of previous infection." There is no remarkable difference in the epizootiological patterns of the equine 1 and equine 2 viruses. In equine populations with little, if any, herd immunity, outbreaks of the disease are generally explosive in character, with the disease spreading very rapidly through the population. Attack rates of 100% may be expected in young susceptible horses with either virus. Since these viruses are widespread throughout the world and vaccination is a common practice most outbreaks are among horses 2 years old or younger. Early in 1963 the equine 2 virus (A/equine/Miami/1/63) was first recognized in the United States. During the period from mid-January through June it spread to all parts of the United States. The horse population of the United States, as is the case in other countries of the world, is extremely mobile, and as horses moved from one race track to another and from show to show the disease went with them. The intensity of outbreaks, particularly at race tracks, was clearly illustrated by the number of "scratches" (horses withdrawn from scheduled races) that were recorded. The epizootic curve obtained in this manner was analogous to the epidemic curves shown by absenteeism at schools and factories.

Since there are two antigenically distinct viruses involved in causing influenza among horses, it has not been uncommon to have two epizootics of respiratory disease occurring in the same population within a very short time of each other. It is also clear as reported by Tumová et al. (1972) that both viruses may occur simultaneously in a stable of horses. Whether these viruses infect any one horse simultaneously has not been determined. There has been no record of two antigenically distinct type A influenza viruses circulating in the human population at the same time. When a new strain or subtype has appeared the old subtype has disappeared, which has not been the case with equine and avian influenza viruses.

The equine viruses have been quite stable, but there has been antigenic variation observed in viruses isolated in South America (Pereira et al., 1972) and Japan (Kono et al., 1972). In both cases viruses similar, but not identical, to the A/equine/Miami/1/63 virus were isolated and characterized.

No unique mechanism has been proposed for the interepizootic maintenance of equine influenza viruses. Gerber (1970) referred to the possibility that an asymptomatic carrier state might exist. Since horses are so mobile, it would appear that the virus is maintained simply by bringing infected horses in contact with horses with various levels of immunity. Those horses with no immunity can be expected to become infected and have severe signs of disease, while those with some level of immunity may become infected and have mild or no signs of disease and still transmit the virus to other animals.

Gerber (1970) reported that donkeys and mules are infected with these viruses, and the features of the disease are similar to those in horses. The extent to which these and other equines are involved under natural conditions is not known. Antibody against the equine 2 virus has been found in horses in Mongolia, an isolated population that has little, if any, opportunity to contact horses from any other area. Although Chincoteague ponies have been experimentally infected with a type B influenza virus of human origin (Kasel *et al.*, 1968) and type B viruses have been reported from horses in Italy (Compagnucci *et al.*, 1969), there are no other indications that type B influenza viruses infect and/or cause disease in equines or other species other than man.

The two most important factors in the rapid spread of equine influenza are the short (1–3 days) incubation period and the characteristic frequent and strong cough. The cough provides conditions for efficiently spreading the virus by the airborne route over at least 35 meters. Considerable amounts of virus are found in the nasal and pharyngeal secretions. Although these virus-laden secretions may be deposited on equipment, utensils, etc., it appears that inanimate vectors play a minor role in transmission in relation to the airborne and direct contact routes. Other animals, including man, do not appear to be important factors in the mechanical spread of the disease.

There has been no seasonal prevalence of the disease that can be directly related to climatic conditions. Gerber (1970) agreed with others that there was no seasonal incidence. Increased prevalence may be associated with racing "seasons" or show "seasons" when horses are congregated for those activities. Climatic factors may be important indirectly in facilitating transmission of the virus. Assembly of large numbers of horses in stables to protect them from harsh climatic conditions serves to bring horses close together in a static air environment, increasing the chances of transmission.

Surveillance for this infection and disease is facilitated by the fact that in most parts of the world most of the horses are probably companion or recreational animals for man. Therefore, animal to human relationships are close, and owners, trainers, and caretakers are likely to recognize the disease very quickly. This is particularly true of race horses and show horses. Where the horse is important as a work animal, e.g., a draft animal on farms or a military mount, the disease is likely to be detected readily because of the effect upon the ability of the animal to work. Once clinical signs of the disease are observed virological and serological diagnostic tests are available in most parts of the world. Serological surveys are probably of little value because of the widespread use of vaccines. The experience with the equine influenza viruses has been such that outbreaks of disease attract attention quickly and demand a resolution to the problem.

The economic importance of equine influenza has not been defined on a nationwide or worldwide basis. There are no data to indicate the annual incidence. It is clear however, that the disease is responsible for considerable economic losses. Perhaps the most important loss is associated with outbreaks of the disease among racing horses. Horses with the disease are not able to work (run) and require a rather extended period of time for recuperation. Such losses can be reduced considerably by the use of equine influenza vaccines that are available (see Section V,A).

C. Avian

The epizootiologic features of avian influenza are poorly understood. If consideration is confined to one virus in one species, for example, fowl plague among chickens or one of several viruses among turkeys, then specific epizootiologic patterns can be defined. For the most part the precise source of infection for outbreaks or avian influenza that have been studied have not been determined. There is great speculation that wild or free-flying species are important in the spread of these viruses. Descriptions of these various outbreaks commonly make reference to the fact that the origin of infection was undetermined (Lang *et al.,* 1965; Smithies *et al.,* 1969a,b; Kleven *et al.,* 1970; Hwang *et al.,* 1970). In an attempt to determine the role that man might play in the spread of the virus, Homme *et al.* (1970) found that a caretaker spread the infection from one flock of 400 infected turkeys to another flock the same size. The infection was spread to a third flock, in sequence, but not to a fourth flock during a 56 day period. The disease seems to spread rapidly within a turkey flock, under natural conditions. Flocks range in size from 2000 to 20,000 birds with one to several flocks on one farm. The infection spreads through a flock quickly upon introduction and then subsides and disappears and may not involve other flocks on the same farm if proper quarantine procedures are employed. Quarantine procedures, mainly concerned with destroying the infected chickens and eliminating the movement of people between flocks, have been effective in controlling the spread of fowl plague (Stubbs, 1965).

Turkey management practices are such that there is periodic depopulation of flocks and farms, a procedure which interrupts the disease cycle and prevents influenza infections from becoming enzootic. Conversely, influenza has been enzootic among quail (*Coturnix*) reared under intense confinement conditions in Italy (Rinaldi *et al.*, 1967b; Mandelli *et al.*, 1968). There were no depopulation procedures, and the disease seemed to be perpetuated by the constant introduction of newly hatched birds.

One of the most striking aspects about influenza among domestic avian species in North America, is the nearly complete confinement to turkeys. Despite the widespread presence of the viruses among turkeys as well as various wild species, chickens seem to have escaped infection. There has been considerable effort expended to determine whether chickens are infected with influenza viruses in southeastern United States and in California. It is not likely, because of the widespread presence of these viruses, that chickens can escape infection indefinitely.

The role of wild birds in the dissemination of influenza viruses to domestic species and among wild species has not been determined. Wild birds probably played a role in the spread of fowl plague in the past (Stubbs, 1965). While both viruses and antibodies have been demonstrated in several wild avian species, there is no evidence for disease among them due to those viruses (except the terns in South Africa), and there is no direct evidence that wild birds have been the source of infection for or been infected by domestic birds.

Easterday *et al.* (1968) demonstrated antibody in the serum of several wild geese in North America, and Winkler *et al.* (1972) reported that about 5% of 1400 geese sera had antibody against one or more of the North American avian influenza viruses. Subsequent to that time Dasen and Laver (1970) and Downie and Laver (1973) have demonstrated antibody and the virus in shearwaters on the Great Barrier Reef. Slemons *et al.* (1973) described the recovery of several influenza viruses from a variety of exotic birds imported into the United States. Slemons *et al.* (1974) also reported on the isolation and identification of several influenza viruses from wild ducks in California. On the opposite side of the Pacific, Soviet workers, Zakstel'skaja *et al.* (1972) and Slepuskin *et al.* (1972), have reported the presence of antibody to several influenza viruses in the sera of wild birds in the far east of the U.S.S.R. Among the pet birds influenza viruses have been isolated from myna birds, parakeets (Easterday and Tumová, 1972b), and parrots (B. C. Easterday, unpublished data, 1973). There is evidence of infection among the guinea fowls in Hungary (Tanyi, 1972) and in Minnesota (A. Bahl, personal communication, 1974). G. C. Schild (personal communication, 1973) reported the isolation of a Hong Kong-like influenza virus from terns in the Norwegian waters.

While it is clear that there are infections among many wild avian species, so far the significance of these findings in the epizootiology of influenza among avian species and the role of the wild birds in the natural history of influenza in all species, particularly man, remains undetermined.

With these influenza viruses so widely scattered and constantly circulating among so many avian species, there is no reason to believe that there is a unique system for the interepizootic maintenance of these viruses. They seem to be circulating almost constantly and so far there has been no evidence of a panzootic among birds. There are indications that some birds, particularly turkeys, may become persistently infected with some of the viruses. Homme *et al.* (1970), Bankowski and Conrad (1966), and Lang *et al.* (1968a) reported on the recovery of the virus for a period of 21–36 days after exposure. Robinson (1971) was able to recover virus 2 months after infection.

Bird to bird transmission appears to require relatively close contact. Narayan *et al.* (1969b) described contact transmission among turkeys kept together on the floor, but there was no transmission to turkeys housed in cages 1 meter above the floor in the same room. Bankowski and Conrad (1966) described contact infections among turkeys in adjacent pens. If the population is reasonably compact, providing for very close contact among individuals, it appears that the infection will spread readily through that population (Homme *et al.*, 1970). The transmission rate is markedly reduced when birds are not confined closely. There has been some suggestion of the possibility of vertical transmission from infected hen turkeys to their offspring via the egg. While infection on turkey breeding farms has been frequent, there is no direct evidence for the presence of the virus in the eggs from infected hens.

Experimental transmission by the contact route has been demonstrated for a number of the avian viruses among several avian species. Turkeys are readily infected by exposure to aerosols of virus. There was a suggestion that severe cold conditions made the disease more severe among turkeys (Homme and Easterday, 1970). However, when turkeys were infected with viruses isolated from turkeys and subjected to extremes of hot and cold, under experimentally controlled conditions, along with water and food deprivation, there were no differences among those turkeys and their counterpart controls properly fed and kept under optimal temperature and humidity conditions.

There is no organized system or concentrated effort in the United States for surveillance of influenza virus infections among birds. Although techniques, particularly the gel diffusion test described by Beard (1970), are available for testing large numbers of bird sera, no organized system for collection and testing has been adopted. During the period (1972–1973) that the emergency control program for Newcastle disease was in operation in California, there was considerable effort expended to collect material and isolate and identify Newcastle disease virus (NDV). Hemagglutinating agents that were isolated and determined to be other than NDV were tested for the presence of the type A influenza virus RNP. As a result, several influenza viruses were recovered from a variety of imported exotic avian species and from wild ducks shot by hunters (Slemons *et al.,* 1973, 1974). There is an organized effort in the Soviet Union to improve influenza surveillance especially among wild avian species by utilizing the system, procedures, techniques, and collected materials that have been established for surveillance of arthropod-borne viruses.

In the concentrated turkey-producing areas of North America, the flock owners and veterinarians are acutely aware of the influenza problem in turkeys, and diagnostic laboratories are commonly requested to assist in the virological and serological diagnosis of influenza. Surveillance among wild species is much more difficult and requires close cooperation of a testing laboratory and ornithologists or other wildlife and natural resources personnel. The sampling of birds killed by hunters and netting and the sampling of flightless young are procedures that have been utilized in the surveillance of these viruses in the United States and other parts of the world. It is a very laborious and expensive procedure to do such surveillance, but it is also important to determine the extent to which influenza viruses are disseminated among our animal species. The viruses that have been isolated from wild species are for the most part the result of *ad hoc* efforts of relatively few investigators.

The economic importance of these viruses has not been determined. During the time fowl plague virus circulated in the United States there were extensive losses among chickens because of the very high mortality rate. While economic loss is difficult to define precisely, it is clear that the effect on the reproductive tract among breeding turkeys has been costly. In many cases it has been necessary to slaughter the breeding flocks because the egg production has been so adversely and irreversibly affected. The slaughter salvage does not offset the investment in the building of the breeding flock. The appearance of a virulent influenza virus among any of the domestic avian species, particularly among chickens in the very concentrated areas, could result in a catastrophic loss.

D. Interspecies Infections

No animal to animal interspecies infections have been identified or described under natural conditions. The isolation of the Hong Kong influenza virus from pigs in Taiwan in 1970 (Kundin, 1970) was the first direct evidence of human to animal transmission. Subsequently it has been shown that Hong Kong influenza virus antibody is common in pig sera in many parts of the world (Styk *et al.,* 1971a; Harkness *et al.,* 1972). About 6% of all swine serum tested in Wisconsin contained antibody to Hong Kong influenza virus (Kundin and Easterday, 1972). The Hong Kong influenza virus has been unique and ubiquitous throughout the world in its ability to infect several species, e.g., swine, cattle, chickens, dogs, cats, and some wild species (Paniker and Nair, 1970; Nikitin *et al.,* 1972; G. C. Schild, personal communication, 1973; Zhezmer *et al.,* 1973; D. K. Lvov, personal communication, 1974).

Pigs have been infected experimentally with the Hong Kong virus without signs of disease (Styk *et al.,* 1971b; Kundin and Easterday, 1972). Other animals that have been infected experimentally with viruses of human origin include dogs with A₂ (H2N2), B, and Hong Kong (H3N2) viruses (Todd and Cohen, 1968; Paniker and Nair, 1972; E. D. Kilbourne and J. M. Kehoe, unpublished data, 1972); cats (Paniker and Nair, 1970, 1972); monkeys (Paniker and Nair, 1972); gibbons (Johnsen *et al.,* 1971); baboons (Kalter *et al.,* 1969); swine and calves (Easterday, 1965); and cattle via the intramammary route (Mitchell *et al.,* 1953).

Transmission of the animal viruses to man so far has been more difficult to demonstrate. A virus similar to fowl plague virus (Brescia strain Hav1N1), closely related hemagglutinin and identical neuraminidase, was isolated in the United States from a man who was seriously ill after returning from a part of the world where he might have contacted the virus (DeLay *et al.,* 1967; Campbell *et al.,* 1970). Schnurrenberger *et al.* (1970) have described serological evidence for infection of swine producers, veterinarians, and slaughter workers with swine influenza virus. Kluska *et al.* (1961) and B. Tumová and J. Menšik (personal communication, 1967) have also reported that human beings have become infected with the swine influenza virus. There are many reports of finding antibody against animal influenza viruses in the serum of human beings, but such antibodies are not necessarily an indication of past infection with those strains (Schild and Stuart-Harris, 1965; Davenport *et al.,* 1968; Gorbunova and Pysina, 1968; Masurel, 1969).

Human beings have been infected experimentally with viruses of swine origin. The A/swine/Taiwan/7310/70 virus (H3N2), closely related to the A/Hong Kong/68 virus (H3N2), caused clinical reactions that were milder than those in volunteers exposed to the A/Hong Kong/68 virus. Two swine influenza viruses (A/swine/Wis/1/66 and A/swine/Manitoba/674/67, both Hsw1N1) had low infectivity for the volunteers. Of the 27 volunteers exposed, 7 were infected, 5 excreted virus, 4 had mild signs, and 2 had rises in antibody (Beare *et al.,* 1971).

There is no evidence that man has been infected under natural conditions with either of the equine influenza viruses or that horses have become infected with human influenza viruses. It has been shown, experimentally, however, that horses can be infected with influenza viruses of human origin and that human beings can be infected with the equine influenza viruses (Couch *et al.*, 1969; Kasel and Couch, 1969; Kasel *et al.*, 1969). Blaškovič *et al.* (1969) have shown that horses may be infected experimentally with the Hong Kong influenza virus.

With regard to animal to animal experimental infections, several species of birds have been infected with a viruses recovered from turkeys but the degree of transmissibility, the severity of the disease, and the nature of the antibody response are quite species dependent. Other examples of experimental interspecies infections are described by Webster and Laver in Chapter 10.

V. Control

A. Vaccination

The only vaccines that are commercially available for any animal species are those for horses against the equine 1 and 2 influenza viruses. These vaccines contain inactivated viruses and no less than 2 doses, given parenterally, are recommended. The experience with equine influenza in various parts of the world has been favorable, and vaccination is recommended for all horses that are "traveling" and have frequent contact with groups of horses (Bryans *et al.*, 1966a; Bryans, 1972; Fontaine and Fontaine, 1973; Frerichs *et al.*, 1973). There are numerous reports on the preparation, testing, and efficacy of vaccines for swine influenza; however, such vaccine has never been available commercially for use in pigs (Easterday, 1970).

Various kinds of vaccines have been used against fowl plague (Stubbs, 1965). A. Rinaldi (personal communication, 1968) used a β-propiolactone-inactivated vaccine to vaccinate quail in an effort to increase levels of maternal antibody in newly hatched birds. An inactivated vaccine against the A/turkey/Ont/7732/66 virus was made and tested by Narayan *et al.* (1970) and found to induce a very short duration of protection. Beard and Easterday (1973) have described the use of an avirulent virus (A/turkey/Oregon/71) with the Hav1 hemagglutinin that provides complete protection of chickens against fowl plague. The major problem in attempting to provide a vaccine against avian influenza is the fact that there are at least eight different hemagglutinins among the influenza viruses affecting birds.

B. Chemotherapy

There is no substance available that has been used routinely in the specific treatment of influenza among the animal species. Adamantanamine has been used in infections in horses (Bryans *et al.*, 1966b), in quail (A. Rinaldi, personal communication, 1968), and in turkeys (Lang *et al.*, 1970). In each case it has been effective in reducing the severity and losses with these infections.

References

Andrews, C. H. (1950). *N. Engl. J. Med.* **242**, 197.
Bankowski, R. A., and Conrad, R. D. (1966). *World's Poultry Congr., Proc., 13th, 1966* pp. 371–379.
Beard, C. W. (1970). *Bull. W.H.O.* **42**, 779.
Beard, C. W., and Easterday, B. C. (1965). *Amer. J. Vet. Res.* **26**, 174.
Beard, C. W., and Easterday, B. C. (1973). *Avian Dis.* **17**, 173.
Beare, A. S., Schild, G. C., Hall, T. S., and Kundin, W. D. (1971). *Lancet* **1**, 305.
Becker, W. B. (1966). *J. Hyg.* **64**, 309.
Blakemore, F., Glover, R. E., and Taylor, E. L. (1941). *Proc. Roy. Soc. Med.* **34**, 611.
Blaškovič, D., Szánto, J., Kapitáncik, J., Lesso, J., Lackovič, V., and Skarda, R. (1966). *Acta Virol. (Prague)* **10**, 513.
Blaškovič, D., Kapitáncik, B., Sabó, A., Styk, B., Vrtiak, O., and Kaplan, M. (1969). *Acta Virol. (Prague)* **13**, 499.
Blaškovič, D., Jamrichová, O., Rathová, V., Kocisková, D., and Kaplan, M. M. (1970). *Bull. W.H.O.* **42**, 767.
Bryans, J. T. (1964). *101st Annu. Meet., Amer. Vet. Med. Ass., 1964* pp. 112–120.
Bryans, J. T. (1972). *Symp. Ser. Immunobiol. Stand.* **20**, 311.
Bryans, J. T., and Gerber, H. (1972). *In* "Equine Medicine and Surgery" (E. J. Catcott and J. F. Smithcors, eds.), 2nd ed., pp. 17–22. Amer. Vet Publ., Wheaton, Illinois.
Bryans, J. T., Doll, E. R., Wilson, J. C., and McCollum, W. H. (1966a). *J. Amer. Vet. Med. Ass.* **148**, 413.
Bryans, J. T., Zent, W. W., Grunert, R. R., and Broughton, D. C. (1966b). *Nature (London)* **212**, 1542.
Cameron, T. P., Alford, R. H., Kasel, J. A., Harvey, E. W., Byrne, R. J., and Knight, V. (1967). *Proc. Soc. Exp. Biol. Med.* **124**, 510.
Campbell, C. H., Webster, R. G., and Breese, S. S. (1970). *J. Inf. Dis.* **122**, 513.
Compagnucci, M., Martone, F., and Bonaduce, A. (1969). *Boll. Ist. Sieroter. Milan.* **48**, 305.
Couch, R. B., Douglas, R. G., Riggs, S., Knight, V., and Kasel, J. A. (1969). *Nature (London)* **224**, 512.
Csontos, L., and Miklovich-Kis Csatári, M. (1967a). *Acta Vet. (Budapest)* **17**, 107.

Csontos, L., and Miklovich-Kis Csatári, M. (1967b). *Acta Vet. (Budapest)* **17,** 115.

Dasen, C. A., and Laver, W. G. (1970). *Bull. W.H.O.* **42,** 885.

Davenport, F. M., Hennessy, A. V., and Minuse, E. (1968). *J. Immunol.* **100,** 581.

DeLay, P. D., Casey, H. L., and Tobiash, H. S. (1967). *Pub. Health Rep.* **82,** 615.

Dinter, Z., and Bakos, K. (1950). *Berlin. Menchen. Tiereztl. Wochenschr.* **63,** 101.

Dorset, M., McBryde, C. N., and Niles, W. B. (1922). *J. Amer. Vet. Med. Ass.* **62,** 162.

Dowdle, W. R., Yarbrough, W. B., and Robinson, R. Q. (1964). *Pub. Health Rep.* **79,** 398.

Downie, J. C., and Laver, W. G. (1973). *Virology* **51,** 259.

Easterday, B. C. (1965). "Exposure of Calves and Pigs to Aerosols of Types A and B Influenza Viruses," Comm. Dis. Cent. Surveillance Rep. No. 5, p. 17. Center for Disease Control, Atlanta, Georgia.

Easterday, B. C. (1970). *In* "Diseases of Swine" (H. W. Dunne, ed.), 3rd ed., pp. 127–157. Iowa State Univ. Press, Ames.

Easterday, B. C., and Tumová, B. (1972a). *In* "Diseases of Poultry" (M. S. Hofstad *et al.,* eds.), 6th ed., pp. 670–700. Iowa State Univ. Press, Ames.

Easterday, B. C., and Tumová, B. (1972b). *Advan. Vet. Sci. Comp. Med.* **16,** 201.

Easterday, B. C., Trainer, D. O., Tumová, B., and Pereira, H. G. (1968). *Nature (London)* **219,** 523.

Fontaine, M., and Fontaine, M. P. (1973). *Proc. Int. Conf. Equine Infect. Dis., 3rd, 1972* pp. 487–502.

Frerichs, G. N., Burrows, R., and Frerichs, C. C. (1972). *Proc. Int. Conf. Equine Infect. Dis., 3rd, 1972* pp. 503–509.

Gardenier, A. A., (1900). "The Successful Stockman and Manual of Husbandry." King-Richardson Co., Springfield, Massachusetts.

Gerber, H. (1970). *Proc. Int. Conf. Equine Dis., 2nd, 1969* pp. 63–80.

Gorbunova, A. S., and Pysina, T. V. (1968). *Bull. W.H.O.* **39,** 271.

Harkness, J. W., Schild, G. C., Lamont, P. H., and Brand, C. M. (1972). *Bull. W.H.O.* **46,** 709.

Hayes, M. H. (1904). "Friedberger and Fröhner's Veterinary Pathology" (authorized translation). W. T. Keener & Co., Chicago, Illinois.

Heller, L., Espmark, A., and Viriden, P. (1956). *Arch. Gesamte Virusforsch.* **7,** 120.

Hodgins, J. E., and Haskett, T. H. (1901). "The Veterinary Science. The Anatomy, Diseases and Treatment of Domestic Animals." 31st ed. Veterinary Science Co., Detroit, Michigan.

Homme, P. J., and Easterday, B. C. (1970). *Avian Dis.* **14,** 278.

Homme, P. J., Easterday, B. C., and Anderson, D. P. (1970). *Avian Dis.* **14,** 240.

Hoyle, L. (1968). *Virol. Monogr.* **4,** 1.

Hwang, J., Lief, F. S., Miller, C. W., and Mallinson, E. T. (1970). *J. Amer. Vet. Med. Ass.* **157,** 2106.

Johnsen, D. O., Wooding, W. L., Tanticharoenyos, P., and Karnjanaprakorn, C. (1971). *J. Infec. Dis.* **123,** 365.

Jungherr, E. L., Tyzzer, E. E., Brandly, C. A., and Moses, H. E. (1946). *Amer. J. Vet. Res.* **7,** 250.

Kalter, S. S., Heberling, R. L., Vice, T. E., Lief, F. S., and Rodriguez, A. R. (1969). *Proc. Soc. Exp. Biol. Med.* **132,** 357.

Kasel, J. A., and Couch, R. B. (1969). *Bull. W.H.O.* **41,** 447.

Kasel, J. A., Byrne, R. J., and Havey, E. W. (1968). *Nature (London)* **219,** 968.

Kasel, J. A., Fulk, R. V., and Harvey, E. W. (1969). *J. Immunol.* **103,** 369.

Kelser, R. A. (1927). "Manual of Veterinary Bacteriology." Williams & Wilkins. Baltimore, Maryland.

Kleven, S. H., Nelson, R. C., Deshmukh, D. R., Moulthrop, J. I., and Pomeroy, B. S. (1970). *Avian Dis.* **14,** 153.

Kluska, V., Macku, M., and Menšik, J. (1961). *Czech. Pediat (Prague)* **16,** 408.

Kono, Y., Ishikawa, K., Fukunaga, Y., and Fujino, M. (1972). *Nat. Inst. Anim. Health Quart.* **12,** 183.

Koppel, Z., Vrtiak, J., Vasil, M., and St. Spiesz, Št. (1956). *Veterinarstvi* **6,** 267.

Kundin, W. D. (1970). *Nature (London)* **228,** 857.

Kundin, W. D., and Easterday, B. C. (1972). *Bull. W.H.O.* **47,** 489.

Lang, G., and Wills, C. G. (1965). *Arch. Gesamte Virusforsch.* **19,** 81.

Lang, G., Ferguson, A. E., Connell, M. C., and Wills, C. G. (1965). *Avian Dis.* **9,** 495.

Lang, G., Rouse, B. T., Narayan, O., Ferguson, A. E., and Connell, M. C. (1968a). *Can. Vet. J.* **9,** 22.

Lang, G., Narayan, O., Rouse, B. T., Ferguson, A. E., and Connell, M. C. (1968b). *Can. Vet. J.* **9,** 151.

Lang, G., Narayan, O., and Rouse, B. T. (1970). *Arch. Gesamte Virusforsch.* **32,** 171.

McBryde, C. N. (1927). *J. Amer. Vet. Med. Ass.* **71,** 368.

McKenzie, B. E., Easterday, B. C., and Will, J. A. (1972). *Amer. J. Pathol.* **69,** 239.

Mandelli, G., Rinaldi, A., Nardelli, L., Cervio, G., Cessi, D., and Valeri, A. (1968). *Proc. Soc. Ital. Sci. Vet. Grado* pp. 26–29.

Masurel, N. (1969). *Lancet* **1,** 907.

Menšik, J. (1960). *Ved. Pr. Vyzk. Ustavu Vet. CSAZV (Cesk. Akad. Zemed. Ved.) Brne* **1,** 99.

Menšik, J. (1962). *Ved. Pr. Vyzk. Ustavu Vet. Lek. Brne* **2,** 31.

Mitchell, C. A., Walker, R. V. L., and Bannister, G. L. (1953). *Can. J. Comp. Med.* **17,** 97.

Mitchell, C. A., Guerin, L. F., and Robillard, J. (1967). *Can. J. Comp. Med. Vet. Sci.* **31,** 103.

Nakamura, R. M. (1967). Ph.D. Thesis, University of Wisconsin, Madison.

Nakamura, R. M. (1972). *J. Infec. Dis.* **126,** 210.

Nakamura, R. M., Easterday, B. C., and Nicoletti, P. (1969). *J. Amer. Vet. Med. Ass.* **154,** 909.

Nakamura, R. M., Easterday, B. C., Pawlisch, R., and Walker, G. L. (1972). *Bull. W.H.O.* **47,** 481.

Narayan, O., Lang, G., and Rouse, B. T. (1969a). *Arch. Gesamte Virusforsch.* **26,** 149.

Narayan, O., Lang, G., and Rouse, B. T. (1969b). *Arch. Gesamte Virusforsch.* **26,** 166.

Narayan, O., Rouse, B. T., and Lang, G. (1970). *Can. J. Comp. Med.* **34,** 72.

Nayak, D. P., Kelly, G. W., and Underdahl, N. R. (1964). *Cornell Vet.* **54,** 160.

Nayak, D. P., Twiehaus, M. J., Kelley, G. W., and Underdahl, N. R. (1965). *Amer. J. Vet. Res.* **26**, 1271.

Nikitin, T., Cohen, D., Todd, J. D., and Lief, F. S. (1972). *Bull. W.H.O.* **47**, 471.

Olesiuk, O. M., Snoeyenbos, G. H., and Roberts, D. H. (1967). *Avian Dis.* **11**, 203.

Paniker, C. K. J., and Nair, C. M. G. (1970). *Bull. W.H.O.* **43**, 859.

Paniker, C. K. J., and Nair, C. M. G. (1972). *Bull. W.H.O.* **47**, 461.

Pereira, H. G., Tumová, B., and Law, V. G. (1965). *Bull. W.H.O.* **32**, 855.

Pereira, H. G., Takimoto, S., Piegas, N. S., and Ribeiro Do Valle, L. A. (1972). *Bull. W.H.O.* **47**, 465.

Pirtle, E. C. (1973). *Amer. J. Vet. Res.* **34**, 83.

Renshaw, H. W. (1970). M.S. Thesis, University of Wisconsin, Madison.

Rinaldi, A., Cervio, G., and Mandelli, G. (1965). *Estratto Selez. Vet.* **6**, 430.

Rinaldi, A., Cervio, G., and Mandelli, G. (1966a). *Boll. Ist. Sieroter. Milan.* **45**, 255.

Rinaldi, A., Cervio, G., and Mandelli, G. (1966b). *Estratto Selez. Vet.* **7**, 336.

Rinaldi, A., Nardelli, L., Pereira, H. G., Mandelli, G. C., Gandolfi, R., and Cervio, G. (1967a). *Atti Soc. Ital. Sci. Vet.* **21**, 867.

Rinaldi, A., Nardelli, L., Pereira, H. G., Mandelli, G. C., Cessi, D., and Cervio, G. (1967b). *Atti Soc. Ital. Sci. Vet.* **21**, 872.

Rinaldi, A., Nardelli, L., Pereira, H. G., Mandelli, G. C., Cervio, G., and Valeri, A. (1968). *Proc. Soc. Ital. Sci. Vet. Grado* pp. 26–29.

Roberts, D. H. (1964). *Vet. Rec.* **76**, 470.

Robinson, J. H. (1971). M. S. Thesis, University of Wisconsin, Madison.

Rott, R., and Schafer, W. (1960). *Zentralbl. Veterinermed.* **7**, 237.

Rouse, B. T., Lang, G., and Narayan, O. (1968). *J. Comp. Pathol. Ther.* **78**, 525.

Rowan, M. K. (1962). *Brit. Birds* **55**, 103.

Schafer, W. (1955). *Z. Naturforsch. B* **10**, 81.

Schild, G. C., and Stuart-Harris, C. H. (1965). *J. Hyg.* **63**, 479.

Schnurrenberger, P. R., Woods, G. T., and Martin, R. J. (1970). *Amer. Rev. Resp. Dis.* **102**, 356.

Scott, J. P. (1941). *Vet. Ext. Quart.* pp. 1–19.

Shope, R. E. (1931a). *J. Exp. Med.* **54**, 349.

Shope, R. E. (1931b). *J. Exp. Med.* **54**, 373.

Shope, R. E. (1941a). *J. Exp. Med.* **74**, 41.

Shope, R. E. (1941b). *J. Exp. Med.* **74**, 49.

Shope, R. E. (1943a). *J. Exp. Med.* **77**, 111.

Shope, R. E. (1943b). *J. Exp. Med.* **77**, 127.

Shope, R. E. (1955). *J. Exp. Med.* **102**, 567.

Slemons, R. D., and Easterday, B. C. (1972). *Bull. W.H.O.* **47**, 521.

Slemons, R. D., Cooper, R. S., and Orsborn, J. S. (1973). *Avian Dis.* **17**, 746.

Slemons, R. D., Johnson, D. C., Orsborn, J. S., and Hays, F. (1974). *Avian Dis.* **18**, 119.

Slepuskin, A. N., Pysina, T. V., Gonsovsky, F. K., Sazonov, A. A., Isachenko, V. A., Sokolova, N. N., Polivanov, V. M., Lvon, D. V., and Zakstel'skaja, L. Ja. (1972). *Bull. W.H.O.* **47**, 527.

Smith, W., Andrewes, C. H., and Laidlaw, P. P. (1933). *Lancet* **2**, 66.

Smithies, L. K., Radloff, D. B., Friedell, R. W., Albright, G. W., Misner, V. E., and Easterday, B. C. (1969a). *Avian Dis.* **13**, 603.

Smithies, L. K., Emerson, F. G., Robertson, S. M., and Ruedy, D. D. (1969b). *Avian Dis.* **13**, 606.

Sovinova, O., Tumova, B., Poustka, F. and Nemec, J. (1958). *Acta Virol. (Prague)* **2**, 52.

Stubbs, E. L. (1965). *In* "Diseases of Poultry" (H. E. Biester and L. H. Schwarte, eds.), 5th ed., pp. 813–822. Iowa State Univ. Press, Ames.

Styk, B., Sabó, A., Blaškovič, D., Masárová, P., Russ, G., and Hána, L. (1971a). *Acta Virol. (Prague)* **15**, 211.

Styk, B., Sabó, A., and Blaškovíč, D. (1971b). *Acta Virol. (Prague)* **15**, 221.

Tanyi, J. (1972). *Acta Vet. (Budapest)* **22**, 125.

Todd, J. D., and Cohen, D. (1968). *Amer. J. Epidemiol.* **87**, 426.

Tumová, B., Easterday, B. C., and Stumpa, A. (1972). *Amer. J. Epidemiol.* **95**, 80.

Urman, H. K., Underdahl, N. R., and Young, G. A. (1958). *Amer. J. Vet. Res.* **19**, 913.

Uys, C. J., and Becker, W. B. (1967). *J. Comp. Pathol. Ther.* **77**, 167.

Van Es, L. (1932). "The Principles of Animal Hygiene and Preventive Veterinary Medicine." Wiley, New York.

Waddell, G. H., Teigland, M. B., and Sigel, M. M. (1963). *J. Amer. Vet. Med. Ass.* **143**, 587.

Walker, G. L. (1971). M. S. Thesis, University of Wisconsin, Madison.

Walker, R. V. L., and Bannister, G. L. (1953). *Can. J. Comp. Med. Vet. Sci.* **17**, 248.

Wells, R. J. H. (1963). *Vet. Rec.* **75**, 783.

Winkler, W. G., Trainer, D. O., and Easterday, B. C. (1972). *Bull. W.H.O.* **47**, 507.

Woods, G. T., and Simpson, A. (1964). *Vet. Med. & Small Anim. Clin.* **59**, 303.

World Health Organization. (1971). *Bull. W.H.O.* **45**, 119.

Youatt, W. (1843). "The Horse." Porter & Coates, Philadelphia, Pennsylvania.

Young, G. A., and Underdahl, N. A. (1949a). *Cornell Vet.* **39**, 105.

Young, G. A., and Underdahl, N. A. (1949b). *Cornell Vet.* **39**, 120.

Young, G. A., and Underdahl, N. A. (1950a). *Cornell Vet.* **40**, 24.

Young, G. A., and Underdahl, N. A. (1950b). *Cornell Vet.* **40**, 201.

Zakstel'skaja, L. Ja., Isachenko, V. A., Osidze, N. G., Timofeeva, C. C., Slepuskin, A. N., and Sokolova, N. N. (1972). *Bull. W.H.O.* **47**, 497.

Zhezmer, V. Y., Lvov, D. K., Isachenko, V. A., and Zakstelskaja, L. Ja. (1973). *Vop. Virusol.* **1**, 94.

15

Epidemiology of Influenza

E. D. Kilbourne

I. Introduction

The epidemiology of viral infections, and particularly that of influenza, is determined and influenced by the triad of virus, host, and environment and by the interactions of these virtually inseparable components. Therefore, it is appropriate that the epidemiology of influenza, which less anthropocentrically can be viewed as the natural history of the virus, is considered in this last chapter in this book after extensive analyses in preceding chapters of viral replication and genetics and the disease that results from virus–host interaction.

The initial interaction between virus and host target cell is subject to influence from both external and internal (host) environments, and infection may in fact be inhibited at this step. If infection is established, then subsequent environmental influences can still affect the host, or more properly the virus–host complex, to modulate the progress or outcome of infection

483

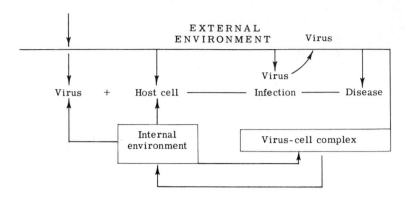

Fig. 15.1. Interrelationships of virus, host target cell, and internal and external environments in infection

(Fig. 15.1). One frequent, but not inevitable, outcome is the progression of infection to disease. In a multicellular host, cells and virus-susceptible tissues comprise in totality an internal environment in which specific and nonspecific immune factors may be elaborated that may favorably or unfavorably affect the outcome of infection. The virus-infected cell complex can also use this internal environment to stimulate antibody- or interferon-forming cells, or, perhaps, to damage them through products of cells altered by virus replication, or to influence the effect of external virus. In productive infections, a final step essential for virus survival is release of virus into the external environment. All of these factors will be considered in the following analysis of the epidemiology of influenza viruses.

No discussion of antigenic variation (Chapter 10), immunity (Chapter 12), the disease in man or animals (Chapters 8 and 10), or diagnostic serology (Chapter 11) can be divorced from epidemiological implications. Epidemiology, therefore, permeates this book, and this chapter rests heavily upon its predecessors and represents a synthesis and summary related to them in part. It must also be clear (Chapter 1) that influenza is unique among human diseases in the antigenic variability of its infective agent. This cardinal attribute of the virus has resulted in the persistence of the disease into modern times as the last great unconquered plague (Kilbourne, 1963).

Epidemiology, based as it is on correlative data and on the outcome of complex interactions among host, virus, and environment, is an inexact science, and therefore admits of differences in interpretation. When to inexactitude is added ignorance of basic facts—as is the case with influenza—then the partially speculative and hypothetical nature of this chapter is explained, and perhaps forgiven. Again, the peculiar importance of understanding the molecular biology of the virus itself will be emphasized. Clearly, the shifting balance of virus and host is most reasonably viewed as virus rather than host determined, because the virus changes demonstrably and frequently and man relatively little (Kilbourne, 1973a), although environment may be critical at times in influencing epidemicity.

II. History

The modern history of influenza began in 1933 with the isolation of influenza A virus from man by Smith *et al.* (1933). The immediately antecedent demonstration by Shope of a similar virus in swine (Shope, 1931) was another landmark, and in retrospect probably represented the indirect, postponed isolation of the human virus responsible for the pandemic of 1918–1919. The relevance of the much earlier recovery of an influenza A virus from poultry in 1901 (then known as fowl plague virus) has been appreciated only recently with a revival of interest in animal influenza (Pereira *et al.,* 1965; and Chapter 10).

With the viruses, in hand, as antigens, interesting ventures in retrospective seroarchaeology have been conducted by study of antibody distribution in different age groups of the population. In this way, the prevalence in humans alive in 1918 of antibodies to swine influenza virus has suggested the common identity of the swine virus of the present with the human virus of the past. Human longevity has also permitted a glimpse of the nineteenth century by demonstrating that the "new" Asian (H2N2) virus of 1957, or an antigenically related virus, may have been circulating in 1889–1890 (Mulder and Masurel, 1958). The presence of antibodies to the virus of equine/2 subtype in very old people adds fuel to the fires of speculation on the possible animal origin of human influenza viruses.

Before the possibility of specific etiological studies, the definition of influenza was dependent entirely upon epidemiological and clinical data. However, the disease as described in the past is so strikingly similar to that of modern times, in both its epidemic and clinical characteristics, that it is only reasonable to ascribe a causal relationship of virus biologically similar to contemporary influenza viruses to the epidemics of the past. This viewpoint seems even more valid now that it has been clearly established (notably in 1957 and 1968) that a contemporary influenza virus might cause pandemic disease.

The uniquely virulent nature of the 1918 pandemic appears to set it apart from those later epidemics demonstrably associated with influenza A viruses. Consequently, it has been postulated that the virus must have been quite different and perhaps unrelated to present day influenza viruses. However, the typical case of disease in 1918 differed not at all from typical cases described in all other recorded epidemics (Burnet and Clark, 1942, p. 88; Kilbourne, 1960), and the high case fatality rate is credibly explained on the basis of secondary bacterial infection (Kilbourne, 1960).

The historical approach to the study of disease has its limitations, and one can easily misread the past. Suffice it to say that influenza as we now know it was described as long ago as 1510 (Francis and Maassab, 1965), although the pandemic of 1889 may have marked the beginning of a "new and more vigorous development of the disease than had ever previously been recorded" (Creighton, 1894, cited by Burnet and Clark, 1942). The scholarly reviews of Creighton (1894), Vaughan (1921), Jordan (1927), Burnet and Clark (1942), Francis (1958), and Francis and Maassab (1965) are available for those interested in the details of past epidemics. An anecdotal but interesting account of the impact of the 1918 pandemic on the United States has been written for the layman by Hoehling (1961).

III. Influenza A, B, and C—An Epidemiological Comparison

Unless qualified, virtually everything written about influenza refers implicitly to the disease associated with influenza A virus. This is understandable in view of the considerably greater importance of influenza A viruses in human disease, their exclusive role in animal disease, and the far more intensive study of the viruses of the influenza A type that have been carried out. The taxonomy and comparative biology of influenza A, B, and C and their causative viruses have been assessed in Chapter 1 (summarized in Table 1.3) and will not be repeated here except in relation to their comparative epidemiology. Influenza A stands apart from influenza B and C in its occurrence in pandemic as well as interpandemic epidemic and endemic phases. No nonhuman natural hosts for influenza B and C viruses have been identified, although both viruses are capable of infecting subhuman species.

A. Intrinsic Viral Virulence

Most evidence points to a rank order of virulence of influenza A, B, and C viruses that coincides with the alphabetical order of their type designations. Influenza A is more often associated with primary influenza viral pneumonia and fatal infections in adults, and more severe disease attends infantile and childhood infections with influenza A viruses (F. Denny, A. Monto, and J. Chin, in Fox and Kilbourne, 1973, Influenza Workshop IV). Although influenza A and B occurred with equal frequency at the Children's Hospital in Washington, D.C. (Brandt, in Fox and Kilbourne, 1973, Influenza Workshop IV), influenza A virus was isolated from 4% of patients ill enough to require hospitalization, and influenza B virus from 1%.

Nevertheless, comparisons of intrinsic viral virulence are fraught with difficulty because few populations are immunologically virgin with respect to experience with any of the influenza viruses, so that less severe disease may reflect relatively greater specific host resistance rather than decreased virulence of the infecting virus.

The fact that influenza B and C viruses are subject to less extensive antigenic variation than those of type A provides them with less opportunity to confront immunologically inexperienced populations; therefore, most infections observed are probably modified in part by preexisting specific antibody. A notable exception was a study of Eskimo children (Maynard *et al.*, 1967), most of whom were devoid of antibody to either influenza A (A/Taiwan/1/64) or influenza B (B/Alaska/1/66) viruses and in whom influenza A and B occurred simultaneously. In patients infected with influenza A virus alone, 75% had signs of lower respiratory tract disease as indicated by rales and tracheobronchitis, while only 20% of influenza B patients were so affected. When coincident epidemics of A and B occur (reviewed by Kilbourne *et al.*, 1951), the ratio of influenza A to influenza B infections is 2:1 or 3:1. However, these data do not necessarily bear on relative virulence per se, but rather on such factors as *transmissibility,* a separate viral property that will be discussed subsequently.

The special question of virulence of pandemic viruses will be discussed in Section IV,A,4,a. It will be noted here, however, that unless individual case fatalities or case severity are considered, extremes of virus severity will be more liable to come to attention during widespread outbreaks, even if their *rate* of occurrence is low.

If experimental host range and replication at higher temperature are measures of virulence, then by these criteria, also, influenza A virus is most virulent, and influenza C virus least virulent (see Table 1.3, Chapter 1).

B. Relative Prevalence

As sampling and surveillance techniques have improved, it has become clearer that influenza A and B infections occur in every month of every year, whether or not such years are identified as "epidemic" on the basis of overt outbreaks of disease. It is especially pertinent that serological conversions and viral isolations attesting to this phenomenon have been demonstrated in free living populations under natural conditions (Dingle *et al.,* 1964; W. R. Dowdle, personal communication).

Epidemic prevalence of both influenza A and B appears to be related to an immediately prior decline in population antibody levels, or more specifically to an increase in the percent of those in the population experiencing significant (fourfold or greater) decline in serum antibody to either influenza A or B virus (Dingle *et al.,* 1964; Hayslett *et al.,* 1962) (Fig. 15.2). The biennial periodicity of influenza A and a less frequent recurrence of influenza B are not invariable in their patterns, but do seem to define adequately the epidemicity of influenza A and B on a regional basis in industrialized societies (Fig. 15.3).

Because the clinical attack rate of influenza B may be as high as 75% in institutional populations (Moffet *et al.,* 1962) and parallels A infection rates in children with respiratory disease (Brandt, in Fox and Kilbourne, 1973, Influenza Workshop IV), the lesser frequency of influenza B seems not to reflect lesser infection rates of the population, but more probably is a consequence of viral antigenic variation of lesser frequency and magnitude. Even so, a 3 year study of families in a "virus watch" program in Seattle disclosed a reinfection rate of 52% for influenza B and only 36% for influenza A, but viral isolation techniques for influenza A were "insensitive" (Hall *et al.,* 1973).

Although infection with influenza C virus must be highly prevalent as determined by serological surveys (Minuse *et al.,* 1954; Taylor, 1951) and

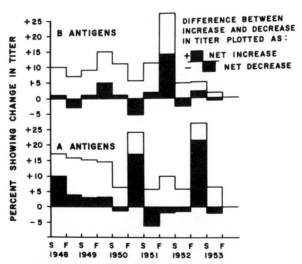

Fig. 15.2. Influenza "antibody balance." Changes in antibody titer during consecutive 6-month intervals plotted to show net percentage of individuals who showed fourfold or greater increases or decreases in titer. (From Dingle *et al.,* 1964.)

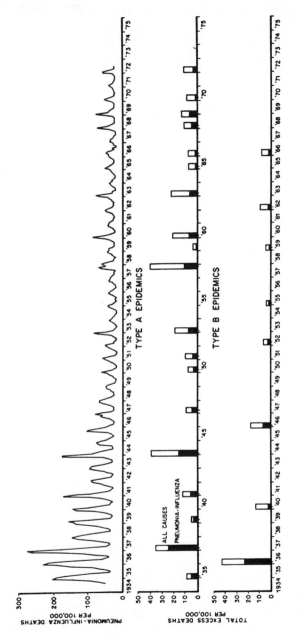

Fig. 15.3. Pneumonia–influenza death rates by month and excess mortality during epidemic periods, United States, 1934–1972. (Influenza-Respiratory Disease Surveillance. U.S. Department of Health, Education and Welfare, Public Health Service, Report No. 88. Center for Disease Control, 1973, p. 8.)

antibodies to influenza C are found in all age groups except young children (Hilleman *et al.,* 1953), epidemic disease clearly and unequivocally associated with influenza C virus has rarely been identified. The concordance of influenza C with influenza A (Taylor, 1951; Francis *et al.,* 1950) or with influenza B (DeMeio *et al.,* 1955) has further confounded evaluation of the role of this virus in human disease. While in military populations influenza B outbreaks were of 3 to 4 weeks in duration, the isolation of influenza C viruses before, during, and after these influenza B epidemics extended over a period of 17 weeks (DeMeio *et al.,* 1955), suggesting a more endemic relationship to the population. The failure to produce febrile disease with the virus in adult women subjected to experimental inoculation probably reflects the presence of preexisting antibody in these subjects (Quilligan *et al.,* 1954), and leaves unanswered the pathogenic potential of the virus in the immunologically virgin adult. Influenza C accounts for less than 1% of acute respiratory disease in children (Hilleman *et al.,* 1962) and less than 2% of such illnesses in young adults (Mogabgab, 1963).

C. Ecological Relationships of Influenza A, B, and C Viruses

Although influenza A variants appear to contest with one another for survival in the human respiratory tract, so that only a single antigenic subtype predominates at any one time in the human population, the survival of such variants appears little affected by the contemporaneous presence in man of the two antigenically heterologous viruses of influenza B and C. Indeed, as mentioned above, coincident epidemics of A and B, A and C, or B and C are not uncommon, and it is probable that dual infection of the same individual can occur simultaneously (evidence reviewed by Kilbourne *et al.,* 1951). Simultaneous infection of hamsters with influenza A and B virus can be achieved experimentally, with viral interference being manifested only by a decrease in the antibody response to each agent compared to the response observed with single infections (Kilbourne *et al.,* 1951).

It can be inferred that those environmental conditions that foster the transmission of one virus type similarly affect circulation of the others, and that on occasion such conditions override the possible mutual interference of viruses competing for the same target cells, and probably for the same cell receptors (see Chapter 3).

The mystery of influenza A virus' precarious existence in man (at least without major alteration) must be addressed in the light of the capacity of influenza B and C to "make a go of it" without recourse to chameleonlike changes of great magnitude.

IV. Influenza A: Pandemic, Epidemic, and Endemic Disease

Influenza A, caused by virus of any given subtype, can occur in pandemic (worldwide), epidemic (regionally restricted) or endemic form. In overt community epidemics, the disease is easily recognized by its explosive nature (especially in institutional or semi-closed populations) and by its characteristic but not pathognomonic clinical picture of acute prostrating but briefly sustained febrile disease, in which aching and systemic symptomology are disproportionate to the moderate respiratory signs. When such cases are encountered en masse, there can be no doubt about the diagnosis. In this situation, almost every febrile respiratory disease in the adult can be assumed to be influenza. In individual sporadic cases, the disease is not easily distinguished from other infections of the upper and middle respiratory tract, adenovirus infection, parainfluenza, or streptococcal pharyngitis in adults and these and respiratory syncytial virus infections in children. Indeed, the frequent confusion of diagnosis in nonepidemic periods led to over-reporting of "influenza," and therefore, important as the disease is, it is no longer reportable in most countries, including the United States. Accurate records of morbidity, therefore, are not available, so that the impact and prevalence of the disease must be assessed by sampling of the population by questionnaires and serological studies. The predictable influence of influenza on excess (pneumonia-associated) mortality makes such excess mortality a valuable indicator of the presence of influenza in the community. Analysis of excess mortality rates has been the principal surveillance method used by the United States Public Health Service for the detection of influenza in recent years. (See Section IV,A,4, and IV,D for further discussion of mortality and methods of surveillance.)

Although the virus is subject to demonstrable mutation throughout the period of its prevalence, the evidence is persuasive that variations in epidemic pattern from pandemic to endemic are determined essentially by the immunological status of the population rather than by a progressive attenuation of virulence of the virus after its initial pandemic introduction.

A. Pandemic Influenza

With the control of the other great plagues of man (plague, cholera, yellow fever, smallpox) by environmental sanitation and vaccination, pandemic influenza remains as an embarassing anachronism in this last quarter of the 20th Century. If the battle has not yet been won, it is chiefly because the nature of the enemy is constantly changing. The magnitude of periodic antigenic change or shift in the virus has been described (Chapters 1, 10, and

12). Uniquely among infectious agents, the influenza virus can change sufficiently to circumvent immunity previously acquired by contact of the human host with antecedent influenza A viruses. Whether or not it is proper to speak of newly introduced pandemic viral subtypes as "changed" depends on whether they are viewed as direct lineal descendants of the immediately preceding subtype, or whether in fact they represent new viruses—either truly novel or new to man. All influenza A viruses are identified as such through the commonality of their internal antigens (Chapters 2 and 11). But antibodies to these polypeptides do not participate in immune reactions. Extreme variation in the antigenic nature of the external glycoproteins (hemagglutinin and neuraminidase) through which host immune reactions are mediated is sufficient for the creation of an effectively "new" virus that is not significantly neutralized by antibody to earlier human subtypes.

The association of different subtypes with pandemics in the twentieth century is sketched in Fig. 15.4. Only the introductions of virus in 1946, 1957, and 1968 have been studied during the period of modern virology. There-

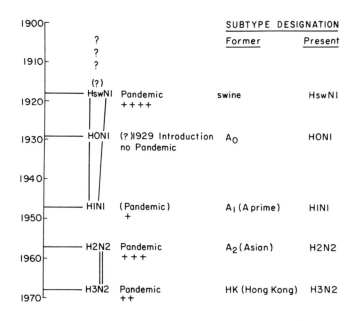

Fig. 15.4. Chronology of major influenza A virus subtype changes in the 20th century, showing old and new terminology. Antigenic relatedness is shown by single connecting lines, close relationship by double vertical lines. Approximated severity of pandemics is indicated by +, mild, to ++++, severe, scale. From Kilbourne (1973a). *J. Infec. Dis.* **127,** 478–487. Copyright 1973, The University of Chicago Press. Reproduced by permission.

fore, the time of introduction of the H0N1 subtype is speculative, and the association of a virus antigenically similar to the present day swine influenza virus with the 1918 pandemic has been inferred from retrospective serological studies. It will be seen that the minimal requirement for the generation of a pandemic seems to be major change in the H (hemagglutinin) antigen, although in 1957 both external antigens, H and N (neuraminidase), changed markedly (H1N1 to H2N2). The severity of the 1957 epidemic compared to the less dramatic global dissemination of virus in 1946–1947, and the somewhat lesser impact of the Hong Kong (H3N2) virus in 1968, may reflect this fact (Table 15.1). The magnitude of antigenic differences of the H2 (1957) and H3 (1968) hemagglutinins is defined in the summary of plaque neutralization tests shown in Table 15.2. The test viruses employed were recombinants containing only the H antigens in common so that the results are not influenced by cross-reactions through the common (N2) neuraminidase antigen of the subtypes.

Since 1946, pandemics associated with appearance of new influenza A virus subtypes have occurred at approximately decennial (actually 11 year) intervals, a pattern apparently at variance with the 28–29 year intervals marking the immediately preceding pandemics of 1889 and 1918 (see Table 15.3). The best records available are from mortality statistics of the United

Table 15.1 Antigenic Variation and Pandemic Severity[a]

Year	Virus[b]	Change[c]	Extent of change	Result
1918	HswN1	?	?	Pandemic (severe)
1928	H0 N1	H	++	(?) Pandemic
		N	+	(?) Year of H0N1 introduction
1946	H1 N1	H	++	Pandemic (mild)
		N	+	
1957	H2 N2	H	+++	Pandemic (severe)
		N	+++	
1968	H3 N2	H	+++	Pandemic (moderate)
		N	0	

[a] Modified from Kilbourne (1973a). *J. Infec. Dis.* **127**, 478–487. Copyright 1973, University of Chicago Press. Reproduced by permission.

[b] Single vertical lines indicate slight antigenic relatedness. Double vertical lines indicate close antigenic similarity. Dashed lines indicate relatedness only through anamnestic response.

[c] H, hemagglutinin; N, neuraminidase.

Table 15.2 Magnitude of Antigenic Differences (in Hemagglutinins) of Major (Pandemic) and Minor (Interpandemic) Mutants in Plaque Neutralization Tests[a]

	Virus		
Antiserum	H2(57)N1	H2(67)N1	H3(68)N1
H2N2(57)	10,240[b]	2,560	<10
H2N2(67)	320	10,240	<10
H3N2	<10	<10	5,120

[a] Homotypic titers are underlined.

[b] Highest dilution of antiserum causing 50% reduction in plaque number.

Table 15.3 Periods of Possible Pandemic Occurrence of Influenza in Recent History

Date	Unquestioned pandemic	Pandemic interval (years)	Major epidemic interval (years)
1847			
1855			8
1875			20
1889	+		14
1900			11
1918	+	29	18
1929			11
1946	+	28	17
1957	+	11	11
1968	+	11	11

[a] Including undisputed pandemics of and major (possible pandemic) outbreaks with high excess mortality. For example, the mortality in England and Wales and in Victoria in 1899–1900 was almost as high as observed with 1889–1891 pandemic [League of Nations' data cited by Burnet and Clark (1942)]. Thirty "pandemics" occurred between 1510 and 1930; the mean interpandemic interval for this period is 14 years [data from Francis and Maassab (1965), interpretation the author's].

Kingdom, United States, and League of Nations epidemiological reports. In the absence of the direct etiological studies possible since isolation of influenza A virus in the early 1930's, excess mortality rates and the limited application of seroarchaeology (*vide supra*) are the blunt instruments available for dissection of the past. If to the undisputed pandemics are added major epidemics (with excessive mortality), then a less striking divergence of "pandemic" periodicity from that recently noted is revealed (Table 15.3, last column). Indeed, if the major epidemics of 1900–1929 are considered to be evidence of introduction of new viral subtypes, then the "magic figure," 11, appears once again. Perhaps testing of the sera from human subjects alive during these epidemics with antigens of various animal influenza A viruses may reveal age-related clusters that will answer this important question concerning the "dark" period. These meager data should not be over interpreted. However, if 1899–1900 and 1928–1929 were, in fact, associated with pandemic distribution of virus, then it is striking that they occurred 11 years after the explosive pandemics of 1889 and 1918, respectively, possibly reflecting the more rapid saturation of the population with virus and a faster exhaustion of susceptibles in those great epidemics.

Dependent as influenza is upon direct dissemination from man to man, the rapidity of its spread cannot exceed the speed of human travel and communication, a conclusion first reached by Parsons concerning the pandemic of 1889 (Parsons, cited by Burnet and Clark, 1942).

If approximately decennial periodicity (Figure 15.5) is indeed a phenomenon of recent origin, it may well reflect the growth of commercial aviation and the greater population mobility of the post-World War II period. The present 11 year cycle may represent a plateau following attainment of the maximal feasible dissemination of virus in the human population contingent upon seeding of virus through jet travel. While passenger kilometers flown reached no more than 2,030,000,000 in the 1930's, this figure had increased almost tenfold by 1947, then fourfold more by 1957, and a further fourfold by 1968 (International Civil Aviation Organization, personal communication).

A scheme of the behavior of recent pandemics in relation to major viral antigenic shifts and the subsequent development by the human population of specific antibody is shown in Figure 15.5. At the time of introduction of the hypothetical "A2" variant, the population is immunologically virgin with respect to the new subtype, so that infection of all age groups occurs. Within a 2 year period most of the population throughout the world will have been infected in initial pandemic waves. Predictions concerning the "next pandemic" rest on the flimsy structure of a series of two instances of decennial prevalence (1946–1957 and 1957–1968). The lesser frequency of overt pandemics in the period 1918–1946 may be related to the damping

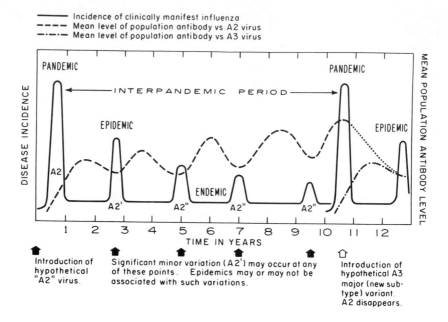

Fig. 15.5. The pattern of influenza pandemics in recent years. Since 1947 an 11 year cycle has recurred. This figure illustrates schematically the relationship between the magnitude of interpandemic epidemics that occur with biennial or triennial frequency and the progressive increase in population antibody specific for the new viral subtype. Hypothetical virus "A2" apparently cannot continue to survive in a population in which most members are specifically immune. At the end of the decade virus "A2" disappears and is replaced by "A3" and the cycle is repeated. Minor antigenic variation of the viruses occurs during each decade, and may be necessary for the virus to survive even 10–11 years.

effect of shared antigenicity of HswN2, H0N1 and H1N1 viruses as a "family" of strains distinct from the later H2N2 and H3N2 viruses (Morita *et al.*, 1972). Although the common neuraminidase (N2) antigen of these latter viruses clearly was insufficient to forestall a pandemic caused by H3N2 virus in 1968, the cumulative effect of its persistence may alter pandemicity in the future.

1. The Disappearance of Influenza A Viral Subtypes from the Human Population

No less remarkable than the sudden appearance of major antigenic variance of influenza A virus as a concomitant of pandemic disease is the seemingly simultaneous disappearance of the antecedent virus from natural circulation. This is all the more remarkable because of the retention and preservation of potentially infective influenza A subtypes of the past in virological and diagnostic laboratories. However, because most such strains are adapted to experimental host systems and at least partially deadapted to man they are improbable sources of epidemics (Kilbourne, 1974). Of course, it is extremely unlikely that all infections with the antecedent virus are halted simultaneously. Indeed, 3 years after introduction of the H2N2 subtype in 1957, WHO epidemiological reports mentioned occasional recoveries in the United States of H1N1 strains. None of these isolations, however, was accomplished under circumstances in which laboratory contamination with H1N1 virus could be excluded (R. Q. Robinson, cited by Isaacs *et al.*, 1962). However, the infection with H1N1 virus of a young English soldier in 1960 appears to have been valid (Issacs *et al.*, 1962), and an H0N1 strain was isolated in 1949 in Alaska 3 years after the beginning of the H1N1 (1946–1957) period (van Rooyen *et al.*, 1949). Evidence of activity of the H2N2 subtype 2 years after appearance of the H3N2 (Hong Kong) virus was demonstrated serologically in isolated Amazonian Indians (Napiorkowski and Black, 1974). Undoubtedly, late in a decade of prevalence a higher proportion of infections are subclinical and recoverability of virus diminishes with increasing antibody in the members of the population. Furthermore, serological documentation of such infections is hampered by the increasing difficulty of demonstrating increases in antibody concentration with higher initial antibody levels (Hirst *et al.*, 1942; Kilbourne *et al.*, 1951). Also, it is clear that surveillance is limited and primarily keyed to the occurrence of overt disease, so that, in part, the "disappearance" of virus reflects its drop below the threshold of contemporary surveillance methods. On the other hand, the fact that the immediately antecedent strain does not *reappear* when circulation of its successor is waning and new susceptibles have been born is evidence for its complete disappearance within a few years of the appearance of the new strain.

2. THE INTRODUCTION OF NEW PANDEMIC STRAINS

Only during the last three pandemic episodes of influenza have the techniques been available to detect the occurrence of major viral antigenic variation apparently characteristic of such episodes. In each of these three instances, new major variants were first isolated in the Far East, and subsequently were found in association with sporadic scattered disease throughout all continents within a 1 year period. The introduction of virus of the 1918 pandemic cannot be similarly documented because only the severity of disease and the occurrence of unusually high mortality in young adults serve as markers. On this basis, influenza of "high virulence" seems to have occurred first on the west coast of Africa (Sierra Leone) in August

1918 and emerged to general notice in the autumn epidemics of that year in all parts of Europe—probably earliest in Spain. However, a severe epidemic had occurred in Chung King in July, suggesting the possibility that "a strain of Asiatic origin reaching France with Chinese laborers or otherwise was responsible for the new type of disease which became visible in May and June" (Burnet and Clark, 1942). The origin of the pandemic of 1889 in central Asia seems undisputed (Burnet and Clark, 1942; Finkler, 1898; Shope, 1958).

Early Seeding of Virus. The data of the previrology pandemics must remain ambiguous because of our inability to distinguish retrospectively between the scattered mild epidemics that characterize the demise of an antigenic subtype and the equally sporadic outbreaks that may occur in the initial period of pandemic introduction of virus if we may draw such inference from recent studies.

Careful virological and serological studies in 1957 and 1968 leave no doubt that pandemic influenza smolders before it bursts into flame. Global dissemination of H2N2 (Asian) influenza virus occurred within 10 months (Fig. 15.6) of its recognition in mainland China (Tang and Liang, 1957), and within 4 months of its introduction the virus had spread throughout the United States (Fig. 15.7). This rapid spread of virus was attended by variable clinical attack rates of 7 to 70%, depending upon the nature of the population and the location of the epidemic in the Southern or Northern Hemisphere [author's interpretation of Dunn's (1958) data]. The occurrence of second waves of epidemics in Asia in September 1957 and in the United Kingdom and the United States in early 1958 (Dowdle *et al.*, 1974) attested to the continued existence of many susceptibles in the population after the initial epidemic introduction of virus. Such closely spaced secondary waves of influenza were observed also in 1889–1890 and 1918–1919 and regionally in 1947–1948 (Meiklejohn and Bruyn, 1949) and are probably characteristic of pandemics (Langmuir, 1961). Serological examinations in Japan demonstrated that about 20% (4.6–38.2%) of health workers had antibody to H2N2 virus after the first epidemic wave, and about 45% (25.7–61.8%) following the second wave (Fukumi, 1961). This experience was typical of other populous areas. It is significant that after the introduction and multiple seedings of the virus in the United States in the summer of 1957, outbreaks were consistently limited to situations in which large numbers of people were crowded together (Langmuir, 1958).

Again in 1968 the Hong Kong (H3N2) virus, after an initial large outbreak in Hong Kong, was rapidly disseminated throughout most of the world. However, a slower kindling to large epidemics was noted than had characterized the first year of H2N2 virus introduction. Cockburn *et al.*

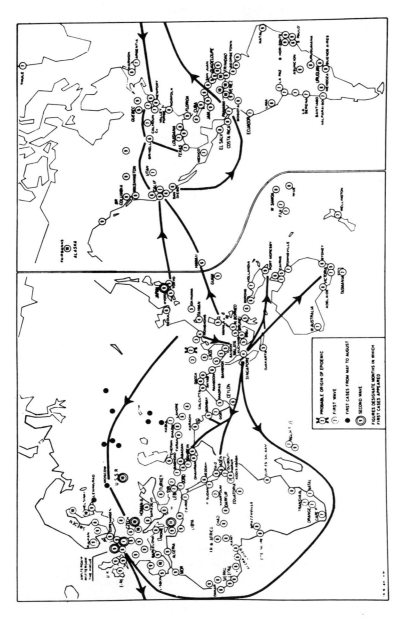

Fig. 15.6. Progress of Asian (H2N2) influenza pandemic, February 1957 to January 1958 From Langmuir (1961).

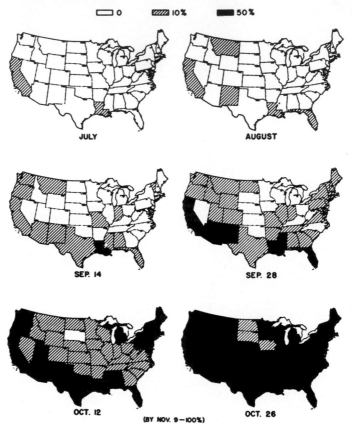

Fig. 15.7. Progressive seeding of the United States with Asian (H2N2) influenza virus in summer-fall of 1957. Percentage of counties reporting influenza outbreaks, July–October 1957. From Trotter *et al.* (1959).

(1969) have pointed out that (1) in Japan the disease failed to spread in August and September despite numerous introductions of virus by travelers, (2) in epidemics in northern and eastern Europe the disease was reported to be mild, and (3) in the Southern Hemisphere no large outbreaks were reported in 1968. The United States appeared to be an exception to the rest of the world in that an epidemic peak associated with significant excess mortality was seen at the end of the year (1968) (Cockburn *et al.,* 1969). Furthermore, in carefully studied populations (e.g., in Seattle), the first viral isolations were made in September without recognized secondary cases at that time; disease reappeared in November in school children, and there were subsequent major attacks in December and January (Fox, in Fox and Kilbourne, 1973, Influenza Workshop IV).

Of special interest was the great variability of transmission and attack rates within very small or isolated populations. The initial introduction of H3N2 virus into the Outer Hebrides in 1969 by foreign fishing vessels resulted in highest morbidity in 31- to 40-year-old persons (presumably those first infected), although 44% of the households were affected (Buchan and Reid, 1972). Feldman (in Fox and Kilbourne, 1973, Influenza Workshop IV) has stressed the apparent randomness of occurrence of influenza in families under serological studies in 1968. While in 3 families all members (15 out of 16) were infected with influenza, in 15 families with a total of 85 persons, only 15% acquired specific antibody. In 9 families comprising 43 individuals, none showed evidence of infection. Nevertheless, the impression in the community was that "everyone was sick." Indolent intrafamilial spread of influenza was also seen in 1957 (Jordan, 1961). The possible existence of transmitters of varying ability to spread virus is discussed in Sections IV,A,4,b and IV,C,3.

3. Factors Affecting Morbidity (Clinical Attack Rates) in Various Pandemics

The evidence summarized thus far appears to indicate no marked differences in initial infection (serological conversion) rates in the first years of recent pandemics. From the least dramatic pandemic of 1946–1947, adequate data are not available for precise comparison with the 1957 and 1968 experiences. However, in carefully studied populations, an unusual incidence of influenza was clearly evident (Brown et al., 1958; Meiklejohn and Bruyn, 1949), although excess mortality did not approach the earlier nonpandemic year of 1943–1944 (Collins, 1957), an observation possibly related to the occurrence of the 1947 epidemic unusually late in the winter season (Sartwell and Long, 1948). As emphasized earlier, significant differences in symptomatology of the "average" case have not been observed in comparisons of pandemics, or even of cases of interpandemic disease, although illness in a spectrum from asymptomatic to fatal infection occurred. On the basis of differences in their medical and economic impact, the pandemics of 1946–1947 and of 1957 can be characterized, respectively, as mild and severe; yet clinical profiles of disease in these pandemics were virtually indistinguishable (Table 13.1, Chapter 13). On this basis, the ratio of symptomatic to asymptomatic infection may provide a measure of comparative morbidity (Kilbourne, 1960). Unfortunately, this type of assessment requires the prospective study of comparable large populations with intensive serological and clinical surveillance, and satisfactory data are not available. The proved occurrence of asymptomatic infections, even with initial introductions of pandemic virus in the severe modern pandemic of 1957 (Blumenfeld et al., 1959; Jensen et al., 1958; Stallones and Lennette, 1959), affirms that pandemic viral virulence can be nonspecifically host determined. (The importance of host factors in the conversion of infection to severe or fatal disease is discussed in Section IV,A,4,b.

The antigenic relatedness of the pandemic virus to its predecessor is also important in the expression of viral virulence and morbidity. Evidence for the close antigenic relationship of influenza A virus subtypes through both hemagglutinin (H) and neuraminidase (N) antigens in the 1918–1946 period has been cited (above and in Chapter 10) and is illustrated in Table 15.1 and Fig. 15.4. The relationship of H2N2 and H3N2 subtypes to the earlier viruses is demonstrated less readily and is not shown by every serological test. Thus, H1N1 virus, appearing at the end of the 1918–1946 period, may have been damped in its effect to the extent that it was antigenically less different, while the severe effects of H2N2 virus may well reflect its greater dissimilarity from preceding viruses (Kilbourne, 1973a).

A further nuance of antigenic variation of pandemic viruses was demonstrated in 1968 with the appearance of the Hong Kong (H3N2) subtype, in which major change was confined to the hemagglutinin antigen. Evidence from experimental infection in animals pointed to a significant role of anti-neuraminidase antibody in the mediation of immunity (Schulman et al., 1968). Following the demonstration of specific anti-neuraminidase antibody production in man following natural infection (Kilbourne et al., 1968), evidence for its protective effect in human disease was found in experimental infection (Murphy et al., 1972b). Seroepidemiologic studies have suggested a role for anti-neuraminidase antibody in the prevention or modification of natural infection (see also Chapter 12; Slepushkin et al., 1971; Monto and Kendal, 1973).

There seems to be general agreement that the initial impact of the Hong Kong (H3N2) pandemic was less than that of the H2N2 virus pandemic of 1957 (Cockburn et al., 1969; Fukumi, 1969; Zachary and Johnson, 1969; Vicente, 1969; Gear, 1969), although the rates of viral seeding were similar (Cockburn et al., 1969). Yet the virus in the United States caused considerable excess mortality in 1968–1969 (Sharrar, 1969) at a time when epidemics in other areas had a milder initial effect. Among other factors, the lessening of initial pandemic impact may have reflected immediately prior experience in some regions with the antecedent H2N2 virus, as was noted in England and Wales (Roden, 1969) and on the other side of the world as well (Gill et al., 1971). This experience may have been significant as evidence of the influence of residual neuraminidase-specific (anti-N2) antibody in blunting the pandemic in what turned out to be a "great natural experiment" of anti-neuraminidase immunity in man (Schulman and Kilbourne, 1969a). A puzzling difference in age-specific attack rates was recorded in 1957 and 1968, with higher attack rates in young children in 1957 and equal or greater involvement of the middle aged in 1968 (Davis et al., 1970; Buchan and

Reid, 1972; Zachary and Johnson, 1969; Sharrar, 1969). Morbidity assessment by questionnaires of high school students and their families in the same high school in the successive pandemics showed that school children in 1957 experienced significantly higher attack rates than adults at the start of the epidemic; in 1968, initial attack rates were comparable, and an adult was as likely as a school child to have been the first family case (Fig.15.8) (Davis *et al.*, 1970). It is difficult to explain this differing experience on other than immunological grounds. The anomaly here is the 1968–1969 experience because most epidemics are characterized by higher clinical attack rates in the young (Dowdle *et al.*, 1974). In 1968, however, it can be assumed that most teenaged children possessed anti-N2 antibody acquired in the previous H2N2 decade, and thus they more closely resembled adults with respect to relevant epidemiologic background. Indeed, the younger population was probably experiencing more influenza at the end of the H2N2 decade than adults and hence might have been boosted in immunity more recently.

Other evidence of the effect of specific immunity in altering pandemic morbidity is provided indirectly by the lower rate of excess mortality for elderly persons in 1968–1969 than had been noted in earlier epidemics

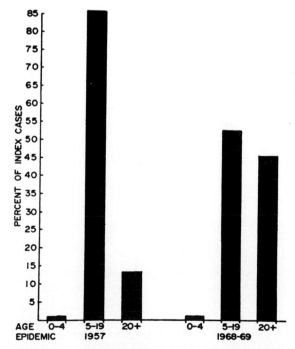

Fig. 15.8. Distribution of index cases of influenza-like illness by age group in study population families, 1957 and 1968–1969. There were 707 index cases in 1957 and 54 index cases in 1968–1969. From Davis *et al.* (1970).

(Housworth and Spoon, 1971). It is probable that this unexpected resistance of this age group to H3N2 influenza virus reflects their possesson of anti-bodies to antigenic determinants of the H3 hemagglutinin acquired at the end of the nineteenth century (Davenport *et al.*, 1969; Masurel, 1969; Fukumi, 1969; Marine *et al.*, 1969).

4. Mortality (Case Fatality Rates) in Various Pandemics

The pandemic of 1918 stands alone in severity in modern history as judged by total influenza-associated mortality. An estimated 20 million people died in 1918–1919, 550,000 deaths in excess of the usual expectancy occurred in the United States (Collins, 1957) (see Fig. 15.9), and the impact on community life was no less than that of the world war with which the epi-demic coincided (see Section IV,E).

The determination of case fatality rates for influenza (the true measure of virulence) is difficult because both numerator (morbidity) and denomina-tor (mortality) are derived from "soft" data. Influenza is not a reportable disease, and mortality is estimated as excess pneumonia-associated mortality

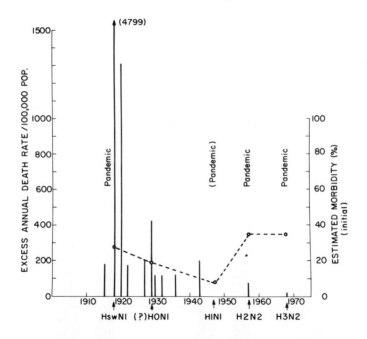

Fig. 15.9. Profile of major epidemics of influenza in the United States during the twentieth century. Open circles estimated morbidity in initial wave; vertical lines, excess annual death rate per 100,000 population. From Kilbourne (1973a). *J. Infec. Dis.* **127,** 478–487. Copyright 1973, University of Chicago Press. Re-produced by permission.

(Collins, 1931; Serfling, 1963). Although this indication of influenza in the community is widely used at present, it is occasionally subject to variation from other causes (Cassell *et al.,* 1968; Housworth and Langmuir, 1974). A crude approximation of case fatality rates in 1918–1919 is 1.1%, based on a global population of 1,699,000,000 (U.S. Survey Chart) and the estimated 20 million death figure. This rate far exceeds the progressively declining figures of recent years (Collins and Lehman, 1957). More meaningful may be the comparisons used by Collins (1931) of pneumonia rates in 1918–1919 and 1928–1929, which were 17.6 and 5.0 per thousand population, respectively.

In comparisons of pandemic mortality, immunological background and environmental factors must be considered just as they are in assessing comparative morbidity, as discussed earlier. The one uncontrollable variable is time or season of occurrence which, in the context of other events, may be critical in determining the fatal outcome of disease.

a. Factors Influencing Mortality—Intrinsic Viral Virulence. Virulence is the reciprocal of host susceptibility, and is not to be equated with disease severity. A virus of low intrinsic virulence may produce severe disease in a highly susceptible host, and a virulent virus may produce asymptomatic infection in a host who is either specifically or nonspecifically resistant. It is evident that comparative and quantitative measurement of virulence among virus strains demands a comparison of their effects (disease) in similar hosts under similar conditions (Kilbourne, 1960). Susceptibility in this context is defined not as vulnerability to the acquisition of infection, but rather as susceptibility to the effects of infection that lead to the development of disease. Peculiarly in the case of viral diseases that may be complicated by secondary bacterial invasion, the ability of the virus to stimulate or pave the way for secondary bacterial infections should be viewed as a sort of "pseudovirulence" which indirectly initiates a worsening of disease. "This result is obviously not a real reflection of intrinsic viral virulence, as the worsening of disease will depend on the nature and vagaries of the bacterial invader" (Kilbourne, 1960).

Even in 1918 all but a comparative few died with secondary bacterial pneumonia (MacCullum, 1919; Wolbach, 1919; Opie *et al.,* 1921). The greater virulence of second waves of pandemic influenza may be related to their occurrence on occasion in midwinter—a time of increased prevalence of respiratory tract pathogens and pneumonia (Kilbourne, 1960). The thesis has been advanced that the greater apparent "virulence" of influenza in 1918–1919 can be explained entirely on the basis of greater prevalence of secondary bacterial pneumonia, the presence of bacterial epidemics in army camps, the high case fatality rate of pneumonia at that time (as high as 45%), and the absence of antibacterial drugs (Kilbourne, 1960). On the other hand, the uniquely high mortality in the young adults may or may not be explicable on this basis, and apparently there was a "much higher incidence of severe (uncomplicated) influenza virus pneumonia (in 1918) in previously healthy patients, than that recorded in 1957/58" (Mulder and Hers, 1972). Nevertheless, several pathologists in 1918–1919 emphasized the relatively high frequency of coexistent chronic endocarditis, especially mitral stenosis, in fatal cases of influenza pneumonia (Straub, 1959, cited by Mulder and Hers, 1972).

Reliable *in vitro* correlations of influenza viral virulence have not been found when such markers as animal pneumotoxicity, neuraminidase activity, viral hemagglutination characteristics, and viral morphology are examined (summarized in Kilbourne, 1960). This is not surprising when one appreciates the polygenic nature of influenza viral virulence (Burnet, 1959; Fraser, 1959; Kilbourne, 1969; Mayer *et al.*, 1973; Beare and Hall, 1971) (see also Chapter 7). Certain biological properties common to the latter day (1957 and 1968) pandemic viruses have been noted, although their relationship to virulence is unclear. These include the relatively high activity of the neuraminidase common to both (Seto *et al.*, 1959; Seta, 1969), their ready isolation in the allantoic sac of the chick embryo without adaptation (Kilbourne, 1959; Coleman and Dowdle, 1969), and their absence of OD phase variation with respect to agglutination of chicken and mammalian erythrocytes (Kilbourne, 1959; Coleman and Dowdle, 1969; Veeraraghavan, 1969).

The probability of some variation in intrinsic viral virulence in nature is not to be discounted, although controlled observations are virtually impossible, and all definitions of disease in the "typical case" suggest a virus that is essentially unvarying in virulence (Chapter 1). However, such episodes as the highly lethal interpandemic outbreak of H1N1 influenza in 1951 in the town of Liverpool (Stuart-Harris, in Fox and Kilbourne, 1973, Influenza Workshop IV; Semple, 1951) and the extraordinarily high mortality of 1943–1944 (another nonpandemic year), which exceeded that of the mild pandemic of 1947 (Langmuir *et al.*, 1964; data of Collins, 1957), do suggest some variation in viral virulence.

The property of viral *transmissibility* is separable from other attributes of influenza virus virulence (Kilbourne, 1960; Schulman and Kilbourne, 1963a) and is especially relevant to pandemic spread. Antigenic novelty alone is probably insufficient to ensure widespread viral dissemination as is witnessed by such evolutionary failures as the 1962 Taiwan influenza B virus (Green *et al.*, 1964) and such interpandemic influenza A viruses as A/Hong Kong/5/72 (Schild *et al.*, 1973) that competed unsuccessfully with contemporary antigenic prototype A/England/42/72 for dominance. A hint that Hong Kong subtype viruses may be exceptionally transmissible is provided by the high frequency of laboratory-acquired infection in 1968 and the unusual ability of the virus to pass from man to animals, especially to swine (summarized in Chapter 9).

b. Host Determinants of Mortality. Prospective and intensive studies in 1957–1958 demonstrated clearly that in that pandemic severe and fatal influenza caused by the virus alone occurred primarily in previously damaged hosts. As the troublesome problem of bacterial pneumonia, so important in 1918–1919, had been modified by antibacterial drugs, the problem of primary influenza virus pneumonia emerged to attention and became proportionately more important. The findings of a combined clinical, pathological, and microbiological study of pneumonia patients in 1957–1958 in the New York Hospital (Louria *et al.,* 1959) are illustrative of findings in other studies conducted in medical centers throughout the world (Eickhoff *et al.,* 1961). The data from the study (summarized in Table 15.4) emphasize the importance of antecedent cardiac disease, especially rheumatic heart disease with mitral stenosis, in the genesis of fatal primary influenza virus pneumonia. Similar experience was reported from Boston (Martin *et al.,* 1959), New Haven (Petersdorf *et al.,* 1959), and other American cities as well as from the Netherlands, where unusually skillful pathological studies were conducted (Mulder and Hers, 1972). This experience was not unique to 1957–1958. A review of all fatal cases of influenza in the period 1937–1958 in which virus, but not bacteria, was demonstrated in the lung, revealed that 15 of 35 had underlying heart disease, while only 2 were described

Table 15.4 The Association of Preexisting Disease (Especially Cardiovascular) with Pulmonary Complications of Influenza[a]

Disease syndrome	No. of patients	No. of patients with chronic disease or pregnancy	No. of patients with cardiovascular disease
Influenza complicated by bacterial pneumonia	15	8	0
Concomitant influenza virus and bacterial pneumonia	9	7	5
Primary influenza virus pneumonia	6	6	6
Totals	30	21	14

[a] From data of Louria *et al.* (1959)

as "normal." The state of 18 was not defined with respect to preexisting disease. Rheumatic heart disease was present in 13 of the 15 patients in which cardiac disease was found (Louria *et al.,* 1959).

In the pandemic of 1968–1969 also, a prospective study in Memphis of pneumonia in influenza patients showed that 73% of influenza patients with pneumonia (including secondary bacterial pneumonia) suffered from underlying disease, including cardiovascular, pulmonary, and renal disease and alcoholism and 7 of 79 were pregnant (Bisno *et al.,* 1971). A relatively low mortality rate was thought to reflect the infrequency of staphylococcal pneumonia and primary influenza virus pneumonia.

The importance of mitral stenosis, and to a lesser extent pregnancy in the last trimester (Eickhoff *et al.,* 1961), in the genesis of primary influenza virus pneumonia suggests that hemodynamic factors rather than the chronic disease state per se are of major importance in pathogenesis of the syndrome. It must be appreciated, however, that the major mortality effected by influenza in all epidemics is determined by secondary bacterial pneumonia rather than by primary (nonbacterial) influenza virus pneumonia.

c. Environmental Determinants.   Interaction between influenza virus and host does not occur *in vacuo,* and like other infections it is influenced by the environment in which it occurs (Fig. 15.1). Definition of such effects in naturally occurring infection obviously is difficult. Certain epidemiological observations are worth noting, however. Although infection with influenza viruses has been documented in every month of the year in the North Temperate Zone, influenza occurs characteristically in winter epidemics, usually in the first quarter of the year. In the Southern Hemisphere, where the seasons are reversed, the epidemic curve of influenza rises in the winter of that part of the world, and so is seasonally influenced. An exception to the generalization concerning winter prevalence is at the time of introduction of new (pandemic) viral subtypes, when summer time or early fall epidemics have occurred frequently (Langmuir, 1961; Dunn, 1958; Tateno *et al.,* 1963; Dowdle *et al.,* 1974).

The term "season" is often equated with "climate," but is actually the composite of several different factors that may influence the occurrence of influenza (Table 15.5). Climate is but one attribute of the season of the year, and it too is multifactorial, comprising both air temperature and humidity. Of equal or greater importance than climate per se is seasonally influenced population behavior. The requirement for space heating in winter seasons results in focal increases in population density (crowding), and school attendance usual in the winter affords a prime opportunity for the dissemination of airborne pathogens. So too the secondary bacterial complications of influenza are subject to seasonal influence related to the higher

Table 15.5   Analysis of Seasonal Effects on
Influenza

Climate
  Air temperature ⎫
  Relative humidity ⎭ outdoor and indoor
Population behavior
  As it affects *travel* (interpersonal contact)
  Population density (school sessions, etc.)
Presence of pathogenic bacteria
  Seasonally-influenced carrier rate will determine
    incidence of secondary bacterial pneumonia and
    mortality
Undefined factors (see text)

---

carrier rate of pneumococci in the winter time (Heffron, 1939) ; as a consequence, mortality but not influenza morbidity may be affected.

i. Effects of Climate.   In family practice, Hope-Simpson (1958) noted a
positive correlation between the incidence of acute respiratory infections and
decline in temperature. A study of five successive winters of differing severity
in the United Kingdom disclosed less influenza, evidenced by fewer sickness
benefit claims, in mild winters than in colder ones (Davey and Reid, 1972).
Tateno *et al.* (1963) correlated low relative humidity with influenza associated deaths. On the other hand, influenza occurs epidemically in the tropics
in the high humidity of Panama (Monto and Olazabal, 1966; Buescher
et al., 1969) or in east Africa (Montefiore *et al.*, 1970). In east Africa,
as in subtropical or temperate areas, the highest frequency of infection was
in populous urban areas (Montefiore *et al.*, 1970). The sparing of isolated
populations has been observed in tropical (Napiorkowski and Black, 1974)
as well as Arctic regions (Philip and Lackman, 1962), indicating the relatively greater importance of population density and communication in the
spread of infection.
   It is not clear whether the effects of climate are principally upon the
virus or upon the host. Influenza virus is probably transmitted in the form
of aerosols in small droplet nuclei. In aerosol suspension the virus is more
susceptible to inactivation at high relative humidity (Hemmes *et al.*, 1960;
Harper, 1961) and survives best in the range of 15–40% relative humidity
(Hemmes *et al.*, 1960). Low relative humidity characterizes the indoor climate in winter. Thus, northern winters combine circumstances for increasing
virus survival in the air and crowding of the population.
   Study of the "winter factor" in a mouse model confirms the influence
of humidity on transmission of virus from mouse to mouse (Schulman and

Kilbourne, 1962). Even when humidity and temperature were carefully controlled in winter and summer, rates of transmission were significantly higher in winter (Schulman and Kilbourne, 1963b), suggesting either that relative humidity before contact may have been important or that another unidentified winter factor was operative. An effect of climate on the host is suggested by the studies of Zhdanov and Ritova (1963), who observed more clinical reactions in experimentally infected human subjects in winter than in summer. Beare *et al.* (1968) found no seasonal effect on experimentally induced influenza, and evidence that chilling influences the disease after its acquisition is lacking.

ii. Socioeconomic Status. To the degree that impoverished populations are crowded, the incidence of influenza may be expected to increase. In addition, a study in Glasgow indicated that although the occurrence of *mortality* was equal in various socioeconomic groups, 74% of the deaths in members of higher social class who were over 65 years of age were ascribed to influenza plus a preexisting chronic condition, while in only 48% of elderly people in the lower class was such a condition found. Therefore, poverty itself constitutes an added environmental burden and increases the risk of mortality (Assaad and Reid, 1971).

5. The Origin of Pandemics

a. Mutability and Antigenic Variability of Influenza Viruses. The distinction between major (pandemic) and minor (interpandemic) antigenic variation of the external antigens of influenza A virus has been considered in preceding chapters and has been treated extensively in Chapter 10. Although minor antigenic variation is credibly explained as the consequence of sequential mutations in the genes coding for hemagglutinin and neuraminidase polypeptides, the magnitude of difference in influenza A viral subtypes as reflected by both antigenic analysis and peptide maps (Laver and Webster, 1971) is difficult to reconcile with a direct mutational origin of one subtype from its predecessor. No evidence exists that the RNA of the influenza virus is unusually mutable, and viral strains handled under cloned and nonselective laboratory conditions are genetically stable. Laboratory passage of virus with homotypic antibody leads to the evolution of distinguishable minor antigenic variants (see Chapter 10), but the proposal of Fazekas de St. Groth (1970) that major subtype variants could similarly be produced has not been verified experimentally.

Except for the intriguing but largely unconfirmed studies of swine influenza by Shope (Chapter 9) and a recent suggestion of the persistence of influenza viral antigen in the brains of patients with postencephalitic Parkinsonism (Gamboa *et al.,* 1974), there is little to suggest that influenza viruses have the potential for persistence and latency. Indeed, even the most temperate viral strains (e.g., nonplaque forming in cell culture) are found to be cytonecrotizing if infected cells are carefully examined by microscopy (Palese *et al.*, 1973). For these reasons, the opportunity for major mutation of virus seems to be limited to the brief (10–11 year) periods of its demonstrable dominance in the human population, and probably does not include a period during which the virus has "gone underground" or become unrecognizable in man. Therefore, it is logical to look beyond man himself for the origin of pandemic (i.e., new subtype) viruses.

b. Animals as a Reservoir of New Influenza Virus Antigens. The hypothesis that animals may be a reservoir for such viruses has been explored intensively in Chapter 10 and it will be paraphrased here only briefly, and to identify points of difference in interpretation of the evidence.

The idea of recombination between human influenza viruses for the acquisition of altered virulence was introduced by Burnet as a possible explanation for the "special virulence" of the second wave of the 1918–1919 pandemic (Burnet, in Herter lectures, Johns Hopkins University, 1957, cited in Burnet, 1973). It has been suggested that the Asian (H2N2) subtype originated in an animal reservoir in Asia (Mulder and Masurel, 1958; Andrewes, 1959), and later Rasmussen (1964) suggested that the Asian (H2N2) subtype virus with its unusually active neuraminidase might have been so derived by recombination with a human virus. Genetic interaction with Asian and avian viruses was demonstrated *in vitro* by Rasmussen (1964) and by Tumová and Pereira (1965). Kilbourne (1968), having demonstrated recombination between human and equine influenza virus, proposed that all major antigenic changes might be derived by recombination of human and animal influenza A viruses. This hypothesis afforded an explanation (Kilbourne, 1973a) for the interspecific transfer of virus that apparently occurs so rarely in nature (Chapter 14). Webster and his colleagues have reinforced the credibility of interspecific recombination by carrying out *in vivo* recombination in domestic animals (Webster *et al.*, 1971; and Chapter 10). An extension of the human–animal virus recombinational hypothesis states that "in fact, there are no true animal strains of influenza virus, but that those strains that we have isolated are artifacts of the domestic propinquity of animals and man. Thus, the graveyard of old (human) influenza may be the barnyard, and animal influenza may indeed be a product of domestication" (Kilbourne, 1973a). The domestication of swine dates back to 7000 BC (Protsch and Berger, 1973). Other scientists (see Chapter 10) have been more impressed with the recovery of influenza A viruses from wild birds (Pereira *et al.*, 1965; Webster and Laver, Chapter 10) and emphasize a reverse relationship of influenza virus origin.

It is clear, however, that the assignment of the avian influenza A viruses to one or another avian species is fraught with difficulty. Identification of viruses as "turkey" or "chicken" strains reflects only the species in which the infection was first recognized (Chapter 9) and such nomenclature has been forsaken for the less specific designation "avian." Indeed, the nature of the disease in birds is so variable both in lethality and pathogenesis (Chapter 14 and Easterday and Couch, 1975, Influenza Workshop VI) that it is difficult to believe that avian species are usual or definitive hosts for the influenza A viruses.

The antigenic relationships of human and animal influenza A viruses have been reviewed elsewhere (Chapters 10 and 14) and are summarized in Table 15.6. It should be pointed out that while the earlier human viral subtypes, such as H0N1, have disappeared, common antigens in the neuraminidase have lingered on to the present in avian influenza strains (Schild *et al.,* 1969). Depending on one's bias, the evidence of common or related antigens in human and animal viruses can be read as flow of virus in one direction or another. The chronology of viral isolation is not particularly helpful, because until recently sampling and identification of animal strains has been sporadic and incomplete, at best. However, during the period of modern virology, it is notable that shared viral antigens have been identified

Table 15.6   Antigenic Relationships of External Antigens of Animal and Human Influenza A Viral Subtypes[a]

Animal virus	Isolation date	Human virus[b]	Isolation date	Comment
HswN1	1930	HswN1	+[c]	Close similarity of present swine virus and human agent of 1918[c]
Hav1N1	1902	H0 N1	1933	Related through N1 neuraminidase (avian viruses)
Hav4N1	?	H1 N1	1946	
Hav5N1	1959			
Hav6N1	?			
Hav6N2	1963	H2N2	1957	Related through N2 neuraminidase
Hav7Neq2	1963	H3N2	1968	Avian and equine viruses related to H3 hemagglutinin and to each other
Heq2Neq2	1963			

[a] Lesser antigenic relationships between Heq2 and H2 (summarized by Davenport *et al.,* 1967) and Heq1 and H2 (Kilbourne, 1968) and Heq1 and H3 (E. D. Kilbourne, unpublished) have been noted.

[b] Single vertical lines show antigenic relatedness. Double vertical lines show close antigenic relatedness or identity.

[c] Not isolated from man. Identification as a human virus of 1918 is on serologic evidence.

first in man (e.g., N2 in 1957) and later in animals (in Hav6N2 in 1963; Pereira *et al.*, 1967). The equine viruses both related to human H2 and H3 were first isolated after the appearance of H2 antigen in man in 1957. Viruses antigenically indistinguishable from human H3N2 virus have been isolated from a large number of animal species since the initial appearance of the virus in man in 1968 (Chapter 14). No prospective observations of transfer of animal viruses to man in epidemic form have yet been made.

c. Recombinational Recapture of Influenza A Hemagglutinin and Neuraminidase Antigens.   The epizootology of animal influenza A viruses differs importantly from the epidemiology of human influenza in the parallel persistence of multiple subtypes in animal populations. Found principally in domestic animals in close contact with man, these viruses provide a reservoir of antigens that are novel with respect to human disease. Because interspecific infection between man and animals rarely occurs (except recently in unidirectional fashion with Hong Kong virus from man to animals) a mechanism must be postulated for the successful transfer of animal viruses with epidemic potential to man. Thus, genetic determinants both of human virulence and transmissibility (separable factors) (Schulman and Kilbourne, 1963a) must be acquired by the animal virus, and even virulence alone is polygenic (Kilbourne, 1969). Direct mutation to human virulence seems improbable, but genetic interchange by recombination or reassortment between human and animals viruses (in animal or man) could yield progeny of "new" (i.e., animal) hemagglutinin–neuraminidase phenotype but possessing other genes of human virus origin necessary for efficient replication in man (Fig. 15.10).

Evidence is now persuasive that wild birds may be infected in nature with influenza A viruses, and at least one antigen (Nav5) not yet identified in man or domestic species has been found in an Australian shearwater (Downie and Laver, 1973). The question, perhaps academic, arises whether such viruses produce indigenous infections in free-flying birds or whether

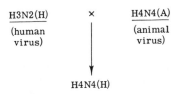

Fig. 15.10.   "Instant adaptation" of antigenically novel animal virus to man. Recombination of human and animal viruses need not result in antigenic hybridization. Progeny virus may bear both hemagglutinin and neuraminidase of animal virus together with genes (H) required for human virulence. Such a virus could then cross the species barrier. From Kilbourne (1973).

such infections are derived from domestic fowl during the contact of wild and domestic avian species that indisputably occurs (Easterday and Couch, 1975, Influenza Workshop VI). Further studies are needed of wild animals and birds as viral reservoirs and their ecologic relationship to domestic species.

Arguments for the origin of most or all influenza viruses in man can be marshalled as follows: (1) There are three antigenically distinct types of human influenza virus, A, B and C, but only influenza A has become established in lower species. This implies ancient infection of man with a primordial ancestral virus before differentiation of the virus into types. (Influenza B and C viruses are more temperate, nonpanvirulent agents that may be further on the path of differentiation to obligate human restriction than A.) If this analysis is correct, then a long association of man and the influenza viruses is implied. (2) Most evidence suggests unidirectional movement of influenza viruses from man into lower animals, and birds and only rarely in the opposite direction. (3) The occasional high mortality induced by the avian viruses in birds does not suggest that they are viruses that have had a long relationship to the species as a definitive host. Where analogues of other viruses are represented in human and animal species (e.g., pox viruses, herpesviruses, enteroviruses, adenoviruses), such common animal species as the mouse, rat, guinea pig, and rabbit appear not to have their own natural infection with orthomyxoviruses.

From these premises I postulate that most or possibly all animal influenza viruses have originated in man. As occasional rare events at various times in the past, domesticated animals in close proximity to man have been infected with human influenza A viruses. In some instances, adaptation and establishment of the virus in the animal species has occurred, as was probably the case with swine influenza virus in 1918 (Shope, 1935–1936; Laidlaw, 1935) and may be occurring now with Hong Kong virus in swine. Such strains clearly become deadapted to man in the process (Beare *et al.*, 1971) and are rarely sources of human infection. As another very rare event, simultaneous infection of animal or man with the currently predominant human strain and this "animal" virus (Fig. 15.10) could produce a human virulent virus capable also of sequential transmission in man, but with the new (animal) external viral proteins to which antibody no longer exists in the human population (Fig. 15.11). This virus then produces pandemic disease in man *if an ecologic niche is available.* That is, if the current strain is declining in prevalence and the new virus can compete effectively for the target cells of the human respiratory tract. Possibly, many such "pandemic candidate" viruses now exist, awaiting only the critical opportunity for entry (reentry) into the human population.

Reasoning from the evidence of the twentieth century, the minimal requirement of the pandemic new subtype virus is the possession of a hemag-

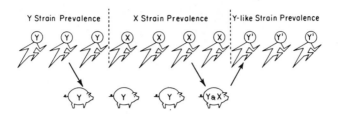

Fig. 15.11. Hypothetical scheme for the development of pandemic influenza strains. As a rare event human influenza A virus (strain Y) infects a domestic animal, and the strain becomes established and perpetuated in series in that species as an "animal" influenza virus. In the meantime strain Y disappears from man at the end of its period of prevalence. Human strain X (a later prevalent subtype) as a very uncommon event may infect an animal infected with "animal" strain Y. The ensuing recombination of viruses may produce progeny virus antigenically like Y but endowed with capacity for replication in man acquired from human virus X. Virus Y' appears as a "new" human virus. No time scale is indicated. Such events might be separated by hundreds or thousands of years. From Kilbourne (1973b).

glutinin antigen to which most of the human population lacks antibody. The neuraminidase may or may not be novel, but pandemic severity may be less as discussed earlier in this chapter.

d. Pandemics and the Recycling of Antigens. The previous experience of elderly people with antigens of the Asian virus of 1957 and the Hong Kong viral antigen of 1968 is indicated by the presence of serum antibodies to these recent strains and the secondary type of antibody response that follows administration of H2N2 and H3N2 vaccines (Davenport *et al.,* 1969; Masurel, 1969; Fukumi, 1969; Marine *et al.,* 1969). The presence of antibodies to equine 2 virus in the elderly (Voth and Feldman, 1963; Minuse *et al.,* 1965; Davenport *et al.,* 1967; Masurel, 1969; Marine and Workman, 1969) has been interpreted as heterologous response to the Hong Kong (H3N2) virus, rather than homologous response to the equine strain with which it shares common antigenic determinants (Marine and Workman, 1969). This conclusion appears to be borne out by the use of a photometric technique that distinguishes between heterologous and homologous antibodies in hemagglutination-inhibition tests (Davenport *et al.,* 1969). Thus, evidence points to the probability that a Hong Kong-like virus may have circulated in man in the past, possibly causing epidemic disease in 1900. Similar serological study suggests that the pandemic virus of 1889 resembled the Asian (H2N2) virus of 1957. Taken together with the Hong Kong data, these findings suggests a recycling of hemagglutinin antigen at 60–70 year intervals (Davenport *et al.,* 1969; Masurel, 1969). Furthermore, Mulder and Masurel (summarized by Masurel, 1969) have described the closely related viruses isolated during the 1918–1957 period as being representative of a "swine (virus) era," now superceded by a reiterated period of "A2" prevalence represented by the H2N2 and H3N2 viruses (see Fig. 15.12).

The foregoing evidence and interpretation have at least two important implications: (1) that major subtype variants can be derived directly from antecedent human subtypes and (2) that perhaps the antigenic variations of the hemagglutinin are limited, a conclusion that is not unreasonable if critical conformation and structure of the antigen are required for its insertion into the virion and expression of its function of binding to the host cell.

With reference to theories of the animal origin of pandemic subtypes, it does seem unlikely that in both of its appearances (1900 and 1968) the Hong Kong prototype was derived from the horse. As Davenport and his associates (1969) state the case: "Whatever the source or sources of pandemic strains, the antibody spectrum of the human population . . . acts as a limiting influence on the spread of strains antigenically like their predecessors. Large and ordered gaps in the age distribution of antibodies oriented to strains of remote periods of past prevalence favor the spread of 'old anti-

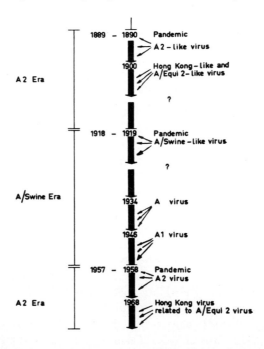

Fig. 15.12. Hypothetical recycling of A2 (H2N2)-like and Hong Kong (H3N2)-like viruses. From Masurel (1969).

genic acquaintances' once they arise. Hence, given the appropriate variant by genetic limitations, recycling is encouraged."

Only intensive prospective studies of future pandemics will test the validity of the recycling and the recombinational hypotheses, all points of which are not necessarily in conflict. If reappearance of a "swine era" is next on the schedule (Masurel and Marine, 1973), the high susceptibility of swine to the present Hong Kong subtype could facilitate retrieval of this antigen from its present reservoir. The truth may lie in a combination of these hypotheses, with the lesser variation of the 1918–1957 era representing serial mutations of virus and the greater changes, such as that of 1957, the introduction of recombinants. The periodicity of a series of two reappearances is not compelling.

e. Pandemicity and the Phenomenon of Viral Disappearance. The remarkable disappearance of old subtype variants has been discussed (Section IV,A,1). To state that the virus is crowded out by a rising tide of antibody in the human population (Fig. 15.5) is simply descriptive and begs the question. Other viruses survive in highly immune populations without recourse to antigenic change (see Chapter 1). The periodic disappearance of influenza A viruses suggests that they live in rather precarious balance with man as intensely obligate parasites, and that their survival is dependent on a large number of susceptibles in the population. The very nature of their initial introduction into a universally susceptible population with consequent rapid exhaustion of susceptibles (because high density infection begets more effective transmission) (Fig. 15.13) may determine the brevity of their subsequent persistence. It is likely that the terminal part of the interpandemic period is associated not only with less disease but with less infection and

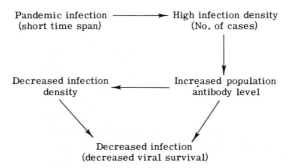

Fig. 15.13. Pandemic infection produces rapid attainment of high infection density in population. Consequent increase in population of specific antibody to the virus decreases chances for virus survival directly, by decreasing infection of the immune, and indirectly, by decreasing infection density (number of cases) and therefore dissemination of virus.

viral transmission. In short, pandemics continue to occur as pandemics because they *began* as pandemics.

B. Interpandemic Influenza

Many aspects of influenza are common to both pandemic and interpandemic periods and therefore have been discussed earlier in this chapter. Only the special characteristics of influenza virus infection in the interpandemic period will be stressed here. The interpandemic period is a time of complex mutual adaptation of man and virus following initial saturation of the human population with virus during the 2 to 3 years after introduction of a new viral subtype. Minor but significant changes in the antigenic composition of the virus are occurring as the population is responding immunologically to its presence. Although regional epidemics of influenza occur in 2–3 year cycles, the virus is present during most of the year in most communities as a cause of sporadic and often unrecognized endemic infection that may or may not be associated with disease. The pattern is one of declining disease incidence and gradual increase in population antibody, as has been somewhat simplistically presented in Fig. 15.5. The declining epidemicity illustrated is correct as an overall global view, but even early regional or national patterns may deviate from this scheme. For example, influenza morbidity in Hungary had a reverse pattern in 1969, 1970, and 1971 with a progressive increase in morbidity with time. In part, this anomalous pattern may have reflected the pattern, characteristic of Europe in general, of more severe H3N2 virus impact in the second rather than the first winter of Hong Kong virus prevalence, and in part the occurrence in 1971 of two discrete epidemics starting at two separate foci and caused by two different antigenic variants (Barb and Takatsy, 1973). Such anomalous experiences are not surprising, and one would hardly expect completely congruent epidemic phases when the chances for minor but deterministic differences in environment, circumstances of viral introduction, and immediate prior experience with influenza are considered.

1. Nature of the Virus in the Interpandemic Period

The minor viral antigenic variation (antigenic drift) observed in the interpandemic period has been well characterized in Chapter 10 as the probable result of sequential point mutations in the viral RNA, with variation occurring both in hemagglutinin and neuraminidase (Schulman and Kilbourne, 1969b). Although antigenic inhomogeneity of viral particles probably begins with the introduction of the new subtype, little significant variation was noted in the first 2–3 years after pandemic introduction of virus in 1947, 1957, and 1968. Antigenic variation alone is probably inadequate to ensure survival of the virus. In the case of the 1971 Hungarian epidemics, the new antigenic variant fared unsuccessfully in competition with the old (Barb and Takatsy, 1973). The Hong Kong (H3N2) variants, A/Hong Kong/5/72 and A/Hong Kong/107/72 of 1972 "never made it" while another variant, A/England/42/72, differing in no greater degree from its predecessor, prevailed on a global scale (Schild *et al.*, 1973). The general antigenic homogeneity of isolates from epidemics of influenza A in 1935–1955 was stressed by Jensen (1957), but the divergence between viral pairs isolated in the same year was also noted. Jensen (1957) also described variation in serological reactivity among 10 isolates from a single epidemic, but variation was assessed by a single serological test in which variation and response may not have been related to antigenic variation but to differences in antigen and antibody avidity. However, the interesting point was made that each individual in the study had a unique antibody profile when his sera were tested against a variety of influenza A viruses from different years.

Not only does the virus change antigenically, but perhaps also in virulence, as has been described earlier in the Liverpool epidemic of 1950–1951 (Semple, 1951). The problems in fixing responsibility for more severe disease on antigenic variation or intrinsic viral virulence have also been discussed.

Variability in the reaction of viruses in the same antigenic subgroup with antibody was noted by Van der Veen and Mulder (1950) and was thought to represent a variation in viral "phase" termed PQR (see Chapter 11). It is now clear that influenza viral isolates comprise mixtures in variable proportion of particles which, while antigenically identical, may differ in other properties, including avidity for antibody. These variations in viral (antigenically reactive) "phase" can be explained in genetic terms as a selection of viral clones, differing in reactivity with both antibody and nonspecific inhibitor, that can be isolated as pure populations (Choppin and Tamm, 1964). Genetic dimorphism (Mowshowitz and Kilbourne, 1975) has been observed with other viral properties, including morphology and the ratio of hemagglutinin to neuraminidase protein per particle (summarized by Mowshowitz and Kilbourne, 1975) (Table 15.7). The significance of such variation in relation to the pathogenicity or epidemiology of the virus is unknown. The fact is that influenza virus isolates in early passage comprise two morphological types, filamentous and spherical (Choppin *et al.*, 1960; Kilbourne and Murphy, 1960), and throat washings from a number of patients contained "+" (inhibitor sensitive) and "−" (inhibitor resistant) particles demonstrable on early passage (Tamm, 1964). It may be that these phenomena are analogous to the balanced polymorphism of animals and provide the virus with still greater genetic diversity and adaptability (Mowshowitz and Kilbourne, 1975). The "−" particles that are less effectively bound by antibody might aid viral survival in partially immune popu-

Table 15.7 Genetic Dimorphism of Influenza Virus[a]

Viral serotypes	Dimorphic property	Functional significance	Reference
H3N2 Heq1N2 H0N2	NA activity	Viral release and replication	Mowshowitz and Kilbourne, 1975
H0N2 (PR8/Eng)	NA activity	Viral release and replication	Palese and Schulman, 1974
H$_{fpv}$N$_{turkey}$	NA activity	Viral release and replication	Webster and Campbell, 1972
H0N2 (NWS/RI/5)	NA activity	Viral release and replication	Kilbourne et al., 1967 Webster et al., 1968
H2N2	Morphology	?	Choppin et al., 1960
H2N2 H0N1	Morphology	?	Kilbourne and Murphy, 1960
H0N1	Morphology	?	Burnet and Lind, 1957
H2N2	Receptor affinity	Cellular, inhibitor and antibody binding, replication	Choppin and Tamm, 1960

[a] From Mowshowitz and Kilbourne (1975).

lations and might be expected to prevail at the end of pandemic periods. No clear-cut evidence exists concerning this point. The answer will depend on the direct identification of such clones on first passage of human material to forestall selection or later mutation within laboratory host systems. Obviously, extensive sampling must be made as well. Variation not related to specific markers was observed by Dowdle et al. (1974) in H2N2 strains isolated toward the end of the decade of their prevalence. These strains were more difficult to isolate and had different reactivity with red blood cells than had earlier strains. The difficulty in recovering such strains from man may have reflected the presence of specific antibody in throat secretions of the partially immune or may have been a valid reflection of more intense human adaptation.

The morphology of the virus and the amount of hemagglutinin represented on the viral surface are subject to phenotypic modification related to intracellular hemagglutinin cleavage that may be host dependent—at least in *in vitro* systems (Chapter 2). Such modification might affect interspecies transfer of virus.

Endogenous autorecombination involving salvage of mutations in incomplete or inactivated viral particles has been invoked as a partial explanation of the mutability of influenza viruses in the interpandemic period (Kilbourne, 1973c).

2. THE NATURE OF THE INFECTION IN THE INTERPANDEMIC PERIOD— CHANGE IN POPULATION IMMUNOLOGICAL PHENOTYPE

Early after pandemic introduction of virus, it seems able to survive without significant antigenic change until a critical point is reached of relative depletion of nonimmune subjects. Although reinfection can occur with virus that is antigenically unchanged (Sigel *et al.*, 1950), survival of virus beyond 4–5 years appears to depend on antigenic mutation. Significant antigenic difference was not observed with H2N2 (Asian) virus circulating in 1957 and 1959, yet reinfection documented by serial serological observations was remarked in such disparate populations as Navajo school children and urban medical students (Hayslett *et al.*, 1962). The pattern of serological response and illness in the Navajo children is shown in Table 15.8. Whereas 44 of 58 infections were symptomatic in 1957–1958, less than half (12 of 26) were ill in 1959–1960. Mean population antibody levels rose during this period, and two discrete infections were documented in 9 of 77 school children under observation. These infections were separated by 2-year intervals. In another study conducted during successive winters, infection in the first winter conferred complete protection against infection with or without illness in the second. In both epidemics about half of those with serological evidence of infection had reported illness (Miller *et al.*, 1973). Thus, the biennial periodicity of epidemics appears to reflect periodic waning of population immunity when measured in such microepidemiological studies (see also Fig. 15.2). However, mass surveys based on testing of large numbers of serum specimens confirm the fluctuation in antibody levels against influenza A virus (Widelock *et al.*, 1965). A graded increase in mean population antibody levels during interpandemic decades has been observed in many areas, including large countries (Broun *et al.*, 1960) and small countries, such as

Table 15.8 A Serial Study of Respiratory Illness and Specific Antibody Response to H2N2 Influenza Virus in 77 Navajo School Children[a]

Clinical diagnosis	1956–1957	1957–1958	1958–1959	1959–1960
Influenza	0	18	3	0
Upper respiratory infection	9	16	15	9
Total illnesses[b]	9	34	18	9
Percent illness	(12)	(44)	(22)	(12)
Incidence of antibody increases to H2N2 virus (%)	(0)	(58)	(14)	(26)

[a] Data from Hayslett *et al.* (1962).
[b] For which children sought medical attention.

Table 15.9   Differing Response of Subjects to Same H2N2 Influenza Vaccine Administered at Year 0 and Year 5 of Interpandemic Period[a]

Year	Hemagglutination-inhibition antibody titer		Average fold response	Number of subjects with 4-fold or antibody rise
	Initial	Final		
1957	1.1[b]	1.8	2.0	16/83 (19%)
1962	2.3	4.4	4.2	9/12 (75%)

[a] From data of Kilbourne and Christenson (1963).
[b] Natural log (ln) of reciprocal serum dilution at end point.

Finland (Pyhala and Kleemola, 1973). Another measure of the changing immune state of the population is response to artificial immunization with the prevalent virus. As shown in Table 15.9, antibody responses to vaccines of the same composition and dose in 1957 and 1962 elicited a far greater number of responses in these adult subjects later in the H2N2 decade than in the immunologically virgin population of 1957 (Kilbourne and Christenson, 1963).

The interplay of viral variation and change in population specific immunity (immunological phenotype) is schematized in Fig. 15.14 in which sequential (minor) changes in viral antigen(s) reflects the selection of mutants least affected by prevalent antibody and hence better equipped to survive and multiply. The present interpandemic period has already seen epidemiologically significant variation; in 1972, in 1973 (A/Port

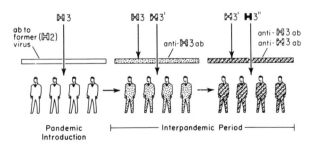

Fig. 15.14.   Selection of antigenic mutants as a function of population antibody. New pandemic viral subtype H3 transcends barrier of antibody to unrelated previously prevalent virus H2 and readily infects the population. When critical percentage of the population has been infected with H3, survival of H3 is impeded, and antigenically changed mutant H3', and later H3", have survival advantage (minor antigenic variation or antigenic "drift").

Chalmers/1/73), and at this writing (1975) multiple and different antigenic variants are appearing as was the case at the end of the H2N2 era (Dowdle *et al.,* 1974). Nevertheless, it appears that despite such variation, epidemics are less severe. The influenza-pneumonia associated excess mortality of the 1973 epidemic in the United States reached 1000 per week (Center for Disease Control, 1973), but thus far in 1975 has not exceeded 750 (Center for Disease Control, 1975). Whether or not 1979 is the next year of major mutation may depend on whether, as in the 1918–1946 period, a common neuraminidase antigen persists in the virus, causing it to confront a population in which immunizing experience with the antigen goes back to 1957.

3. ENDEMIC AND SUBCLINICAL INFECTION

The expression of infection as a clinically apparent disease or inapparent infection obviously depends on the threshold of clinical perception. There are no pathognomonic symptoms of influenza, and clinical recognition of the individual case is strongly influenced by its observation in the context of an epidemic. As emphasized earlier, influenza virus infection, even in the immunologically inexperienced, can occur without symptoms. Such silent infections are part of the epidemiological chain, and as they increase in proportion with rising population immunity (Bell *et al.,* 1961; Farník and Bruj, 1966) may facilitate virus spread because they do not immobilize the infected person. [However, viral shedding by such partially immune individuals may be reduced in magnitude and duration (see Chapter 12; also Fox and Kilbourne, 1973, Influenza Workshop IV).]

When looked for by serological testing, "off season" infections have been demonstrated (Dingle *et al.,* 1964; Hall *et al.,* 1973), and virus has been isolated in every month of the year (W. R. Dowdle, personal communication).

In nonepidemic periods, "silent" or asymptomatic influenza virus infections may be clinically heralded by their sequel of secondary bacterial pneumonia (Maxwell *et al.,* 1949; Stuart-Harris *et al.,* 1949; Kilbourne, 1961). In 1960, influenza was not recognized as an epidemic in New York City, but infection was serologically documented in the general population, increased (pneumonia-related) mortality occurred in older people, and viral isolations were obtained from patients hospitalized with pneumonia (Kilbourne, 1961; Kaye *et al.,* 1962).

Before the frequency of subclinical and endemic infection was appreciated, the mechanism of survival of influenza virus as an obligate human parasite was a mystery. There now seems no need to postulate secondary hosts or animal reservoirs to explain the interpandemic persistence of the virus.

4. CONGENITAL EFFECTS OF INFLUENZA

Congenital effects of influenza are discussed in Chapter 13. A recent review (MacKenzie and Houghton, 1974) concludes that "probably no direct association exists between maternal influenza infections and either congenital malformations or subsequent neoplasms in childhood."

5. GENETIC DETERMINANTS OF INFECTION

The evidence first published by McDonald and Zuckerman (1962) suggesting a higher prevalence of influenza in patients with blood group O and supported by other studies has not been confirmed in the single prospective study reported (Evans *et al.*, 1970).

C. Determinants of Transmission of Infection

1. ENVIRONMENTAL FACTORS

Influenza is a contagious disease that is transmitted directly from person to person by expulsion of the virus from the respiratory tract. The relative contribution of direct contact infection, mediated by touch or large droplets, and true aerosol infection by virus in small droplet nuclei is difficult to assess. However, infection rates have been significantly reduced by the environmental effects of ultraviolet irradiation (McLean, 1961) (presumably effective only on aerosol suspensions), and pathological evidence suggests initial or early involvement of pulmonary alveolar cells (Hers and Mulder, 1961)— a site accessible only to small (less than 5 μm) particles. Experimental infections have been induced by both methods in man (mainly intranasal installation or aerosol) (summarized in Fox and Kilbourne, 1973, Influenza Workshop IV). Probably a single particle can infect through aerosol inhalation (Couch, in Fox and Kilbourne, 1973, Influenza Workshop IV).

2. HOST FACTORS

Not only is the immune subject less liable to the acquisition of infection (Couch *et al.*, 1971), but he is probably less effective as a transmitter of influenza in that he sheds less virus. Magnitude and duration of viral shedding are directly related to the severity of illness in experimental infections (Couch *et al.*, 1971; Murphy *et al.*, 1973). Secondary infections are rarely observed with the experimental disease, so that the epidemiological significance of these observations is not clear. However, transmission of infection from recipients of live virus vaccine to contacts has occurred 2 days after infection of vaccinees (Slepushkin, in Fox and Kilbourne, 1973, Influenza Workshop IV). Although it does not prevent infection, anti-neuraminidase antibody may be effective in reduction of viral shedding (Murphy *et al.,* 1972b; Couch *et al.,* 1974) and in prevention of transmission from mouse to mouse (Schulman *et al.,* 1968). (Details concerning viral shedding patterns in man have been presented in Chapter 13.)

The incubation period of influenza is 1 to 7 days and is probably virus dose related. Infection appears to be transmitted during the symptomatic period in relation to the demonstrable presence of infectious virus in the respiratory tract, usually for 3 to 4 days after the onset of illness (Chapter 13). The transmission of virus through aerosols and the ubiquity of viral carriers during epidemics make it difficult to document the sequence of spread or transmission except in truly closed populations. An apparently focal outbreak in a hospital ward is illustrated in Fig. 15.15. The origin of the epidemic appeared to be a single patient, with the first secondary case appearing 24 hours after her admission in a patient in an adjacent bed.

The generally higher incidence of infection in children renders them important sources of spread of virus in the community. It has been suggested

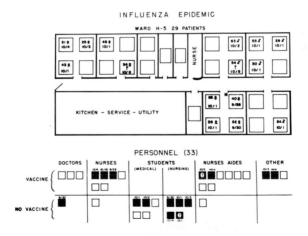

Fig. 15.15. Topography of Ward H5 and make-up of ward personnel. Shaded blocks represent individual patients and personnel who developed influenza symptoms. The date of appearance of symptoms is indicated within or above the blocks. The location of the initial case is indicated by an asterisk. From Blumenfeld *et al.* (1959).

that selective immunization of school children can reduce epidemic spread (Monto *et al.,* 1969; and Figure 12.4, Chapter 12).

3. Viral Determinants

Viral virulence and transmissibility are separable factors (Schulman and Kilbourne, 1963a; Easterday, in Fox and Kilbourne, 1973, Influenza Workshop IV), and in experimental animals strain related differences in transmissibility have been shown, and the trait is transferrable by genetic recombination (Schulman, 1970a).

Obviously, little information is available concerning viral dose in nature. The occasionally indolent and sporadic spread of virus in family groups may indicate that the effective output of virus from the primary case is small, or it may suggest variability in individual persons in their capacity to transmit infection, as is the case with mice (Schulman and Kilbourne, 1963b). There is no doubt that the explosiveness of epidemics and the incidence of influenza is influenced by population density, with highest clinical attack rates occurring in semi-closed and institutional populations (Jordan, 1961). Sustained exposure of partially immune mice to infected cagemates resulted in infection of 12–15% of the animals, despite their solid resistance to a single challenge in an aerosol chamber (Schulman, 1970b). It is likely that the probability of infection in man similarly depends on circumstances conducive to repeated reexposure to virus.

D. Surveillance

It has been pointed out that influenza is not a reportable disease because its rather nonspecific symptoms are easily confused with those of other diseases so that it tends to be over-reported. Consequently, only those methods that measure the overt epidemic impact of the infection have been useful. These include absenteeism from school and industry and, less commonly, sampling of the population by telephone surveys. A reliable but sometimes insensitive barometer of the presence of influenza in the community is the occurrence of excess (greater than the expected number) of deaths—either total or ascribed to pneumonia.

Isolation of the virus is not commonly undertaken and is beyond the capability of the average microbiology laboratory. Serological surveillance can be effectively carried out by the average laboratory, but has not been widely done, nor are diagnostic tests for individual cases generally available to physicians. Selective attempts at viral isolation from pneumonia patients have been rewarding in detecting influenza in the community at times when other indices failed (Kilbourne, 1961). Virus culture of children has been proposed as an economical and selective surveillance method (Levine *et al.*, 1974).

The definitive surveillance method is serological, and the newly improved methods for such seroepidemiological surveillance have been presented in Chapter 11. Only through an increase in such surveillance can the natural history of the disease be defined adequately. Continual and continuing surveillance is uniquely important for influenza in order that new antigenic variants be perceived quickly.

E. Socioeconomic Impact of Influenza

In its pandemic visitations influenza has obvious and dramatic effects on community life. The manifold impact of the 1968–1969 epidemic in a single city (Milwaukee), as assessed by multiple indices, is shown in Fig. 15.16.

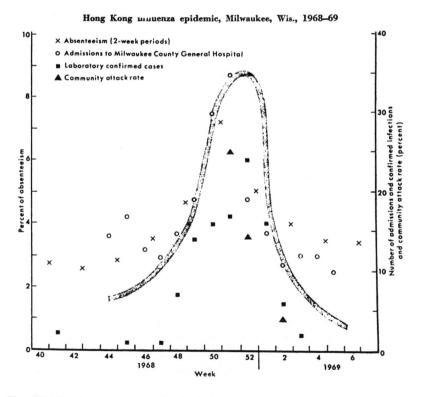

Fig. 15.16. Impact of pandemic influenza in one American city judged by multiple indices. From Piraino *et al.* (1970).

The impact of influenza as an epidemic disease in which most individual cases are not serious is perhaps greater than the sum of its parts. Preparation for the pandemic of 1957 by public health agencies revealed divergent reactions of public health workers and physicians. Public health officials viewed influenza as "constituting a threat to the community," but influenza was interpreted by practicing physicians as "not constituting a threat to the individual" (Rosenstock *et al.,* 1960).

Public concern during the notorious pandemic of 1918 reflected not only the greater mortality of that epidemic, but also the ignorance of the time regarding its causation and the absence of specific vaccines—a state dramatically illustrated by headlines culled from this period in a single city (Fig. 15.17).

Kavet has reviewed the economic impact of influenza in the United States in interpandemic and pandemic years. In 1963, 1966, and 1969, total costs, including earning loss, ranged between $1.7 billion and $3.9 billion per year, while direct (medically related) costs were less than 20% of these amounts. When the population covered by Medicare (those 65 years of age or older) was examined, it was estimated that the epidemic of 1968–1969 resulted in additional disbursements of $86.6 million for physicians' services, in- and out-patient services, and diagnostic procedures. The total direct cost to the Medicare program was $228 million and the average cost was $98.56 per Medicare case in this relatively severe epidemic. Such cost estimates are incomplete, as they omit the cost of out-patient drugs, deductibles and coinsurance, and other indirect costs of morbidity and mortality (Kavet, in Fox and Kilbourne, 1973, Influenza Workshop IV). In an 8-year period in the United Kingdom, 113 million days were lost because of influenza, and in 1969–1970 influenza accounted for 28.8 million pounds sterling of a total of 383 million pounds sterling in direct payments to sick people (Schild, in Fox and Kilbourne, 1973, Influenza Workshop IV).

F. Control of Influenza

1. CHEMOPROPHYLAXIS

As is the case with most other viral diseases, effective chemotherapy has not been developed for influenza. However, the synthetic drug, amantadine (L-amantanamine hydrochloride) is effective in preventing infection of animals (Grunert *et al.,* 1965) and man (Stanley *et al.,* 1965; Togo *et al.,* 1968) with influenza A viruses by interference with the penetration step of viral replication. A related compound, rimantadine, was found to be more effective in mice in preventing infection and reduced the infectiousness of treated

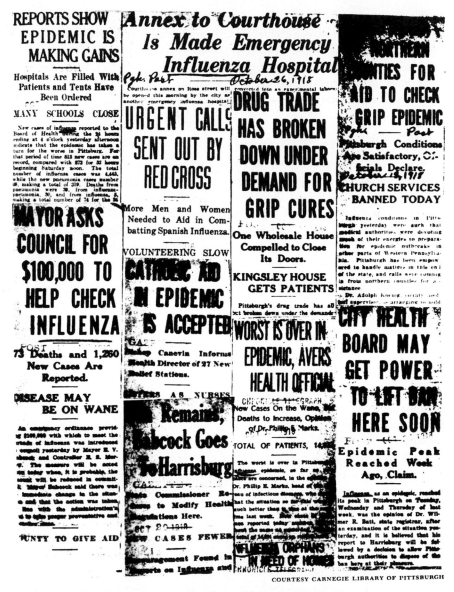

COURTESY CARNEGIE LIBRARY OF PITTSBURGH

Fig. 15.17. Newspaper headlines in 1918 in Pittsburgh—commentary on the impact of the pandemic. From Hoehling (1961).

mice which had acquired infection (Schulman, 1968). In man, the early prophylactic administration of amantadine to household contacts of index cases of influenza reduced the incidence of clinical influenza from 14.1 to

3.6%. The incidence of subclinical infection was also reduced in treated contacts (Galbraith *et al.*, 1969). In large epidemics this compound therefore might be of value in the interruption of viral spread. However, the need for twice daily doses over an unpredictable period of time and the occurrence of toxicity in the elderly precludes general application of this interesting drug in the control of influenza.

2. ARTIFICIAL IMMUNIZATION

Space does not permit a detailed discussion here of the development of vaccines for influenza. The principle was established in the late 1930's (reviewed by Salk *et al.*, 1945) that the parenteral administration of inactivated influenza virus could significantly reduce the incidence of disease in subjects exposed to experimental or naturally acquired infections. The complex and interlocking reasons why artificial immunization has never been effectively employed on a wide scale have been reviewed in detail (Kilbourne *et al.*, 1974) and include viral antigenic variation, impurity and poor standardization of past vaccines, and variability in demand and supply related to differing perceptions of risk by public health officials and variability in their recommendations to the public and to the medical profession.

Present day commercial vaccines are 50–90% effective (Leibovitz *et al.*, 1971) in reducing morbidity, depending on the closeness of antigenic fit of vaccine and challenge (wild-type) viruses, the recency of immunization, the dose of vaccine employed, and whether or not it is administered to immunologically experienced or inexperienced persons. The potential of parenterally administered inactivated influenza vaccine is illustrated by the remarkable record of 70–90% efficacy achieved by annual vaccination in United States military populations over a 26 year period (Davenport, 1961, 1973). In the military, as a relatively small homogeneous and controlled population of healthy persons, the goal of immunization has been the prevention of morbidity. In civilian life, the vaccine has been recommended chiefly in the United States for the selective immunization of the elderly and the chronically diseased in an effort to reduce pneumonia-associated mortality. However, in 1969–1970 insufficient vaccine was produced (22 to 24 million doses) to provide immunization for the more than 46 million of the population who were over 65 years of age or affected with chronic diseases (i.e., the target population). Although these persons, comprising 23% of the population, received 50% of the vaccine given, only one-quarter were vaccinated due to deficiencies in the implementation of this policy (Kavet, in Kilbourne *et al.*, 1974, Influenza Workshop V).

Despite the increased purity and potency of present vaccines, mass immunization in nonpandemic years is presently unjustified on the basis of the short-lived immunizing effect and variable reaction rate, especially in young children. Selective immunization of children has been proposed because of their importance as vectors of infection (Francis, 1967) (see Chapter 12, Section II,C). Both actual experience (Monto *et al.*, 1969) and theoretical models (Elveback, in Kilbourne *et al.*, 1974, Influenza Workshop V) support this approach to the induction of herd immunity. However, other experiences in the 1968–1969 pandemic, referred to earlier in this chapter, indicated a lower relative incidence in school age children than in other years—so that this approach may not be uniformly effective.

It is possible that the efficacy and duration of immunity can be increased by the use of live virus vaccine administered by the respiratory route to simulate natural infection. The early pioneering work of Smorodintsev *et al.* (1961) has been followed recently by the ingenious use of temperature-sensitive (Murphy *et al.*, 1972a) and cold-adapted (Maassab, 1968) mutants that have reduced virulence, probably associated with their inability to multiply at the higher temperature of the lower respiratory tract. A related approach in which either natural or induced infection is the definitive immunizing step is the use of viral neuraminidase-specific vaccine for the induction of partial immunity that does not preclude subsequent infection. (At this writing, these approaches remain experimental and none addresses the problem of anticipation of antigenic variation. A summary of present and potential vaccines is presented in Table 15.10.)

It is interesting to speculate on what might be achieved by simultaneous worldwide mass immunization, even with the present imperfect vaccines—an economic and logistical feat that is staggering to envision. If indeed influenza A virus is exquisitely dependent upon a large proportion of susceptibles in the population for its survival, and time is required for the evolution of new variants, then such immunization might prematurely terminate the present decennial cycles. Would the consequence then be an acceleration of the introduction of major subtype variants and more frequent pandemics? Because we know nothing of the origin of such variants or the timetable of their emergence, the answer obviously is unknown. However, if pandemic strains do arise in animals by recombination, or otherwise, then control of this reservoir is not impossible. A rational approach in this direction will depend upon a better knowledge of influenza in animals than we now possess. Surely in domestic animals control might be achieved eventually through artificial immunization (Kilbourne, 1975) or even selective eradication of infected animals in the manner that is so effective in the control of brucellosis and bovine tuberculosis. One approaches the prospect of "eradication" in biology with temerity, but it is not an impossible goal.

Table 15.10   Types of Influenza Vaccines—Actual and Potential[a]

I. Inactivated or noninfective
- A. Whole virus—formalin-inactivated
    1. Conventional empirically selected[b]
    2. Recombinant for high yield characteristic[b]
    3. Recombinant antigenic hybrid specific for neuraminidase antigen
    4. Any of the above plus adjuvant
- B. Disrupted or "split" virus[b]
    1. Presently made from (1) or (2) above
    2. Contains all viral proteins but are usually less toxic and less antigenic
- C. Isolated purified antigens
    1. Hemagglutinin
    2. Neuraminidase   } May require adjuvant
    3. Above in combination

II. Live virus (infective)
- A. Empirically selected by passage and spontaneous attenuation[c]
- B. Selected mutants
    1. Inhibitor-resistant (thought to correlate with attenuation)[b]
    2. Temperature sensitive (ts)
    3. Cold-adapted
- C. Recombinant
    1. Hybrid derived from virulent (wild type) and avirulent viruses, usually intermediate in virulence
    2. Properties of (2) and (3) (selected mutants) can be transferred to new serotype by recombination
    3. Any of above variants can be conferred with "high yield" genes by recombination (2) (whole virus-formalin-inactivated)

---

[a] From Kilbourne (1975).
[b] Currently in use and commercially available.
[c] In intermittent use in U.S.S.R. for many years.

References

Andrewes, C. H. (1959). *In* "Perspectives in Virology" (M. Pollard, ed.), p. 184. Wiley, New York.

Assaad, F. A., and Reid, D. (1971). *Bull. W.H.O.* **45**, 113.

Barb, K., and Takatsy, G. Y. (1973). *Bull. W.H.O.* **49**, 21.

Beare, A. S., and Hall, T. S. (1971). *Lancet* **2**, 1271.

Beare, A. S., Bynoe, M. L., and Tyrrell, D. A. J. (1968). *Brit. Med. J.* **4**, 482.

Beare, A. S., Hall, T. S., Schild, G. C., and Kundin, W. D. (1971). *Lancet* **1**, 305.

Bell, J. A., Craighead, J. E., James, R. G., and Wong, D. (1961). *Amer. J. Hyg.* **73**, 84.

Bisno, A. L., Griffin, J. P., van Epps, K. A., Niell, H. B., and Rytel, M. W. (1971). *Amer. J. Med. Sci.* **261**, 251.

Blumenfeld, H. L., Kilbourne, E. D., Louria, D. B., and Rogers, D. E. (1959). *J. Clin. Invest.* **38**, 199.

Broun, G. O., Muether, R. O., Shrader, E. L., Bawell, M. B., Legier, M., Pope, M. D., and Schmidt, R. R. (1958). *Arch. Intern. Med.* **101**, 203.

Broun, G. O., Oligschlaeger, D., Legier, M. S., and Schmidt, R. R. (1960). *Arch. Intern. Med.* **106**, 496.

Buchan, K. A., and Reid, D. (1972). *Health Bull.* **30**, 183.

Buescher, E. L., Smith, T. J., and Zachary, I. H. (1969). *Bull. W.H.O.* **41**, 387.

Burnet, F. M. (1959). *In* "Viruses" (F. M. Burnet and W. M. Stanley, eds.), Vol. 3, pp. 275–306. Academic Press, New York/London.

Burnet, F. M. (1973). *Med. J. Aust., Spec. Suppl.* 1, p. 3.

Burnet, F. M., and Clark, E. (1942). *In* "Influenza" (C. W. Ross, ed.), Monograph No. 4 of the Walter and Eliza Hall Institute. Macmillan, New York.

Burnet, F. M., and Lindt, P. E. (1957). *Arch. Virusforsch.* **7**, 413.

Cassell, E. J., Wolter, D. W., Mountain, J. D., Diamond, J. R., Mountain, I. M., and McCarroll, J. R. (1968). *Amer. J. Pub. Health* **58**, 1653.

Center for Disease Control. (1973). "Morbidity and Mortality Weekly Report," Vol. 22, p. 134. U.S. Dept. of Health, Education and Welfare, Atlanta, Georgia.

Center for Disease Control. (1975). "Morbidity and Mortality Weekly Report" Vol. 24, p. 105. U.S. Dept. of Health, Education and Welfare, Atlanta, Georgia.

Choppin, P. W., and Tamm, I. (1960). *J. Exp. Med.* **112**, 895.

Choppin, P. W., and Tamm, I. (1964). *Cell Biol. Myxovirus Infect., Ciba Found. Symp., 1964* p. 218.

Choppin, P. W., Murphy, J. S., and Tamm, I. (1960). *J. Exp. Med.* **112**, 945.

Cockburn, C. W., Delon, P. J., and Ferreira, W. (1969). *Bull. W.H.O.* **41**, 345.

Coleman, M. T., and Dowdle, W. R. (1969). *Bull. W.H.O.* **41**, 415.

Collins, S. D. (1931). *Pub. Health Rep.* **46**, 1909.

Collins, S. D. (1957). *U.S., Pub. Health Serv., Pub. Health Monogr.* **48**.

Collins, S. D., and Lehman, J. L. (1957). *Pub. Health Rep.* **72**, 771.

Couch, R. B., Douglas, R. G., Jr., Fedson, D. S., and Kasel, J. A. (1971). *J. Infec. Dis.* **124**, 473.

Couch, R. B., Kasel, J. A., Gerin, J. L., Schulman, J. L., and Kilbourne, E. D. (1974). *J. Infec. Dis.* **129**, 411.

Creighton, C. (1894). "A History of Epidemics in Britain." Cambridge Univ. Press, London and New York.

Davenport, F. M. (1961). *Amer. Rev. Resp. Dis.* **83**, No. 2, 146.

Davenport, F. M. (1973). *Med. J. Aust., Spec. Suppl.* 1, p. 33.

Davenport, F. M., Hennessey, A. V., and Minuse, E. (1967). *J. Exp. Med.* **126**, 1049.

Davenport, F. M., Minuse, E., Hennessey, A. V., and Francis, T., Jr. (1969). *Bull. W.H.O.* **41**, 453.

Davey, M. L., and Reid, D. (1972). *Brit. J. Prev. Soc. Med.* **26**, 28.

Davis, L. E., Caldwell, G. G., Lynch, R. E., Bailey, R. E., and Chin, T. D. Y. (1970). *Amer. J. Epidemiol.* **92**, 240.

DeMeio, J. L., Woolridge, J. E., Whiteside, J. E., and Seal, J. R. (1955). *Proc. Soc. Exp. Biol. Med.* **88**, 436.

Dingle, J. H., Badger, G. F., and Jordan, W. S. (1964). "Illness in the Home." Western Reserve Univ. Press, Cleveland, Ohio.

Dowdle, W. R., Coleman, M. T., and Gregg, J. B. (1974). *Progr. Med. Virol.* **17**, 91.

Downie, J. C., and Laver, W. G. (1973). *Virology* **51**, 259.

Dunn, F. L. (1958). *J. Amer. Med. Ass.* **166**, 1140.

Easterday, B. C., and Couch, R. B. (1975). *J. Infec. Dis.* **131**, 602.

Eickhoff, T. C., Sherman, I. L., and Serfling, R. E. (1961). *J. Amer. Med. Ass.* **176**, 776.

Evans, A. S., Shephard, K., and Richards, V. (1970). *Lancet* **2**, 1364.

Farník, J., and Bruj, J. (1966). *J. Infec. Dis.* **116**, 425.

Fazekas de St. Groth, S. (1970). *Arch. Environ. Health* **21**, 293.

Finkler, D. (1898). *In* "Twentieth Century Practice of Medicine," Vol. 15, p. 1. Wm. Wood, New York.

Fox, J. P., and Kilbourne, E. D. (1973). *J. Infec. Dis.* **128**, 361.

Francis, T., Jr. (1958). *In* "Preventive Medicine in World War II" (J. B. Coates, Jr., E. C. Hoff, and P. M. Hoff, eds.), Vol. IV. Office of the Surgeon General, Department of the Army, US Govt. Printing Office, Washington, D.C.

Francis, T., Jr. (1967). *Med. Clin. N. Amer.* **51**, 781.

Francis, T., Jr., and Maassab, H. F. (1965). *In* "Viral and Rickettsial Infections of Man" (F. L. Horsfall, Jr. and I. Tamm, eds.), 4th ed., p. 689. Lippincott, Philadelphia, Pennsylvania.

Francis, T., Jr., Quilligan, J. J., Jr., and Minuse, E. (1950). *Science* **112**, 495.

Fraser, K. B. (1959). *Virology* **9**, 202.

Fukumi, H. (1961). *Amer. Rev. Resp. Dis.* **83**, No. 2, 10.

Fukumi, H. (1969). *Bull. W.H.O.* **41**, 469.

Galbraith, A. W., Oxford, J. S., Schild, G. C., and Watson, G. I. (1969). *Lancet* **2**, 1026.

Gamboa, E. T., Wolf, A., Yahr, M. D., Harter, D. H., Duffy, P. E., Barden, H., and Hsu, K. C. (1974). *Arch. Neurol. (Chicago)* **31**, 226.

Gear, J. H. S. (1969). *Bull. W.H.O.* **41**, 409.

Gill, P. W., Babbage, N. F., Gunton, P. E., Flower, W., and Garrett, D. A. (1971). *Med. J. Aust.* **2**, 53 (July 3).

Green, I. J., Hung, S. C., Yu, P. S., Lee, G. W., and Pereira, H. G. (1964). *Amer. J. Hyg.* **79**, 107.

Grunert, R. R., McGahen, J. W., and Davies, W. L. (1965). *Virology* **26**, 262.

Hall, C. E., Cooney, M. K., and Fox, J. P. (1973). *Amer. J. Epidemiol.* **98**, 365.

Harper, G. J. (1961). *J. Hyg.* **59**, 479.

Hayslett, J., McCarroll, J. R., Brady, E., Dueschle, K., McDermott, W., and Kilbourne, E. D. (1962). *Amer. Rev. Resp. Dis.* **85**, 1.

Heffron, R. (1939). "Pneumonia." The Commonwealth Fund, Oxford Univ. Press, London and New York.

Hemmes, J. H., Winkler, K. C., and Kool, S. M. (1960). *Nature (London)* **188**, 430.

Hers, J. F. P., and Mulder, J. (1961). *Amer. Rev. Resp. Dis.* **83**, No. 2, 84.

Hilleman, M. R., Werner, J. H., and Gauld, R. L. (1953). *Bull. W.H.O.* **8**, 613.

Hilleman, M. R., Hamparian, V. V., Ketler, A., Reilly, C. M., McClelland, L., Cornfeld, D. and Stokes, J., Jr. (1962). *J. Amer. Med. Ass.* **180**, 445.

Hirst, G. K., Rickard, E. R., Whitman, L., and Horsfall, F. L., Jr. (1942). *J. Exp. Med.* **75**, 495.

Hoehling, A. A. (1961). "The Great Epidemic." Little, Brown, Boston, Massachusetts.
Hope-Simpson, R. E. (1958). *Proc. Roy. Soc. Med.* **51**, 267.
Housworth, J., and Langmuir, A. D. (1974). *Amer. J. Epidemiol.* **100**, 40.
Houseworth, W. J., and Spoon, M. (1971). *Amer. J. Epidemiol.* **94**, 348.
Isaacs, A., Hart, R. J. C., and Law, V. G. (1962). *Bull. W.H.O.* **26**, 253.
Jensen, K. E. (1957). *J. Immunol.* **78**, 373.
Jensen, K. E., Dunn, F. L., and Robinson, R. Q. (1958). *Progr. Med. Virol.* **1**, 165.
Jordan, E. O. (1927). "Epidemic Influenza; A Survey." Amer. Med. Ass., Chicago, Illinois.
Jordan, W. S. (1961). *Amer. Rev. Resp. Dis.* **83**, No. 2, 29.
Kaye, D., Rosenbluth, M., Hook, E., and Kilbourne, E. D. (1962). *Amer. Rev. Resp. Dis.* **85**, 9.
Kilbourne, E. D. (1959). *J. Clin. Invest.* **38**, 266.
Kilbourne, E. D. (1960). *Ciba Found. Study Group* **4**, 58.
Kilbourne, E. D. (1961). *Amer. Rev. Resp. Dis.* **83**, 265.
Kilbourne, E. D. (1963). *In* "Preventive Medicine and Public Health" (W. G. Smillie and E. D. Kilbourne, eds.), p. 192. Macmillan, New York.
Kilbourne, E. D. (1968). *Science* **160**, 74.
Kilbourne, E. D. (1969). *Bull. W.H.O.* **41**, 643.
Kilbourne, E. D. (1973a). *J. Infec. Dis.* **127**, 478.
Kilbourne, E. D. (1973b). *Natur. Hist.* **82**, 72.
Kilbourne, E. D. (1973c). *J. Infec. Dis.* **128**, 668.
Kilbourne, E. D. (1974). *Science* **184**, 414.
Kilbourne, E. D. (1975). *Acta Med. Scand. Suppl.* No. 576.
Kilbourne, E. D., and Christensen, W. N. (1963). *Amer. Rev. Resp. Dis.* **87**, 899.
Kilbourne, E. D., and Murphy, J. S. (1960). *J. Exp. Med.* **111**, 387.
Kilbourne, E. D., Anderson, H. C., and Horsfall, F. L., Jr. (1951). *J. Immunol.* **67**, 547.
Kilbourne, E. D., Lief, F. S., Schulman, J. L., Jahiel, R. I., and Laver, W. G. (1967). *Perspectives Virol.* **5**, 87.
Kilbourne, E. D., Christensen, W. N., and Sande, M. (1968). *J. Virol.* **2**, 761.
Kilbourne, E. D., Chanock, R. M., Choppin, P. W., Davenport, F. M. Fox, J. P., Gregg, M. B., Jackson, G. G., and Parkman, P. D. (1974). *J. Infec. Dis.* **129**, 750.
Laidlaw, P. P. (1935). *Lancet* **1**, 1118.
Langmuir, A. D. (1958). *Ann. Intern. Med.* **49**, 483.
Langmuir, A. D. (1961). *Amer. Rev. Resp. Dis.* **83**, No. 2, 2.
Langmuir, A. D., Henderson, D. A., and Serfling, R. E. (1964). *Amer. J. Pub. Health* **54**, 563.
Laver, W. G., and Webster, R. G. (1971). *Virology* **44**, 317.
Leibovitz, A., Coultrip, R. L., Kilbourne, E. D., Legters, L. J. Smith, C. D. Chin, J., and Schulman, J. L. (1971). *J. Infec. Dis.* **124**, 481.
Levine, M. M., Togo, Y., and Wald, E. (1974). *Amer J. Epidemiol.* **100**, 272.
Louria, D. B., Blumenfeld, H. L., Ellis, J. T., Kilbourne, E. D., and Rogers, D. E. (1959). *J. Clin. Invest.* **38**, 213.
Maassab, H. F. (1968). *Nature (London)* **219**, 645.
MacCallum, W. G. (1919). "The Pathology of the Pneumonia in the United States Army camps during the winter of 1917–1918," Monograph No. 10. Rockefeller Inst. Med. Res, New York.
McDonald, J. C., and Zuckerman, A. J. (1962). *Brit. Med. J.* **2**, 89.

MacKenzie, J. S., and Houghton, M. (1974). *Bacteriol. Rev.* **38**, 356.

McLean, R. L. (1961). *Amer. Rev. Resp. Dis.* **83**, No. 2, 36.

Marine, W. M., and Workman, W. M. (1969). *Amer. J. Epidemiol.* **90**, 406.

Marine, W. M., Workman, W. M., and Webster, R. G. (1969). *Bull. W.H.O.* **41**, 475.

Martin, C. M., Kunin, C. M., Gottlieb, L. S., Barnes, M. W., Liu, C., and Finland, M. (1959). *Arch. Intern. Med.* **103**, 515.

Masurel, N. (1969). *Bull. W.H.O.* **41**, 461.

Masurel, N., and Marine, N. (1973). *Amer. J. Epidemiol.* **97**, 44.

Maxwell, E. S., Ward, T. G., and van Metre, T. E., Jr. (1949). *J. Clin. Invest.* **28**, 307.

Mayer, V., Schulman, J. L., and Kilbourne, E. D. (1973). *J. Virol.* **11**, 272.

Maynard, J. E., Feltz, E. T., Wulff, H., Fortuine, R., Poland, J. D., and Chin, T. D. Y. (1967). *J. Amer. Med. Ass.* **200**, 927.

Meiklejohn, G., and Bruyn, H. B. (1949). *Amer. J. Pub. Health* **39**, 44.

Miller, D. L., Reid, D., Diamond, J. R., Pereira, M. S., and Chakraverty, P. (1973). *J. Hyg.* **71**, 535.

Minuse, E., Quilligan, J. J., Jr., and Francis, T., Jr. (1954). *J. Lab. Clin. Med.* **43**, 31.

Minuse, E., McQueen, J. L., Davenport, F. M., and Francis, T., Jr. (1965). *J. Immunol.* **94**, 563.

Moffet, H. L., Cramblett, H. G., Middleton, G. K., Black, J. P., Schulenberger, H. K., and Yongue, A. M. (1962). *J. Amer. Med. Ass.* **182**, 834.

Mogabgab, W. J. (1963). *Ann. Intern. Med.* **59**, 306.

Montefiore, D., Drozdov, S. G., Kafuko, G. W., Faninka, O. A., and Soneji, A. (1970). *Bull. W.H.O.* **43**, 269.

Monto, A. S., and Kendal, A. P. (1973). *Lancet* **1**, 623.

Monto, A. S., and Olazabal, F., Jr. (1966). *Amer. J. Epidemiol.* **83**, 101.

Monto, A. S., Davenport, F. M., Napier, J. A., and Francis, T., Jr. (1969). *Bull. W.H.O.* **41**, 537.

Morita, M., Suto, T., and Ishida, N. (1972). *J. Infec. Dis.* **126**, 61.

Mowshowitz, S., and Kilbourne, E. D. (1975). *In* "Negative-Strand Viruses" (R. D. Barry and B. W. J. Mahy, eds.). Academic Press, New York.

Mulder, J., and Hers, J. F. P. (1972). "Influenza." Wolters-Noordhoff, Gröningen, The Netherlands.

Mulder, J., and Masurel, N. (1958). *Lancet* **1**, 810.

Murphy, B. R., Chalhub, E. G., Nusinoff, S. R., and Chanock, R. M. (1972a). *J. Infec. Dis.* **126**, 170.

Murphy, B. R., Kasel, J. A., and Chanock, R. M. (1972b). *N. Engl. J. Med.* **286**, 1329.

Murphy, B. R., Chalhub, E. G., Nusinoff, S. R., Kasel, J., and Chanock, R. M. (1973). *J. Infec. Dis.* **128**, 479.

Napiorkowski, P. A., and Black, F. L. (1974). *Lancet* **2**, 1390.

Opie, E. L., Blake, F. G., Small, J. C., and Rivers, T. M. (1921). "Epidemic Respiratory Disease: The Pneumonias and Other Infections of the Respiratory Tract Accompanying Influenza and Measles." Kimpton, London.

Palese, P., and Schulman, J. L. (1974). *Virology* **57**, 227.

Palese, P., Bucher, D., and Kilbourne, E. D. (1973). *Appl. Microbiol.* **25**, 195.

Pereira, H. G., Tumová, B., and Law, V. G. (1965). *Bull. W.H.O.* **32**, 855.

Pereira, H. G., Tumová, B., and Webster, R. G. (1967). *Nature (London)* **215**, 982.

Petersdorf, R. G., Fusco, J. J., Harter, D. H., and Albrink, W. S. (1959). *Arch. Intern. Med.* **103**, 266.

Philip, R. N., and Lackman, D. B. (1962). *Amer. J. Hyg.* **75**, 322.

Piraino, F. F., Brown, E. M., and Krumbiegel, E. R. (1970). *Pub. Health Rep.* **85**, 140.

Protsch, R., and Berger, R. (1973). *Science* **179**, 235.

Pyhala, R., and Kleemola, M. (1973). *Scand. J. Infec. Dis.* **5**, 273.

Quilligan, J. J., Jr., Minuse, E., and Francis, T., Jr. (1954). *J. Lab. Clin. Med.* **43**, 43.

Rasmussen, A. F., Jr. (1964). *In* "Newcastle Disease Virus" (R. P. Hanson, ed.), p. 313. Univ. of Wisconsin Press, Madison.

Roden, A. T. (1969). *Bull. W.H.O.* **41**, 375.

Rosenstock, I. M., Hochbaum, G. M., and Leventhal, H. (1960). *U.S., Pub. Health Serv., Publ.* **766**.

Salk, J. E., Pearson, H. E., Brown, P. N., Smyth, C. J., and Francis, T., Jr. (1945). *Amer. J. Hyg.* **42**, 307.

Sartwell, P. E., and Long, A. P. (1948). *Amer. J. Hyg.* **47**, 135.

Schild, G. C., Pereira, H. G., and Shetler, C. H. (1969). *Nature (London)* **222**, 1299.

Schild, G. C., Henry-Aymard, M., Pereira, M. S., Chakraverty, P., Dowdle, W., Coleman, M., and Chang, W. K. (1973). *Bull. W.H.O.* **48**, 269.

Schulman, J. L. (1968). *Proc. Soc. Exp. Biol. Med.* **128**, 1173.

Schulman, J. L. (1970a). *In* "Aerobiology" (I. H. Silver, ed.), p. 248. Academic Press, New York.

Schulman, J. L. (1970b). *Progr. Med. Virol.* **12**, 128.

Schulman, J. L., and Kilbourne, E. D. (1962). *Nature (London)* **195**, 1129.

Schulman, J. L., and Kilbourne, E. D. (1963a). *J. Exp. Med.* **118**, 257.

Schulman, J. L., and Kilbourne, E. D. (1963b). *J. Exp. Med.* **118**, 267.

Schulman, J. L., and Kilbourne, E. D. (1969a). *Bull. W.H.O.* **41**, 425.

Schulman, J. L,. and Kilbourne, E. D. (1969b). *Proc. Nat. Acad. Sci. U.S.* **63**, 326.

Schulman, J. L., Khakpour, M., and Kilbourne, E. D. (1968). *J. Virol.* **2**, 778.

Semple, A. B. (1951). *Proc. Roy. Soc. Med.* **44**, 794.

Serfling, R. E. (1963). *Pub. Health. Rep.* **78**, 494.

Seto, J. T. (1969). *Bull. W.H.O.* **41**, 489.

Seto, J. T., Hickey, B. J., and Rasmussen, A. F., Jr. (1959). *Proc. Soc. Exp. Biol. Med.* **100**, 672.

Sharrar, R. G. (1969). *Bull. W.H.O.* **41**, 361.

Shope, R. E. (1931). *J. Exp. Med.* **54**, 373.

Shope, R. E. (1935–1936). *Harvey Lect.* **31**, 183.

Shope, R. E. (1958). *Pub. Health Rep.* **73**, 165.

Sigel, M. M., Kitts, A. W., Light, A. B., and Henle, W. (1950). *J. Immunol.* **64**, 33.

Slepushkin, A. N., Schild, G. C., Beare, A. S., Chinn, S., and Tyrrell, D. A. J. (1971). *J. Hyg.* **69**, 571.

Smith, W., Andrewes, C. H., and Laidlaw, P. P. (1933). *Lancet* **2**, 66.

Smorodintsev, A. A., Chalkina, O. M., Burov, S. A., and Ilyin, N. A. (1961). *J. Hyg., Epidemiol., Microbiol. Immunol.* **5**, 60.

Stallones, R. A., and Lennette, E. H. (1959). *Amer. J. Pub. Health* **49**, 656.

Stanley, E. D., Muldoon, R. E., Akers, L. W., and Jackson, G. G. (1965). *Ann. N.Y. Acad. Sci.* **130**, 44.

Straub, M. (1959). *Ned. Tijdschr. Geneesk.* **103**, 1208.

Stuart-Harris, C. H., Laird, J., Tyrrell, D. A., Kelsall, M. H., and Franks, Z. C. (1949). *J. Hyg.* **47**, 434.

Tamm, I. (1964). *Cell. Biol. Myxovirus Infec., Ciba Found: Symp., 1964* p. 240.

Tang, F. F., and Liang, Y. K. (1957). *Proc. Int. Meet. Biol. Stand., 3rd Opatija* p. 89.

Tateno, I., Suzuki, S., Nakamura, S., Kitamoto, O., Togashi, M., and Sato, T. (1963). *Jap. J. Exp. Med.* **33**, 159.

Taylor, R. M. (1951). *Arch. Gesamte Virusforsch.* **4**, 485.

Togo, Y., Hornick, R. B., and Dawkins, A. T. (1968). *J. Amer. Med. Ass.* **203**, 1089.

Trotter, Y., Dunn, F. L., Drachman, R. H., Henderson, D. A., Pizzi, M., and Langmuir, A. D. (1959). *Amer. J. Hyg.* **70**, 34.

Tumová, B., and Pereira, H. G. (1965). *Virology* **27**, 253.

Van der Veen, J., and Mulder, J. (1950). *Onderz. Meded. Inst. Praev. Geneesk* No. 6.

van Rooyen, C. E., McClelland, L., and Campbell, E. K. (1949). *Can. J. Pub. Health* **40**, 447.

Vaughan, W. T. (1921). *Amer. J. Hyg., Monogr.* No. 1.

Veeraraghavan, N. (1969). *Bull. W.H.O.* **41**, 489.

Vicente, M. (1969). *Bull. W.H.O.* **41**, 408.

Voth, D. W., and Feldman, H. A. (1963). *Amer. J. Pub. Health* **53**, 1512.

Webster, R. G., and Campbell, C. H. (1972). *Virology* **48**, 528.

Webster, R. G., Laver, W. G., and Kilbourne, E. D. (1968). *J. Gen. Virol.* **3**, 315.

Webster, R. G., Campbell, C. H., and Granoff, A. (1971). *Virology* **44**, 317.

Widelock, D., Schaeffer, M., and Millian, S. J. (1965). *Amer. J. Pub. Health* **55**, 578.

Wolbach, S. B. (1919). *Bull. Johns Hopkins Hosp.* **30**, 104.

Zachary, I. G., and Johnson, K. M. (1969). *Amer. J. Trop. Med. Hyg.* **18**, 1048.

Zhdanov, V. M., and Ritova, V. V. (1963). *Fed. Proc., Fed. Amer. Soc. Exp. Biol.* **22**, 1800.

Index

H

H